Tuberculosis

& Nontuberculous Mycobacterial Infections

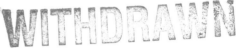

Tuberculosis
& Nontuberculous Mycobacterial Infections

FIFTH EDITION

Edited by

David Schlossberg, MD, FACP

Professor of Medicine
Temple University School of Medicine
Philadelphia, Pennsylvania
Medical Director
Tuberculosis Control Program
Philadelphia Department of Health
Philadelphia, Pennsylvania

McGraw-Hill
Medical Publishing Division

New York   Chicago   San Francisco   Lisbon   London   Madrid   Mexico City   Milan
New Delhi   San Juan   Seoul   Singapore   Sydney   Toronto

Tuberculosis & Nontuberculous Mycobacterial Infections, Fifth Edition

Copyright © 2006 by the McGraw-Hill Companies, Inc. All rights reserved. Printed in the United States of America. Except as permitted under the United States Copyright Act of 1976, no part of this publication may be reproduced or distributed in any form or by any means, or stored in a database or retrieval system, without the prior written permission of the publisher.

Previous editions copyright © 1999 by W.B. Saunders Company; copyright © 1994, 1988, by Springer-Verlag; copyright © 1983, by Praeger.

1 2 3 4 5 6 7 8 9 0   DOC/DOC   0 9 8 7 6 5

ISBN: 0-07-143913-7

This book was set in Times by International Typesetting and Composition.
The editors were James Shanahan, Karen Edmonson, and Regina Y. Brown.
The production supervisor was Sherri Souffrance.
The cover designer was Aimee Nordin.
The indexer was Alexandra Nickerson.
R.R. Donnelley was printer and binder.

This book is printed on acid-free paper.

Library of Congress Cataloging-in-Publication Data
Tuberculosis and nontuberculous mycobacterial infections / edited by David Schlossberg—
    5th ed.
        p. ; cm.
    Includes bibliographical references and index.
    ISBN 0-07-143913-7 (hardcover)
    1. Tuberculosis. 2. Mycobacterial diseases. I. Schlossberg, David.
    [DNLM: 1. Tuberculosis. 2. Mycobacterium Infections. WF 200 T8792 2005]
RC311.T824 2005
616.99′5—dc22
                                                                    2005052241

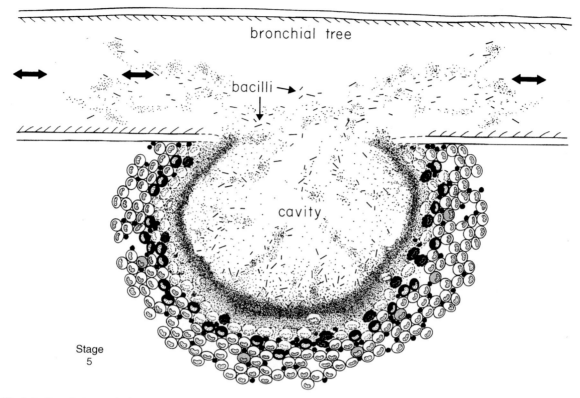

bronchial tree

bacilli →

cavity

Stage
5

Fig. 2-4. Stage 5: A recently formed small cavity discharging liquefied caseous material into a bronchus. In this liquefied material, the bacilli have multiplied profusely and extracellularly. With such large numbers of bacilli, there is an increased likelihood of a mutation resulting in antimicrobial resistance. Also, the large quantities of bacilli and their antigens in the liquefied caseum overwhelm a formerly effective CMI, causing progression of the disease and the destruction of local tissues, including the wall of an adjacent bronchus. The liquefied caseous material is then discharged into the airways, so that the bacilli disseminate to other parts of the lung and to the environment. (Reprinted with permission from Dannenberg AM Jr, Rook GAW. Pathogenesis of pulmonary tuberculosis: an interplay of tissue-damaging and macrophage-activating immune responses—dual mechanisms that control bacillary multiplication. In: Bloom BR, ed. *Tuberculosis: Pathogenesis, Protection, and Control.* Washington, DC: American Society for Microbiology; 1994:459–483. Reproduced by permission of ASM Press, Washington, DC.)

by bacillary dormancy. In addition to dormancy, the flat part of the curves in Fig. 2-2 also represents a balance between bacillary growth and destruction.

During the second (symbiotic) stage, and at its end, the lungs of Lurie's susceptible rabbits contained 20–30 times more bacilli than did the lungs of his resistant rabbits (Fig. 2-2). Most of these bacilli were probably located in developing tubercles. Unexpectedly, the susceptible hosts inhibited further bacillary growth just as effectively as did the resistant hosts (Fig. 2-2). CMI could not be responsible, because the susceptible hosts developed only

weak CMI, and at this stage of the disease, the good CMI of the resistant hosts was not yet fully developed. The marked inhibition of bacillary growth in both strains of rabbits must therefore be due to another mechanism, i.e., the tissue-damaging DTH that occurs in the third stage of tuberculosis.

As stated above, such DTH kills the nonactivated macrophages in which the bacilli are growing, thereby eliminating the intracellular environment that is favorable to such growth. This concept was advocated by several research groups,[39–45] and had been predicted many

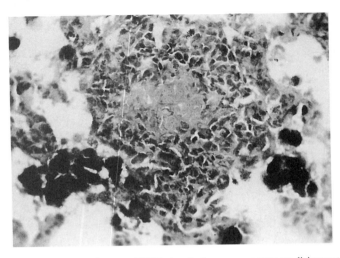

Fig. 2-5. A tissue-section of a 10-day (rabbit) pulmonary BCG lesion. In the caseous center are disintegrated β-galactosidase-negative epithelioid cells and more than 10 faintly stained tubercle bacilli. Around the caseous center are viable, young β-galactosidase-negative mononuclears, dendritic cells, macrophages, and lymphocytes from the bloodstream, which control the fate of tuberculous lesions. Alveolar macrophages, staining 3+ and 4+ for β-galactosidase have accumulated in the surrounding alveolar area, rather far from the bacilli in the center. Although this lesion was produced by the intravenous injection of tubercle bacilli, tubercles produced by the inhalation of bacilli should show the same pattern. Specifically, bacilli are released from pulmonary alveolar macrophages that failed to control bacillary multiplication. These bacilli and host cytokines chemotactically attract new nonactivated macrophages from the bloodstream, which cannot control the multiplication of tubercle bacilli in their cytoplasm until they become activated by antigen-specific T lymphocytes. X300. (Reprinted with permission from Shima K, Dannenberg AM Jr, Ando M, et al. Macrophage accumulation, division, maturation, and digestive and microbicidal capacities in tuberculous lesions. I. Studies involving their incorporation of tritiated thymidine and their content of lysosomal enzymes and bacilli. *Am J Pathol.* 1972;67:159–180.)

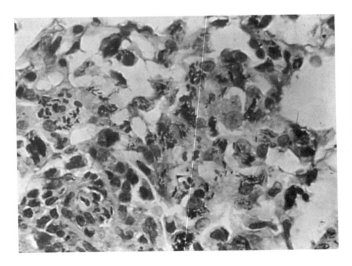

Fig. 2-6. A tissue section of a tuberculous lesion from one of Lurie's genetically susceptible rabbits, 2 weeks after the inhalation of virulent human-type tubercle bacilli. The nonactivated macrophages from the blood stream contain numerous, rod-shaped, acid-fast bacilli. Two weeks is near the end of Stage 2, the stage of symbiosis: The bacilli have grown logarithmically within these nonactivated macrophages with no apparent damage to the cells. X690. (Reprinted with permission from Lurie MB, Zappasodi P, Tickner C. On the nature of genetic resistance to tuberculosis in the light of the host-parasite relationships in natively resistant and susceptible rabbits. *Am Rev Tuberc Pulm Dis.* 1955;72:297–329. Official Journal of the American Thoracic Society. Copyright 1990. Reprinted with permission from Elsevier.)

years ago.[46,47] In fact, Robert Koch (the discoverer of the tubercle bacillus) described it before DTH and CMI were in our vocabulary.[48]

But, why did the susceptible rabbits, which are known to develop weak CMI responses (i.e., activate macrophages poorly),[6] stop the logarithmic growth of the bacillus just as effectively as did the resistant rabbits? The answer is that two immune mechanisms (CMI and tissue-damaging DTH) control the growth of tubercle bacilli. Lurie's susceptible rabbits developed weak CMI, but they developed strong tuberculin reactions, especially when numerous tubercle bacilli were present in their bodies: A large number of bacilli provides a greater antigenic stimulus than does a smaller number. When the bacillary growth curves became level (Fig. 2-2), the susceptible rabbits often had tuberculin reactions approximately equal to those of resistant rabbits.[6] The caseous centers of the lesions were larger in the susceptible rabbits than in resistant rabbits, apparently because more bacilli-laden macrophages had been present and were killed.[30]

The tubercle bacillus can survive in solid caseous material, but it cannot multiply, probably due to the anoxic conditions, reduced pH, and the presence of inhibitory fatty acids.[47,49] In fact, some bacilli may survive for years in solid caseous tissue. In this dormant state, the bacilli are not metabolizing and therefore are not sensitive to antimicrobial therapy.[50]

Thus, the host locally destroys its own tissues to control the uninhibited growth of bacilli within nonactivated macrophages, which otherwise would be lethal to the host.[46,47] Only after such control is established can CMI, producing highly activated macrophages around the caseous focus, prevent the progression of the disease (Fig. 2-7).

Caseous necrosis in tuberculosis is a DTH reaction produced by T cells, especially cytotoxic T cells[39–45,51–53] (Table 2-1). Contributing to this necrosis are clotting factors (anoxia), cytokines (e.g., tumor necrosis factor),[50,54–57] reactive oxygen, and nitrogen intermediates[58–62] (from macrophages and other cells); and possibly antigen-antibody complexes, complement, and toxic products released from dead bacilli.

Tuberculin-like products seem to play a major role in the caseous process. These products,[63] and other antigens,[64–66] seem to be secreted or released from the live and perhaps dead intracellular tubercle bacilli. T-cell sensitivity (DTH) to tuberculin-like products probably occurs before T-cell sensitivity to the other antigens of the bacillus, because the release of other antigens may require

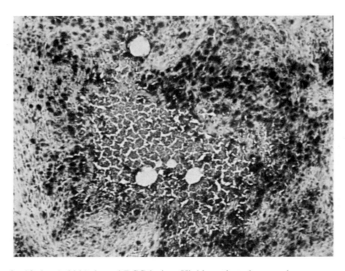

Fig. 2-7. A tissue section of a 12-day (rabbit) dermal BCG lesion. Highly activated macrophages surround the caseous center. This figure illustrates another aspect of effective cell-mediated immunity, namely, that large numbers of activated (β-galactosidase-positive) macrophages accumulate around the caseous focus. Therefore, bacilli released from dead and dying macrophages will now be ingested by macrophages that are able to inhibit intracellular bacillary growth. X90. (Reprinted with permission from Shima K, Dannenberg AM Jr, Ando M, et al. Macrophage accumulation, division, maturation, and digestive and microbicidal capacities in tuberculous lesions. I. Studies involving their incorporation of tritiated thymidine and their content of lysosomal enzymes and bacilli. *Am J Pathol.* 1972;67:159–180.)

Table 2-1. Causes of Tissue Damage and Caseous Necrosis

Cytotoxic T Cells and Natural Killer Cells
Involving apoptosis and other mechanisms

Anoxia
Produced by thrombosis—macrophages produce
  clotting factors

Toxic Cell Products
Reactive oxygen and nitrogen intermediates; certain
  cytokines, such as tumor necrosis factor (TNF);
  hydrolytic enzymes; and complement

Toxic Bacillary Products
Intact tubercle bacilli are nontoxic, but, when they are
  broken down, toxic products, such as "cord factor"
  (trehalose dimycolate), may be released

Overview
Caseous necrosis is initiated by a tissue-damaging, DTH
  reaction to high local concentrations of tuberculin-like
  bacillary products. Th1-type lymphocytes are responsible
  for the specificity of this reaction.

Source: Reprinted with permission from Dannenberg AM Jr,
Tomashefski JF Jr. Pathogenesis of pulmonary tuberculosis.
In Fishman AP, ed-in-chief, *Fishman's Pulmonary Diseases
and Disorders*, 3rd ed. New York, NY: McGraw-Hill; 1998:
2447–2471.

killing and lysis of this microorganism. Thus, tuberculin-like proteins and other early-released bacillary products probably play major roles in stopping the logarithmic microbial growth of the symbiotic stage, whereas in later stages of the disease, the necrosis that these proteins produce may be more harmful than beneficial. (See Development of Better Vaccines in Part II.)

If cytotoxic DTH is directed against tuberculin-like products of the bacillus on the surface of bacilli-laden macrophages, why is there so much damage to adjacent tissues? An answer to this question was suggested in an article from our laboratory.[67] In all inflammatory reactions, the vascular endothelium, usually in the postcapillary venule, is activated by cytokines that up-regulate ICAM-1, ELAM-1, VCAM-1, and other adhesion molecules,[67–72] as well as major histocompatibility complex (MHC) class I and MHC class II molecules.[67,73] Such activated endothelial cells, therefore, would then be capable of presenting tuberculin-like antigens to cytotoxic T cells, which in turn could injure the endothelium and thereby initiate the clotting cascade. Increased sensitivity to the toxic

effects of TNF seems to be involved,[74] as well as other factors.[75] Local thrombosis would follow endothelial cell injury,[76] and the thrombosis would cause ischemia and necrosis to nearby tissues.

The Fourth Stage of Tuberculosis: Interplay of Cell-Mediated Immunity and Tissue-Damaging Delayed-Type Hypersensitivity

During the fourth stage, the caseous tuberculous lesion may become clinically apparent, at least by radiograph, or it may be arrested with little visible evidence remaining, except for a positive tuberculin skin test. The fate of the lesion is mainly controlled by cell-mediated immunity. If CMI is weak, as in Lurie's susceptible rabbits, the bacilli escaping from the edge of the caseous centers again multiply intracellularly in poorly activated macrophages. Again, such infected macrophages are killed by tissue-damaging DTH, and the caseous center enlarges (Fig. 2-3A).

If the lesion is regressing, as in Lurie's resistant rabbits, the bacilli escaping from the caseous center are ingested and destroyed or inhibited by the highly activated macrophages that have accumulated perifocally (Figs. 2-3B and 2-7). These macrophages were previously activated[77] by the strong CMI that develops in these resistant hosts.

In each case, the number of viable bacilli is stationary (Fig. 2-2) (a) because of bacillary dormancy and slow death in the caseous material of the tubercle, and (b) because of a balance between growth of bacilli in some macrophages and their destruction by other macrophages. Also, the tubercle bacillus might become dormant in some macrophages with no growth or destruction.

Histologically, the tuberculous lesions are quite different in the resistant and susceptible rabbits. The lesions in the *resistants* have less necrosis and many strongly activated macrophages (mature epithelioid cells). Those in the *susceptibles* have more necrosis and many weakly activated macrophages (immature epithelioid cells). Large numbers of perifocal mature epithelioid cells, i.e., strongly activated macrophages (Fig. 2-7), enable the resistant host to control the disease.[6,8] Thirty years ago, Lurie had no histochemical test for activated macrophages capable of destroying tubercle bacilli, but he identified them histologically as mature epithelioid cells. We found that such cells contained high levels of β-galactosidase[78–80] and other histochemically-demonstrable marker enzymes.[78]

In the resistant rabbits and in the majority of immunocompetent adult human beings, the caseous center of the lesion becomes surrounded by many such microbicidal macrophages (activated by T-cell lymphokines) (Fig. 2-7). The bacilli that escape the caseous center are, therefore, ingested and destroyed. Eventually, the tubercle is walled off, the caseous center inspissates, and the disease is arrested, usually for a lifetime. The few bacilli that enter the lymphatics or the bloodstream are rapidly destroyed at their site of lodgment by accelerated tubercle formation, i.e., a rapid CMI response producing many locally activated macrophages (Fig. 2-7)[4,80–83] with relatively little caseous necrosis.

In the susceptible rabbits and in human infants and immunosuppressed persons, the caseous center is surrounded by many poorly activated macrophages, which permit the bacillus to grow intracellularly.[5,6,8] These macrophages are usually killed because of tissue-damaging DTH, and the caseous center enlarges. Thus, throughout the fourth stage of this disease in susceptible rabbits, DTH stops the intracellular growth of tubercle bacilli in the poorly activated macrophages, and this process results in further caseous necrosis.

In susceptible rabbits infected with virulent bovine-type tubercle bacilli, the bacilli lodging in the draining tracheobronchial lymph nodes, and often elsewhere are not destroyed. The same is true for human beings infected with virulent human-type bacilli who develop only weak CMI. In both cases, multiple progressing caseous tubercles of hematogenous origin develop throughout the body, especially in the lungs, and the host eventually succumbs.[5–8]

In hosts with such poor CMI, most of the secondary lesions in the lungs originate from bacilli in the caseous tracheobronchial lymph nodes. The lymph from these nodes drains the bacilli into the great veins leading to the right side of the heart, from which the bacilli are distributed directly into the lungs. Bacilli entering the bloodstream from primary pulmonary lesions are carried via the pulmonary veins to the left side of the heart, from which these bacilli are distributed throughout the body, but not directly into the lungs.

The Fifth Stage of Tuberculosis: Liquefaction and Cavity Formation

Unfortunately, even if CMI is well developed, progression of the disease may still occur in resistant hosts including immunocompetent adult human beings. Such progression is caused by liquefaction and cavity formation, which perpetuate the disease in mankind.[5,6,8,46,84]

The liquefied material is frequently, but not always, an excellent growth medium for the tubercle bacillus.[6,46,85] In liquefied caseum, the bacillus often multiplies extracellularly, for the first time during the course of the disease, sometimes reaching tremendous numbers (Fig. 2-8). Because of the presence of DTH, this large bacillary load is toxic to tissues and frequently causes the wall of a nearby bronchus to become necrotic. If the bronchial wall ruptures, a cavity is formed. Then, the bacilli and the liquefied caseous material are discharged into the airways and are distributed to other parts of the lung and also to the outside environment.

The liquefied caseous material contains tuberculin-like proteins. When this material is aspirated into the alveoli,

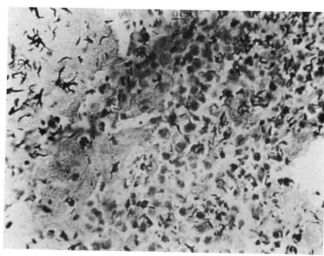

Fig. 2-8. A tissue section of the wall of a cavity from a genetically resistant rabbit, 8 weeks after the inhalation of human-type tubercle bacilli. The liquefied caseous tissue (right) and liquefying caseous tissue (left) are swarming with, rod-shaped, acid-fast bacilli. The bacilli are inhibited in solid caseous tissue before it liquefies. X600. (Reprinted with permission from Lurie MB, Zappasodi P, Tickner C. On the nature of genetic resistance to tuberculosis in the light of the host-parasite relationships in natively resistant and susceptible rabbits. *Am Rev Tuberc Pulm Dis*. 1955;72:297–329. Official Journal of the American Thoracic Society.)

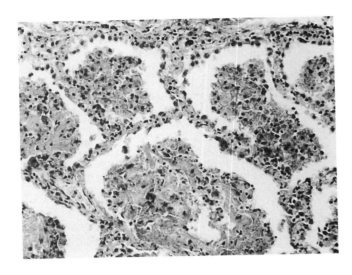

Fig. 2-9. A tissue section of an area of tuberculous pneumonia in the lung of a 47-year-old man. A large proportion of the cellular exudate in the alveolar spaces has undergone caseous necrosis, and infiltrating cells thicken the intervening alveolar septa. (Copyright 1999. The Alan Mason Chesney Medical Archives of the Johns Hopkins Medical Institutions. All rights reserved.)

an exudate results. If the aspiration is extensive, caseous bronchopneumonia results (Fig. 2-9). The bacilli need not multiply in the exudate, because the high concentration of tuberculin-like antigens in the liquefied caseum is usually sufficient to cause this form of the disease.

Mutant bacilli resistant to antimicrobial agents may arise among the large number of bacilli in the liquefied caseum of the inner cavity wall. For this reason, tuberculosis is usually treated with several antimicrobials simultaneously. Liquefied caseous foci and cavities do not occur in Lurie's susceptible rabbits,[6,8] and are not common in infants and in fully immunosuppressed individuals infected exogenously with *M. tuberculosis*.[5,86]

Macrophages do not survive in solid caseous material, and even when the caseum liquefies, the entering macrophages do not function effectively.[6] Possibly, they have been passively sensitized to tuberculin and other antigens, which are present in high (lethal) concentrations. Possibly, the entering macrophages are killed by toxic fatty acids originating from host cells, or the bacilli, or both.[47,49] Thus, even activated macrophages, produced by well-developed CMI, are completely ineffective in controlling the extracellular multiplication of bacilli within a cavity.

The cause of liquefaction is largely unknown. See Refs. 85, 87 and 88 for reviews of the subject, and Refs. 88–90 for recent experiments on cavity formation in rabbits. Hydrolytic enzymes,[85] and DTH to the tuberculin-like products of the bacillus[87,91] are involved (Table 2-2). At present, no therapeutic agents exist to prevent liquefaction; but, if developed, such agents would greatly aid antimicrobial therapy in reducing the number of viable bacilli and in controlling the disease.

Clinical Tuberculosis

Pulmonary tuberculosis, once developed in human beings, often shows a composite picture.[5,46,47,84] Tuberculosis is a local disease influenced by the local concentration of antigen, the amount of local macrophage

Table 2-2. Causes and Results of Liquefaction

Causes
Delayed-type hypersensitivity to tuberculin-like
  bacillary products
Hydrolytic enzymes: proteases, DNases and RNases,
  and probably lipases

Results
Extracellular multiplication (sometimes tremendous)
  of the bacilli, resulting in antimicrobial
  drug-resistant mutants
Erosion of bronchial walls, resulting in spread of
  bacilli through the air passages to other parts of
  the lung and to other persons.

Source: Reprinted with permission from Dannenberg AM Jr, Tomashefski JF Jr. Pathogenesis of pulmonary tuberculosis. In Fishman AP, ed-in-chief, *Fishman's Pulmonary Diseases and Disorders*, 3rd ed. New York, McGraw-Hill; 1998:2447–2471.

Table 2-3. Basic Types of Pulmonary Tuberculosis

Types of Lesions

Encapsulated caseous, liquefied, or calcified nodules
Proliferative type of pulmonary lesions
Exudative type of pulmonary lesions
Cavities

Types of Disease

Small discrete tubercles of hematogenous origin;
  focally localized or scattered diffusely throughout
  both lungs (miliary tuberculosis)
Liquefied caseous lesions with cavity formation and
  bronchogenic spread
Progressive, locally destructive lesions

Source: Modified from Rich AR. *The Pathogenesis of Tuberculosis*, 2nd ed. Springfield, Illinois: Charles C. Thomas; 1951.

activation, and the number of local lymphocytes with receptors for the tuberculin-like products of the bacillus. The host handles each lesion almost as if other lesions did not exist. Thus, lesions in one area of the lung may liquefy and progress, while lesions in another area of the same lung may stabilize or may regress. Even parts of a single lesion may progress, while other parts of the same lesion remain stable or regress. Finally, the disease as a whole may fluctuate between periods of exacerbation and remission (Table 2-3).

Tuberculosis in Common Laboratory Animals

The rabbit is the only common laboratory animal in which the disease closely resembles the typical chronic cavitary type found in the majority of human beings.[6,92–94]

Mice show less tuberculin sensitivity and less caseous necrosis than do human beings and rabbits; and liquefaction and cavity formation do not occur at all in mice (Table 2-4).[92,93]

The guinea pig, a species with good DTH, is the most susceptible of the group[6,92–94] and usually develops a blood-disseminated disease similar to that in infants and immunosuppressed persons. Cavity formation is not common in guinea pigs, but can occur.[36]

Lurie infected both his inbred resistant and susceptible strains of rabbits by the inhalation of virulent tubercle bacilli.[6] These studies are the main ones on record in which the onset, development, and progression or healing of primary pulmonary tubercles have been studied histopathologically. They provide insights, not obtainable by any other means into host-parasite interactions that also occur in the human disease.

When evaluated at 5 and 12 months, pulmonary lesions caused by the inhalation of virulent human-type bacilli were regressing in both the resistant and the susceptible rabbits. At those times, the *susceptibles* showed distinct primary lesions and often, metastatic lesions of hematogenous origin; and the *resistants* showed either small almost healed primary lesions or larger (primary) cavitary lesions. In these resistant animals, no grossly visible metastatic lesions were found, even though some bacilli must have spread from the cavitary lesions into the airways.[6]

In both strains of rabbits, the pulmonary lesions produced by the inhalation of virulent bovine-type bacilli did not heal, but caused progressive disease.[6,32,33] The *susceptibles* died of a disease spread via the hematogenous route, and the *resistants* died of a disease spread via the airways by the bacilli-containing liquefied caseum discharged from pulmonary cavities.[6,8,32] Lurie's susceptible rabbits did not form cavities.[6]

Table 2-4. Tuberculosis in Various Animal Species

| | Response | | | |
Species	Susceptibility	Tuberculin Sensitivity	Amount of Caseation	Cavity Formation
Mice	++	+	+	0
Guinea pigs	+++++	+++	+++++	+
Rabbits*	++	++	+++++	++++
Humans	++	+++++	+++++	++++

*Rabbits are fairly resistant to human-type tubercle bacilli, but rather susceptible to the bovine-type tubercle bacilli. The other species are more equally susceptible to both types.

Source: Adapted from Francis[93] and reproduced in Refs.1 and 92.

Animal studies have also confirmed the genetic basis of susceptibility to tuberculosis. The resistant C57BL/6 and BALB/c mouse strains survived much longer than did the susceptible C3H, CBA, and DBA/2 mouse strains.[95] Studies of genetic linkages in mice have found a possible susceptibility locus on chromosome 1, containing the intracellular pathogen resistance gene (*ipr 1*).[96] Other loci have also been discovered, suggesting that resistance to tuberculosis is complex.[97]

Multiple genetic differences existed among Lurie's resistant and susceptible rabbits.[6,98] Unfortunately, these strains are now extinct. However, a strain of inbred rabbits, recently developed by Jeanette Thorbecke, was found to be more susceptible to tuberculosis than commercial outbred New Zealand White rabbits.[99] (The outbred rabbits are almost as resistant as Lurie's inbred resistant strains.[89]) When compared to the commercial rabbits, the Thorbecke rabbits had larger tuberculous lesions that showed more bacilli, fewer mature epithelioid cells, and more extensive caseous necrosis. Their tuberculin skin tests were smaller.

Human Susceptibility to Tuberculosis

The average number of infectious particles of one to three bacilli that human beings must inhale before converting their tuberculin skin test is unknown. Estimates vary from 5 to 200. However, only 1 in 10 persons who convert their tuberculin skin test will develop active tuberculosis during their lifetime. The majority of these persons completely arrest the infection.

This arrestment, however, depends on a fully functional cell-mediated immune response. Persons coinfected with HIV, or immunosuppressed from other causes, are more likely to develop clinical disease from exogenously inhaled tubercle bacilli and also from endogenous (latent) tubercle bacilli that were inhaled years previously. Five to 10% of tuberculin-positive HIV-infected individuals reactivate their disease in a given year. In contrast, 5 to 10% of tuberculin-positive non-HIV-infected individuals reactivate their disease in their entire lifetime.

Even in the absence of immunosuppression, a spectrum of human susceptibility to tuberculosis clearly exists. Monozygotic twins show higher concordance rates of the disease than do dizygotic twins.[6] Population-based studies of susceptibility to tuberculosis have identified several genetic polymorphisms that may be associated with an increased risk of developing active tuberculosis, including genes for *NRAMP1* (natural-resistance-associated macrophage protein 1), the vitamin-D receptor, and the major histocompatibility complex.[100–106]

PART II. IMMUNOLOGY OF TUBERCULOSIS

Comment

In this part, we briefly review the innate and acquired (adaptive) immune factors that play a role in tuberculosis. The reader is referred to textbooks of immunology (e.g., Ref. 107) for more details than those given here. Additional references were published in our chapter in the last edition of this book. The immunology of mouse tuberculosis is reviewed in Refs. 108–110.

Overview of the Immunology of Tuberculosis

Cell mediated immunity (CMI) and delayed type hypersensitivity (DTH) play key roles in the pathogenesis of tuberculosis.[27–29] The tubercle bacillus apparently is *not* injurious to the host until the time when both of these immune responses begin to develop.

CMI can be defined as a beneficial host response characterized by an expanded population of specific T lymphocytes (Th1 cells), which, in the presence of microbial antigens, produce cytokines locally. These cytokines attract monocytes/macrophages from the bloodstream into the lesion and activate them. Interferon gamma (IFN-γ) and tumor necrosis factor alpha (TNF-α) are major macrophage-activating cytokines. IFN-γ also induces interleukin 2 (IL-2) receptors in monocyte/macrophages[111–113] following which IL-2, from T lymphocytes exposed to specific antigens, becomes an additional activating cytokine for these phagocytes. Activated macrophages produce reactive-oxygen and reactive-nitrogen intermediates,[58–61] lysosomal enzymes, and other factors that kill and digest tubercle bacilli.

Acquired cellular resistance (ACR) is characterized by the presence of a local population of activated (microbicidal) macrophages, produced by CMI, i.e., by the cytokines of antigen-stimulated lymphocytes.[114] Macrophages enter the tuberculous lesion in a nonimmune, nonactivated state. They readily ingest the bacillus and provide a favorable intracellular environment for its multiplication. These macrophages become activated and develop their microbicidal ability only where the bacillary antigens are located (Figs. 2-10 and 2-11). The greater the local accumulation of highly activated macrophages, the greater will be the host's ability to destroy tubercle bacilli (Fig. 2-7).

In this chapter we include ACR in our definition of CMI, even though, in the absence of antigen, CMI (i.e., an expanded specific T-cell population) can exist without ACR (i.e., without locally activated macrophages).

DTH is immunologically the same process as CMI, involving Th1-type T cells and their cytokines.

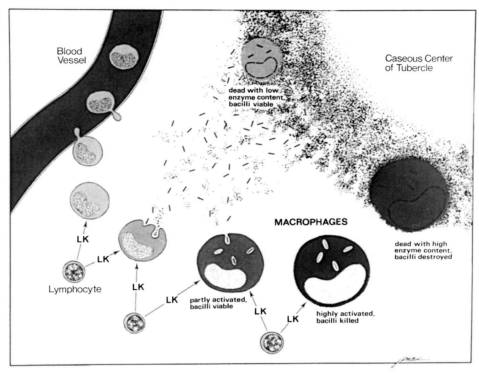

Fig. 2-10. Cell mediated immunity (CMI) producing local activation of macrophages in a tuberculous lesion. Mononuclear phagocytes are attracted from the bloodstream and are activated locally by lymphocytes and their lymphokines (LK), probably the most efficient mechanism, by endotoxin-like bacillary products, and also by ingestion of dead cells and tissue debris. The lymphokines, now called cytokines, e.g., IFN-γ and tumor necrosis factor, are produced when lymphocytes, mainly T cells with antigen-specific receptors are stimulated by the bacillus and its products. Only activated macrophages seem capable of destroying the tubercle bacillus. (Reprinted with permission from Dannenberg AM Jr. Pathogenesis of pulmonary tuberculosis in man and animals: protection of personnel against tuberculosis. In: Montali RJ, ed. *Mycobacterial Infections of Zoo Animals*. Washington, DC: Smithsonian Institution Press; 1978:65–75.)

The difference between CMI and DTH is the concentration of antigen required. CMI requires a relatively large amount of antigen to elicit a host reaction. However, DTH requires only a minute quantity. In a tuberculin-positive individual, skin tests can be elicited with first strength, i.e., 1 TU (Tuberculin Unit), containing 0.00002 mg of purified protein derivative (based on PPD-S, the PPD standard). At higher concentrations necrosis may develop.

In this chapter, we use the term "tissue-damaging DTH" for the immunologic reaction that causes necrosis. Such necrosis develops locally wherever the tuberculin-like antigens from the bacilli reach excessive concentrations, and these concentrations occur locally wherever a large number of tubercle bacilli or their products exist.

Synergism between CMI and DTH in the control of facultative intracellular microorganisms has been a subject of debate for most of the twentieth century. From the bacillary growth curves (Fig. 2-2) and a histologic study of the lesions,[6,27,30,32] it is quite apparent that both CMI and DTH inhibit the multiplication of tubercle bacilli equally well. However, CMI does so by activating macrophages to kill the bacilli they ingest; and tissue-damaging DTH does so by destroying bacilli-laden, non-activated macrophages and nearby tissues, thereby eliminating the intracellular environment, which is so favorable for bacillary growth.

Thus, both tuberculin-positive hosts with good CMI and tuberculin-positive hosts with poor CMI can arrest

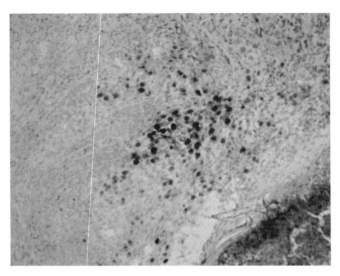

Fig. 2-11. A tissue section of a 21-day rabbit dermal BCG lesion, showing a group of activated macrophages (epithelioid cells) stained darkly for the lysosomal enzyme, β-galactosidase. We use β-galactosidase activity as a histochemical marker for activated macrophages that are capable of destroying tubercle bacilli.[80,115,116] Although perifocal tuberculous granulation tissue contains thousands of macrophages, only those macrophages in locations where tubercle bacilli, and their products, are present become activated and develop the power to destroy the bacillus. In other words, cell-mediated immunity is mainly a local phenomenon. The darker the macrophage is stained for β-galactosidase, the more it resembles Lurie's mature epithelioid cell, a cell that has destroyed tubercle bacilli.[6,116] X150. (Reprinted with permission from Dannenberg AM Jr. Cellular hypersensitivity and cellular immunity in the pathogensis of tuberculosis: specificity, systemic and local nature, and associated macrophage enzymes. *Bacteriol Rev.* 1968;32:85–102. Reproduced by permission of ASM Press, Washington, DC.)

bacillary growth. But, the host with poor CMI does so with much damage to its own tissues. Eventually, the host with good CMI may recover, but the host with poor CMI will die from excessive tissue destruction.

Tissue-damaging DTH causing local necrosis stops the initial bacillary growth within nonactivated macrophages. Such cytotoxic DTH can never take the place of CMI, because the bacilli that escape from the edge of necrotic areas are ingested by perifocal macrophages. If the perifocal macrophages have been sufficiently activated by CMI, they can destroy the ingested bacilli. If these macrophages have *not* been sufficiently activated by CMI, the bacilli will again grow intracellularly until the macrophages are killed by tissue-damaging DTH, thereby enlarging the caseous necrotic area.

Nonactivated macrophages containing many bacilli are frequently killed by this tissue-damaging DTH reaction, but it is not known whether nonactivated macrophages containing only a few bacilli can be activated sufficiently by T-cell lymphokines to prevent further intracellular bacillary multiplication. The main function of CMI is to activate the surrounding uninvolved macrophages

(Fig. 2-7).[27–29,80] These, now activated, perifocal macrophages ingest and destroy the bacilli escaping from the edges of the caseous center as well as bacilli released when macrophages are killed by DTH (Fig. 2-12).

Phagocytosis and Killing of Tubercle Bacilli by Macrophages

Macrophage Receptors

In order to recognize a microorganism, these phagocytes must first recognize patterns on its surface. The pattern recognition receptors (PRR) of macrophages and dendritic cells include mannose receptors, complement receptors, fibronectin receptors, and Toll-like receptors—all of which are involved in the host's innate immune response.

Extensive studies have recently been made on Toll-like receptors (TLRs),[107–110,117] This receptor family is comprised of at least 10 members that recognize various mycobacterial cell-wall components, including lipoproteins and glycolipids (e.g., lipoarabinomannan). Engagement of human macrophage TLRs by the 19κDa mycobacterial

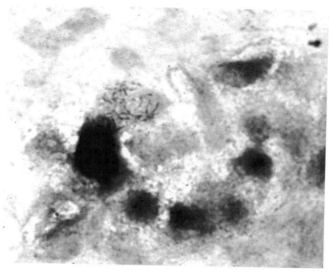

Fig. 2-12. Macrophages stained for β-galactosidase activity and acid-fast bacilli in a BCG lesion of a rabbit injected intradermally 21 days earlier. One of these macrophages shows negligible β-galactosidase activity. It contains numerous bacilli and has ruptured. Another macrophage (just adjacent) shows high β-galactosidase activity. It contains no bacilli, but is apparently ingesting the bacilli released from the ruptured cell. This figure illustrates effective cell-mediated immunity, specifically, that highly activated macrophages can ingest and destroy, bacilli released from ineffectual macrophages.[116] X740. (Reprinted with permission from Dannenberg AM Jr. Cellular hypersensitivity and cellular immunity in the pathogenesis of tuberculosis: specificity, systemic and local nature, and associated macrophage enzymes. *Bacteriol Rev.* 1968;32:85–102. Reproduced by permission of ASM Press, Washington, DC.)

lipoprotein activates NFκB, induces IL-12 secretion, and increases the transcription of inducible nitric oxide synthase[118] all of which participate in killing or inhibiting tubercle bacilli. TLR-knockout mice produced conflicting results,[119–121] possibly due to differences in the infecting dose or differences in the innate immune mechanisms of humans and mice.

After acquired immunity develops, macrophages recognize antibody-opsonized microorganisms by FC receptors and by complement C3b receptors.[76,107]

Fate of Mycobacteria within Macrophages

Because of the receptors just mentioned, *M. tuberculosis* is easily bound to macrophages and internalized into phagosomes. Ordinarily, such phagosomes fuse with lysosomes, undergo acidification, and receive an abundance of lysosomal enzymes that can degrade the microorganisms. However, *M. tuberculosis* subverts phagosome-lysosome fusion and subsequent maturation of the phagosome into an acidic, microbicidal and hydrolytic compartment. *M. tuberculosis* also resists degradation by lysosomal enzymes. Although the bacillus inhibits the entry of many microbicidal factors into the phagosome,[122]

it allows nutrients, such as iron carried by transferrin, to enter.[9,11,123]

The intracellular growth of virulent tubercle bacilli is currently an active field of investigation. One interesting finding is a mycobacterial eukaryotic-like serine/threonine protein kinase G (PknG) that modulated signal transduction pathways for the trafficking of host-cell organelles,[124] thereby inhibiting lysosome-phagosome fusion. Tetrahydrobenzothiophene specifically inhibited PknG and is a promising candidate for developing another class of antimicrobials to combat tuberculosis.[124]

In mice, isocitrate lyase (ICL) is produced by inhibited mycobacteria within activated macrophages, but ICL is *not* produced in multiplying mycobacteria within nonactivated macrophages.[9,125] This lysase enables the bacillus to persist on the fatty acids released from lipids and thereby avoid being destroyed by the microbicidins of activated macrophages.[9,125] ICL is present in mycobacteria but not in mammalian hosts, and therefore is still another potential target for new antimicrobials.

Macrophage defenses include the formation of reactive nitrogen intermediates (RNI) and reactive oxygen intermediates (ROI) to which *M. tuberculosis* is exquisitely susceptible.[126] In mice, chemical inhibition of nitric oxide synthase (NOS) or the deletion of the NOS gene exacerbate tuberculosis.[127–129] The proteasomes of the tubercle bacillus are also involved in its resistance against host RNI, possibly by activating transcription factors for bacillary genes that produce RNI-resistance products.[130,131]

Innate Immunity and Its Relation to Acquired (Adaptive) Immunity

In innate immunity, the host recognizes substances that are present in the pathogen, but not in the host itself. Such foreign substance recognition, also existing in invertebrates, is used in higher animals to upregulate the costimulatory molecules of antigen-presenting cells (APCs). These costimulatory molecules must be upregulate for the antigen-specific immune response of T lymphocytes to occur in vertebrates. Most self-antigens do not upregulate costimulatory molecules on APCs. Therefore, autoimmune reactions are rare. Not only are there costimulatory surface molecules, but there are also coinhibitory surface molecules that control and limit the specific immune response. Coinhibition to self-antigens seems to be defective in some autoimmune diseases. The intricacies of APC, T-cell and B-cell interactions have been clearly presented by Matzinger.[132]

In acquired immunity, APCs first recognize lipopolysaccharides and other microbial products by means of innate receptors.[107] Then, the APCs up regulate their B7 costimulatory factors and their MHC class I and class II surface molecules. Both B7s and MHC are needed for the APCs to present antigens to T cells. The T-cell ligand CD28 binds to B7, and the antigen-specific α/β T-cell receptor binds to the antigen-MHC complex. These T cells then become activated and clonally expand, producing the antigen-specific immunity found in vertebrates. The activated T cells also secrete various cytokines and express other surface molecules, e.g., ligands for CD40, a major costimulatory molecule, and ligands for Fas, a major cell-surface death receptor.

A major cytokine activating the innate immune pathway of host resistance is the IL-12 produced by macrophages and dendritic cells (DCs) stimulated by microbial products. IL-12 activates both natural killer (NK) cells and Th1 lymphocytes. Subsequently, IL-12 induces IL-10 production in lymphocytes and phagocytes, and the IL-10 in turn inhibits or regulates IL-12 production.[133] IL-10 also activates Th2 lymphocytes. Patients infected with HIV are often deficient in their ability to produce IL-12, and this deficiency seems to play a role in the susceptibility of these patients to tuberculosis.[133]

Antigen-Presenting Cells (APCs) and the Major Histocompatibility Complex (MHC)

The main APCs for T cells are the dendritic cells (Table 2-5)[107,134–136] located in the marginal zones of lymph nodes. They are produced in the bone marrow, reside in various tissues, and mature by a two-step process: Initially for antigen-processing and subsequently for T-cell stimulation. The main APCs for B cells are the DCs in the lymphoid follicles. Macrophages, B cells and other cells[137] can also present antigens, but they do so less effectively than DCs.

DC subsets determine the type and the extent of the acquired (adaptive) immune response. The differentiation of immature DCs into a particular subset is influenced by the organ in which the infectious agent resides.[132]

DCs circulate in the blood and are recruited to sites of inflammation,[138] such as tuberculous lesions. Not only do DCs initiate and enhance the immune response, but "tolerogenic" DCs exist that turn off or suppress the immune response.[139] The use of in vitro expanded DCs as adjuvants to increase host immune responses is beginning to find clinical application.

APCs present antigens to most T cells as specific peptides in the context of the MHC, which means that a given T cell will recognize the antigen only when its peptide fragments are bound to a self-MHC molecule. In general, MHC class I molecules present peptides (generated in the APC cytosol) to (cytotoxic) CD8 T cells, and MHC class II molecules present peptides, (from proteins degraded in APC endosomes) to (helper) CD4 T cells. CD stands for clusters of differentiation, specifically cell surface molecules recognized by monoclonal antibodies with the designated number. The MHC class I molecules can react with stimulatory, as well as inhibitory receptors, on T cells. Thus, the immune response is carefully controlled.

MHCs differ from person to person. Therefore, the response to various antigens also differs from person to person—in part depending on the affinity of a person's own MHC molecules for each antigenic peptide. Thus, some people will produce a strong immune response to the antigens of the tubercle bacillus, and other people will produce a weaker response.

Mycolic acid and lipoarabinomannan are cell-wall components of the tubercle bacillus. Such lipid and glycolipid antigens have recently been found to be presented to T cells in association with CD1 surface molecules[140–143a] rather than in association with MHC class I and II molecules. CD1-restricted T cells appear to play an important role in the control of many microbial infections, especially those caused by the tubercle bacillus.[142–146]

Table 2-5. Major Cell Types Involved in Specific and Nonspecific Host Defense Reactions against the Tubercle Bacillus

Macrophages

Macrophages are the effector cells of the mononuclear phagocyte system. They are produced in the bone marrow, circulate as monocytes in the bloodstream, and are called macrophages when they emigrate from the blood into the tissues. Nonactivated monocyte/macrophages allow tubercle bacilli to multiply within them. Highly activated macrophages destroy or inhibit tubercle bacilli.

Lymphocytes (T cells and B cells)

T cells, from the thymus, and B cells, from the bone marrow in mammals or bursa in birds, provide immunologic specificity to the host's defense against tubercle bacilli. In tuberculous lesions, antigen-activated T cells activate macrophages by producing cytokines.

T cells have been subdivided in a variety of ways based on (a) their surface markers (CD4 and CD8 T cells), (b) their receptors (α/β, γ/δ and CD1), (c) the cytokines they produce (Th1 and Th2 cells), and (d) their functions (helper, regulatory and cytotoxic T cells).

Antigen-activated B cells produce antibodies, especially when they differentiate into plasma cells. In tuberculous lesions, antigen-antibody reactions hasten the local accumulation of dendritic cells, macrophages and antigen-specific T cells, i.e., antibodies enhance the local cell-mediated immune response.

Antigen-Presenting Cells (APCs)

Dendritic cells are the main APCs. Dendritic cells migrate from the site of infection to the draining lymph nodes, where they initiate the immune response by presenting antigens to the recirculating lymphocytes that enter these nodes. Dendritic cells and macrophages and B cells can also present antigens to lymphocytes within tuberculous lesions.

Natural Killer (NK) Cells

NK cells, both local and circulating, are an important early defense against intracellular microorganisms (viruses, bacteria, fungi, and protozoa). In tuberculosis, NK cells can kill bacilli-laden macrophages and can produce interferon-gamma, which activates macrophages and stimulates a Th1 cytokine immune response.

Source: Adapted from Dannenberg AM Jr, Tomashefski JF Jr. Pathogenesis of pulmonary tuberculosis. In Fishman AP, ed-in-chief. *Fishman's Pulmonary Diseases and Disorders*, 3rd ed. New York, McGraw-Hill; 1998:2447–2471.

Such CD1-restricted T cells can lyse macrophages infected with virulent *M. tuberculosis*.[143] These CD1 T cells also produce high levels of IFN-γ,[143] a major Th1 cytokine that activates macrophages so that they can destroy or inhibit the growth of tubercle bacilli.[147,148]

In humans infected with *M. tuberculosis*, circulating CD8 T cells have been identified that are classically restricted (MHC class Ia)[149,150] and also nonclassically restricted (Group 1 CD1[151] and HLA-E (HLA Ib)[152]).

Lymphocytes: T cells, CD4 cells, CD8 cells, $\gamma\delta$ T cells, B cells

Overview

Lymphocytes provide the immunologic specificity for the host's CMI and DTH responses to tubercle bacilli. Lymphocyte *memory* is synonymous with an expanded specific lymphocyte population that enables a rapid recall of local CMI and DTH at sites where endogenous or exogenous tubercle bacilli infect the host. The major types of lymphocytes (listed in Table 2-5) are described in more detail in this section.

Lymphocytes originate in the bone marrow and follow two paths of differentiation.[107] *T lymphocytes*, usually called *T cells*, enter the thymus, where they develop their antigen-specific receptors by DNA rearrangements. In contrast, *B lymphocytes*, usually called *B cells*, develop their antigen-specific receptors in the bone marrow. When exposed to the antigen for which they have a receptor, these T and B cells respond by clonal proliferation, greatly increasing their number. In tuberculosis, T cells appear to have two main functions: (a) killing poorly activated macrophages in which the bacilli are multiplying, and (b) producing cytokines that activate macrophages so that these macrophages can now kill or inhibit ingested bacilli.

B Cells

B cells produce antibodies, especially when they differentiate into plasma cells. Plasma cells are frequently found in tuberculous lesions. B cells when activated also increase the production of IFN-γ by NK cells (see next section). NK cells can kill antibody-coated, bacilli-laden macrophages by ADCC (antibody-dependent cell-mediated cytotoxicity).

T Cells

T cells can be divided into two subsets, Th1 and Th2, on the basis of the cytokines they produce, although some T cells show a mixed, i.e., heterogeneous, cytokine pattern. Th1 and Th2 have also been called type 1 and type 2, respectively. Th1 cells suppress Th2 cells, and Th2 cells suppress Th1 cells.

The *Th1 subset* produces IL-2, which causes T-cell proliferation, as well as IFN-γ and tumor necrosis factor beta (TNF-β), both of which activate macrophages. IFN-γ down-regulates the Th2 response. The *Th2 subset* produces IL-4, IL-5, IL-6, IL-9, IL-10, and IL-13, which promote antibody production by B cells. IL-4, IL-10 and IL-13 down-regulate the Th1 response.

Macrophages produce IL-12, a major Th1 activator, and later they produce IL-10, a major Th1 inhibitor. Th2 cells also seem to have a role in keeping the Th1 response from becoming excessive. Costimulatory surface markers play major roles in determining whether the Th1 or Th2 cytokine pattern predominates. Cytotoxic CD8 lymphocytes can also be divided into Th1 and Th2 subsets on the basis of the cytokines they produce.

CD4 Cells

MHC class II-restricted CD4 lymphocytes are key players in the immune response against tuberculosis, because they produce IFN-γ and other activating cytokines. HIV-infected persons with reduced CD4 cells have increased susceptibility to tuberculosis and a more severe disease.[153] In mice, the critical importance of CD4 cells was confirmed by depletion (with CD4-specific antibodies),[154] adoptive transfer,[155,156] and knockout procedures.[157]

CD8 cells

The primary role of CD8 lymphocytes is cell-mediated cytotoxicity, but they also produce IFN-γ which activates macrophages.[108–110] Mice deficient in either CD8 cells[158] or MHC class I-restricted cells[159] are less able to control infection with *M. tuberculosis*. CD8 cells can kill infected cells by producing perforin, granzymes and Fas ligand. Perforin punches holes in the cell membranes, and granzymes and Fas ligand cause apoptosis.[160,160a]

Additional information on the role of CD8 T cells in tuberculosis can be found in Refs. 108, 161–164. For information on CD1-restricted CD8 cells see Antigen Presenting Cells (discussed earlier).

Gamma-Delta T cells

These lymphocytes have receptors that are composed of γδ chains rather than the usual αβ chains.[165] γδ T cells seem to have a much wider influence on the host's response to microorganisms than was previously expected, because they affect functions of NK cells, B cells and other T cells, in part by producing IFN-γ and other cytokines.[165,166]

γδ T cells are activated before αβ T cells and have been postulated to play an early role in host defense against tuberculosis.[167,168] At least some of the γδ T cells have receptors that combine directly with intact antigens without the usual processing and presentation by dendritic cells. γδ T cells are present in high percentages in mucosal epithelium and play a role in bronchial sensitivity to antigens.[169,170]

γδ T cells expressing the Vγ2Vδ2 T-cell receptor are the majority of circulating γδ T cells in humans and nonhuman primates, but are absent in mice.[108,109] The Vγ2Vδ2 T cells recognize small organic phosphate antigens, such as aminobisphosphonates. Such phospho-ligands occur in *M. tuberculosis*. In macaques infected intravenously with BCG, Vγ2Vδ2 T cells are present 3 to 5 weeks later in lung and intestinal mucosa, but not in lymph nodes. After BCG reinfection, this T-cell subset expands in 4 to 6 days to levels 2 to 9 times as large as those seen during primary infection. Similarly, BCG-vaccinated macaques had a rapid recall of Vγ9Vδ2 T cells in bronchoalveolar lavages after a challenge with virulent *M. tuberculosis*.[171]

Humans with active *M. tuberculosis* infection, or health-care professionals recently exposed to patients with tuberculosis, have increased numbers of γδ T cells in their blood.[172–178]

Natural Killer (NK) Cells

NK cells (see Table 2-5) comprise 5 to 10% of the peripheral blood lymphocyte population. They proliferate in response to both macrophage and T-cell derived cytokines. NK cells have the morphology of large granular lymphocytes and are currently defined as cytotoxic cells that do not express surface CD3 or many other T-cell receptors, but do express CD56.

The NK cells have both MHC class I and non MHC-requiring receptors, whereas the cytotoxic T (CD8) cells recognize only specific antigenic peptides in association with MHC class I molecules. In fact, engagement of surface receptors on NK cells with MHC class I molecules on host cells usually turns off, rather than activates, the lytic machinery of the NK cells. Cells infected by viruses and other intracellular microorganisms have reduced or absent MHC class I expression and will be lysed by NK cells, whereas healthy cells, expressing normal levels of MHC I, will not be lysed. Since NK cells can kill infected host cells without prior sensitization, they are considered part of the innate immune system.[179] In tuberculosis, NK cells are an early source of IFN-γ, which activates macrophages and enhances Th1 immunity.

NK T cells have T-cell receptors that recognize CD1 molecules rather than MHC molecules.[107] Since they respond to lipid and glycolipid antigens, they probably play a role in the early host response to tubercle bacilli.

Only a few studies have been made on NK cells and mycobacteria. *Human* peripheral blood mononuclear cells (PBMC) kill more intracellular *M. tuberculosis* when cocultured with NK cells.[180] Also, human NK cells, stimulated in vitro with IL-12 activate macrophages to inhibit the intracellular growth of *Mycobacterium avium*.[181] In *mice*, NK-cell depletion enhances the growth of *M. avium*.[182]

Role of Antibodies in Tuberculosis

Antibodies have never been thought to play a significant role in the pathogenesis of tuberculosis, because the passive transfer of antibodies to uninfected animals had no observable effect on the course of a subsequent infection with tubercle bacilli.[6,183]

However, recent studies in our laboratory[69] suggest a role for antibodies that had not previously been considered. Namely, in hosts with good cell-mediated immunity, an antigen-antibody reaction causes a more rapid infiltration of DTH and CMI-producing cells into sites where tubercle bacilli are located. In other words, antibodies enhance the local cell-mediated host response.[69]

Circulating antibodies to the various antigens of the tubercle bacillus exist in all tuberculin-positive individuals,[184–186] including BCG-vaccinated hosts and healthy persons with inapparent tuberculous lesions. Such antibodies rapidly combine with tubercle bacilli from exogenous or endogenous infection. The resulting antigen-antibody reaction produces chemotaxins, e.g., the C5 component of complement and probably chemokines. These chemotaxins rapidly bring dendritic cells, macrophages and the expanded antigen-specific memory T-cell population to sites of bacillary lodgment. The rapidity with which DTH and CMI are locally produced can prevent many developing microscopic tubercles from reaching clinically apparent size. In brief, antibodies are beneficial in tuberculosis whenever an expanded antigen-specific T-cell population exists.

Cytokines: Chemokines, IL-12, TNF-α, and IFN-γ[187–189]

Cytokines are proteins made by cells that affect the behavior of other cells, which are usually close by.[107] They can be considered local hormones and include the interleukins (ILs), interferons (IFNs) and tumor necrosis factors (TNFs). Chemokines are chemotactic cytokines. Macrophage chemoattractant (activating) protein 1 (MCP-1) is a major chemokine that plays a role in the formation of tuberculous lesions.[68,69] Three key cytokines, IL-12, TNF-α and IFN-γ, will be discussed further, because their critical roles have been documented in mouse tuberculosis.

Interleukin 12

IL-12 is a cytokine that is produced primarily by phagocytes, including dendritic cells, in response to ingested microorganisms.[190] IL-12 activates both NK cells and Th1 lymphocytes causing them to produce IFN-γ and TNF. Therefore, IL-12 is a key cytokine in the cell-mediated immune response to tubercle bacilli.

IL-12 is a covalent dimer of 35 kDa and 40 kDa peptides (p35 & p40). Mice deficient in p40 were more susceptible to *M. tuberculosis* than those deficient in p35.[191] The administration of IL-12 to mice increased their survival time with this disease.[192,193] Supplemental IL-12 was also beneficial to one patient with *Mycobacterium abscessus* and one patient with drug-resistant *M. tuberculosis*.[194,195]

Tumor Necrosis Factor-Alpha (TNF-α)

TNF-α is predominantly secreted by monocytes and tissue macrophages. It is a powerful inducer of the inflammatory response and plays a critical role in host resistance to tuberculosis.[196,197] TNF-knockout mice, TNF-receptor knockout mice, and mice receiving antiTNF antibody all have more severe disease.[198–200]

On the other hand, TNF therapy was beneficial to mice infected with BCG.[201]

Patients with rheumatoid arthritis or Crohn's disease, who were treated with antiTNF-α monoclonal antibodies, showed a high incidence of reactivation tuberculosis, and greater dissemination of the disease.[202,203]

On the other hand, the cachexia found in advanced cases of human tuberculosis[204] and the severity of mycobacterial meningitis[205,206] are at least partly due to TNF-α. Ultimately, in both animals and humans, it is the balance of various cytokines that is of critical importance in the control of tuberculosis.[200–207]

Interferon-Gamma (IFN-γ)

IFN-γ is secreted by CD4 and CD8 T cells as well as NK cells.[208–210] IFN-γ knockout mice had impaired activation of macrophages with low levels of nitric oxide synthase. In these mice, bacillary growth was not contained, and rapid death occurred. Although IFN-γ was necessary to contain the infection, it did not clear the infection in mice or in humans.

Humans with IFN-γ-receptor defects have higher rates of atypical mycobacterial disease.[105,211] Because of the critical role of IFN-γ in host resistance, patients with multidrug-resistant tuberculosis have been treated with adjunctive IFN-γ by aerosol with some benefit.[211,212]

Systemic Immunity

Greater numbers of T lymphocytes with specific receptors for the antigens of the tubercle bacillus are present in the blood and lymphoid tissues of individuals infected with virulent or avirulent tubercle bacilli than in the blood and tissues of individuals who have never been exposed to such bacilli. The clonal expansion of these antigen-specific T cells is the basis of the immunizing process. When these *immune* individuals are exposed to exogenous or endogenous tubercle bacilli, greater numbers of these antigen-specific T cells accumulate at sites where the bacilli are deposited. The large number of local T cells produce high concentrations of cytokines that accelerate the local accumulation and activation of macrophages, so that the bacillus is destroyed before it multiplies appreciably. The developing lesion usually remains small and heals rapidly. Such accelerated tubercle formation is the reason why small secondary tubercles of hematogenous, lymphogenous and bronchogenic origins do not usually progress in immunocompetent adult human beings.

In immune disease-free individuals, the only systemic immunity may be the expanded antigen-specific T cell population. In that case, macrophages are activated at an accelerated rate at sites wherever exogenous tubercle bacilli are deposited. Thus, immunity in tuberculosis is a local, not a systemic, phenomenon.

Turnover of Macrophages in the Tuberculous Lesions[213]

Macrophages have a continual turnover in the caseous tuberculous lesions. Numerous macrophages enter these lesions, and numerous macrophages die there or leave via the lymphatics. In spite of this turnover, numerous macrophages accumulate in the lesions and become activated. Both the macrophage turnover rate and the accumulation of activated macrophages peak when CMI—DTH first develops. At that time, large numbers of bacilli, lymphocytes, and macrophages are present and much local cytokine production occurs. Before DTH develops, relatively few lymphocytes with specific receptors for the antigens of tubercle bacilli are present to produce cytokines. (Clonal expansion has not yet occurred.) Later, after most of the bacilli and their antigens have been destroyed, the stimulus for cytokine production is greatly reduced, so that relatively few macrophages enter, become activated, and die or leave.

Duration and Specificity of Cell-Mediated Immunity (CMI) and Its Recall Upon Reinfection

The following principles were established in mice by Mackaness and his associates,[81–83] briefly reviewed in Reference 80.

After an intravenous injection of BCG, acquired cellular resistance decreases with time. Such resistance, however, can be rapidly recalled to full strength by reinjection of BCG. From the first exposure, the host retains increased numbers of (clonally-expanded) T cells with specific receptors for these antigens. Upon reexposure to BCG antigens, these T cells rapidly produce lymphokines, which cause local macrophage and lymphocyte accumulation and activation.

The injection of other types of facultative intracellular bacilli (e.g., listeria or salmonella) does not rapidly recall immunity to BCG, however, once macrophages have been activated in local sites by BCG, the specific antigen, these macrophages can nonspecifically destroy a variety of facultative intracellular microorganisms in the same local sites. The specificity of cell-mediated immunity resides entirely in the T lymphocyte, not in the macrophage. Macrophages kill facultative intracellular microorganisms only nonspecifically.

The Mackaness group administered the immunizing and recalling BCG intravenously. In this case, most of the bacilli were deposited in the liver and spleen, where many local sites containing activated macrophages developed. Such macrophages could readily destroy other types of facultative intracellular bacilli that were deposited in the liver and spleen by a subsequent intravenous injection.

The number of specific T cells in the blood and tissues decreases with time, and a positive tuberculin reaction may even disappear. These events may occur if the tubercle bacilli and their antigens have been eliminated from the host. Nonetheless, a large number of specific T cells still remain in the host, so that, upon reinfection, specific CMI and DTH, i.e., tuberculin sensitivity, are rapidly recalled.

Prognostic Significance of the Tuberculin Skin Test

The size of the dermal tuberculin reaction is of little or no prognostic significance, either during the disease or after it is arrested. During the disease, a large reaction may signify a host of high native and acquired resistance to tuberculosis, because such resistant hosts are able to accumulate large numbers of lymphocytes and macrophages, both in tuberculous lesions and at the site of tuberculin injection. A large tuberculin reaction may also signify a host of low native and acquired resistance, because the lesions of such susceptible hosts contain numerous bacilli that provide a high dose of antigen for sensitization.

A large tuberculin reaction, remaining years after the primary disease has healed, probably signifies that a few dormant bacilli are still present in inapparent caseous foci. Such bacilli seem to be released from time to time and then are rapidly destroyed, which gives a booster effect to the whole immune system, including the level of tuberculin sensitivity.

Booster Effect of a Repeat Tuberculin Skin Test

Persons who have recently been infected with the tubercle bacillus can, in time, become tuberculin-negative with or without antimicrobial treatment. In many of these persons, a recall of tuberculin sensitivity is produced by the antigens in tuberculin (PPD) that was injected for skin testing. When retested with intermediate strength PPD, a person who was negative three weeks earlier may now be tuberculin positive as a result of the booster effect of tuberculin itself.[214,215] The previous injection of PPD had expanded the tuberculin sensitive T cell population, i.e., memory T cells, to a level where the number of these cells is now sufficient to produce a positive tuberculin test. Details on this booster effect of tuberculin are reviewed in Ref. 216.

A Negative Tuberculin Test in Patients with Active Tuberculosis

Individuals who are ill with this disease may have a negative tuberculin skin test. When they are recovering, however, they again develop a positive skin test. Compartmentalization could be the cause of this skin-test anergy. The pulmonary tuberculous lesions may collect most of the antigen-specific circulating T-cells, so that few are available to participate in the dermal tuberculin reaction. This concept receives support from the fact that lymphocytes from diseased tissues obtained by bronchoalveolar lavage, or from pleural exudates, contain a greater proportion of antigen-specific T cells, secrete greater quantities of lymphokines, and show a greater tendency to proliferate, in the presence of specific antigens, than do the T lymphocytes in peripheral blood.[114,217–219]

Tuberculin-negative patients with active tuberculosis also have a greater number of suppressor monocytes and lymphocytes in their peripheral blood.[217–225] This fact, however, does not prove that T cells within tuberculous lesions are suppressed. In such lesions, the composition of the cell population is different from that present in peripheral blood, as indicated by studies of the cells in both blood and pleural fluids from patients with tuberculous pleurisy.

In peripheral blood of such patients, mononuclear cells produce transforming growth factor-beta (TGF-β) and IL-10, which are, at least in part, responsible for the immunosuppressive effects on tuberculin sensitivity, as are reactive nitrogen intermediates, free fatty acids, and phospholipids.[223,224]

In summary, many patients with active tuberculosis have a negative PPD skin test. This immunosuppression was correlated with a decrease in the ability of their peripheral blood lymphocytes to undergo clonal expansion and to produce IFN-γ and IL-2 when these cells were cultured in vitro with PPD.[217,226] The suppressive effect is in part due to the production of TGF-β and IL-10 by circulating mononuclear cells.

Whether such studies on peripheral blood mononuclear cells can predict the future course of the disease remains to be determined. At least during effective antimicrobial therapy, the return of a positive PPD skin test and the return of increased PPD-induced peripheral blood lymphocyte blastogenesis and IFN-γ production are good prognostic signs.[226]

Improved Diagnostic Tests for Active Tuberculosis

The tuberculin skin test cannot reliably differentiate between DTH from a progressive tuberculous lesion and DTH from environmental mycobacteria or BCG vaccination or a nonprogressive arrested lesion. Since the secreted antigen ESAT-6 is produced by virulent human-type tubercle bacilli and not by BCG or by many environmental mycobacteria, an in vitro diagnostic test on human peripheral blood mononuclear cells (PBMC) was developed and evaluated in Ethiopia.[227,228] This test measures the amount of IFN-γ produced by PBMC after 5 days in culture and stimulation with ESAT-6.

At the beginning of this study, the amount of IFN-γ produced by PBMC from tuberculin-positive household contacts of active (sputum-positive) tuberculous persons was determined.[229] Two years later these contacts were evaluated for clinically active tuberculosis. The household contacts who developed clinially active tuberculosis in two years were those whose PBMC originally produced high levels of IFN-γ, whereas those contacts whose PBMC originally produced low levels of IFN-γ remained healthy. Parallel studies with tuberculin (PPD) as the in vitro antigen showed no difference between these two groups. Evidently, the contacts with early progressive tuberculosis could be identified by an increase in the number of circulating lymphocytes capable of responding to ESAT-6.

This was the first study in which a laboratory test could distinguish tuberculin-positive persons with progressive early tuberculous lesions, who should be treated with antimicrobials, from persons with nonprogressive lesions, who would not need antimicrobial therapy. If further studies confirm these results, the ESAT-6 in vitro test would be a major addition to the control of this disease.

Effect of Vaccines on the Establishment of Pulmonary Tuberculous Lesions

Vaccination *cannot* prevent the establishment of an infection with the tubercle bacillus.[230] It can only prevent progression of the disease after a microscopic tubercle is established. In vaccinated (usually tuberculin-positive)

individuals, the inhaled virulent tubercle bacillus is ingested by an alveolar macrophage. These highly activated cells usually destroy the inhaled tubercle bacillus before it has a chance to multiply in both, vaccinated and nonvaccinated individuals. One or two years after vaccination with BCG, all but a small residual of the BCG has been eliminated. At that time, one would expect vaccinated and nonvaccinated individuals to show no difference in the number of alveolar macrophages or in their microbicidal abilities. Thus, both vaccinated and nonvaccinated hosts would initially destroy the same number of inhaled virulent bacilli, or initially allow the same number to multiply.

When first inhaled, a bacillary unit of 1 to 3 bacilli, which is the only quantity that can stay suspended in the air stream long enough to reach the alveolar spaces, contains insufficient antigen to stimulate the immune system. However, once this bacillary unit begins to multiply, enough antigen is present to be recognized by lymphocytes. From this point on, vaccinated and nonvaccinated individuals show different responses. Vaccinated hosts show accelerated tubercle formation, i.e., a rapid local accumulation of lymphocytes and macrophages and a rapid activation of these cells. This accelerated immune response often arrests the early focus of infection, thereby preventing its development into clinical disease.[31] In nonvaccinated hosts, lymphocyte and macrophage activation develops at a much slower pace, so that clinical disease occurs more frequently. See Reference 69.

Differences exist between humans and rabbits in their minute arrested tuberculous lesions. Humans are so sensitive to the tuberculin products of the bacillus that even microscopic tuberculous lesions soon caseate. In practically all tuberculin-positive human beings, without clinically apparent disease, a calcified arrested caseous lesion, usually 0.5 to 1.0 mm in size can been found at necropsy many years later.[230] The tuberculin sensitivity of rabbits is much less than the tuberculin sensitivity of humans. Therefore, in rabbits, following the inhalation of virulent human-type tubercle bacilli, many microscopic tuberculous lesions resolve without caseation or calcification and become undetectable at a later time. In both humans[230] and rabbits,[31] however, BCG vaccination reduces the progress of tuberculous lesions once they are established.

Development of Better Vaccines for Tuberculosis (see Chap. 9)

The challenge to researchers engaged in vaccine development for tuberculosis is to find (a) antigens that are more potent than BCG in producing T-cell populations that activate macrophages to destroy the bacillus (CMI), and (b) antigens that are less potent than BCG in producing T-cell populations that cause caseous necrosis and liquefaction, which we define *pathologically* as tissue-damaging DTH. In other words, a vaccine is needed that produces a higher "CMI : tissue-damaging DTH" ratio than do currently available BCG vaccines.

Both CMI and DTH are immunologic processes produced by T lymphocytes with specific receptors for the various antigens of the tubercle bacillus. These specific T cells attract macrophages and other lymphocytes to sites of antigen deposition. There, the macrophages and T lymphocytes activate each other, as well as other members of their own cell type.

Tissue necrosis (DTH) is apparently necessary to stop the logarithmic growth of tubercle bacilli within nonactivated macrophages. Would, therefore, vaccines that produce little or no tuberculin sensitivity be able to stop such logarithmic intracellular growth? The answer seems to be "Yes".

In the British Medical Research Council trials, one lot of vole bacillus vaccine produced a high incidence of tuberculin-positivity and another lot did not. Yet, both lots showed equally high protective potency against tuberculosis.[231] This and other studies with different strains of BCG[232] clearly demonstrate that the antigens causing appreciable tuberculin-positivity were not required for the protection of human beings.

When applied to the pathogenesis of tuberculosis, these findings indicate that the killing of nonactivated macrophages, in which the bacilli are growing intracellularly in a logarithmic fashion, is not only due to tuberculin-like antigens. It can apparently be produced by a DTH response to other antigens of the bacillus when these antigens are in a sufficiently high concentration. In fact, in the mouse model, lymphocytes transferring protective immunity can be dissociated from those that transfer tuberculin sensitivity.[156]

A vaccine superior to present strains of BCG would be one that produces strong CMI with little or no sensitivity to tuberculin. Favorable antigenic fractions of the tubercle bacillus, probably certain proteins complexed with certain carbohydrates and lipids, would stimulate CMI with minimal tissue-damaging DTH; whereas detrimental antigens, probably the tuberculoproteins that produce the tuberculin reaction, would produce more tissue-damaging DTH (caseation and liquefaction) with less CMI.

Tuberculoproteins that cause the tuberculin reaction have never been shown to be protective.[6,233,234] In fact, they can produce severe necrosis in the tuberculin-positive host if their concentration exceeds that which is safe for a given host.[84] Other fractions may be effective immunogens without producing tuberculin sensitivity. These principles, however, still remain to be established. The roles of the carbohydrate fractions of these bacilli and of the proteins secreted by living tubercle bacilli need further investigation.[235]

Additional insight has recently been gained into the adjuvanticity of tuberculosis vaccines.[68] In dermal BCG lesions, the percentage of mononuclear cells containing cytokine, especially chemokine, mRNA and protein was highest during the first 3 days. This finding suggests that the most effective tuberculosis vaccines would not only contain the most appropriate mycobacterial antigens, but would also contain mycobacterial adjuvants that recruit the largest number of macrophages, lymphocytes and dendritic cells into local sites of antigen deposition.

It is possible that recombinant BCG vaccines will be better than existing BCG vaccines.[236–240] To produce such vaccines, the DNAs for additional antigens are added to the BCG genome. These antigens may increase the virulence of the BCG, so careful evaluation in animal models should be performed before human trials are begun.

DNA vaccines are those in which the DNAs of one or more mycobacterial antigens are incorporated into a plasmid and usually injected intramuscularly. Such DNA vaccines increased the immunity of mice and guinea pigs to virulent tubercle bacilli, but not more than did BCG; and the immunity produced was shorter lived.[236,239] DNA vaccines or vaccines incorporating mycobacterial protein, lipid, and/or glycolipid antigens (in adjuvants) may be useful in HIV patients, because such vaccines cannot cause tuberculosis in immunosuppressed individuals.

A substantial percentage of the world's human population is already tuberculin-positive from inhaling virulent tubercle bacilli. Therefore, postinfection immunization to prevent endogenous and exogenous reinfection would be especially useful. Subunit vaccines are probably the safest type to use for this purpose.[239,240]

Finally, combination vaccines, which consist of BCG and one or more booster immunizations with important mycobacterial antigens, including those produced by DNA vaccines,[241] will probably provide the most effective protection against active disease.[236,239–242] The antigens in such boosters would expand the appropriate T-lymphocyte population almost as well as if these antigens had been incorporated into the live vaccine itself. They would, however, probably require one or more repeat injections.

Refs. 236, 239, 240, 243–246 briefly review some of the newly developed vaccines for tuberculosis that were evaluated in mice and guinea pigs.

Because BCG may persist in the host for years, recombinant BCG vaccines containing specific antigens from various viral, bacterial and parasitic microorganisms are currently being evaluated.[247]

Advantages of Vaccines Containing Little or no Tuberculin-Like Antigens

There are many benefits in eliminating tuberculin-like antigens from BCG (Table 2-6).[248] First, vaccinated individuals would not be appreciably tuberculin-positive, so that tuberculin testing of such persons would still be a useful procedure for diagnosing infection with virulent tubercle bacilli.

Second, such a vaccine could even be given to tuberculin-positive individuals with less harm, and probably with true benefit. It would expand the T-cell population responding to protective antigens of the tubercle bacillus and not expand the T-cell population responding to antigens like tuberculin that are often detrimental. Thus, existing latent or even active foci of tuberculosis would be less apt to progress, because a population rich in beneficial T cells and macrophages would surround them.

Third, because it produces little or no DTH, a vaccine without tuberculin-like antigens could be given more than once to create high levels of immunity, especially in high risk groups.

Fourth, when available, such a vaccine might replace isoniazid (INH) in preventive therapy of persons who recently became tuberculin positive. Substituting such a

Table 2-6. Advantages of Tuberculosis Vaccines Producing Strong CMI and Weak Tissue-Damaging DTH (especially those producing little or no tuberculin sensitivity)

To prevent clinical tuberculosis (prophylaxis)
To treat clinical tuberculosis (immunotherapy)
To vaccinate PPD-positive persons without possible harm
To further enhance immunity by repeated vaccinations
    (not advised with current BCG vaccines)

Source: Adapted from Dannenberg AM Jr: Controlling tuberculosis. The pathologist's point of view. From the 5th Forum in Microbiology on "Killing of Intracellular Mycobacteria: Dogmas and Realities." *Res Microbiol (formerly, Ann Inst Pasteur).* 1990;141:192–196, 262–263. Copyright 1990. Reprinted with permission from Elsevier.

vaccine for INH would eliminate the danger of INH hepatotoxicity and INH bacillary resistance.

PART III. CONCLUSIONS

(a) Activated macrophages can kill ingested tubercle bacilli. Under normal conditions, i.e., before the infection begins, most of the alveolar macrophages are nonspecifically activated.

(b) During the infection, tubercle bacilli multiply logarithmically in nonactivated macrophages. Their cytoplasm provides a very fertile "soil" for such bacillary growth.

(c) The tissue-damaging DTH to the antigens of the bacilli, is the main mechanism by which the host stops the bacillary growth in nonactivated macrophages. DTH does so by killing these macrophages and nearby tissues. Tubercle bacilli do not multiply appreciably in the resulting solid caseous necrotic material.

(d) This favorable result occurs at the expense of host tissues. As bacilli escape from the edge of the caseous focus, they are ingested by immature non-activated macrophages from the bloodstream. In the cytoplasm of these nonactivated cells the bacilli again find fertile soil in which to grow. And, again, the DTH reaction of the host will kill the bacilli-laden macrophages and nearby tissues. If the sequence continues, so much viable lung tissue is sacrificed that the host will die.

(e) Only CMI can stop the continued destruction of host tissues caused by the DTH reaction to bacillary antigens, especially tuberculin-like antigens. Immunologically specific T cells and their lymphokines, especially IFN-γ, which characterize the CMI reaction, produce a perifocal mantle of highly activated macrophages around the caseous center. These macrophages ingest and destroy the bacilli that escape from the edge of the caseous center. Continued destruction of host tissue is no longer required to stop the multiplication of the bacillus, because the bacillus now resides in highly activated macrophages.

(f) If developed, recombinant BCG strains that produce little or no sensitivity to tuberculin should be more effective than currently available BCG strains. Such a BCG vaccine would expand the T cell population capable of producing CMI with less expansion of the T cell population capable of producing DTH (caseous necrosis). Lesions caused by virulent bacilli in such vaccinated hosts would therefore contain more T cells from the memory population that cause activated macrophages (CMI) and relatively few tuberculin-reactive T cells that cause tissue necrosis and liquefaction with little CMI.

(g) When solid caseous tissue liquefies, the tubercle bacillus again finds a fertile soil in which to multiply logarithmically. For the first time during the course of the disease, the bacillus can now multiply extra-cellularly and frequently reaches tremendous numbers. Such numbers may not be controlled even in a highly immune host. Due to the presence of DTH, the bacilli and/or their tuberculin-like products often cause extensive necrosis. One or more bronchi are eroded, a cavity forms, and the bacilli can spread throughout the airways to other parts of the lung and to the outside environment. Also, antimicrobial-resistant mutants may arise among the numerous actively growing bacilli.

(h) Therapeutic agents that reduce the amount of liquefaction would be of considerable help in the treatment of tuberculosis and in limiting the spread of this disease to other persons. Yet, to our knowledge, little or no research to develop such agents is currently underway.

The pathogenesis of tuberculosis (Part I) with respect to the bacillary multiplication is summarized in Table 2-7. The major research advances in immunology that have direct bearing on the pathogenesis of tuberculosis are summarized in the whole of Part II. Three of these research advances are especially pertinent, namely, interactions between innate immunity and acquired immunity,

interactions among the cytokines, and the role of apoptosis as a control mechanism of both inflammatory and immune responses.

ACKNOWLEDGMENTS

Max B. Lurie, with whom Dr. Dannenberg spent 12 years at the University of Pennsylvania, established many of these principles of pathogenesis of tuberculosis. His insight into the mechanisms of this disease was both penetrating and comprehensive.

The authors appreciate the superb editorial assistance of Ilse M. Harrop and Rena Ashworth, and the financial support of grant HL-71554 and contract NIAID-DMID 03-09 from the National Institutes of Health.

Figures 2-1, 2-3 and 2-4 were drawn by Roberta R. Proctor and Lester J. Dyer, and Fig. 2-10 by Joseph M. Dieter, Jr.

REFERENCES

1. Dannenberg AM Jr. Pathogenesis of pulmonary tuberculosis in man and animals: protection of personnel against tuberculosis. In: Montali RJ, ed. *Mycobacterial Infections of Zoo Animals.* Washington, DC: Smithsonian Institution Press; 1978:65–75.

2. Centers for Disease Control. Guidelines for preventing the transmission of *Mycobacterium tuberculosis* in healthcare facilities. *MMWR Morb Mortal Wkly Rep.* 1994; 43:1–132.

3. Centers for Disease Control. A strategic plan for the elimination of tuberculosis in the United States. *MMWR Morb Mortal Wkly Rep.* (April 21, Suppl. S-3), 1989;38:1–25.

4. Dannenberg AM Jr. Immune mechanisms in the pathogenesis of pulmonary tuberculosis. *Rev Infect Dis.* 1989;11(Suppl 2):S369–S378.

5. Dannenberg AM Jr, Tomashefski JF Jr. Pathogenesis of pulmonary tuberculosis. In Fishman AP, ed-in-chief *Fishman's Pulmonary Diseases and Disorders*, 3rd ed. New York, NY: McGraw-Hill; 1998:2447–2471.

6. Lurie MB. *Resistance to Tuberculosis: Experimental Studies in Native and Acquired Defense Mechanisms.* Cambridge, MA: Harvard University Press; 1964.

7. Riley RL, Mills CC, O'Grady F, et al. Infectiousness of air from a tuberculosis ward. Ultraviolet irradiation of infected air: comparative infectiousness of different patients. *Am Rev Respir Dis.* 1962;85:511–525.

8. Lurie MB, Dannenberg AM Jr. Macrophage function in infectious disease with inbred rabbits. *Bacteriol Rev.* 1965;29:466–476.

9. Russell DG. Mycobacterium tuberculosis: here today, and here tomorrow. *Nat Rev Mol Cell Biol.* 2001;2: 569–577.

Table 2-7. Multiplication of Tubercle Bacilli and the Host Immune Response

---

No Multiplication of bacilli: no disease, no CMI, no DTH

Bacilli Dormant in caseous focus: arrested disease, good CMI, strong, weak, or nearly absent DTH

Intracellular Multiplication of bacilli: caseous foci, hematogenous spread, poor CMI, often good DTH

Extracellular Multiplication of bacilli: cavity formation, bronchial spread, caseous bronchopneumonia, good CMI, sometimes overwhelmed, usually good DTH

10. Schlesinger LS. Role of mononuclear phagocytes in M. tuberculosis pathogenesis. *J Med Invest*. 1996;44: 312–323.

11. Pieters J. Entry and survival of pathogenic mycobacteria in macrophages. *Microbes Infect*. 2001;3:249–255.

12. Sreevatsan S, Pan X, Stockbauer KE, et al. Restricted structural gene polymorphism in the *Mycobacterium tuberculosis* complex indicates evolutionarily recent global dissemination. *Proc Natl Acad Sci USA*. 1997;94:9869–9874.

13. Fleischmann RD, Alland D, Eisen JA, et al. Whole-genome comparison of *Mycobacterium tuberculosis* clinical and laboratory strains. *J Bacteriol*. 2002;184:5479–5490.

14. Brosch R, Gordon SV, Marmiesse M, et al. A new evolutionary scenario for the *Mycobacterium tuberculosis* complex. *Proc Natl Acad Sci USA*. 2002;99:3684–3689.

15. Brodin P, Eiglmeier K, Marmiesse M, et al. Bacterial artificial chromosome-based comparative genomic analysis identifies *Mycobacterium microti* as a natural ESAT-6 deletion mutant. *Infect Immun*. 2002;70:5568–5578.

16. Manabe Y, Scott C, Bishai W: Naturally attenuated, orally administered *Mycobacterium microti* is more effective than *Mycobacterium bovis* BCG as a tuberculosis vaccine. *Infect Immun*. 2002;70:1566–1570.

17. Behr MA, Small PM. A historical and molecular phylogeny of BCG strains. *Vaccine*. 1999;17:915–922.

18. Behr MA, Wilson MA, Gill WP, et al. Comparative genomics of BCG vaccines by whole-genome DNA microarray. *Science*. 1999;284:1520–1523.

19. Behr MA, Small PM. Has BCG attenuated to impotence? (letter). *Nature*. 1997;389:133–134.

20. Mitchison D, Bhatia L, Radhakrishna S, et al. The virulence in the guinea-pig of tubercle bacilli isolated before treament from South Indian patients with pulmonary tuberculosis. *Bull World Health Organ*. 1961;25:285–312.

21. Dickinson JM, Lefford MJ, Lloyd J, et al. The virulence in the guinea-pig of tubercle bacilli from patients with pulmonary tuberculosis in Hong Kong. *Tubercle*. 1963;44:446–451.

22. Comstock GW, O'Brien RJ. Tuberculosis. In: Evans AS, Brachman PS, eds. *Bacterial Infections of Humans: Epidemiology and Control*. New York, NY: Plenum Medical; 1991:745–771.

23. Manca C, Tsenova L, Bergtold A, et al. Virulence of a *Mycobacterium tuberculosis* clinical isolate in mice is determined by failure to induce Th1 type immunity and is associated with induction of IFN-alpha/beta. *Proc Natl Acad Sci USA*. 2001;98:5752–5757.

24. Manca C, Tsenova L, Barry CE 3d, et al. *Mycobacterium tuberculosis* CDC1551 induces a more vigorous host response in vivo and in vitro, but is not more virulent than other clinical isolates. *J Immunol*. 1999;162:6740–6746.

25. Manabe YC, Dannenberg AM Jr, Tyagi SK, et al. Different strains of *Mycobacterium tuberculosis* cause various spectrums of disease in the rabbit model of tuberculosis. *Infect Immun*. 2003;71:6004–6011.

26. Dannenberg AM Jr, Burstone M, Walter PC, et al. A histochemical study of phagocytic and enzymatic functions of rabbit mononuclear and polymorphonuclear exudate cells and alveolar macrophages. I. Survey and quantitation of enzymes, and states of cellular activation. *J Cell Biol*. 1963;17:465–486.

27. Dannenberg AM Jr. Delayed-type hypersensitivity and cell-mediated immunity in the pathogenesis of tuberculosis. *Immunol. Today*. 1991;12:228–233.

28. Dannenberg AM Jr. Immunopathogenesis of pulmonary tuberculosis. *Hosp Pract*. 1993;28:33–40(Off Ed: 51–58).

29. Dannenberg AM Jr, Rook GAW. Pathogenesis of pulmonary tuberculosis: an interplay of tissue-damaging and macrophage-activating immune responses—dual mechanisms that control bacillary multiplication. In: Bloom BR, ed. *Tuberculosis: Pathogenesis, Protection, and Control*. Washington, DC: American Society for Microbiology; 1994:459–483.

30. Lurie MB, Zappasodi P, Tickner C. On the nature of genetic resistance to tuberculosis in the light of the host-parasite relationships in nately resistant and susceptible rabbits. *Am Rev Tuberc Pulm Dis*. 1955;72:297–329.

31. Dannenberg AM Jr. Lurie's tubercle-count method to test TB vaccine efficacy in rabbits. *Front Biosci*. 1998;3: 27–33. http://www.bioscience.org/1998/v3/c/dannenbe/list.htm.

32. Allison M, Zappasodi P, Lurie MB. Host-parasite relationships in natively resistant and susceptible rabbits on quantitative inhalation of tubercle bacilli. *Am Rev Resp Dis*. 1962;85:553–569.

33. Dannenberg AM Jr. Pathogenesis of pulmonary *Mycobacterium bovis* infection: Basic principles established by the rabbit model. In: *Third International Conference on Mycobacterium bovis*. Cambridge, UK: July 13–16, 2000. *Tuberculosis*. 2001;81:87–96.

34. Leonard EJ, Yoshimura T. Human monocyte chemoattractant protein-1 (MCP-1). *Immunol. Today*. 1990;11: 97–101.

35. Shima K, Dannenberg AM Jr, Ando M, et al. Macrophage accumulation, division, maturation, and digestive and microbicidal capacities in tuberculous lesions. I. Studies involving their incorporation of tritiated thymidine and their content of lysosomal enzymes and bacilli. *Am J Pathol*. 1972;67:159–180.

36. Smith DW, Harding GE. Animal model of human disease. Pulmonary tuberculosis. Animal model: Experimental airborne tuberculosis in the guinea pig. *Am J Pathol*. 1977; 89:273–276.

37. Pabst MJ, Gross JM, Brozna JP, et al. Inhibition of macrophage priming by sulfatide from *Mycobacterium tuberculosis*. *J Immunol*. 1988;140:634–640.

38. Brozna JP, Horan M, Rademacher JM, et al. Monocyte responses to sulfatide from *Mycobacterium tuberculosis:* inhibition of priming for enhanced release of superoxide, associated with increased secretion of interleukin-1 and tumor necrosis factor alpha, and altered protein phosphorylation. *Infect Immun*. 1991;59:2542–2548.

39. Kaufmann SHE: In vitro analysis of the cellular mechanisms involved in immunity to tuberculosis. *Rev Infect Dis*. 1989;11([Suppl 2):S448–S454.

40. Bryk R, Lima CD, Erdjument-Bromage H, et al. Metabolic enzymes of mycobacteria linked to antioxidant defense by a thioredoxin-like protein. *Science.* 2002;295:1073–1077.

41. Kaufmann SHE. CD8+ T lymphocytes in intracellular microbial infections. *Immunol. Today.* 1988;9:168–174.

42. Ottenhoff TH, de Vries RRP. Antigen reactivity and autoreactivity: Two sides of the cellular immune response induced by mycobacteria. *Curr Top Microbiol Immunol.* 1990;155:111–121.

43. Boom WH, Wallis RS, Chervenak KA. Human *Mycobacterium tuberculosis*-reactive CD4+ T-cell clones. Heterogeneity in antigen recognition, cytokine production, and cytotoxicity for mononuclear phagocytes. *Infect Immun* 1991;59:2737–2743.

44. Kaleab B, Ottenhoff T, Converse P, et al.. Mycobacterial-induced cytotoxic T cells as well as nonspecific killer cells derived from healthy individuals and leprosy patients. *Eur J Immunol.* 1990;20:2651–2659.

45. Lowrie DB. Is macrophage death on the field of battle essential to victory, or a tactical weakness in immunity against tuberculosis? *Clin Exp Immunol.* 1990;80:301–303.

46. Canetti G. *The Tubercle Bacillus.* New York, NY: Springer Publishing Company; 1955.

47. Poole JCF, Florey HW. Chronic inflammation and tuberculosis. In: Florey HW, ed. *General Pathology.* Philadelphia, PA: WB Saunders; 1970:1183–1224.

48. Koch R. Fortsetzung der Mittheilungen über ein Heilmittel gegen Tuberculose (Continuation of the communication concerning a treatment for tuberculosis). *Dtsch Med Wochenschr.* 1891; Jan 15:101–102.

49. Hemsworth GR, Kochan I. Secretion of antimycobacterial fatty acids by normal and activated macrophages. *Infect Immun.* 1978;19:170–177.

50. Rook GAW. Mycobacteria, cytokines and antibiotics. *Pathol Biol (Paris).* 1990;38:276–280.

51. Kumararatne DS, Pithie AS, Drysdale P, et al. Specific lysis of mycobacterial antigen-bearing macrophages by class II MHC-restricted polyclonal T cell lines in healthy donors or patients with tuberculosis. *Clin Exp Immunol.* 1990;80:314–323.

52. Ottenhoff TH, Ab BK, van Embden JD, et al. The recombinant 65-kD heat shock protein of *Mycobacterium bovis* Bacillus Calmette-Guérin/*M. tuberculosis* is a target molecule for CD4+ cytotoxic T lymphocytes that lyse human monocytes. *J Exp Med.* 1988;168:1947–1952.

53. Rock KL. A new foreign policy: MHC class I molecules monitor the outside world. *Immunol Today.* 1996;17:131–137.

54. Rook GAW. Role of activated macrophages in the immunopathology of tuberculosis. *Br Med Bull.* 1988;44:611–623.

55. Jaattela M. Biologic activities and mechanisms of action of tumor necrosis factor-alpha/cachectin. *Lab Invest.* 1991;64:724–742.

56. Filley EA, Rook GAW. Effect of mycobacteria on sensitivity to the cytotoxic effects of tumor necrosis factor. *Infect Immun.* 1991;59:2567–2572.

57. Rook GAW, al Attiyah R. Cytokines and the Koch phenomenon. *Tubercle.* 1991;72:13–20.

58. Klebanoff SJ. Phagocytic cells: Products of oxygen metabolism. In: Gallin JI, Goldstein IM, Snyderman R, eds. *Inflammation: Basic Principles and Clinical Correlates.* New York, NY: Raven Press; 1988:391–444.

59. Stuehr DJ, Marletta, MA. Induction of nitrite/nitrate synthesis in murine macrophages by BCG infection, lymphokines, or interferon-gamma. *J Immunol.* 1987;139:518–525.

60. Moncada S, Palmer RM, Higgs EA. Nitric oxide: physiology, pathophysiology, and pharmacology. *Pharmacol Rev.* 1991;43:109–142.

61. Green SJ, Nacy CA, Meltzer MS. Cytokine-induced synthesis of nitrogen oxides in macrophages: a protective host response to Leishmania and other intracellular pathogens. *J Leukoc Biol.* 1991;50:93–103.

62. Laskin DL, Pendino KJ. Macrophages and inflammatory mediators in tissue injury. *Annu Rev Pharmacol Toxicol.* 1995;35:655–677.

63. Long ER. *The Chemistry and Chemotherapy of Tuberculosis.* Balitmore, MD: Williams & Wilkins; 1958:106–108, 122–124.

64. Kaufmann SHE. Leprosy and tuberculosis vaccine design. *Trop Med Parasitol.* 1989;40:251–257.

65. Abou-Zeid C, Smith I, Grange JM, et al. The secreted antigens of *Mycobacterium tuberculosis* and their relationship to those recognized by the available antibodies. *J Gen Microbiol.* 1988;134(Pt 2):531–538.

66. Andersen P, Askgaard D, Ljungqvist L, et al. Proteins released from *Mycobacterium tuberculosis* during growth. *Infect Immun.* 1991;59:1905–1910.

67. Abe Y, Sugisaki K, Dannenberg AM Jr. Rabbit vascular endothelial adhesion molecules: ELAM-1 is most elevated in acute inflammation, whereas VCAM-1 and ICAM-1 predominate in chronic inflammation. *J Leukoc Biol.* 1996;60:692–703.

68. Sugisaki K, Dannenberg AM Jr, Abe Y, et al. Nonspecific and immune-specific up-regulation of cytokines in rabbit dermal tuberculous (BCG) lesions. *J Leukoc Biol.* 1998;63:440–450.

69. Shigenaga T, Dannenberg AM Jr, Lowrie DB, et al. Immune responses in tuberculosis: Antibodies and CD4-CD8 lymphocytes with vascular adhesion molecules and cytokines (chemokines) cause a rapid antigen-specific cell infiltration at sites of Bacillus Calmette-Guérin reinfection. *Immunol.* 2001;102:466–479.

70. Tsuruta J, Sugisaki K, Dannenberg AM Jr, et al. The cytokines NAP-1 (IL-8), MCP-1, IL-1 beta, and GRO in rabbit inflammatory skin lesions produced by the chemical irritant sulfur mustard. *Inflammation* 1996;20:293–318.

71. Kupper TS, Groves RW. The interleukin-1 axis and cutaneous inflammation. *J Invest Dermatol.* 1995;105(1 Suppl): 62S–66S.

72. Kansas GS. Selectins and their ligands: current concepts and controversies. *Blood.* 1996;88:3259–3287.

73. Pober JS, Cotran RS. The role of endothelial cells in inflammation. *Transplantation.* 1990;50:537–544.

74. Filley EA, Bull HA, Dowd PM, et al. The effect of *Mycobacterium tuberculosis* on the susceptibility of human cells to the stimulatory and toxic effects of tumour necrosis factor. *Immunology*.1992;77:505–509.

75. Lindner H, Holler E, Ertl B, et al. Peripheral blood mononuclear cells induce programmed cell death in human endothelial cells and may prevent repair: role of cytokines. *Blood*. 1997;89:1931–1938.

76. Majno G, Joris I. *Cells, Tissues, and Disease*. Cambridge, MA: Blackwell Science; 1996.

77. Nathan C. Mechanisms and modulation of macrophage activation. *Behring Inst Mitt*. 1991;88:200–207.

78. Dannenberg AM Jr, Meyer OT, Esterly JR, et al. The local nature of immunity in tuberculosis, illustrated histo-chemically in dermal BCG lesions. *J Immunol*. 1968;100: 931–941.

79. Ando M, Dannenberg AM Jr, Sugimoto M, et al. Histochemical studies relating the activation of macrophages to the intracellular destruction of tubercle bacilli. *Am J Pathol*. 1977;86:623–633.

80. Dannenberg AM Jr. Cellular hypersensitivity and cellular immunity in the pathogensis of tuberculosis: specificity, systemic and local nature, and associated macrophage enzymes. *Bacteriol Rev*. 1968;32:85–102.

81. Mackaness GB. The immunology of antituberculous immunity. *Am Rev Respir Dis*. 1968;97:337–344.

82. North RJ. Cell-mediated immunity and the response to infection. In: McCluskey RT, S. Cohen S, eds. *Mechanisms of Cell-mediated Immunity*. New York, NY: John Wiley and Sons; 1974:185–219.

83. Collins FM, Campbell SG. Immunity to intracellular bacteria. *Vet Immunol Immunopathol*. 1982;3:5–66.

84. Rich AR. *The Pathogenesis of Tuberculosis*, 2nd ed. Springfield, Illinois: Charles C. Thomas; 1951.

85. Dannenberg AM Jr, Sugimoto M. Liquefaction of caseous foci in tuberculosis. *Am Rev Respir Dis*. 1976;13:257–259.

86. Barnes PF, Bloch AB, Davidson PT, et al. Tuberculosis in patients with human immunodeficiency virus infection. *N Engl J Med*. 1991;324:1644–1650.

87. Yamamura Y. The pathogenesis of tuberculous cavities. *Adv Tuberc Res*. 1958;9:13–37.

88. Yoder MA, Lamichhane G, Bishai WM. Cavitary tuber-culosis: The "Holey Grail" of disease transmission. *Curr Sci*. 2004;86:74–81.

89. Converse PJ, Dannenberg AM Jr, Estep JE, et al. Cavitary tuberculosis produced in rabbits by aerosolized virulent tubercle bacilli. *Infect Immun*. 1996;64:4776–4787.

90. Converse PJ, Dannenberg AM Jr, Shigenaga T, et al. Pulmonary bovine-type tuberculosis in rabbits: Bacillary virulence, inhaled dose effects, tuberculin sensitivity, and *Mycobacterium vaccae* immunotherapy. *Clin Diagn Lab Immunol*. 1998;5:871–881.

91. Yamamura Y, Ogawa Y, Maeda H, et al. Prevention of tuberculous cavity formation by desensitization with tuberculin-active peptide. *Am Rev Respir Dis*.1974;109: 594–601.

92. Dannenberg AM Jr. Pathogenesis of Tuberculosis: native and acquired resistance in animals and humans. In: *Microbiology—1984*. Washington, DC: American Society for Microbiology; 1984:344–354.

93. Francis J. *Tuberculosis in animals and man. A study in comparative pathology*. London: Cassell and Company; 1958:293–318.

94. Dannenberg AM Jr, Collins FM. Progressive pulmonary tuberculosis is not due to increasing numbers of viable bacilli in rabbits, mice and guinea pigs, but is due to a con-tinuous host response to mycobacterial products. *Tuberculosis*. 2001;81:229–242.

95. Medina E, North RJ. Resistance ranking of some common inbred mouse strains to *Mycobacterium tuberculosis* and relationship to major histocompatibility complex haplotype and Nramp-1 genotype. *Immunology*. 1998;93: 270–274.

96. Pan H, Yan BS, Rojas M, et al. *Ipr1* mediates innate immunity to tuberculosis. *Nat Med*. 2005;434:709–711.

97. Kramnik I, Demant P, Bloom BR. Susceptibility to tuber-culosis as a complex genetic trait: analysis using recombinant congenic strains of mice. *Novartis Found Symp*. 1998;217:120–131, discussion 132–137.

98. Lurie MB, Zappasodi P, Dannenberg AM Jr, et al. On the mechanism of genetic resistance to tuberculosis and its mode of inheritance. *Am J Human Genet*. 1953;4: 302–314.

99. Dorman S, Hatem CL, Tyagi SK, et al. Susceptibility to tuberculosis: Clues from studies with inbred and outbred New Zealand White rabbits. *Infect Immun*. 2004;72: 1700–1705.

100. Bellamy R, Ruwende C, Corrah T, et al. Variations in the NRAMP1 gene and susceptibility to tuberculosis in West Africans. *N Engl J Med*.1998;338:640–644.

101. Bellamy R, Ruwende C, Corrah T, et al. Tuberculosis and chronic hepatitis B virus infection in Africans and variation in the vitamin D receptor gene. *J Infect Dis*. 1999;179:721–724.

102. Selvaraj P, Narayanan PR, Reetha AM. Association of functional mutant homozygotes of the mannose binding protein gene with susceptibility to pulmonary tuberculosis in India. *Tuber Lung Dis*. 1999;79:221–227.

103. Selvaraj P, Narayanan PR, Reetha AM: Association of vitamin D receptor genotypes with the susceptibility to pulmonary tuberculosis in female patients & resistance in female contacts. *Indian J Med Res*. 2000;111: 172–179.

104. Wilkinson RJ, Patel P, Llewelyn M, et al. Influence of polymorphism in the genes for the interleukin (IL)-1 receptor antagonist and IL-1beta on tuberculosis. *J Exp Med*. 1999;189:1863–1874.

105. Casanova J-L, Abel L. Genetic dissection of immunity to mycobacteria: the human model. *Annu Rev Immunol*. 2002;20:581–620.

106. Malik S, Schurr E. Genetic suseptibility to tuberculosis. *Clin Chem Lab Med*. 2002;40:863–868.

107. Janeway CA Jr., Travers P, Walport M, et al. *Immunobiology: The Immune System in Health and Disease.* 5th ed. New York, NY: Garland Publishing; 2001.

108. Flynn JL, Chan J. Immunology of tuberculosis. *Annu Rev Immunol.* 2001;19:93–129.

109. Kaufmann SHE. Immunity to intracellular bacteria. In: Paul WE, ed. *Fundamental Immunology.* 5th ed. Philadelphia, PA: Lippincott Williams & Wilkins; 2003:1229–1261.

110. North RJ, Jung, YJ. Immunity to tuberculosis. *Annu Rev Immunol.* 2004;22:599–623.

111. Toossi Z, Sedor JR, Lapurga JP, et al. Expression of functional interleukin 2 receptors by peripheral blood monocytes from patients with active pulmonary tuberculosis. *J Clin Invest.* 1990;85:1777–1784.

112. Wahl SM, McCartney-Francis N, Hunt DA, et al. Monocyte interleukin 2 receptor gene expression and interleukin 2 augmentation of microbicidal activity. *J Immunol.* 1987;139:1342–1347.

113. Holter W, Goldman CK, Casabo L, et al. Expression of functional IL 2 receptors by lipopolysaccharide and interferon-gamma stimulated human monocytes. *J Immunol.* 1987;138:2917–2922.

114. Barnes PF, Fong SJ, Brennan PJ, et al. Local production of tumor necrosis factor and IFN-gamma in tuberculous pleuritis. *J Immunol.* 1990;145:149–154.

115. Dannenberg AM Jr, Meyer OT, Esterly JR, et al. The local nature of immunity in tuberculosis, illustrated histochemically in dermal BCG lesions. *J Immunol.* 1968;100:931–941.

116. Ando M, Dannenberg AM Jr, Sugimoto M, et al. Histochemical studies relating the activation of macrophages to the intracellular destruction of tubercle bacilli. *Am J Pathol.* 1997;86:623–634.

117. Means TK, Wang S, Lien E, et al. Human toll-like receptors mediate cellular activation by *Mycobacterium tuberculosis. J Immunol.* 1999;163:3920–3927.

118. Brightbill HD, Libraty DH, Krutzik SR, et al. Host defense mechanisms triggered by microbial lipoproteins through Toll-like receptors. *Science.* 1999;285:732–736.

119. Shim TS, Turner OC, Orme IM. Toll-like receptor 4 plays no role in susceptibility of mice to *Mycobacterium tuberculosis* infection. *Tuberculosis (Edinb).* 2003;83:367–371.

120. Reiling N, Holscher C, Fehrenbach A, et al. Toll-like receptor (TLR)2- and TLR4-mediated pathogen recognition in resistance to airborne infection with *Mycobacterium tuberculosis. J Immunol.* 2002;169:3480–3484.

121. Abel B, Thieblemont N, Quesniaux VJ, et al. Toll-like receptor 4 expression is required to control chronic *Mycobacterium tuberculosis* infection in mice. *J Immunol.* 2002;169:3155–3162.

122. Armstrong JA, Hart PD. Response of cultured macrophages to *Mycobacterium tuberculosis,* with observations on fusion of lysosomes with phagosomes. *J Exp Med.* 1971;134:713–740.

123. Russell DG, Mwandumba HC, Rhoades EE. *Mycobacterium* and the coat of many lipids. *J Cell Biol.* 2002;158:421–426.

124. Walburger A, Koul A, Ferrari G, et al. Protein kinase G from pathogenic mycobacteria promotes survival within macrophages. *Science.* 2004;304:1800–1804.

125. McKinney JD, Hîner zu Bentrup K, Muñoz-Elias EJ, et al. Persistence of *Mycobacterium tuberculosis* in macrophages and mice requires the glyoxylate shunt enzyme isocitrate lyase. *Nature,* 2000;406:735–738.

126. Long R, Light B, Talbot JA. Mycobacteriocidal action of exogenous nitric oxide. *Antimicrob Agents Chemother.* 1999;43:403–405.

127. MacMicking JD, North RJ, LaCourse R, et al. Identification of nitric oxide synthase as a protective locus against tuberculosis. *Proc Natl Acad Sci USA.* 1997;94:5243–5248.

128. Scanga CA, Mohan VP, Tanaka K, et al. The inducible nitric oxide synthase locus confers protection against aerogenic challenge of both clinical and laboratory strains of *Mycobacterium tuberculosis* in mice. *Infect Immun.* 2001;69:7711–7717.

129. Scanga CA, Mohan VP, Joseph H, et al. Reactivation of latent tuberculosis: variations on the Cornell murine model. *Infect Immun.* 1999;67:4531–4538.

130. Darwin KH, Ehrt S, Gutierrez-Ramos JC, et al. The proteasome of *Mycobacterium tuberculosis* is required for resistance to nitric oxide. *Science.* 2003;302:1963–1966.

131. Pieters J, Ploegh H. Chemical warfare and mycobacterial defense. *Science.* 2003;302:1900–1902.

132. Matzinger P. The danger model: a renewed sense of self. *Science.* 2002;296:3015.

133. Trinchieri G. Cytokines acting on or secreted by macrophages during intracellular infection (IL-10, IL-12, IFN-γ). *Curr Opin Immunol.* 1997;9:17–23.

134. Steinman RM. The dendritic cell system and its role in immunogenicity. *Annu Rev Immunol.* 1991;9:271–296.

135. Banchereau J, Steinman RM. Dendritic cells and the control of immunity. *Nature.* 1998;392:245–252.

136. Austyn JM. New insights into the mobilization and phagocytic activity of dendritic cells. *J Exp Med.* 1996;183:1287–1292.

137. Sprent J. Antigen presenting cells-Professionals and amateurs. *Curr Biol.* 1995;5:1095.

138. Brown KA, Bedford P, Macey M, et al. Human blood dendritic cells: binding to vascular endothelium and expression of adhesion molecules. *Clin Exp Immunol.* 1997;107:601–607.

139. Steinman RM, Hawiger D, Nussenzweig MC. Tolerogenic dendritic cells. *Annu Rev Immunol.* 2003;21:685–711.

140. Beckman EM, Brenner MB. MHC class I-like, class II-like and CD1 molecules: distinct roles in immunity. *Immunol Today.* 1995;16:349–352.

141. Porcelli SA. The CD1 family: a third lineage of antigen-presenting molecules. *Adv Immunol.* 1995;59:1–98.

142. Porcelli SA, Morita CT, Modlin RL. T-cell recognition of nonpeptide antigens. *Curr Opin Immunol.* 1996;8:510–516.

143. Jullien D, Stenger S, Ernst WA, et al. CD1 presentation of microbial nonpeptide antigens to T cells. *J Clin Invest.* 1997;99:2071–2074.

143a. Brigl M, Brenner MB. CD1: antigen presentation and T cell function, *Annu Rev Immunol.* 2004;22:817–890.

144. Porcelli SA, Modlin RL. The CD1 system: antigen-presenting molecules for T cell recognition of lipids and glycolipids. *Annu Rev Immunol.* 1999;17:297–329.

145. Beckman EM, Melian A, Behar SM, et al. CD1c restricts responses of mycobacteria-specific T cells. Evidence for antigen presentation by a second member of the human CD1 family. *J Immunol*; 157:2795–2803.

146. Moody DB, Ulrichs T, Muhlecker W, et al. CD1c-mediated T-cell recognition of isoprenoid glycolipids in *Mycobacterium tuberculosis* infection. *Nature.* 2000;404:884–888.

147. Nathan C. Mechanisms and modulations of macrophage activation. *Behring Inst Mitt.* 1991;88:200–207.

148. Denis M. Interferon-gamma-treated murine macrophages inhibit growth of tubercle bacilli via the generation of reactive nitrogen intermediates. *Cellu Immunol.* 1991;132:150–157.

149. Turner J, Dockrell HM. Stimulation of human peripheral blood mononuclear cells with live *Mycobacterium bovis* BCG activates cytolytic CD8+ T cells in vitro. *Immunology.* 1996;87:339–342.

150. Lewinsohn DM, Zhu L, Madison VJ, et al. Classically restricted human CD8+ T lymphocytes derived from *Mycobacterium tuberculosis*-infected cells: definition of antigenic specificity. *J Immunol.* 2001;166:439–446.

151. Rosat JP, Grant EP, Beckman EM, et al. CD1-restricted microbial lipid antigen-specific recognition found in the CD8+ alpha beta T cell pool. *Immunol.* 1999;162:366–371.

152. Heinzel AS, Grotzke JE, Lines RA, et al. HLA-E-dependent presentation of Mtb-derived antigen to human CD8+ T cells. *J Exp Med.* 2002;196:1473–1481.

153. Chaisson RE, Slutkin G. Tuberculosis and human immunodeficiency virus infection. *J Infect Dis.* 1989;159:96–100.

154. Muller I, Cobbold SP, Waldmann H, et al. Impaired resistance to *Mycobacterium tuberculosis* infection after selective in vivo depletion of L3T4+ and Lyt-2+ T cells. *Infect Immun.* 1987;55:2037–2041.

155. Orme IM, Collins FM. Protection against *Mycobacterium tuberculosis* infection by adoptive immunotherapy. Requirement for T cell-deficient recipients. *J Exp Med.* 1983;158:74–83.

156. Orme IM, Collins FM. Adoptive protection of the *Mycobacterium tuberculosis*-infected lung. Dissociation between cells that passively transfer protective immunity and those that transfer delayed-type hypersensitivity to tuberculin. *Cell Immunol.* 1984;84:113–120.

157. Caruso AM, et al. Mice deficient in CD4 T cells have only transiently diminished levels of IFN-gamma, yet succumb to tuberculosis. *J Immunol.* 1999;162:5407–5416.

158. Sousa AO, Mazzaccaro RJ, Russell RG, et al. Relative contributions of distinct MHC class I-dependent cell populations in protection to tuberculosis infection in mice. *Proc Natl Acad Sci USA.* 2000;97:4204–4208.

159. Rolph MS, Raupach B, Kobernick HH, et al. MHC class Ia-restricted T cells partially account for beta2-microglobulin-dependent resistance to *Mycobacterium tuberculosis. Eur J Immunol.* 2001;31:1944–1949.

160. Hirsch CS, Toossi Z, Johnson JL, et al. Augmentation of apoptosis and interferon-gamma production at sites of active *Mycobacterium tuberculosis* infection in human tuberculosis. *J Infect Dis.* 2001183:779–788.

160a. Cooper AM, D'Sousa C, Frank AA, et al. The course of *Mycobacterium tuberculosis* infection in the lungs of mice lacking expression of either perforin- or granzyme-mediated cytolytic mechanisms. *Infect Immun.* 1997;65:1317–1320.

161. Flynn JL, Goldstein MM, Triebold KJ, et al. Major histocompatibility complex class I-restricted T cells are required for resistance to *Mycobacterium tuberculosis* infection. *Proc Natl Acad Sci USA.* 1992;89:12013–12017.

162. Cho S, Mehra V, Thoma-Uszynski S, et al. Antimicrobial activity of MHC class I-restricted CD8+ T cells in human tuberculosis. *Proc Natl Acad Sci USA.* 2000;97:12210–12215.

163. Serbina NV, Liu CC, Scanga CA, et al. CD8+ CTL from lungs of *Mycobacterium tuberculosis*-infected mice express perforin in vivo and lyse infected macrophages. *J Immunol.* 2000;165:353–363.

164. Behar SM, Dascher CC, Grusby MJ, et al. Susceptibility of mice deficient in CD1D or TAP1 to infection with *Mycobacterium tuberculosis. J Exp Med.* 1999;189:1973–1980.

165. Hayday AC. $\gamma\delta$ Cells: A right time and a right place for a conserved third way of protection. *Annu Rev Immunol.* 2000;18:975–1026.

166. Boismenu R, Havran WL. An innate view of $\gamma\delta$ T cells. *Curr Opin Immunol.* 1997;9:57–63.

167. Ladel CH, Blum C, Dreher A, et al. Protective role of gamma/delta T cells and alpha/beta T cells in tuberculosis. *Eur J Immunol.* 1995;25:2877–2881.

168. D'Souza CD, Cooper AM, Frank AA, et al. An anti-inflammatory role for gamma delta T lymphocytes in acquired immunity to *Mycobacterium tuberculosis. J Immunol.* 1997;158:1217–1221.

169. Lahn M, Kanehiro A, Takeda K, et al. MHC Class I-dependent Vγ4+ pulmonary T cells regulate $\alpha\beta$ T cell-independent airway responsiveness. *Proc Natl Acad Sci USA.* 2002;99:8850–8855.

170. Hahn Y-S, Taube C, Jin N, et al. Vγ4+ $\gamma\delta$ T cells regulate airway hyperreactivity to methacholine in ovalbumin-sensitized and challenged mice. *J Immunol.* 2003;171:3170–3178.

171. Shen Y, Zhou D, Qiu L, et al. Adaptive immune response of Vgamma9Vdelta2+ T cells during mycobacterial infections. *Science.* 2002;295:2255–2258.

172. Balbi B, Valle MT, Oddera S, et al. T-lymphocytes with gamma delta+ V delta 2+ antigen receptors are present in increased proportions in a fraction of patients with tuberculosis or with sarcoidosis. *Am Rev Respir Dis.* 1993;148:1685–1690.

173. Chen ZW, Letvin NL. Vgamma2Vdelta2+ T cells and antimicrobial immune responses. *Microbes Infect.* 2003;5:491–498.

174. Ito M, Kojiro N, Ikeda T, et al. Increased proportions of peripheral blood gamma delta T cells in patients with pulmonary tuberculosis. *Chest.* 1992;102:195–197.

175. Ueta C, Tsuyuguchi I, Kawasumi H, et al. Increase of gamma/delta T cells in hospital workers who are in close contact with tuberculosis patients. *Infect Immun.* 1994;62:5434–5441.

176. Li B, Rossman MD, Imir T, et al. Disease-specific changes in gamma-delta T cell repertoire and function in patients with pulmonary tuberculosis. *J Immunol.* 1996;157:4222–4229.

177. Carvalho AC, Matteelli A, Airo P, et al. Gamma-delta T lymphocytes in the peripheral blood of patients with tuberculosis with and without HIV coinfection. *Thorax.* 2002;57:357–360.

178. Gioia C, Agrati C, Casetti R, et al. Lack of CD27-CD45RA-V gamma 9V delta 2+ T cell effectors in immunocompromised hosts and during active pulmonary tuberculosis. *J Immunol.* 2002;168:1484–1489.

179. Raulet DH. Natural killer cells. In: Paul WE, ed. *Fundamental Immunology.*, 5th ed. Philadelphia, PA: Lippincott Williams & Wilkins; 2003:365–391.

180. Yoneda T, Ellner JJ. CD4(+) T cell and natural killer cell-dependent killing of *Mycobacterium tuberculosis* by human monocytes. *Am J Respir Crit Care Med.* 1998;158:395–403.

181. Bermudez LE, Wu M, Young LS. Interleukin-12-stimulated natural killer cells can activate human macrophages to inhibit growth of *Mycobacterium avium. Infect Immun.* 1995;63:4099–4104.

182. Harshan KV, Gangadharam PR. In vivo depletion of natural killer cell activity leads to enhanced multiplication of *Mycobacterium avium* complex in mice. *Infect Immun.* 1991;59:2818–2821.

183. Reggiardo Z, Middlebrook G. Failure of passive serum transfer of immunity against aerogenic tuberculosis in rabbits. *Proc Soc Exp Biol Med.* 1974;145:173–175.

184. Lind A, Ridell M. Immunologically based diagnostic tests: Humoral antibody methods. In: Kubica GP, Wayne LG, eds. *The Mycobacteria: A Sourcebook.* New York, NY: Marcel Dekker; 1984:221–248.

185. Daniel TM. Rapid diagnosis of tuberculosis: laboratory techniques applicable in developing countries. *Rev Infect Dis.* 1989;11([Suppl 2):S471–S478.

186. Daniel TM. Antibody and antigen detection for the immunodiagnosis of tuberculosis: why not? What more is needed? Where do we stand today? *J Infect Dis.* 1998;158:678–680.

187. Fitzgerald KA, O'Neill LAJ, Gearing AJH, et al. *The Cytokine FactsBook.* 2nd ed. San Diego, CA: Elsevier Academic Press; 2001.

188. Vaddi K, Keller M, Newton RC. *The Chemokine FactsBook.* San Diego, CA: Academic Press; 1997.

189. Nathan C. Points of control in inflammation. *Nature.* 2002;420:846–852.

190. Trinchieri G. Interleukin-12 and the regulation of innate resistance and adaptive immunity. *Nat Rev Immunol.* 2003;3:133–146.

191. Cooper AM, Kipnis A, Turner J, et al. Mice lacking bioactive IL-12 can generate protective, antigen-specific cellular responses to mycobacterial infection only if the IL-12 p40 subunit is present. *J Immunol.* 2002;168:1322–1327.

192. Flynn JL, Goldstein MM, Triebold KJ, et al. IL-12 increases resistance of BALB/c mice to *Mycobacterium tuberculosis* infection. *J Immunol.* 1995;155:2515–2524.

193. Nolt D, Flynn JL. Interleukin-12 therapy reduces the number of immune cells and pathology in lungs of mice infected with *Mycobacterium tuberculosis. Infect Immun.* 2004;72:2976–2988.

194. Greinert U, Ernst M, Schlaak M, et al. Interleukin-12 as successful adjuvant in tuberculosis treatment. *Eur Respir J.* 2001;17:1049–1051.

195. Holland SM. Cytokine therapy of mycobacterial infections. *Adv Intern Med.* 2000;45:431–452.

196. Roach DR, Bean AG, Demangel C, et al. TNF regulates chemokine induction essential for cell recruitment, granuloma formation, and clearance of mycobacterial infection. *J Immunol.* 2002;168:4620–4627.

197. Mohan VP, Scanga CA, Yu K, et al. Effects of tumor necrosis factor alpha on host immune response in chronic persistent tuberculosis: possible role for limiting pathology. *Infect Immun.* 2001;69:1847–1855.

198. Flynn JL, Goldstein MM, Chan J, et al. Tumor necrosis factor-alpha is required in the protective immune response against *Mycobacterium tuberculosis* in mice. *Immunity.* 1995;2:561–572.

199. Kindler V, Sappino AP, Grau GE, et al. The inducing role of tumor necrosis factor in the development of bactericidal granulomas during BCG infection. *Cell.* 1989;56:731–740.

200. Bean AG, Roach DR, Brisco H, et al. Structural deficiencies in granuloma formation in TNF gene-targeted mice underlie the heightened susceptibility to aerosol *Mycobacterium tuberculosis* infection, which is not compensated for by lymphotoxin. *J Immunol.* 1999;162:3504–3511.

201. Roach DR, Briscoe H, Baumgart K, et al. Tumor necrosis factor (TNF) and a TNF-mimetic peptide modulate the granulomatous response to *Mycobacterium bovis* BCG infection in vivo. *Infect Immun.* 1999;67:5473–5476.

202. Keane J, Gershon S, Wise RP, et al. Tuberculosis associated with infliximab, a tumor necrosis factor alpha-neutralizing agent. *N Engl J Med.* 2001;345:1098–1104.

203. Maini R, St. Clair EW, Breedveld F, et al. Infliximab (chimeric antitumour necrosis factor alpha monoclonal antibody) versus placebo in rheumatoid arthritis patients receiving concomitant methotrexate: a randomised phase III trial. ATTRACT Study Group. *Lancet.* 1999;354:1932–1939.

204. Law KF, Jagirdar J, Weiden MD, et al. Tuberculosis in HIV-positive patients: cellular response and immune activation in the lung. *Am J Respir Crit Care Med.* 1996;153:1377–1384.

205. Tsenova L, Bergtold A, Freedman VH, et al. Tumor necrosis factor alpha is a determinant of pathogenesis and disease progression in mycobacterial infection in the central nervous system. *Proc Natl Acad Sci USA.* 1999;96:5657–5662.

206. Tsenova L, Sokol K, Freedman VH, et al. A combination of thalidomide plus antibiotics protects rabbits from mycobacterial meningitis-associated death. *J Infect Dis.* 1998;177:1563–1572.

207. Bekker LG, Moreira AL, Bergtold A, et al. Immunopathologic effects of tumor necrosis factor alpha in murine mycobacterial infection are dose dependent. *Infect Immun.* 2000;68:6954–6961.

208. Lalvani A, Brookes R, Wilkinson RJ, et al. Human cytolytic and interferon gamma-secreting CD8+ T lymphocytes specific for *Mycobacterium tuberculosis. Proc Natl Acad Sci USA.* 1998;95:270–275.

209. Orme IM, Roberts AD, Griffin JP, et al. Cytokine secretion by CD4 T lymphocytes acquired in response to *Mycobacterium tuberculosis* infection. *J Immunol.* 1993;151:518–525.

210. Wang J, Wakeham J, Harkness R, et al. Macrophages are a significant source of type 1 cytokines during mycobacterial infection. *J Clin Invest.* 1999;103:1023–1029.

211. Dorman SE, Holland SM. Mutation in the signal-transducing chain of the interferon-gamma receptor and susceptibility to mycobacterial infection. *J Clin Invest.* 1998;101:2364–2369.

212. Condos R, Rom WN, Schluger NW. Treatment of multidrug-resistant pulmonary tuberculosis with interferon-gamma via aerosol. *Lancet.* 1997;349:1513–1515.

213. Dannenberg AM Jr. Macrophage turnover, division and activation within developing, peak and "healed" tuberculous lesions produced in rabbits by BCG. *Tuberculosis.* 2003;83:251–260.

214. Thompson NJ, Glassroth JL, Snider DE Jr, et al. The booster phenomenon in serial tuberculin testing. *Am Rev Respir Dis.* 1979;119:587–597.

215. Comstock GW, Woolpert SF. Tuberculin conversions: true or false? *Am Rev Respir Dis.* 1978;118:215–217.

216. Menzies D. Interpretation of repeated tuberculin skin tests. Boosting, conversion and reversion. *Am J Respir Crit Care Med.* 1999;159:15–21.

217. Tsuyuguchi I. Regulation of the human immune response in tuberculosis. *Infect Agents Dis.* 1996;5:82–97.

218. Barnes PF, Mistry SD, Cooper CL, et al. Compartmentalization of a CD4+ T lymphocyte subpopulation in tuberculous pleuritis. *J Immunol.* 1989;142:1114–1119.

219. Rohrbach MS, Williams DE. T-lymphocytes and pleural tuberculosis. *Chest.* 1986;89:473–474.

220. Toossi Z, Gogate P, Shiratsuchi H, et al. Enhanced production of TGF-beta by blood monocytes from patients with active tuberculosis and presence of TGF-beta in tuberculous granulomatous lung lesions. *J Immunol.* 1995;154:465–473.

221. Gong JH, Zhang M, Modlin RL, et al. Interleukin-10 downregulates *Mycobacterium tuberculosis*-induced Th1 responses and CTLA-4 expression. *Infect Immun.* 1996;64:913–918.

222. Ellner JJ. Immunosuppression in tuberculosis. *Infect Agents Dis.*1996;5:62–72.

223. Maw WW, Shimizu T, Sato K, et al. Further study on the roles of the effector molecules of immunosuppressive macrophages induced by mycobacterial infection in expression of their suppressor function against mitogen-stimulated T cell proliferation. *Clin Exp Immunol.* 1997;108:26–33.

224. Hirsch CS, Toossi Z, Othieno C, et al. Depressed T-cell interferon-gamma responses in pulmonary tuberculosis: analysis of underlying mechanisms and modulation with therapy. *J Infect Dis.* 1999;180:2069–2073.

225. Hirsch CS, Hussain R, Toossi Z, et al. Cross-modulation by transforming growth factor beta in human tuberculosis: suppression of antigen-driven blastogenesis and interferon gamma production. *Proc Natl Acad Sci USA.* 1996;93:3193–3198.

226. Ellner JJ. Regulation of the human immune response during tuberculosis. *J Lab Clin Med.* 1997;130:469–475.

227. Demissie A, Ravn P, Olobo J, et al. T-cell recognition of *Mycobacterium tuberculosis* culture filtrate fractions in tuberculosis patients and their household contacts. *Infect Immun.* 1999;67:5967–5971.

228. Ravn P, Demissie A, Eguale T, et al. Human T cell responses to the ESAT-6 antigen from *Mycobacterium tuberculosis. J Infect Dis.* 1999;179:637–645.

229. Doherty TM, Demissie A, Olobo J, et al. Immune responses to the *Mycobacterium tuberculosis*-specific antigen ESAT-6 signal subclinical infection among contacts of tuberculosis patients. *J Clin Microbiol.* 2002;40:704–706.

230. Sutherland I, Lindgren I. The protective effect of BCG vaccination as indicated by autopsy studies. *Tubercle.* 1979;60:225–231.

231. Comstock GW. Identification of an effective vaccine against tuberculosis. *Am Rev Respir Dis.* 1998;138:479–480.

232. Fine PE. The BCG story: lessons from the past and implications for the future. *Rev Infect Dis.* 1989;11(Suppl 2): S353–S359.

233. Reggiardo Z, Middlebrook G. Delayed-type hypersensitivity and immunity against aerogenic tuberculosis in guinea pigs. *Infect Immun.* 1974;9:815–820.

234. Crowle AJ. Immunization against tuberculosis: what kind of vaccine? *Infect Immun.* 1988;56:2769–2773.

235. Seibert FB. A theory of immunity in tuberculosis. *Perspect Biol Med.* 1960;3:264–281.

236. Andersen P. TB vaccines: progress and problems. *Trends Immunol.* 2001;22:160–168.

237. Horowitz MA, Harth G, Dillon BJ, et al. Recombinant bacillus Calmette-GuÇrin (BCG) vaccines expressing the *Mycobacterium tuberculosis* 30-kDa major secretory protein induce greater protective immunity against tuberculosis than conventional BCG vaccines in a highly susceptible animal model. *Proc Natl Acad Sci USA.* 2000;97:13853–13858.

238. Ohara N, Yamada T. Recombinant BCG vaccines. *Vaccine.* 2001;19:4089–4098.

239. Britton WJ, Palendira U. Improving vaccines against tuberculosis. *Immunol Cell Biol.* 2003;81:34–45.

240. Collins HL, Kaufmann SHE. Prospects for better tuberculosis vaccines. *Lancet Infect Dis.* 2001;1:21–28.

241. Lowrie DB. DNA vaccination: an update. *Methods Mol Med.* 2003;87:377–390.

242. Brooks JV, Frank AA, Keen MA, et al. Boosting vaccine for tuberculosis. *Infect Immun.* 2001;69:2714–2717.

243. Kaufmann SHE. How can immunology contribute to the control of tuberculosis? *Nat Rev Immunol.* 2001;1:20–30.

244. Young DB, Stewart GR. Tuberculosis vaccines. *Br Med Bull.* 2002;62:73–86.

245. Orme IM, McMurray DN, Belisle JT. Tuberculosis vaccine development: recent progress. *Trends Microbiol.* 2001;9:115–118.

246. Rook GAW, Seah G, Ustianowski A. *M. tuberculosis:* immunology and vaccination. *Eur Respir J.* 2001;17: 537–557.

247. O'Donnell MA. The genetic reconstitution of BCG as a new immunotherapeutic tool. *Trends Biotechnol.* 1997;15: 512–517.

248. Dannenberg AM Jr: Controlling tuberculosis. The pathologist's point of view. From the 5th Forum in Microbiology on "Killing of Intracellular Mycobacteria: Dogmas and Realities." *Res Microbiol (formerly, Ann Inst Pasteur).* 1990;141:192–196, 262–263.

3

Laboratory Diagnosis and Susceptibility Testing

Glenn D. Roberts
Gary W. Procop

INTRODUCTION

Clinical microbiology laboratories currently have a number of methods available that will provide for a more accurate and rapid laboratory diagnosis of tuberculosis. Molecular methods are a part of the diagnostic algorithm in many laboratories and they have dramatically shortened the time to diagnosis; however, the sensitivity of all methods is dependent on the selection and collection of an appropriate clinical specimen source. It is important for the clinician to request the specimen(s) that will most likely contain *Mycobacterium tuberculosis*; this ensures that the laboratory has the best opportunity to detect and identify this important microorganism. The control of tuberculosis is dependent on a number of factors and the laboratory plays an important role in making a definitive diagnosis in as short a time as possible, depending on the competency of the laboratory.

SPECIMEN COLLECTION

The specimens submitted for mycobacterial culture include a wide variety of different body fluids and tissues from various sites. When pulmonary tuberculosis is suspected, the most common specimen submitted for culture is sputum. Collection is preferable in the early morning and patients should be instructed to expectorate a deep respiratory specimen with no nasal secretions or saliva. Ideally, the sputum should be obtained on 3 consecutive days. 5–10 ml of sample each time is appropriate. Specimens with less volume than this amount should be processed and a notation made on the report that "less than optimal amount was submitted." Sample collection with swabs should be discouraged because the amount of material collected is limited and negative culture results may be misleading. For patients who are unable to produce sputum, hypertonic saline (5–15%) can be nebulized for induction. When nebulization is ineffective or an immediate diagnosis is needed, bronchoscopy or bronchoalveolar lavage are the next best choices, because

these procedures provide additional material for study (washing, brushing, and biopsy specimen) and can help one obtain a rapid diagnosis of tuberculosis. Pooled respiratory tract specimens are unacceptable due to bacterial overgrowth and contamination.

For children and some adult patients who are unable to expectorate sputum, gastric lavage is a specimen of alternative choice, although it may not be as good as induced sputum for culturing.[1] These specimens should be processed within 4 hours, because the gastric acidity is potentially harmful to the mycobacteria. If rapid processing is not possible, gastric aspirates must be neutralized with sodium carbonate or another buffer salt to a pH of 7.0.

The diagnosis of renal tuberculosis is made by culturing 3–5 first morning midstream urine specimens. A pooled urine specimen is inappropriate because pooling increases bacterial contamination and decreases the recovery rate for mycobacteria.

Mycobacterial culture of stool specimens is usually not thought to be of value because intestinal tuberculosis cases are rare. This type of culture is usually requested to detect mycobacteria in AIDS patients.

If extrapulmonary tuberculosis is suspected, several specimen sources may be cultured, including blood, cerebrospinal fluid, pleural fluid, pericardial fluid, peritoneal fluid, purulent aspirates, joint fluids, biopsy tissues such as synovial or pleural biopsy, lymph nodes, and liver and bone marrow.

Generally, all the specimens should be collected in clean, sterile containers and transported to the laboratory in a rapid manner. Specimens must be refrigerated if they cannot be processed immediately; this prevents overgrowth by other bacteria. Specimens should be collected before chemotherapy is initiated; even a few days of therapy may obscure the diagnosis because of the failure to recover mycobacteria.

DECONTAMINATION AND PROCESSING OF SPECIMENS

Some species of mycobacteria are slow-growing and have an extended generation time (20–22 hours) compared with that of common bacterial flora (40–60 minutes); overgrowth of cultures by other bacteria and fungi can occur in specimens obtained from nonsterile sources. The high lipid content of the cell wall makes mycobacteria more resistant to strong acids and alkalis compared with other bacteria. This property has been used to develop the decontamination procedures to eliminate common bacterial flora while ensuring the mycobacteriae viability. Specimens that require decontamination include sputum, urine, and bronchial and gastric aspirates among others.

A number of alkaline digestion-decontamination solutions are commonly used for eliminating bacteria from contaminated specimens. Benzalkonium (Zephiran) chloride with trisodium phosphate or 4% NaOH is usually effective in reducing contamination. If specimens are transported promptly, often collections, N-acetyl-L-cysteine (NALC) – 2% NaOH is a suitable alternative. Excessive amounts of mucus may interfere with centrifugation-concentration procedures. Dithiothreitol (Sputolysin, Calbiochem, LaJolla, CA) or NALC should be added to the alkali solution as a mucolytic agent. A centrifugation speed of at least $3000 \times g$ is necessary to counteract the buoyant quality of the cell-wall lipids and to permit optimal sedimentation and concentration of mycobacteria.[2] All liquid specimens should be centrifuged prior to culturing. If the sterility of the specimen is questioned, aliquots of the specimen should be cultured onto bacteriologic media and incubated prior to culturing for mycobacteria.

CULTURE OF MYCOBACTERIA

Solid Media

The growth requirements of mycobacteria on artificial media include simple compounds such as potassium, magnesium, phosphorus, and sulfur. Ammonium salts or egg ingredients provide a nitrogen source, and glucose or glycerol, supply a carbon source. The optional pH range for growth is 6.5–7.0. Although mycobacterial are strict aerobes, a CO_2 concentration of between 5 and 10% is necessary for their primary recovery on solid media. The incubation conditions should include high humidity and a temperature of 35°–37°C for noncutaneous sources.

Traditional mycobacterial culture media include egg-based, agar-based, liquid, and selective media. Examples of egg-based media are Löwenstein-Jensen (L-J), Petragnani, and American Thoracic Society (ATS) media. Among them, Petragnani medium is the most inhibitory to contaminating bacteria because of the high content of malachite green (an antibacterial agent). All are complex media and include whole eggs, potato flour, salts, glycerol, and malachite green. L-J is the most common egg-based medium used for primary culture. It has been noted that it has a lesser recovery rate (40%) compared with 7H11 agar-based medium (81%), and therefore it is not recommended as a primary mycobacterial recovery media by some authors.[3] Middlebrook 7H10 and 7H11 are well-defined

agar-based media containing agar, organic compounds, salts, glycerol, and albumin. 7H11 also contains 0.1% casein hydrolysate, that is incorporated to improve the recovery rate and enhance the growth of mycobacteria exhibiting resistance to isoniazid (INH). Selective media are made with the base media plus the addition of antimicrobials to inhibit contaminating bacteria that survived the decontamination procedure. Among them, L-J Gruft medium contains penicillin, nalidixic acid, and malachite green. Middlebrook selective 7H11 (S7H11) contains carbenicillin, polymyxin B, trimethoprim lactate, amphotericin B, and malachite green.

After processing, 0.25 ml of the sediment from the decontaminated specimen is inoculated onto the surface of solid media contained in tubes; 0.5 ml is inoculated onto the media contained in culture plates, or both. The caps on media in tubes should be left slightly loose to provide adequate aeration of the culture. Culture plates should be placed in CO_2-permeable polyethylene plastic bags and sealed by heat pressure. All media should be incubated for up to 8 weeks at 35°C; the first 3–4 weeks of incubation should be in an atmosphere of 5–10% CO_2.

Specimens yielding positive acid-fast smears and negative cultures for mycobacteria after 8 weeks of incubation on solid media should be incubated for an additional 8 weeks. Young cultures (0–4 weeks old) should be examined twice weekly for visible evidence of growth. Older cultures (4–8 weeks old) should be examined at least once weekly. When colonies resembling mycobacteria are observed, an acid-fast smear and subculture for identification and susceptibility testing should be made. Nucleic acid probe testing can be performed on colonies as soon as they appear, and the definitive identification can be made if results are consistent with *Mycobacterium tuberculosis* complex (*Mycobacterium tuberculosis, Mycobacterium bovis, Mycobacterium africanum, Mycobacterium microti,* and *Mycobacterium canetti*).

Broth Media

Because the growth rate of *M. tuberculosis* complex on solid agar media is slow, it is recommended that broth media also be used for primary culturing. The BACTEC 460 TB System (Becton Dickinson Diagnostic Instruments Systems, Sparks, MD) uses liquid Middlebrook 7H12 medium containing ^{14}C-labeled palmitic acid for the radiometric detection of growth. This medium has been considered as one "gold standard" since the early 1980's. The sediment from processed specimens (0.5 ml) is inoculated to a BACTEC 12B bottle, and when the organism grows, $^{14}CO_2$ is released into the head space of the bottle and is detected by a sensor in the BACTEC 460 System. The time required for recovery of mycobacteria with this system is much less than that for solid agar culture. For *M. tuberculosis* complex, the average time for recovery in the BACTEC TB system is approximately 10–12 days and is faster for acid-fast smear-positive specimens.[3–5] One advantage for this system is that DNA probe identification and antibiotic susceptibility testing can be performed from this system.

Currently, in addition to the BACTEC 460 TB System, three commercial systems are available for the recovery of mycobacteria. All have been evaluated for their ability to recover mycobacteria from clinical specimens and determine the antimicrobial susceptibility or resistance profile of an organism. All appear to be suitable alternatives to the BACTEC 460 TB system.

The ESP Culture II System for mycobacterial recovery is a modification of the blood culture system (Trek Diagnostic Systems, Cleveland, OH) and consists of a bottle containing a modification of Middlebrook 7H9 broth and oleic acid, albumin, dextrose, catalase (OADC) enrichment in addition to the automated hardware. Bottles contain the medium and a cellulose sponge, which is thought to increase the surface area for growth. Each bottle is supplemented with an antibiotic mixture used to prevent bacterial contamination. The ESP system is automated and measures a change in oxygen consumption.

Recovery rates for *M. tuberculosis* were 85.27 and 89% for the ESP II System when compared to the BACTEC 460 TB System where rates were 85.27 and 92% in two studies, respectively.[6,7] Recovery times for *M. tuberculosis* in the ESP II System were 15.5 and 14.5 days, respectively for two studies.[6,7] This system, when used with a solid medium, is as reliable as the BACTEC 460 TB System for the recovery of *M. tuberculosis*. Studies have shown that the overall recovery rate for mycobacteria, and specifically for *M. tuberculosis*, was equivalent to the BACTEC system; the difference was slight.

The BacT/Alert MB (bioMeriéux, Durham, NC) uses bottles containing modified Middlebrook 7H9 medium and growth factors. Numerous studies have shown that the BacT/Alert MB System for mycobacterial recovery is satisfactory but should be used in combination with a solid medium as is true for all of the automated systems. Recovery rates for *M. tuberculosis* were 98.7, 96.7, and 91.3%, respectively for the BacT/Alert MB in three studies.[8–10] Recovery rates for the BACTEC 460 were 89.8, 96.7, and 90.0%, respectively when compared.

In general the mean recovery time for the BacT/Alert MB was 11.6 and 17.8 days, respectively for acid-fast smear positive and negative specimens, respectively. Recovery times for the BACTEC 460 TB System ranged from 2–24 days with a mean recovery time of 8.0 days and 16.9 days for acid-fast smear positive and negative specimens, respectively. The BacT/Alert MB System is considered to be comparable to the "gold standard" BACTEC 460; however, recovery rates and times are less and longer, respectively. The major advantage of the BacT/Alert MB System is that there is no radioactivity associated with the procedure.

The MGIT tube system (Becton Dickinson, Sparks, MD) contains a 7H9-based medium with enrichment, antibiotics, and an oxygen-labile fluorescent indicator at the bottom of each tube. As mycobacteria grow and use oxygen, the indicator compound is excited and the resulting fluorescence can be visually examined with an ultraviolet source. It was designed to replace the BACTEC 460 TB System to eliminate the use of ^{14}C. The MGIT System is automated and continuous monitors tubes inoculated with clinical specimens for evidence of growth. It is suggested that the MGIT 960 is a suitable alternative to the BACTEC 460. However, published results vary in the in their conclusions as to recovery rates and times for *M. tuberculosis*. Recovery rates of 91.5,[11] 88,[12] and 88%[13] for the MGIT are reported when compared to 95.7,[11] 90,[12] and 90.5%[13] for the BACTEC 460 TB System. The reading times are different for the two systems and the MGIT 960 is read more often. Recovery times for the MGIT 960 ranged from 12.5 to 13.4 days for acid-fast smear positive and negative specimens, respectively[11] while another study reported recovery times of 12.5 and 19.6 days for smear positive and negative specimens, respectively.[13] The MGIT 960 has a higher contamination rate ($\geq10\%$) when compared to the BACTEC 460 TB System and this could result in a decrease in the recovery rate by this system.

STAINING PROCEDURES AND BIOCHEMICAL IDENTIFICATION

Staining followed by microscopic observation is applied to both direct smear examinations of patient specimens and organisms growing from the culture. If an organism is present in sufficient numbers, this is the most rapid procedure for the detection of mycobacteria in clinical samples. It has been estimated that at least 10^5 organisms/ml of sputum must be present to be detected by staining of a smear, and the sensitivity of the smear is related to the type of infection (i.e., advanced cavitary disease), relative centrifugal force used to concentrate the specimen, and other factors. Overall, the acid-fast smear used with clinical specimens is not an adequate diagnostic tool. Further, it does not provide information concerning the identification or viability of the organism, since all species of mycobacteria are acid-fast.

Two procedures are commonly used for acid-fast staining: carbol-fuchsin methods, including the Ziehl-Neelsen and Kinyoun procedures, and a fluorochrome method using auramine O or auramine-rhodamine dyes.

The Ziehl-Neelsen and Kinyoun staining procedures differ in their staining principles. The former procedure requires heating the carbol-fuchsin to penetrate the mycobacterial cell wall. The latter is a *cold* staining method using an increased amount of phenol in the solution to enhance penetration of the cell wall. Both methods stain the mycobacterial cells red against a methylene blue counterstain. The stained smears must be viewed using a 100x oil-immersion objective.

Auramine O-stained mycobacteria are bright yellow against a dark background and are easily visualized using a 25x objective. Modification of the auramine O technique includes the use of rhodamine, which gives a golden appearance to the cells. Auramine-rhodamine is the method of choice for clinical specimens, including tissue sections when trying to detect for mycobacteria.

Fluorochrome staining has the advantage of being more sensitive than carbolfuchsin techniques. Fluorochrome-stained smears can be scanned using a 25x objective, whereas an oil-immersion objective is required for viewing smears stained with carbol-fuchsin. A disadvantage of all these different staining methods is the indiscriminate staining of nonviable organisms. Therefore, mycobacteria rendered nonviable by chemotherapy may be stained. It has been noticed that blood present in the sputum can sometimes cause false-positive auramine stains. In addition, variable staining of *Mycobacterium fortuitum* occurs. Because of the ease of reading, specificity, and sensitivity, it is recommended that a fluorochrome staining method of detecting acid fast bacilli (AFB) in clinical specimens be used. If desired, a carbol-fuchsin procedure may then be used for confirming questionable fluorochrome results. It is also extremely important to perform a culture. Clinicians should be aware that the presence of mycobacteria as seen on direct examination does not establish the specific diagnosis of tuberculosis. Also, weakly decolorized acid-fast stains sometimes yield positive results (i.e., the organism appears "acid-fast")

with nonmycobacteria such as *Rhodococcus, Nocardia, Legionella micdadei*, and cysts of Cryptosporidium, *Isospora*, and Cyclospora.

Traditionally, the identification of *M. tuberculosis* complex has relied on acid-fastness, niacin production, nitrate reduction, and inactivation of catalase at 68°C. Generally, the recovery time for *M. tuberculosis* complex varies; on solid media, colonies can be observed as short a time as 12 days or as long as 4–6 weeks with an average of about 3–4 weeks. The colonies are rough, *cauliflower-like*, and colorless. Unlike most mycobacterial species, *M. tuberculosis* complex lacks the enzyme to convert free niacin-to-niacin ribonucleotide, and niacin accumulates in the medium resulting in a positive niacin test result. *Mycobacterium tuberculosis* complex possesses nitro reductase and yields a positive result using nitrate reduction testing. Among mycobacteria, the quantity of catalase produced and its stability at 68°C is species-dependent. *Mycobacterium tuberculosis* complex produces a column measuring less than 50 mm in the quantitative catalase production test performed with L-J slants. This organism also produces heat-labile catalase that is inactivated after 20 minutes of exposure to 68°C.[14]

CHROMATOGRAPHIC IDENTIFICATION

Although the subculturing and subsequent biochemical testing is a time-honored traditional method for species identification, it requires at least several weeks. The Sherlock Mycobacteria Identification System (MIDI, Newark, DE) procedure utilizes high-performance liquid chromatography (HPLC),[13] a procedure advocated by many laboratories. The long-chained cell wall, fatty acids, and mycolic acids extracted from mycobacteria are species-specific and yield different chromatographic peaks when separated by HPLC. The number of peaks, heights, and their position are used for identification of mycobacteria. High performance liquid chromatography can distinguish the Bacille Calmette-Guérin (BCG) strain of *Mycobacterium bovis* from *M. tuberculosis* complex. Furthermore, HPLC is shown to be able to discriminate other bacteria such as the genera *Nocardia, Gordona, Rhodococcus*, and *Corynebacterum*.[15–20]

Identification by Nucleic Acid Probe

Since the beginning of the 1990's, nucleic acid probes have been used for the identification of mycobacteria. At present, these commercially available probes (AccuProbe, Gen-Probe, Inc., San Diego, CA) can identify *M. tuberculosis* complex, *Mycobacterium kansasii, Mycobacterium avium-intracellulare*, and *Mycobacterium gordonae*. After lysis of mycobacterial cells, an acridinium ester-labeled, single-stranded DNA probe binds with the ribosomal ribonucleic acid (rRNA) of the target organism and forms a stable DNA-rRNA hybrid. After chemically degrading the unhybridized DNA-acridinium ester probes, the acridinium present on the DNA-rRNA hybrid is detected when chemiluminescence of the acridinium ester is measured in a luminometer.

The *M. tuberculosis* complex nonisotopic probe demonstrated a sensitivity and specificity of 100% when compared with its isotopic predecessor.[21] The procedure is quick and can be finished in an hour. Originally, this probe test was designed to be used for culture confirmation of organisms growing on solid media. However, this test has been successfully used with BACTEC 12B medium and MGIT System.[22–24] To do this, mycobacteria growing in the culture broth vials are concentrated by centrifugation, organisms are lysed, and subjected for nucleic acid probe hybridization. The combination of nucleic acid probe identification and BACTEC 12B culture system makes the *M. tuberculosis* complex culture times and reporting times as short as 15.5 days[25] or 16.4 to 10 days,[26,27] depending on the study reported. The only drawback reported is the false-positive reactions caused by a few isolates of *M. terrae*-like organisms and *M. celatum*.[28] However, this problem can be eliminated by extending the selection time to 8 or 10 minutes.[28] Clinical laboratories use the nucleic acid probes alone or in combination with other identification methods,[16,29] including nucleic acid sequencing.[30,31]

ANTIMICROBIAL SUSCEPTIBILITY TESTING OF *M. TUBERCULOSIS* COMPLEX

The reemergence of *M. tuberculosis* complex as a cause of disease and the increasing percentage of cases with drug resistance has made antimicrobial susceptibility testing more important.[32] Susceptibility tests should be performed on all isolates of *M. tuberculosis* complex recovered from previously untreated patients and also on isolates from patients on therapy who have positive acid-fast smears or cultures after 2 months of treatment. Patients at increased risk for drug resistance also include those with a history of treatment failure for tuberculosis, contacts of patients with resistant tuberculosis, and residents of high-prevalence areas including countries outside of the United States.

The traditional susceptibility test method is a 1% agar proportion method. Resistance is defined as mycobacteria with greater than 1% of the population exhibiting growth in the presence of the lowest concentration of drug tested. Based on clinical experience, a correlate has been found between the 1% resistance *in vitro* to *in vivo* chemotherapeutic failure. Organisms are inoculated onto 7H10 or 7H11 agar plates containing the various antibiotic concentrations and incubated, results may be obtained after 14–21 days.

Another method is based on the BACTEC 460 TB system that provides a result much earlier. An organism is inoculated into BACTEC 12B bottles containing antimicrobials, and the susceptibility is detected by failure of the test organism to produce $^{14}CO_2$ in the presence of an antibiotic. This method not only correlates well with that of 1% proportion method (90–100% agreement) but also significantly shortens the turnaround time of antibiotic susceptibility testing (4–7 days compared with 14–21 days).[5] Antimicrobials currently available for testing include streptomycin, isoniazid, rifampin, ethambutol, pyrazinamide, kanamycin, capreomycin, rifabutin, and ciprofloxacin (or other quinolones).

The more recently introduced commercially—available automated systems can also perform antimycobacterial susceptibility testing.[33–36] The National Committee of Clinical Laboratory Standards document, "Susceptibility Testing of *Mycobacteria Nocardiae* and Other Aerobic Actinomycetes; approved Standard M-24" indicates that the MGIT 960 and ESP II Systems have been approved by the FDA for use in susceptibility testing.[37] It appears that all three automated systems are suitable alternatives to the BACTEC 460 TB System for susceptibility testing of *M. tuberculosis* complex.

More recently, as some of the molecular mechanisms of drug resistance have become clear,[38–40] detection of molecular targets, such as mutations, have been studied. Some offer promise because they can potentially shorten the turnaround time from weeks to days and they may be subject to automation. One of the more thoroughly studied targets for drug resistance to rifampin is *rpo*B, which encodes the β-subunit of RNA polymerase, *kat*G, *inh*A, *Imab*A, and *ahp*C are genes associated with isoniazid resistance. A real-time PCR assay has been developed to detect *inh*A and *rpo*B genes.[41] Resistance and detection targets on other drugs include streptomycin (*rps*L and *rrs*), ethambutol (*emb*CAB), and fluoroquinolones (*gyr*A). Although the advantages of genetic testing of antibiotic susceptibility are obvious, the conventional methods may not soon be fully replaced. The clinical correlation of genetic testing to clinical treatment outcomes must still be determined before this testing is routinely used.

MOLECULAR METHODS FOR DETECTION OF *M. TUBERCULOSIS* COMPLEX

Because of the slow-growing nature of *M. tuberculosis* complex, prompt detection and identification has been a challenge for clinical microbiology laboratories. Extensive studies have shown that nucleic acid amplification methods are promising and may be a good solution to the problem.[42,43]

These methods include target, probe, and signal amplification systems. Ribosomal RNA or different parts of genomic DNA are selected as targets. Although many "laboratory-developed" assays reported by academic scientists show promise; commercial tests have also demonstrated good performance. These systems have less carryover contamination, are more amenable to quantification, provide very high specificity, and are capable of being automated.[44] They include the Amplified *Mycobacterium tuberculosis* Direct (AMTD) test by Gen-Probe and the Amplicor *M. tuberculosis* test by Roche Diagnostic Systems (Branchburg, NJ). The Food and Drug Administration (FDA) approve both the AMTD and Amplicor M. tuberculosis tests. However, the AMTD is approved for use with both acid-fast smear positive and negative respiratory tract specimens.

The AMTD test uses a transcription-mediated amplification (TMA) system. It is an isothermal test and uses a single temperature during the amplification step. The target is the 16S RNA. After the nucleic acids are released from mycobacterial cells by sonication, specimens are heated to disrupt the secondary structure of the rRNA. At a constant 42°C temperature, the test generates multiple copies of the mycobacterial RNA. The *M. tuberculosis complex*-specific sequences are then detected by the Gen-Probe chemiluminescent-labeled DNA probes, and results are measured in a luminometer. The test has several advantages: It detects rRNA, that theoretically exists in concentrations several thousand-fold more than that found in genomic DNA of the organism, so the sensitivity is high; and it uses a single temperature and a single-tube format, which makes the test easier to perform and contamination less likely to occur. Because the amplification products are RNA, that is more labile than DNA, the risk of carryover is reduced. Specimens used for testing should be obtained from untreated patients. It has been shown that the test result can remain positive after cultures become negative during therapy.[45] The usefulness of the system on nonrespiratory specimens has been studied by different investigators. Specimens included urine, feces, tissue, pleural exudates, cerebrospinal fluids, ascitic fluid, and bone marrow.

Generally, the specificity was high (97.7–100%) whereas the sensitivity was greater than or equal to 83.9%.[46–48] A recent review of AMTD is presented by Piersimoni[49] presents the most current information available.

Users of the AMTD test should be aware that a false positive test, although rare, might occur in patients infected with *Mycobacterium celatum.*[28]

The Roche Amplicor *M. tuberculosis* test is a polymerase chain reaction (PCR)-based assay. Instead of detecting rRNA, it detects the rRNA gene in the genome (DNA). After amplification using biotinylated oligonucleotide primers, the products are hybridized with a specific probe that is bound to a Microwell plate. The avidin-horseradish peroxidase (Av-HRP) conjugate and the substrates are then added for color development. The kit is approved for use with acid-fast, smear-positive respiratory specimens. Bergmann and Woods evaluated the method using 956 respiratory tract specimens from 502 patients and compared results with those of the culture and the medical history.[50] They found that although the specificity was very high (99.5–100%), the sensitivity was 97.6 and 40% for AFB smear-positive and -negative specimens, respectively. The results reported by Bennedsen, in 1996 were similar, with a sensitivity of 91.4 and 60.9% for AFB smear-positive and -negative specimens, respectively.[51] Even for those culture-positive, smear-negative samples, the sensitivity of this test is reported as 46%.[52] So far, smear-positive samples are optimal and the method is not recommended for use with nonrespiratory specimens.[53] Therefore, although the AMTD and Amplicor *M. tuberculosis* tests use different amplification techniques and are manufactured by different companies, both methods are rapid and specific. The sensitivity of AMTD is similar to or slightly greater than that of Amplicor.[54] There have been numerous reports on the use of the Amplicor *M. tuberculosis* test on detection and identification of *M. tuberculosis* in BACTEC 12B and ESP II broth cultures. Piersimoni[49] presents a comprehensive review of the performance of this test.

It should be mentioned that although these nucleic acid amplification methods provide rapid results, mycobacterial cultures are still required. Cultures are essential for organism identification (amplification tests give results only for *M. tuberculosis complex* level) as well as antimicrobial susceptibility testing. Further, a survey that evaluated the reliability and performance of nucleic acid amplification for the detection of *M. tuberculosis* complex internationally showed that among the 30 laboratories in 18 countries using different tests (including both in-house and commercial kits) only five laboratories were able to identify correctly the presence or absence of mycobacterial nucleic acid in all 20 samples distributed.[55]

These results emphasize the variation of tests and results from laboratory to laboratory and the need for good laboratory practice. Hundreds of "laboratory-developed" assays including real-time PCR[56,57] are present in the literature and most have not been compared.

In general, amplified tests currently are not "stand-alone" tests. They must still be used in conjunction with conventional cultures. When the specimen volume is an issue, conventional cultures are preferred over amplified tests. To date, these methods are not useful to detect *M. tuberculosis* in paraffin block sections. Currently the cost of these tests is excessive and must be considered when their use is entertained. The American Thoracic Society provided a statement in 1997 on the specific uses for these tests and the information is still relevant today.[58] When used on properly selected cases, using appropriate specimens, FDA-approval nucleic acid amplified tests for the detection of *M. tuberculosis* can be powerful diagnostic tools that can have a great impact on patient care and the control of tuberculosis in today's world.

REFERENCES

1. Pomputius WF III, Rost J, Dennehy PH, et al. Standardization of gastric aspirate technique improves yield in the diagnosis of tuberculosis in children. *Pediatr Infec Dis J.* 1997;16(2):222–226.
2. Rickman TW, Moyor NO. Increased sensitivity of acid-fast smears. *J Clin Microbiol.* 1980;11:618.
3. Wilson ML, Stone BL, Hildred MV, et al. Comparison of recovery rates of mycobacteria from BACTEC 12 B vials, Middlebrook 7H11 selective biplates and Lowenstein-Jensen slants in a public health mycobacteriology laboratory. *J Clin Microbiol.* 1995;33:2516–2518.
4. Anargyros P, Astill SJ, Sim IS. Comparison of improved BACTEC and Lowenstein-Jensen media for culture of mycobacteria from clinical specimens. *J Clin Microbiol.* 1990;38:1288–1291.
5. Roberts GD, Goodman NL, Heifets L, et al. Evaluation of the BACTEC radiometric method for recovery of mycobacteria and drug susceptibility testing of *Mycobacterium tuberculosis* from acid-fast smear positive specimens. *J Clin Microbiol.* 1983;18:689–696.
6. Woods GL, Fish G, Plaunt M, et al. Clinical evaluation of Difco culture system II for growth and detection of mycobacteria. *J Clin Microbiol.* 1997;35(1):121–124.
7. Tortli E, Cichero P, Chirillo MG. Multicenter comparison of ESP Culture System II with BACTEC 460TB and with Lowenstein-Jensen medium for recovery of mycobacteria from different clinical specimens, including blood. *J Clin Microbiol.* 1998;36:1378.
8. Manterola GF, Padilla E, Lonca J, et al. Comparison of a nonradiometric System with BACTEC 12B and culture on egg-based media for recovery of mycobacteria from clinical specimens. *Eur J Clin Microbiol Infect Dis.* 1998;17:773.
9. Laverdiere M, Poirier L, Weiss K, Beliveau C, Bedard L, Desnoyers D. Comparative evaluation of the MB/BacT and BACTEC 460 TB systems for the detection of mycobacteria from clinical specimens: clinical relevance of higher recovery rates from broth-based detection systems. *Diagn Microbiol Infect Dis.* 2000;36(1):1–5.
10. Piersimoni C, Scarparo C, Callegaro A, Tosi CP, Nista D, Bornigia S, Scagnelli M, Rigon A, Ruggiero G, Goglio A. Comparison of MB/Bact alert 3D system with radiometric BACTEC system and Lowenstein-Jensen medium for recovery and identification of mycobacteria from clinical specimens: a multicenter study. *J Clin Microbiol.* 2001;39(2):651–657.
11. Scarparo C, Piccoli P, Rigon A, Ruggiero G, Ricordi P, Piersimoni C. Evaluation of the BACTEC MGIT 960 in comparison with BACTEC 460 TB for detection and recovery of mycobacteria from clinical specimens. *Diagn Microbiol Infect Dis.* 2002;44(2):157–161.
12. Cruciani M, Scarparo C, Malena M, Bosco O, Serpelloni G, Mengoli C. Meta-analysis of BACTEC MGIT 960 and BACTEC 460 TB, with or without solid media, for detection of mycobacteria. *J Clin Microbiol.* 2004;42(5):2321–2325.
13. Tortoli E, Cichero P, Piersimoni C, Simonetti MT, Gesu G, Nista D. Use of BACTEC MGIT 960 for recovery of mycobacteria from clinical specimens: multicenter study. *J Clin Microbiol.* 1999;37(11):3578–3582.
14. Kubica GP, Pool Gl. Studies on the catalase activity of acid-fast bacilli: I. An attempt to subgroup these organisms on the basis of their catalase activities at different temperatures and pH. *Am Rev Respir Dis.* 1960;83:737.
15. Glickman SE, Kilburn SO, Butler WR, et al. Rapid identification of mycolic acid patterns of mycobacteria by high-performance liquid chromatography using pattern recognition software and a *Mycobacterium* library. *J Clin Microbiol.* 1994; 32:740–749.
16. Herold CD, Fitzgerald RL, Herold DA. Current techniques in mycobacterial detection and speciation. *Crit Rev Cin Lab Sci.* 1996;33(2):83–138.
17. Butler W, Ahearn D, Kilburn J. High-performance liquid chromatography of mycolic acids as a tool in the identification of *Corynebacterium, Nocardia, Rhodococcus* and *Mycobacterium* species. *J Clin Microbiol.* 1986;23(1):182–185.
18. Thiebert L, Lapierre S. Routine application of high-performance liquid chromatography for identification of mycobacteria. *J Clin Microbiol.* 1993;31(7):1759–1763.
19. DeBriel D, Couderc F, Riegel P, et al. Contribution of high-performance liquid chromatography to the identification of some *Corynebacterium* species by comparison of their corynomycolic acid patterns. *Res Microbiol.* 1992;143(2):191–198.
20. Roberts GD, Bottger EC, Stockman L. Methods for the rapid identification of mycobacterial species. *Clin Lab Med.* 1996;16(3):603–615.

21. Goto M, Oka S, Okuzumi K, et al. Evaluation of acridinium-ester-labeled DNA probes for identification of *Mycobacterium tuberculosis* and *Mycobacterium avium-intracellulare* complex in culture. *J Clin Microbiol.* 1991;29(11):2473–2476.

22. Evans KD, Nakasone AS, Sutherland PA, et al. Identification of *Mycobacterium tuberculosis* and *Mycobacterium avium-intracellulare* directly from primary BACTEC culture by using acridinium-ester-labeled DNA probes. *J Clin Microbiol.* 1992;31:2427–2431.

23. Metchock B, Diem L. Algorithm for the use of nucleic acid probes for identifying *Mycobacterium tuberculosis* from BACTEC 12 B bottles. *J Clin Microbiol.* 1995;33:1934–1937.

24. Alcaide F, Benitez MA, Escriba JM, Martin R. Evaluation of the BACTEC MGIT 960 and the MB/BacT systems for recovery of mycobacteria from clinical specimens and for species identification by DNA AccuProbe. *J Clin Microbiol.* 2000;38(1):398–401.

25. Telenti M, deQuiros JF, Alvarez, et al. The diagnostic usefulness of a DNA probe for *Mycobacterium tuberculosis* complex (Gen-Probe) in BACTEC cultures versus other diagnostic methods. *Infection.* 1994;22:18–23.

26. Ellner PD, Kiehn TE, Cammarata R, et al. Rapid detection and identification of pathogenic mycobacteria by combining radiometric and nucleic acid probe methods. *J Clin Microbiol.* 1988;26(7):1349–1352.

27. Ford E, Snead S, Todd J, et al. Strains of *Mycobacterium terrae* complex which react with DNA probes for *Mycobacterium tuberculosis* complex. *J Clin Microbiol.* 1993; 31(10):2805–2806.

28. Christiansen D, Roberts G, Patel R. *Mycobacterium celatum,* an emerging pathogen and cause of false positive amplified *Mycobacterium tuberculosis* direct test. *Diagn Microbiol Infect Dis.* 2004;49(1):19–24.

29. Bird BR, Denniston MM, Huebner RE, et al. Changing practices in mycobacteriology: A follow-up survey of state and institutional public health laboratories. *J Clin Microbiol.* 1996;34:554–559.

30. Hall L, Doerr K, Wohlfiel S, et al. Evaluation of the MicroSeq system for identification of mycobacteria by 16S ribosomal DNA sequencing and its integration into a routine clinical mycobacteriology laboratory. *J Clin Microbiol.* 2003;41(4):1447–1453.

31. Turenne CY, Tschetter L, Wolfe J, et al. Necessity of quality-controlled 16S rRNA gene sequence databases: identifying nontuberculous mycobacterium species. *J Clin Microbiol.* 2001 Oct;39(10):3637–3648.

32. Heifets LB. Drug susceptibility testing. *Clin Lab Med.* 1996;16(3):641–656.

33. Kontos F, Maniati M, Costopoulos C, et al. Evaluation of the fully automated BACTEC MGIT 960 system for the susceptibility testing of *Mycobacterium tuberculosis* to first-line drugs: a multicenter study. *J Microbiol Methods.* 2004;56(2):291–294.

34. Tortoli E, Benedetti M, Fontanelli A, et al. Evaluation of automated BACTEC MGIT 960 system for testing susceptibility of *Mycobacterium tuberculosis* to four major

35. antituberculous drugs: comparison with the radiometric BACTEC 460TB method and the agar plate method of proportion. *J Clin Microbiol.* 2002;40(2):607–610.

35. Angeby KA, Werngren J, Toro JC, et al. Evaluation of the BacT/ALERT 3D system for recovery and drug susceptibility testing of *Mycobacterium tuberculosis.* Clin Microbiol Infect. 2003;9(11):1148–1152.

36. Bemer P, Bodmer T, Munzinger J, et al. Multicenter evaluation of the MB/BACT system for susceptibility testing of *Mycobacterium tuberculosis.* *J Clin Microbiol.* 2004;42(3):1030–1034.

37. Woods G, Brown-Elliot B, Desmond E, et. al. *Susceptibility Testing of Mycobacteria, Nocardiae, and Other Aerobic Actinomycetes.* Approved Standard M-24-A. Wayne, PA: National Committee for Clinical Laboratory Standards:2003.

38. Blanchard JS. Molecular mechanisms of drug resistance in *Mycobacterium tuberculosis. Annu Rev Biochem.* 1996;65: 215–239.

39. Musser JM. Antimicrobial agent resistance in mycobacteria: Molecular genetic insights. *Clin Microbiol Rev.* 1995;8(4): 496–514.

40. de Viedma G. Rapid detection of resistance in *Mycobacterium tuberculosis:* a review discussing molecular approaches. *Clin Microbiol Infect.* 2003;9(5):349–359.

41. Torres MJ, Criado A, Ruiz M, et al. Improved real-time PCR for rapid detection of rifampin and isoniazid resistance in *Mycobacterium tuberculosis* clinical isolates. *Diagn Microbiol Infect Dis.* 2003;45(3):207–212.

42. Centers for Disease Control and Prevention. Nucleic acid amplification tests for tuberculosis. *Morb Mortal Weekly Rep.* 1996;45(43):950–952.

43. Jonas V, Longiaru M. Detection of *Mycobacterium tuberculosis* by molecular methods. *Clin Lab Med.* 1997;17(1): 119–128.

44. Sandin RL. Polymerase chain reaction and other amplification techniques in mycobacteriology. *Clin Lab Med.* 1996;16(3):617–639.

45. Moore DF, Curry JI, Knott CA, et al. Amplification of rRNA for assessment of treatment response of pulmonary tuberculosis patients during antimicrobial therapy. *J Clin Microbiol.* 1996;34:1745–1749.

46. Gamboa F, Manterola JM, Vinado B, et al. Direct detection of *Mycobacterium tuberculosis* complex in nonrespiratory specimens by Gen-Probe Amplified *Mycobacterium tuberculosis* Direct Test. *J Clin Microbiol.* 1997;35(1): 307–310.

47. Pfyffer GE, Kissling P, Jahn EM, et al. Diagnostic performance of amplified *Mycobacterium tuberculosis* Direct Test with cerebrospinal fluid, other nonrespiratory, and respiratory specimens. *J Clin Microbiol.* 1996;34(4):834–841.

48. Ehlers S, Ignatius R, Regnath T, et al. Diagnosis of extrapulmonary tuberculosis by Gen-Probe Amplified *Mycobacterium tuberculosis* Direct Test. *J Clin Microbiol.* 1996; 34(9):2275–2279.

49. Piersimoni C, Scarparo C . Relevance of commercial amplification methods for direct detection of *Mycobacterium*

tuberculosis complex in clinical samples. *J Clin Microbiol.* 2003;41(12):5355–5365.

50. Bergmann JS, Woods GL. Clinical evaluation of the Roche AMPLICOR PCR *Mycobacterium tuberculosis* Test for detection of *M. tuberculosis* in respiratory specimens. *J Clin Microbiol.* 1996;34(5):1083–1085.

51. Bennedsen J, Thomsen VO, Pfyffer GE, et al. Utility of PCR in diagnosing pulmonary tuberculosis. *J Clin Microbiol.* 1996;34(6):1407–1411.

52. Cartuyvels R, Ridder CD, Jonckheere S, et al. Prospective clinical evaluation of Amplicor *Mycobacterium tuberculosis* PCR test as a screening method in a low-prevalence population. *J Clin Microbiol.* 1996;34(8):2001–2003.

53. Huang T-S, Liu Y-C, Lin H-H, et al. Comparison of the Roche AMPLICOR MYCOBACTERIUM Assay and Digene SHARP signal system with in-house PCR and culture for detection of *Mycobacterium tuberculosis* in respiratory specimens. *J Clin Microbiol.* 1996;34(12):3092–3096.

54. Piersimoni C, Callegaro A, Nista D, et al. Comparative evaluation of two commercial amplification assays for direct detection of *Mycobacterium tuberculosis* complex in respiratory specimens. *J Clin Microbiol.* 1997;35(1): 193–196.

55. Noordhoek GT, vanEmbden JA, Kolk AHJ. Reliability of nucleic acid amplification for detection of *Mycobacterium tuberculosis:* An international collaborative quality control study among 30 laboratories. *J Clin Microbiol.* 1996; 34(10):2522–2525.

56. Drosten C, Panning M, Kramme S. Detection of *Mycobacterium tuberculosis* by real-time PCR using pan-mycobacterial primers and a pair of fluorescence resonance energy transfer probes specific for the *M. tuberculosis* complex. *Clin Chem.* 2003;49(10):1659–1661.

57. Kraus G, Cleary T, Miller N, et al. Rapid and specific detection of the *Mycobacterium tuberculosis* complex using fluorogenic probes and real-time PCR. *Mol Cell Probes.* 2001;15(6):375–383.

58. Catanzaro A, Davidson BL, Fujiwara PI, et al. Rapid diagnostic tests for tuberculosis. *Am J Respir Crit Care Med.* 1997;155:1804–1814.

4

Diagnosis of Latent Tuberculosis Infection

Alfred A. Lardizabal
Lee B. Reichman

OVERVIEW

During 2003, there were a total of 14,871 tuberculosis (TB) cases, 5.1/100,000 population, in the United States. This represents a 1.4% decrease in cases and a 1.9% decline in the rate from 2002. But this decline is the smallest since 1992 when TB incidence peaked in the U.S. And despite a decline in TB nationwide, rates have increased in certain states, and elevated TB rates continue to be reported in certain populations, e.g., foreign born persons and racial/ethnic minorities.[1] This is a trend observed in the U.S. many other industrialized nations with low incidence of TB. In these countries, most new, active cases have occurred among persons who were once infected, contained the infection, and then later developed active disease.[2] Where TB case rates have declined significantly over the past decade. The elimination of TB will increasingly depend on diagnosing and treating latent TB infection (LTBI) to prevent development of disease. This chapter will review the tuberculin skin test and the newer blood tests to detect LTBI.

Tuberculin Skin Testing

Tuberculin skin testing is currently still the most widely used and available test for the diagnosis tuberculous infection. Following infection with *M. tuberculosis*, a cascade of immune responses ensues triggered by activated macrophages and carried out by T cells. Two different cell mediated immunity (CMI) mechanisms result in both protection, mediated by Th1 cytokines (IL-2, IL-12, and IFN-γ), and delayed-type hypersensitivity (DTH) mediated by chemokines.[3] Infection with *M. tuberculosis* results in delayed-type hypersensitivity reaction to antigens derived from the organism which is the basis of the tuberculin skin test. Proper use of the tuberculin skin test requires knowledge of the antigen used, immunologic basis for the reaction to this antigen, and the proper technique of administering and reading the test, and, the results of epidemiologic and clinical experience with the test.

When the material is injected intradermally, a classic delayed hypersensitivity reaction occurs in the infected patient. The initial process of sensitization following infection takes about 6–8 weeks with sensitized T-lymphocytes developing in regional lymph nodes and entering the circulation. Restimulation of these lymphocytes by intracutaneous injection of tuberculin results in the indurated skin reaction of a positive result. The induration is due to cellular infiltration mediated by the sensitized lymphocytes. The reaction is maximal at 48–72 hours and then slowly fades, although it commonly lasts more than 96 hours. Two types of tuberculin preparations have been in use, old tuberculin (OT) and purified protein derivative (PPD).

Tuberculin—Historical Perspective

Tuberculin was developed a decade after Robert Koch discovered the tubercle bacillus and also a method of growing it in pure culture in 1882. He came up with this preparation from heat sterilized cultures of tubercle bacilli that were filtered and concentrated and contained tuberculoproteins. It was initially used and touted as therapeutic. However, the curative value of the preparation was disappointing but it led to the discovery of the tuberculin's diagnostic value. Because the original preparation, known as old tuberculin (OT) was an unrefined product with extraneous material present, a positive reaction lacked the sensitivity to be diagnostic of infection with *M. tuberculosis*. Currently, OT is only available as an immunological reagent for veterinary tuberculosis diagnostics.

PURIFIED PROTEIN DERIVATIVE

Florence Siebert originally developed PPD in 1939 at the Phipps Institute, Philadelphia. It is a precipitate prepared from filtrates of OT with ammonium sulfate or trichloroacetic acid. The reference standard material for all tuberculin is PPD-S (Siebert's Lot 49608).

There are three dosage strengths of PPD available, 1 tuberculin unit (TU), 5 TU and 250 TU. In 1972, the Bureau of Biologics of the Food and Drug Administration mandated that the standard test dose of all Tween-containing PPD tuberculin licensed for use in humans be biologically equivalent to 5 TU of PPD-S.[4] No biological standard is required for 1 TU and 250 TU preparations. Basically, these preparations are not useful in the diagnosis of tuberculous infection. The definition of tuberculous infection is a positive reaction to 5 TU PPD.[5] Tween-80 is added to the PPD diluent to prevent antigenic material from being adsorbed by glass and plastic containers and syringes, thus preventing decreased potency of the preparation. PPD antigen is available in both multiple puncture tests and in the intracutaneous Mantoux test. Multiple puncture tests (i.e., Tine and Heaf) and PPD strengths of 1 TU and 250 TU are not accurate, and should not be used.

Mantoux Test

This test is performed by intradermally injecting 0.1 ml of PPD tuberculin (5 TU) into the skin of the volar aspect of the forearm. A single-dose plastic syringe is used with a 26–27-gauge needle. The injection is done with the needle bevel upward. A wheal 6–10 mm in diameter should result. Proper dosage is important; the larger the dose, the larger the reaction. Weaker doses produce smaller reactions. The test is read in 48–72 hours. Test significance depends on the presence or absence of induration. The presence of induration is determined by touch. The diameter of the induration is measured transversely. Erythema is not considered. The size of induration in millimeters, the antigen strength, and lot number, the date of testing, and the date of reading are all recorded.

Adverse reactions to PPD are unusual. Some sensitive individuals may develop local ulceration and necrosis or vesicle formation. Fever and lymphadenopathy may also occur. Aside from local application of petrolatum jelly, no specific therapy is indicated in these instances.

SIGNIFICANCE OF REACTIVITY

The 5 TU dose is used because of its specificity. But tuberculin is a biological product and the *M. tuberculosis* shares antigens with other nontuberculous mycobacteria, so the 5 TU is not completely specific. The use of large doses such as 250 TU of PPD would result in an increased number of nonspecific reactions.

Figure 4-1[6] shows a bimodal distribution of reactions to 5 TU PPD among Alaskan Eskimos. In this group, a reaction size of 5 mm results in a clear separation between reactors and nonreactors. In Alaska, reactions above 5 mm also correlate well with the findings in individuals in this population group known to have tuberculous disease. There are no known cross-reacting mycobacteria in Alaska. So, for this population, a reaction size greater than 5 mm of induration instead of 10 mm can be considered "positive."

Figure 4-2[7] shows the distribution of reactions of 5 TU PPD in Navy recruits from the state of Georgia. A much different situation is shown from that in Fig. 4-1. There is no clear separation point. In order to clarify this, a frequency distribution curve has been constructed by using 15 mm of induration as the mean. The mirror image

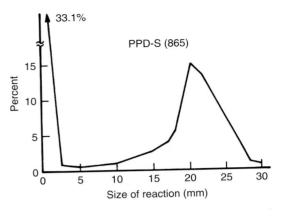

Fig. 4-1. Distribution of reactions to 5 TU purified protein derivative (PPD) among Alaskans tested in 1962. (From Edwards PQ, Comstock GW, Patner CE. Contributions of northern population to the understanding of tuberculin sensitivity. *Arch Environ Health.* 1968;17:507. Copyright 1968. Reprinted with permission of the Helen Dwight Reid Educational Foundation. Published by Heldref Publications, Washington, DC.)

of the distribution to the right of 15 mm is placed to the left of the 15 mm mean (*dotted line*). It has been found[8] that when 5TU PPD is given to patients with cultures positive for *M. tuberculosis*, a symmetrical distribution about a mean of 16–17 mm induration results. From these

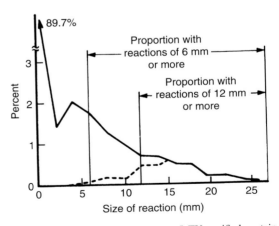

Fig. 4-2. Distribution of reactions to 5 TU purified protein derivative (PPD) among white navy recruits from the state of Georgia with estimate of proportion infected with *M. tuberculosis*. (From: The Tuberculin Test. *Supplement to Diagnostic Standards and Classification of Tuberculosis and Other Mycobacterial Diseases (1974).* New York, NY: American Lung Association; 1974. Official Journal of the American Thoracic Society.)

data, the value of a 15 mm induration has been suggested for distribution curve construction.[9] In Georgia, nontuberculous mycobacteria are found in soil and cross-reactions to tuberculin tests performed with PPD occur. By constructing the distribution curve one can assume that the reactions falling between the solid and dotted lines in Fig. 4-2 are probably due to cross-reactions of nontuberculous mycobacteria. One can also assume that the solid line beyond a 15 mm induration represents true infection and does not included cross-reactions. As demonstrated in Fig. 4-2, if 6 mm induration was taken as indicative of positive reaction, almost no cases of true tuberculous infection would be missed, but a large number of reactions, probably due to nontuberculous mycobacteria, would be included. If a 12 mm induration was used as a cut-off point, the number of nontuberculous reactions included would be less, but several cases of true infection would be missed. Therefore, each geographic area should determine its own cut-off point for a positive reaction depending on the characteristics of the population, the risk for TB infection, and the prevalence of environmental mycobacteria as exemplified in the previous figure. Fig. 4-3 illustrates the distribution of reactors in the New York metropolitan area, a region with a significantly lower prevalence of nontuberculous mycobacteria.

Other factors are important. Persons in close contact with a bacteriologically positive case of TB or with chest radiographic findings consistent with TB are more likely to experience a PPD reaction that is due to a true tuberculous infection than one due to a cross-reaction. One study of an urban population[10] found that variables such as race, socioeconomic status, age, and sex affected the tuberculin skin test reaction rate as regards infection. More positive reactions occurred in nonwhite ethnic groups, in areas of lower socioeconomic status, in men, and with increasing age.

Currently in the United States, a reaction of greater than 5 mm to 5 TU PPD with the Mantoux test after 48 hours is considered positive for those with HIV infection, for those with chest radiographs consistent with old inactive TB, with recent, close contact with infectious TB cases, and for patients with organ transplants and other immunosuppressed patients.

A reaction of greater than 10 mm is positive for recent immigrants (i.e., within the last 5 years) from high prevalence countries; injection drug users; residents and employees of high risk congregate settings such as prisons and jails, nursing homes, hospitals and homeless shelters; Mycobacteriology laboratory personnel; those with clinical conditions in which the risk of TB is increased, such as silicosis, diabetes mellitus, chronic renal failure, hematologic and other malignancies, and weight loss of more than 10% of ideal body weight, gastrectomy, and jejunoileal bypass; and children younger than 4 years of age or infants, children, and adolescents exposed to adults at high risk.

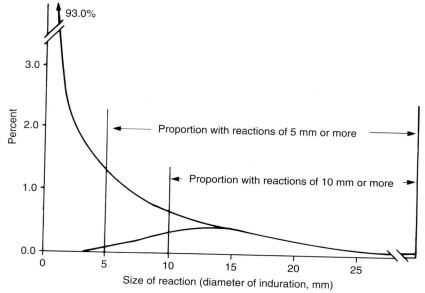

Fig. 4-3. Schema of probable distribution of reactors to 5 TU purified protein derivative (PPD) in the New York metropolitan area.

Table 4-1. Criteria for Tuberculin Positivity, by Risk Group

Reaction ≥5 mm of Induration	Reaction ≥10 mm of Induration	Reaction ≥15 mm of Induration
Human immunodeficiency virus (HIV)-positive persons Recent contacts of TB case patients Fibrotic changes on chest radiograph consistent with prior TB	Recent immigrants (i.e., within the last 5 yr) from high prevalence countries Injection drug users Residents and employees* of the following high-risk congregate settings: prisons and jails, nursing homes, and other long-term facilities for the elderly, hospitals, and other health care facilities, residential facilities for patients with acquired immunity.	Persons with no risk factors for tuberculosis
Patients with organ transplants and other immunosuppressed patients (receiving the equivalent of ≥15 mg/d of prednisone for 1 mo or more)†	Mycobacteriology laboratory personnel Persons with the following clinical conditions that place them at high risk: silicosis, diabetes, mellitus, chronic renal failure, some hematologic disorders (e.g., leukemias and lymphomas), other specific malignancies (e.g., carcinoma of the head or neck) Children younger than 4 yr of age or infants, children, and adolescents exposed to adults at high-risk	

*For persons who are otherwise at low risk and are tested at the start of employment, a reaction of ≥15 mm induration is considered positive

†Risk of TB in patients treated with corticosteroids increases with higher dose and longer duration

Source: Adapted from Centers for Disease Control and Prevention. Screening for TB and TB infection in high-risk populations: recommendations of the Advisory Council for the Elimination of Tuberculosis. *MMWR Morb Mortal Wkly Rep.* 1995;44(No. RR-11):19–34.

In all other persons with no risk factor for tuberculosis, a reaction of greater than 15 mm is considered positive. (Table 4-1)[11]

False Positive Reactions

Inoculation with Bacille Calmette-Guérin (BCG) can be the cause of false positive tuberculin test results; BCG is a live attenuated mycobacterial strain derived from *Mycobacterium bovis*. Several BCG vaccines are available. The vaccines are derived from the original strain but differ in immunogenicity and reactivity. The tuberculin reaction produced by the BCG vaccine cannot be distinguished from that due to *M. tuberculosis* infection. It is best to manage the patient with a previous BCG vaccination without regard to the BCG history, especially because BCG reaction tends to wane with time. The age

at which BCG vaccination is given is important. Tuberculin reactions greater than 10 mm in those vaccinated in infancy should not be attributed to BCG. In persons vaccinated after infancy, positive tuberculin reactions may be due to TB infection or BCG.[12] Immunity to tuberculous infection after BCG vaccination is also still seriously in question.[13] Infection with various nontuberculous or environmental mycobacteria can also cause false positive reactions. For persons with LTBI and normal immune responsiveness, TST sensitivity approaches 100%. These false positive reactions result in lower specificity and a low positive predictive value in persons who have a low probability of LTBI. A lower prevalence of TB infection results in higher false positive reaction and raising the threshold reaction size that separates positive from negative reactors can improve specificity.

False Negative Reactions

A negative reaction to the tuberculin test does not rule out tuberculous infection. A negative reaction can be due to true negativity, that is, an individual's not having tuberculous infection. Various technical factors also result in a falsely negative tuberculin test, however. The tuberculin preparation used must be stored properly. Despite the use of Tween-80, loss of potency can occur from denaturation of the preparation due to heat, light, or bacteria.

Poor technique of administration (e.g., too little antigen injected or too deep an injection) can result in a falsely insignificant reaction. Errors in reading and recording the test can lead to erroneous interpretation.

Various associated conditions can cause a decrease in delayed-type hypersensitivity and cutaneous anergy, resulting in a falsely negative tuberculin test. Conditions associated with anergy include HIV infection, viral infections (e.g., measles, varicella), live virus vaccination, use of immunosuppressive drugs, sarcoidosis, bacterial infections, including fulminant TB, malignancies, particularly lymphoreticular forms, and malnutrition.[13]

HIV infection is particularly important as a cause of cutaneus anergy. About one third of patients with HIV infection and more than 60% of those with acquired immunodeficiency syndrome (AIDS) have a reaction of less than 5 mm to tuberculin despite infection with *M. tuberculosis*.[12] Approximately 50% of HIV-infected patients with active TB have negative tuberculin test results whether 5 mm or 10 mm induration is used.[14] The usefulness of anergy testing in selecting tuberculin-negative, HIV infected persons who might benefit from treatment of latent tuberculous infection (LTBI) has not been demonstrated.

Tuberculin tests indicate infection by the tubercle bacillus. Testing, rather than history, is necessary; however, we have shown that history is notoriously inaccurate (56%) and that a baseline test is required when a patient enters a new health care delivery situation.[15]

BOOSTER EFFECT

Though skin sensitivity usually persists and is life-long, waning can occur, often with age, resulting in an apparent negative reaction. In such instances reactivity can be accentuated with repeated testing (the booster effect).

The booster effect can be a problem with serial tuberculin testing. With serial testing some persons show an increase in the size of their reaction. This can occur in all age groups but does increase with age. In a patient

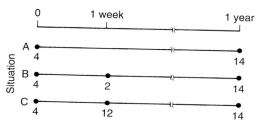

Fig. 4-4. Schematic representation of three booster effect possibilities. (See text for discussion.)

whose reaction has waned, the booster effect can result in an apparent conversion of reaction from negative to positive.[16] For adults who will be screened periodically (e.g., the yearly testing of medical personnel) a two-step procedure for initial skin testing should be used. For those in whom results are negative on the initial test a second test is performed within 1–3 weeks. This second test identifies those in whom boosting is occurring.[17] If the second test result is positive, the person can be considered infected. If the second test result is negative, the person can be considered uninfected. Any subsequent positive reaction in an individual in whom boosting did not occur initially can be considered a true conversion due to infection.

The booster effect is explained in three clinical situations (Fig. 4-4). In situation A, because no repeat testing at the end of 1 week was performed the change in 1 year from 4 mm of induration to 14 mm may or may not represent true conversion. Situation B represents a true conversion (infection), and situation C represents the booster effect, ruling out a true conversion.

SKIN TEST INDICATIONS—TARGETED TUBERCULIN TESTING

Targeted tuberculin testing for LTBI identifies persons at high risk for TB who would benefit by treatment of LTBI. Persons at high risk for TB have either been infected recently with *M. tuberculosis* or have clinical conditions that are associated with an increased risk of progression of LTBI to active TB. Screening of low risk persons and testing for administrative purposes should be replaced with targeted testing. With targeted testing, a decision to tuberculin test is a decision to treat. Table 4-1[11] summarizes the current CDC recommendations and outlines the various risk groups.

Interferon-γ Based Tests

Immunologic diagnosis of *M. tuberculosis* infection has been limited for practical reasons to the tuberculin skin test (TST). TST has been used to detect both LTBI and infection associated with active TB. But concerns about its sensitivity and specificity due to false-positive results after BCG vaccination or exposure to nontuberculous mycobacteria (NTM) have limited its utility. In addition, the TST requires for two encounters with a health care professional, which sometimes causes logistical problems.

The QuantiFERON-TB test (QFT) has recently become available as a test for the detection of *M. tuberculosis* infection. This assay is a whole-blood interferon gamma release assay that is available from Cellestis. (St Kilda, Victoria, Australia). The T cells responsible for conferring protection secrete IFN-γ in response to stimulation with *M. tuberculosis* antigens. Thus, IFN-γ is antigen specific. The profile of cytokine secretion by these T cells is referred to as a Th1-type response and is associated with CMI. Of practical importance is that IFN-γ is released into the surrounding serum is measurable and relatively stable.

Like the TST, QFT measures a component of CMI reactivity to *M. tuberculosis* antigens. Unlike TST, QFT requires a single patient visit, assesses response to both *M. tuberculosis* and nontuberculous mycobacteria simultaneously, and does not boost anamnestic immune responses. The interpretation of the whole-blood interferon gamma assay is less subjective than the TST, and the test is less affected by prior BCG vaccination, and reactivity to nontuberculous mycobacteria than the TST. The Food and Drug Administration approved it in November of 2001 as an aid for detecting LTBI. A second generation test which appears to be more specific (QuantiFERON-TB Gold, discussed further) has been submitted to the FDA for approval.

How the QuantiFERON-TB Test is Performed

IFN-γ is released by stimulation of fresh heparinized venous blood with test antigens. The blood must be stimulated while it is fresh (within 12 hours of collection) and while the lymphocytes are viable. To stimulate the blood, 1 mL aliquots of blood are mixed with four different antigen solutions, and incubated for 16–24 hours at 37°C. The antigens included in the QuantiFERON-TB kits are PPD from *M. tuberculosis* (referred to as "Human tuberculin PPD" by the manufacturer), PPD from *Mycobacterium avium* (referred to as "Avian sensitin"), phytohemaglutinin (referred to as "Mitogen"), and saline (referred to a "Nil control"). Phytohemaglutinin is used as a positive assay control, and saline is used as a negative control. The next generation QuantiFERON-TB Gold utilizes TB specific antigens such as ESAT 6 and CFP 10 instead of human PPD (Discussed later).

After incubation, plasma is collected from each aliquot, and the concentration of IFN-γ is determined by enzyme-linked immunosorbent assay (ELISA). QFT results are based on the proportion of IFN-γ released in response to tuberculin as compared with Mitogen, and response to tuberculin as compared to avian sensitin. Software is available from Cellestis that will assess validity of the ELISA, calculated IFN-γ concentrations, compare IFN-γ concentrations, and provide a report of results.

Calculations include:

$$\% \text{ Tuberculin response} = \frac{(\text{tuberculin} - \text{nil})}{(\text{mitogen} - \text{nil})} \times 100$$

$$\% \text{ Avian difference} = \frac{(\text{avian} - \text{nil}) - (\text{tuberculin} - \text{nil})}{(\text{tuberculin} - \text{nil})} \times 100$$

Because the QFT assay requires fresh whole blood, arrangements should be made with a qualified laboratory before blood is collected for testing. The arrangements should include methods for quality assurance and methods for transporting and stimulating the collected blood within the required 12 hours.

QuantiFERON-TB results suggestive of *M. Tuberculosis*

- % Avian difference ≤10%, and
- (mitogen-nil) and (tuberculin-nil) are both ≥1.5 IU
- % Tuberculin response ≥15% (if increased risk of LTBI) or ≥30% (if low risk of LTBI)

Interpretation of QFT results (Table 4-1) is stratified by estimated risk of infection with *M. tuberculosis*, in a manner similar to that used for interpreting positive cutoff values for the TST. (Table 4-2)[18] Selection of different cutoffs affect the number of people classified as having positive test results. Using 15% as the percentage tuberculin response cutoff for interpreting a QFT test as positive identifies approximately the same number of people than using a TST induration cutoff of 10 mm. Using 30% as the percentage tuberculin response cutoff

Table 4-2. QuantiFERON-TB Results and Interpretation

M-N* (IU/ml)	T-N† (IU/ml)	Avian Difference (%)	Tuberculin Response (%)‡	Report and Interpretation	Interpretation
≤1.5		All other response profiles		Interferon-gamma (IFNγ) response to mitogen is inadequate	Indeterminate
≥1.5		All other response profiles	<15	Percentage tuberculin response is <15 or not significant	Negative: *Mycobacterium tuberculosis* infection unlikely
≥1.5	≥1.5	≤10	≥15 but <30	Percentage tuberculin response is 15–30	Conditionally positive: *Mycobacterium tuberculosis* infection likely if risk is identified, but unlikely in persons who are at low risk
≥1.5	≥1.5	≤10	≥30	Percentage tuberculin response is ≥30	Positive: *Mycobacterium tuberculosis* infection likely

*M-N is the IFN-γ response to mitogen minus the IFN-γ response to nil antigen

†T-N is the IFN-γ response to purified protein derivative from *Mycobacterium tuberculosis* minus the IFN-γ response to nil antigen. QuantiFERON-TB-positive for *M. tuberculosis* infection. If T—N <1.5 IU/ml, the persons are deemed negative for *Mycobacterium tuberculosis* infection, regardless of their percentage tuberculin response and percentage avian difference results

‡A percentage tuberculin response cut-off of 15% is used for persons with identified risk for tuberculosis infection, whereas a cut-off of 30% is used for persons with no identified risk factors

Source: Reproduced from CDC. Guidelines for using the QuantiFERON-TB test for diagnosing latent *Mycobacterium tuberculosis infection. MMWR Morb Mortal Wkly Rep.* 2003;52(RR02):15–18.

for interpreting a QFT test as positive identifies approximately the same number of people than using a TST induration cutoff of 15 mm. The test is considered negative if (mitogen-nil) ≥1.5 IU but (tuberculin-nil) <15% (mitogen-nil). Results are considered indeterminate if (mitogen-nil) <1.5 IU, which may be seen in anergic persons.

COMPARING QFT AND TST

The TST has been used for years as an aid in diagnosing LTBI and includes measurement of the delayed type hypersensitivity response 48–72 hours after intradermal injection of PPD. Although both tests are immunologically based, the TST and QFT do not measure the same components of the immunologic response and are not interchangeable. Assessment of the accuracy of these tests is limited by the lack of a gold standard for confirming LTBI.

As a diagnostic test, QFT 1) requires phlebotomy, 2) can be accomplished after a single patient visit, 3) assesses responses to multiple antigens simultaneously, and 4) does not boost anamnestic immune responses. Compared with TST, QFT results are less subject to reader bias and error. Table 4-3 summarizes these differences.

Several studies conducted comparing QFT and TST have results that show these tests to be moderately concordant.[19,20] In comparing the IFN-γ assay to the TST in persons with varying risk for *Mycobacterium tuberculosis* infection (MTB) infection, Mazurek, et al.[19] showed that the assay was comparable to the TST in its ability to detect LTBI, was less affected by BCG vaccination, discriminated responses due to NTM, and avoided the variability and subjectivity associated with placing and reading the TST. Table 4-4 outlines the interim recommendations for the use of QFT.

ANTICIPATED REFINEMENTS FOR QFT: QuantiFERON-TB Gold

The second generation QuantiFERON-TB Gold (Cellestis Ltd.) assay detects CMI responses in vitro to TB infection by measuring interferon gamma harvested from whole blood incubated with the *M. tuberculosis* specific antigens, ESAT-6 and CFP-10. By using the *specific* tuberculosis proteins, ESAT-6 and CFP-10, which are only made by *M. tuberculosis* complex organisms (*Mycobacterium tuberculosis, Mycobacterium bovis, Mycobacterium africanum*), the QuantiFERON-TB Gold test identifies the presence of T-cells that are totally specific for tuberculosis infection. Neither ESAT-6 nor CFP-10 is present in the TB vaccine organism (BCG) *M. bovis* or in most environmental (nontubercular) mycobacteria with the exception of *Mycobacterium kansasii, Mycobacterium szulgai, and Mycobacterium marinum*. Thus these proteins are precise markers of true MTB infection and unlike the tuberculin skin test (TST or Mantoux test) is completely unaffected by the BCG vaccination status of the individual being tested.

Mori, et al., recently published results after examining the use of these two antigens, ESAT-6, and CFP-10, in a whole blood interferon γ assay as a diagnostic test for TB in BCG vaccinated individuals. Specificity of the test in low risk people was 98.1% and sensitivity in patients with TB infection was 89%. The results showed the test to be highly specific and sensitive and was unaffected by BCG vaccination status.[21] This test was also used to detect recent infection among contacts in a TB outbreak at a Danish high school. Since a majority of contacts were BCG-unvaccinated direct comparison between the TST and QFT could be performed. Analysis revealed an excellent agreement between the two tests was found (94%, kappa value 0.866) and that the blood test was not influenced by the vaccination status of the subjects tested.[22]

The QuantiFERON-TB Gold test is accurate and simple to perform. Small amounts of blood are incubated overnight with the TB specific proteins and IFN-γ levels in plasma are measured the next day. Like the original test, this test uses undiluted whole blood with no need for tedious cell isolation and enumeration.

QuantiFERON-TB Gold has received FDA approval. CDC recommendations regarding its use is expected to follow.

Table 4-3. Comparison between QFT and TST

QFT		TST
In vitro test		In vivo test
Multiple antigens		Single antigen
No boosting	vs	Boosting
1 patient visit		2 patient visits
Minimal inter-reader variability		Inter-reader variability
Results possible in 1 day		Results in 2–3 days

Table 4-4. Interim Recommendations for Applying and Interpreting QuantiFERON-TB (QFT)

Reason for Testing	Population	Initial Screening	Positive Results	Evaluation
Tuberculosis suspect	Persons with symptoms of active TB	Tuberculin skin testing (TST) might be useful; QFT not recommended	Induration ≥5 mm	Chest radiograph, smears, and cultures, regardless of test results
Increased risk for progression to active TB, if infected	Persons with recent contact with TB, changes on chest radiograph consistent with prior TB, organ transplants, or human immunodeficiency virus infection, and those receiving immunosuppressing drugs equivalent of ≥15 mg/day of prednisone for ≥1 month*	TST: QFT not recommended	Induration ≥5 mm	Chest radiograph if TST is positive; treat for latent TB infection (LTBI) after active TB disease is ruled out
	Persons with diabetes, silicosis, chronic renal failure, leukemia, lymphoma, carcinoma of the head, neck, or lung, and persons with weight loss of ≥10% of ideal body weight, gastrectomy, or jejunoileal bypass*	TST: QFT not recommended	Induration ≥10 mm	
Increased risk for LTBI	Recent immigrants, injection-drug users, and residents and employees of high-risk congregate settings (e.g., prisons, jails, homeless shelters, and certain health-care facilities)†	TST or QFT	Induration ≥10 mm: percentage tuberculin response ≥15‡	Chest radiograph if either test is positive; confirmatory TST is optional if QFT is positive; treat for LTBI after active TB disease is ruled out; LTBI treatment when only QFT is positive should be based on clinical judgment and estimated risk
Other reasons for testing among persons at low risk for LTBI	Military personnel, hospital staff, and health-care workers whose risk of prior exposure to patients is low, and U.S.-born students at certain colleges and universities†	TST or QFT	Induration ≥15 mm: percentage tuberculin response ≥30‡	Chest radiograph if either test is positive; confirmatory TST if QFT is positive; treatment for LTBI (if QFT and TST are positive and after active TB disease is ruled out) on the bases of assessment of risk for drug toxicity, TB transmission, and patients

*QFT has not been adequately evaluated among persons with these conditions; It is not recommended for such populations.
†QFT has not been adequately evaluated among persons aged <17 years, or among pregnant women; it is not recommended for such populations.
‡The following additional conditions are required for QFT to indicate *M. tuberculosis* infection: (1) mitogen—nil and tuberculin—nil are both >1.5 IU, and (2) percentage avian difference is ≤10.
Source: Adapted from CDC. Guidelines for using the QuantiFERON-TB test for diagnosing latent *M. tuberculosis infection. MMWR Morb Mortal Wkly Rep.* 2003;52(RR02):15–18.

REFERENCES

1. CDC. *Reported tuberculosis in the United States, 2002.* Atlanta, Georgia: U.S. Department of Health and Human Services, CDC; 2003.
2. Styblo, K. Recent advances in epidemiological research in tuberculosis. *Adv Tuberc Res.* 1980;20:1–63.
3. Orme IM, Cooper AM. Cytokine/chemokine cascades in immunity to tuberculosis. *Immunol Today.* 1999;20:307–312.
4. Edwards PQ. Tuberculin negative? (Editorial). *N Engl J Med.* 1972;286:373–374.
5. American Thoracic Society. Diagnostic standards and classification of tuberculosis and other mycobacterial diseases. *Am Rev Respir Dis.* 1981;123:343–358.
6. Edwards PQ, Comstock GW, Palmer CE. Contributions of northern population to the understanding of tuberculin sensitivity. *Arch Environ Health (Chicago).* 1968;17:507.
7. American Lung Association Committee. *The tuberculin skin test: Supplement to Diagnostic standards and classification of tuberculosis and other mycobacterial diseases.* New York, NY: American Lung Association; 1974.
8. Palmer CE, Edwards LB, Hopwood L, et al. Experimental and epidemiologic basis for the interpretation of tuberculin sensitivity. *J Pediatr.* 1959;55:413–429.
9. American Thoracic Society. The tuberculin skin test. *Am Rev Respir Dis.* 1981;124:356–363.
10. Reichman LB, O'Day R. Tuberculous infection in a large urban population. *Am Rev Respir Dis.* 1978;117:705–712.
11. CDC. Targeted tuberculin testing and treatment of latent tuberculosis infection. *MMWR Morb Mortal Wkly Rep.* 2000;49(RR-6):1–51.
12. Menzies R, Vissandjee B. Effect of Bacille Calmette-Guérin vaccination on tuberculin reactivity. *Am Rev Respir Dis.* 1992;145:621–625.
13. Snider DE. Bacille Calmette-Guérin vaccinations and tuberculin skin tests. *JAMA.* 1985;253:3438–3439.
14. CDC. *Core Curriculum on Tuberculosis,* 4th ed. Washington, D.C. Government Printing Office; 2000.
15. Reichman LB, O'Day R. The influence of a history of a previous test on the prevalence and size of reaction to tuberculin. *Am Rev Respir Dis.* 1977;115:737–741.
16. Thompson NJ, Glasroth JL, Snider DE, et al. The booster phenomenon in serial tuberculin testing. *Am Rev Respir Dis.* 1979;119:587–597.
17. American Thoracic Society. Control of tuberculosis in the United States. *Am Rev Respi Dis.* 1992;146:1623–1633.
18. CDC. Guidelines for using the QuantiFERON-TB test for diagnosing latent *Mycobacterium tuberculosis infection. MMWR Morb Mortal Wkly Rep.* 2003;52(RR02):15–18.
19. Mazurek GH, LoBue PA, Daley CL, et al. Comparison of a whole-blood interferon γ assay with tuberculin skin testing for detecting latent *Mycobacterium tuberculosis* infection. *JAMA.* 2001;286:1740–1747.
20. Streeton JA, Desem N, Jones SL. Sensitivity and specificity of a gamma interferon blood test tuberculosis infection. *Int J Tuberc Lung Dis.* 1998;2:443–450.
21. Mori T, Sakatani M, Yamagishi F, et al. Specific Detection of Tuberculosis Infection with an Interferon–gamma Based Assay Using New Antigens. *Am J Respir Crit Care Med.* 2004;170:59–64.
22. Brock I, Weldingh K, Lillebaek T, et al. Comparison of a New Specific Blood Test and the Skin Test in tuberculosis Contacts. *Am J Respir Crit Care Med.* 2004;170:65–69.

5

Treatment of Latent Tuberculosis Infection

Jonathan E. Golub
George W. Comstock

Two prophylactic measures are available in the control of tuberculosis (TB), and each has its place, depending on the epidemiologic situation. Immunization, or Bacille Calmette-Guérin (BCG) vaccination, is discussed in the chapter BCG and The Search for Newer Vaccines. This chapter discusses treatment of Latent Tuberculosis Infection (LTBI), formerly called Chemoprophylaxis or Preventive Therapy. Treatment of LTBI is directed at persons already infected, particularly those at significant risk of progression to active disease.

TREATMENT OF LATENT TUBERCULOSIS INFECTION (LTBI)

Treatment of LTBI, or preventive therapy for short, started from the observations of an astute clinician. Preventive therapy usually consists of the oral administration of isoniazid (INH). It can be a useful tool, particularly when the risk of infection is low and the infected population is relatively small. During the 1950s in the United States, children with primary TB were considered to need chemotherapy only if they were clinically ill. When INH was added to the armamentarium of streptomycin, para-aminosalicylic acid, and promizole, Dr. Edith Lincoln noted that children hospitalized at Bellevue Hospital in New York City no longer experienced complications of their primary TB; at her suggestion, the U.S. Public Health Service organized a multiclinic controlled trial among 2,750 children with asymptomatic primary TB or a recent tuberculin conversion. Preventive therapy with INH proved to be remarkably effective, producing a 94% reduction in tuberculous complications during a year of preventive treatment and a 70% reduction over the subsequent 9-year period.[1]

Effectiveness

A total of 19 randomized, placebo-controlled trials of preventive therapy with INH that involved a total of more than 135,000 subjects had been reported by 1994.[2] Among these trials, the average reduction in TB was 60% during the period of observation, being somewhat higher during the year of treatment. These results were based on the total study populations regardless of how well medication was taken. The five trials with less than 50% effectiveness included one that used small doses of INH, one in which compliance was poor, and one that included patients who had undergone previous chemotherapy, a group now known not to benefit from additional treatment. When analyses were limited to those who took their medication for most of the treatment year, efficacy approximated 90%. Protection also appears to be long lasting, being demonstrable nearly 20 years after initiation of treatment.[3]

Until recently, the generally accepted regimen for preventive treatment was 5–10 mg of INH per kilogram of body weight, not exceeding a total dose of 300 mg/day, given orally in a single daily dose for 6–12 months. In studies among U.S. veterans and Alaskan villagers, treatment for more than a year did not confer additional benefits.[3,4] Doses lower than 5 mg/kg were found to be less effective.[5,6]

The optimal duration of treatment is a matter of considerable importance. This question was addressed in a large trial in six eastern European countries among persons with untreated inactive TB.[7] Regimens of daily INH for 3, 6, and 12 months were tested against daily placebo for the same durations. The results of 5 years' observation of the total population showed that treatment for 12 months resulted in a 75% reduction in TB, compared with a reduction of 65% in those treated for 6 months, and 21% for those treated for only 3 months; however, when the analysis was restricted to those who took at least 80% of the prescribed regimen, efficacy increased to 93% for the 12-month group but improved only slightly for those treated for 6 and 3 months. In the U.S. Public Health Service trials among household contacts and Alaskan villagers, the optimal duration of treatment appeared to be 9–10 months[1–3] (Fig. 5-1). In the contact trial, irregular treatment was still effective as long as 80% of the 12-month dose (i.e., 9–10 months) was taken within a reasonable time.

Therefore, although a six-month regimen confers significant protection, the currently preferred regimen is nine months of daily isoniazid, at a dosage of 5 mg/kg in the adult, not to exceed 300 mg; for children, the dosage is 10–20 mg/kg, not to exceed 300 mg. Isoniazid can also be administered twice weekly for nine months, at a dosage of 15 mg/kg in the adult, not to exceed 900 mg, and 20–40 mg/kg in children, not to exceed 900 mg; the twice weekly regimen must be given as directly observed therapy (DOT). Rifampin daily for four months is the alternative for patients intolerant of isoniazid or who may have isoniazid-resistant infection (see below). Rifampin dosage is 10 mg/kg for adults, not to exceed 600 mg; for children it is 10–20 mg/kg,

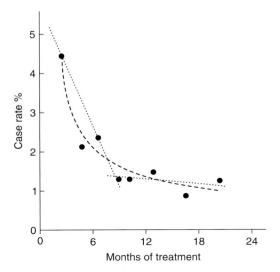

Fig. 5-1. Tuberculosis case rates (%) in the Bethel Isoniazid Studies population according to the number of months INH was taken in the combined programs. *Dots* represent observed values; *dashed line*, the calculated curve (y = a + b/x); and *dotted lines* the calculated values based on the first four and the last five observations (y = a + bx). (*Source:* Comstock, GW. How much isoniazid is needed for prevention of tuberculosis among immunocompetent adults? *Int J Tuberc Lung Dis.* 1999;3:847–850. Reprinted by permission of the International Union against Tuberculosis and Lung Disease.)

not to exceed 600 mg. Rifampin may also be given twice weekly in adults (with DOT), at the same dosage.

Short course preventive therapy regimens containing rifampin and pyrazinamide have been investigated in an effort to shorten the duration of treatment for preventive therapy while maintaining efficacy and minimal toxicity. Among HIV-positive patients, two clinical trials have shown that a 2-month course of rifampin and pyrazinamide was equally efficacious as longer courses of INH.[8,9] Patients were more likely to show compliance with the shorter regimen and tolerability was similar between the rifampin/pyrazinamide and INH arms. A randomized controlled trial among HIV-positive patients in Zambia found no significant difference between TB rates in patients receiving 6 months of INH or 3 months of rifampin/pyrazinamide on a twice weekly dosage regimen, but a moderate difference between these combined groups and those receiving a placebo after an average of 2.7 person years of observation per patient.[10,11] The difference in tuberculosis-free survival between either treatment group and the placebo persisted for four years. Neither regimen had a significant impact on HIV progression or overall mortality.

However, this combination is presently considered too toxic and is not recommended (please see later discussion).

HIV infection has been shown to be a major risk factor for recurrent TB.[12–14] In a randomized clinical trial in Haiti, HIV-infected patients receiving post-treatment INH reported recurrent TB at a rate of 1.4 per 100 person years compared to 7.8 per 100 person years among those receiving placebo.[12] An observational study among gold miners in South Africa found overall TB incidence reduced by 55% among those who received secondary preventive therapy with INH compared to those who did not.[15] Current international guidelines for preventive therapy in HIV-infected individuals do not recommend secondary prophylaxis, but these studies challenge these recommendations.[16]

Global policy regarding INH preventive therapy in patients with HIV infection is contradictory. The WHO and UNAIDS recommend that INH preventive therapy be offered to HIV-infected patients with or at risk for latent TB infection as part of a package of care for the "personal health benefit," but do not endorse INH preventive therapy for public health purposes.[17] Because global policy is lukewarm with respect to INH preventive therapy, few countries have effectively implemented programs for its delivery. Several operational studies in Africa found that uptake of INH preventive therapy was limited, adherence problematic and completion of therapy less than desired.[18,19] These results have further dampened enthusiasm for the use of INH prevention, despite the promising data from the cohort studies cited above. The Pro-Test projects in southern Africa provided operational evidence that HIV voluntary counseling and testing could be used as an effective bridge to INH preventive therapy, with moderate to very good levels of adherence, depending on the setting. These projects did not, unfortunately, include an assessment of the impact of INH prophylactic therapy on TB incidence or survival.[20]

The combination of policies to provide antiretroviral therapy and INH preventive therapy to HIV-infected populations is likely to have a synergistic effect on controlling HIV-related TB.[21] For HIV-infected people who are not candidates for antiretroviral therapy, INH is highly efficacious for preventing TB. INH preventive therapy can also provide an important benefit in patients who are receiving antiretroviral therapy and who remain at increased risk of developing TB. Because TB is capable of causing disease in individuals with seemingly normal immunity, the improvement in immune function that is produced by antiretrovirals cannot eliminate the risk of TB. Specific chemotherapy for latent TB infection will complement antiretroviral therapy that results in immune restoration.

INH preventive therapy has been shown to reduce the incidence of TB in HIV-infected people with latent infection by 60–80%, though no benefit has been proved in tuberculin-negative or anergic individuals.[22] The duration of protection provided by a single course of INH preventive therapy has varied in different settings, with prolonged benefit apparent in clinical trials done in developed and some developing countries, while the effect was lost after 18–48 months in clinical studies done in Zambia and Uganda.[8–11,23] The impact of INH preventive therapy in cohort populations has been assessed in the United States and Brazil.[24,25] In a cohort of more than 2,000 injection drug users with a high prevalence of both HIV and latent infection in Baltimore, USA, a dramatic and significant decline in TB incidence was observed after INH preventive therapy was selectively offered to tuberculin-positive cohort members.[24] Tuberculosis incidence, which had increased five-fold in the several years prior to the intervention, fell to zero within 18 months, and no new cases of TB were diagnosed in the cohort for more than nine years subsequently. In Brazil, individuals in an HIV-infected cohort with access to medical care, including antiretrovirals, had a 62% lower risk of developing TB and a 76% lower risk of dying if they received TB preventive therapy.[25] These cohort studies demonstrate that preventive therapy can have a marked effect on TB risk in populations with access to medical care, and may have community benefit beyond the personal advantages conferred on individual patients.

Benefits and Risks

A committee convened by the American Thoracic Society recommended that certain screening procedures be carried out before starting preventive therapy.[26] The presence of active TB should be ruled out. Persons with previous side effects from INH and those with current acute liver disease should be excluded. Conditions that do not contraindicate preventive therapy but that require special medical assessment include interactions with other medications, daily use of alcohol, previous minor side effects from INH, chronic liver disease, and current or recent pregnancy.

In the most recently revised guidelines, "Targeted Tuberculin Testing and Treatment of Latent Tuberculosis Infection," emphasis has shifted to tuberculin testing only those groups at high risk of progression to active TB disease and those who would benefit by treatment for latent TB infection.[27] Screening of low risk groups and testing for administrative purposes has been discouraged in place of targeted testing. Thus, the decision to test is also a decision to treat, should the test be positive. Moreover, infected persons at increased risk for developing active TB should be offered treatment of latent TB infection regardless of age; therefore, the earlier cutoff of age 35 no longer applies. Persons at high risk for developing TB include those individuals who have been recently infected with *M. tuberculosis* or have a clinical condition associated with an increased risk (see further). The epidemiology of TB in a specific geographic area may define specific high-risk groups in addition to these established and known risk factors.

INH is one of the least toxic of the antituberculosis drugs; most of the reactions are mild and transient. The side effect of principal concern is hepatitis, which is rare in those under the age of 20 but increases with age to a peak of 2% to 3% in the age group 50 to 64 years.[28] Recently, over 11,000 patients who started INH preventive therapy between 1989 and 1995 in a Seattle public health TB clinic were reported to have had very low (0.15%) rates of hepatotoxic reactions, though the risk did increase with age (p = 0.02).[29] This low rate was attributed to careful monitoring of symptoms of toxicity. Deaths due to INH-associated hepatitis have occurred, especially among persons who continued to take the drug after symptoms of hepatitis had appeared. The risk of infected persons developing TB if preventive therapy is not given must be weighed against the risk of hepatitis if it is. For tuberculin reactors with no additional risk factors, a sensitivity analysis suggested that the balance is most strongly in favor of preventive treatment among children and young adults.[30] For persons with additional risk factors, the benefit/risk ratio is increased at all ages.

Case reports of patients receiving combination regimens including rifampin and pyrazinamide have raised concern about the potential increased risk of hepatitis among HIV-negative patients.[31] Recently, a multicenter clinical trial in the United States found an increased risk for grade 3 or 4 hepatoxicity among patients receiving a 2-month regimen of rifampin/pyrazinamide (7.7%) compared to a 6-month regimen of INH (1%; $P < 0.01$).[32] Among 114 patients receiving rifampin/pyrazinamide, four patients developed hepatitis on therapy and another two (5.3%) with symptoms did not report for laboratory testing.[33] Although the authors state that the high completion rates warrant use in high-risk individuals with careful monitoring, no comparison group was included.[34] These and other data regarding rifampin/pyrazinamide regimens for preventive therapy were recently reviewed by TB experts at a meeting held during the 99th International American Thoracic Society Conference in Seattle, Washington, in May, 2003.[31]

The American Thoracic Society and the Centers for Disease Control now recommend that this regimen "should generally not be offered to persons with latent TB infection for either HIV-negative or HIV-infected persons," despite these regimens being recommended in the 2000 ATS guidelines.[27]

Patients need to be motivated to take their medication faithfully and must be warned to stop INH promptly should symptoms of hepatitis develop. Only a month's supply of INH should be given at one time. Each patient or a responsible surrogate should be interviewed each month to be certain no symptoms or other findings suggestive of hepatitis have occurred. The use of laboratory tests for hepatic dysfunction is recommended for persons with suspicious symptoms but not for routine monitoring.

The adoption of similar recommendations in 1974 appears to have decreased markedly the risk of serious hepatitis[35] and to have established preventive treatment with INH as a safe, effective procedure for prevention of TB in individuals and for control of the disease in a community.[29] The cost of preventive treatment, even with monthly monitoring of symptoms, is rarely a major consideration in developed countries in which the program is merely added to existing procedures in TB clinics. In countries with limited resources, scarce antituberculosis medications should be used for prevention only after the needs of TB patients have been met.

Indications

The American Thoracic Society and the Centers for Disease Control and Prevention have recommended that persons with any of the following six risk factors should be considered candidates for preventive therapy, regardless of age, if they have not previously been treated.[27] This recommendation is qualified by the size of induration to an intracutaneous tuberculin test using 5 tuberculin units (TU) of purified protein derivative (PPD) of tuberculin. The criteria for a positive tuberculin test result are given in parentheses. They depend on the probability of infection with *Mycobacterium tuberculosis* and the importance and nature of the risk factor[26]:

- Known or suspected infection with HIV (≥5 mm). HIV infection appears to be by far the most potent risk factor for the development of TB in tuberculin-positive persons. This risk is so high that patients with HIV infection and skin test anergy who have a high probability of having been infected with *M. tuberculosis* should also be considered for preventive therapy. For persons known to be HIV-positive, treatment should be continued for at least 9 months.

- Tuberculin-positive close contacts of persons with infectious TB (≥5 mm).

- Persons whose tuberculin test result has changed from negative to positive within 2 years, with a 10 + mm increase, regardless of age (≥10 mm).

- Tuberculin-positive persons whose chest radiographs suggest untreated fibrotic TB (≥5 mm).

- Intravenous drug abusers with negative tests for HIV infection (≥10 mm).

- Tuberculin reactors (≥10 mm) with one of the following medical conditions that have been reported to increase TB risk: silicosis, diabetes mellitus, hematologic, and reticuloendothelial malignancies such as leukemia or Hodgkin's disease, gastrectomy, cancer of the head and neck, end-stage renal disease, and conditions associated with rapid weight loss or chronic malnutrition.

- Immunosuppression such as chronic corticosteroid administration (≥5 mm).

In addition, persons who do not have any of the preceding risk factors and are in any of the following three categories should also be treated with INH if their tuberculin test results show induration of 10 or more mm:

- Foreign-born persons from high-prevalence countries who have immigrated within the past five years.

- Other residents of high-prevalence areas in the United States (e.g., inner cities, Native American reservations).

- Residents and employees of high-risk congregate settings, including nursing homes, mental institutions, correctional institutions, hospitals, and homeless shelters.

Persons who are not included in any of the preceding groups, and whose tuberculin reactions are 15 mm or larger, should also be considered for preventive therapy. This may occur, for example, in people at low risk who undergo testing upon entry to a high-risk work site such as a hospital.

Treatment of LTBI for Persons Exposed to Drug-Resistant *Mycobacterium Tuberculosis*

INH is the only medication that has been tested in multiple large trials and approved for preventive treatment. When there is strong evidence that infection with an INH-resistant strain of tubercle bacilli has occurred, there is no proven substitute. However, rifampin is a reasonable candidate because it can be taken by mouth and is known to be highly effective in therapeutic regimens. Experience with animals and humans indicates that rifampin will be as effective or more effective than INH and well tolerated, causing few hepatotoxic reactions. Rifampin's side effects include a red-orange coloration of body fluids such as urine, sweat, and tears as well as interactions with a number of other drugs, including methadone, and oral contraceptives. These side effects should not be a problem if patients are carefully instructed about the need for preventive therapy and the action of the drug. Although concern may be expressed about the emergence of resistant organisms when rifampin is given alone, it is reassuring that INH resistance has not been demonstrated when INH has been used alone in preventive treatment.[1]

Exposure to TB cases with organisms resistant to both INH and rifampin is becoming more common, particularly among disadvantaged members of society. Management of persons with such exposures must be based to a considerable extent on clinical and epidemiologic judgment, taking into consideration the infectiousness of the case and closeness, intensity, and duration of exposure.[36] Persons who have competent immune responses and are at only a low risk of having been infected with multiple-resistant organisms should follow the usual recommendations for close TB contacts. If they have a moderate to high likelihood of having been infected with multidrug-resistant *M. tuberculosis* and have a high risk of developing TB as a result of immunosuppression, risk factors for HIV infection, or other conditions known to cause a considerable increase in the risk of developing active disease, multidrug preventive therapy should be considered. This should consist of at least two antituberculosis drugs, depending on the resistance pattern of the organisms from the suspected source case and the patient's ability to tolerate these drugs. Possible regimens would include a regimen of two drugs selected from ethambutol, pyrazinamide, or a quinolone. The drugs should be prescribed for 12 months at standard dosages used in the treatment of disease. Consultation with or referral to a TB specialist is strongly advised.

Treatment of LTBI in Skin-Test Negative Persons

Some persons who are close contacts of patients with active TB may be candidates for treatment of LTBI, even if their skin test is negative. These groups include close contacts of others who had a similar exposure and are now skin-test positive, close contacts who are infants, children or adolescents (treat them until a repeat PPD is negative three months later or until treatment has been given for nine months), and close contacts who are HIV+ or otherwise immunosuppressed.

CONCLUSIONS

Taking pills to prevent disease some time in the indistinct future is an almost incomprehensible concept for many persons, especially those from other cultures. Furthermore, many immigrants have been told that their BCG vaccination has already protected them against TB and see no reason to treat their positive tuberculin tests. To motivate them to start and complete preventive therapy requires understanding their beliefs about TB, its cause, its treatment, and its prevention. That these beliefs vary markedly among ethnic groups has been clearly shown in New York City.[37] Case managers who are attuned to these ethnocentric beliefs have been able to improve the acceptance of and adherence to preventive therapy.[38–40] Their use deserves wider application.

REFERENCES

1. Ferebee SH. Controlled chemoprophylaxis trials in tuberculosis: A general review. *Bibl Tuberc*. 1970;26:28–106.
2. Comstock GW, Woolpert SF. Preventive Therapy. In: *The Mycobacteria: A Sourcebook*. New York, NY: Marcel Dekker; 1994.
3. Comstock GW. How much isoniazid is needed for prevention of tuberculosis among immunocompetent adults? *Int J Tuberc Lung Dis*. 1999;3(10):847–850.
4. Falk A, Fuchs GF. Prophylaxis with isoniazid in inactive tuberculosis: A Veterans Administration Cooperative Study XII. *Chest*. 1978;73(1):44–48.
5. Horwitz O, Magnus K. Epidemiologic evaluation of chemoprophylaxis against tuberculosis. *Am J Epidemiol*. 1974;99(5):333–342.
6. Comstock GW, Hammes LM, Pio A. Isoniazid prophylaxis in Alaskan Boarding schools: A comparison of two doses. *Am Rev Respir Dis.*1969;100(6):773–779.
7. International Union Against Tuberculosis Committee on Prophylaxis. Efficacy of various durations of isoniazid preventive therapy for tuberculosis: five years of follow-up in the IUAT trial. *Bull World Health Organ*. 1982;60(4):555–564.
8. Gordin F, Chaisson RE, Matts JP, et al. Rifampin and pyrazinamide vs isoniazid for prevention of tuberculosis in HIV-infected persons: an international randomized trial. Terry Beirn Community Programs for Clinical Research on AIDS, the Adult AIDS Clinical Trials Group, the Pan American Health Organization, and the Centers for Disease Control and Prevention Study Group. *JAMA*. 2000;283(11):1445–1450.
9. Halsey NA, Coberly JS, Desormeaux J, et al. Randomised trial of isoniazid versus rifampicin and pyrazinamide for prevention of tuberculosis in HIV-1 infection. *Lancet*. 1998;351(9105):786–792.

10. Mwinga A, Hosp M, Godfrey-Faussett P, et al. Twice weekly tuberculosis preventive therapy in HIV infection in Zambia. *AIDS*. 1998;12(18):2447–2457.

11. Quigley MA, Mwinga A, Hosp M, et al. Long-term effect of preventive therapy for tuberculosis in a cohort of HIV-infected Zambian adults. *AIDS*. 2001;15(2):215–222.

12. Fitzgerald DW, Desvarieux M, Severe P, et al. Effect of post-treatment isoniazid on prevention of recurrent tuberculosis in HIV-1-infected individuals: a randomized trial. *Lancet*. 2000;356(9240):1470–1474.

13. Mallory KF, Churchyard GJ, Kleinschmidt I, et al. The impact of HIV infection on recurrence of tuberculosis in South African gold miners. *Int J Tuberc Lung Dis*. 2000;4(5):455–462.

14. Sonnenberg P, Murray J, Glynn JR, et al. HIV-1 and recurrence, relapse, and reinfection of tuberculosis after cure: a cohort study in South African mineworkers. *Lancet*, 2001;358(9294):1687–1693.

15. Churchyard GJ, Fielding K, Charalambous S, et al. Efficacy of secondary isoniazid preventive therapy among HIV-infected Southern Africans: time to change policy? *AIDS*. 2003;17(14):2063–2070.

16. World Health Organization. Preventive therapy against tuberculosis in people living with HIV. *Wkly Epidemiol Rec*. 1999;74(46):385–398.

17. WHO/UNAIDS. Policy Statement on Preventive Therapy Against Tuberculosis in People Living with HIV. Report on a meeting held in Geneva 18–20 February 1998. WHO/TB/98.255.UNAIDS/98.34. 2003.

18. Aisu T, Raviglione MC, van Praag E, et al. Preventive chemotherapy for HIV-associated tuberculosis in Uganda: an operational assessment at a voluntary counseling and testing centre. *AIDS*. 1995;9(3):267–273.

19. Lugada ES, Watera C, Nakiyingi J, et al. Operational assessment of isoniazid prophylaxis in a community AIDS service organization in Uganda. *Int J Tuberc Lung Dis*. 2002;6(4):326–331.

20. Godfrey-Faussett P, Maher D, Mukadi YD, et al. How human immunodeficiency virus voluntary testing can contribute to tuberculosis control. *Bull World Health Organ*. 2002;80(12):939–945.

21. Williams BG, Dye C. Antiretroviral drugs for tuberculosis control in the era of HIV/AIDS. *Science*. 2003;301(5639): 1535–1537.

22. Bucher HC, Griffith LE, Guyatt GH, et al. Isoniazid prophylaxis for tuberculosis in HIV infection: a meta-analysis of randomized controlled trials. *AIDS*. 1999;13(4):501–507.

23. Johnson JL, Okwera A, Hom DL, et al. Duration of efficacy of treatment of latent tuberculosis infection in HIV-infected adults. *AIDS*. 2001;15(16):2137–2147.

24. Graham NM, Galai N, Nelson KE, et al. Effect of isoniazid chemoprophylaxis on HIV-related mycobacterial disease. *Arch Intern Med*. 1996;156(8):889–894.

25. de Pinho AM, Santoro-Lopes G, Harrison LH, et al. Chemoprophylaxis for tuberculosis and survival of HIV-infected patients in Brazil. *AIDS*. 2001;15(16):2129–2135.

26. Bass JB, Jr., Farer LS, Hopewell PC, et al. Treatment of tuberculosis and tuberculosis infection in adults and children. American Thoracic Society and the Centers for Disease Control and Prevention. *Am J Respir Crit Care Med*. 1994;149(5):1359–1374.

27. American Thoracic Society/Centers for Disease Control and Prevention. Targeted tuberculin testing and treatment of latent tuberculosis infection. *Am J Respir Crit Care Med*. 2000;161(4, Pt 2):S221–S247.

28. Kopanoff DE, Snider DE, Jr., Caras GJ. Isoniazid-related hepatitis: a U.S. Public Health Service cooperative surveillance study. *Am Rev Respir Dis*. 1978;117(6):991–1001.

29. Nolan CM, Goldberg SV, Buskin SE. Hepatotoxicity associated with isoniazid preventive therapy: a 7-year survey from a public health tuberculosis clinic. *JAMA*. 1999;281(11): 1014–1018.

30. Rose DN, Schechter CB, Silver AL. The age threshold for isoniazid chemoprophylaxis. A decision analysis for low-risk tuberculin reactors. *JAMA*. 1986;256(19):2709–2713.

31. Centers for Disease Control and Prevention. Update: adverse event data and revised American Thoracic Society/CDC recommendations against the use of rifampin and pyrazinamide for treatment of latent tuberculosis infection—United States, 2003. *MMWR Morb Mortal Wkly Rep*. 2003;52(31):735–739.

32. Jasmer RM, Saukkonen JJ, Blumberg HM, et al. Short-course rifampin and pyrazinamide compared with isoniazid for latent tuberculosis infection: a multicenter clinical trial. *Ann Intern Med*. 2002;137(8):640–647.

33. Stout JE, Engemann JJ, Cheng AC, et al. Safety of 2 months of rifampin and pyrazinamide for treatment of latent tuberculosis. *Am J Respir Crit Care Med*. 2003;167(6): 824–827.

34. Jasmer RM, Daley CL. Rifampin and pyrazinamide for treatment of latent tuberculosis infection: is it safe? *Am J Respir Crit Care Med*. 2003;167(6):809–810.

35. Dash LA, Comstock GW, Flynn JP. Isoniazid preventive therapy: Retrospect and prospect. *Am Rev Respir Dis*. 1980;121(6):1039–1044.

36. Villarino ME, Dooley SW Jr, Geiter LJ. Management of persons exposed to multidrug-resistant tuberculosis. *MMWR Morb Mortal Wkly Rep*. 1992;41(No. RR-11):59–71.

37. Fujiwara PI. Tide pools: what will be left after the tide has turned? *Int J Tuberc Lung Dis*. 2000;4(12 Suppl 2):S111–S116.

38. Goldberg SV, Wallace J, Jackson JC, et al. Cultural case management of latent tuberculosis infection. *Int J Tuberc Lung Dis*. 2004;8(1):76–82.

39. Coly A, Morisky D. Predicting completion of treatment among foreign-born adolescents treated for latent tuberculosis infection in Los Angeles. *Int J Tuberc Lung Dis*. 2004;8(6):703–710.

40. Jackson JC, Chaulk CP. Assessing culture, context, power differences, and psychological development when delivering health care to foreign-born adolescents. *Int J Tuberc Lung Dis*. 2004;8(6):687–688.

6

Chemotherapy of Tuberculosis

A. Edward Khan
Michael E. Kimerling

INTRODUCTION

The treatment of tuberculosis (TB) is increasingly complicated by issues related to patient comorbidities and drug-drug interactions. In this chapter, the principles in the chemotherapy for TB are discussed, and the most current treatment recommendations are noted.[1]

Organism Characteristics

Mycobacterium tuberculosis (MTB), the organism which causes TB, is a slow-growing organism that has the ability to enter a state of dormancy, which allows it to persist in the host despite adequate drug treatment. In a patient with TB, there are three populations of MTB organisms that need to be considered.[2] The first population is the actively growing extracellular organisms. Huge numbers of organisms can grow extracellularly in pulmonary cavities within liquefied caseous debris and it is in this population where drug resistance develops most readily. The second population consists of slow-growing or intermittently growing organisms, which are inside macrophages. There are fewer of these organisms, but the intracellular environment is acidic and many drugs are not active in these conditions. The third population is made up of slow growing organisms, which grow in solid caseous material. This environment is neutral in pH, but the penetration of drugs into this area may be compromised by a poor blood supply.

Rifampin (RIF) is the only drug that is bactericidal against all three populations. Isoniazid (INH), streptomycin, and the other aminoglycosides are bactericidal against extracellular organisms and INH also has bactericidal activity against intracellular organisms. Pyrazinamide (PZA) is bactericidal only against intracellular organisms and works well in an acidic pH. All the other first line TB drugs are bacteriostatic[3] (Table 6-1). Of the alternate drugs, the quinolones have the highest bactericidal activity against MTB.[4]

When formulating a therapeutic regimen for TB, it is important to remember that viable organisms from slow-growing or intermittently-growing populations may persist if drugs are not continued for an adequate period of time. Relapses of TB then occur after chemotherapy is stopped. Bactericidal drugs should be used whenever possible. Drug regimens with two or more bactericidal drugs, including rifampin, should be used when possible since this regimen results in the lowest relapse rates.

Development of Drug Resistance

MTB develops resistance to a drug by random genetic mutation. Resistance to individual drugs occurs infrequently and the rate of mutation has been estimated to be approximately one in 10^6–10^7 organisms.[5] Because the mutations are unlinked, the probability of a single MTB organism developing resistance to two drugs is the product of the drug-specific mutation rate. Since the number of bacilli in a patient with active TB rarely exceeds 10^9, two drugs given simultaneously make the likelihood of spontaneous drug resistance unlikely. Preventive therapy with a single drug is effective because the numbers of organisms in individuals with TB infection, in contrast to those with TB, are small.

Although some genetic mutations which are responsible for mycobacterial drug resistance have been identified, traditional culture methods in the presence of the TB drugs are still needed to confirm the diagnosis and determine MTB drug susceptibility. For many drugs, there are multiple genetic mutations that result in resistance[6]; thus molecular methods which identify mutations at a single site will not detect the other mutations which also confer resistance to that drug.

An important factor leading to drug resistance is adding a single drug to a failing regimen. If a single agent is given sequentially or intermittently in a patient with active disease, drug resistance can emerge. When the bacilli population is large and a single drug is given, the majority of organisms which are susceptible to the drug will be killed, but the small number of organisms which have spontaneously mutated will survive and multiply. Over time, selection of drug resistant organisms will occur. Drug-resistant TB can then be transmitted to contacts that may subsequently develop drug-resistant disease.

Adherence to Therapy

In order to prevent relapse and drug resistance, clinicians must prescribe an adequate regimen and insure that patients adhere to therapy. To insure adherence, directly observed therapy (DOT) should be considered in all cases. DOT means that a health care worker watches the patient swallow each dose of the prescribed antituberculosis drugs. This method of therapy should be considered for all

Table 6-1. Bactericidal First Line Drugs

Drug	Actively Growing Extracellular Organisms	Slowly Growing Intracellular Acid pH Organisms	Slowly Growing Neutral pH Extracellular Organisms
Rifampin	+	+	+
Isoniazid	+	+	−
Streptomycin	+	−	−
Pyrazinamide	−	+	−

patients because there is no way to predict which patients will adhere to treatment.[7] There are many factors that may influence patients' compliance, including the patients' social characteristics, personality, understanding of the illness, understanding of the treatment, patient-practitioner relationship, and the practitioner attitudes.[8]

When DOT is not possible, pills containing a combination of TB medicines can be used to prevent a patient from taking a single drug and thus help prevent the development of drug resistance. Rifamate is a fixed combination of INH (150 mg) and RIF (300 mg) and Rifater is a fixed combination of INH (50 mg), RIF (120 mg), and PZA (300 mg). Patients take multiple pills containing the combination medication in order to achieve the proper dosing. By taking an improper number of pills, combination medications can result in inadequate drug levels and therefore can still result in drug resistance.

Medication monitors are devices that can be used to follow patients who are self-administering their medications. Although these monitors will not prevent a patient from deliberate misuse of the medications, it can aid a patient who wishes to adhere to their therapeutic regimen succeed in doing so.

Drugs

There are five standard first-line drugs used in the treatment of TB. They are isoniazid (INH), rifampin (RIF), ethambutol (EMB), pyrazinamide (PZA), and streptomycin (SM). It is necessary to know the standard dosage and adverse reactions caused by these drugs (Tables 6-2 and 6-3). Patients should be evaluated at least monthly for adverse reactions to these drugs. It is helpful to have a baseline measurement of hepatic enzymes, bilirubin, complete blood count with platelets, and serum creatinine prior to initiating antituberculosis drugs. If ethambutol is included in the regimen, visual acuity, and red-green color perception should be evaluated. Hearing tests should be performed prior to initiation of streptomycin.

First-Line Drugs

Isoniazid

Isoniazid (INH) is metabolized by the liver and is bactericidal. It can be given orally, intramuscularly, or intravenously; is low in cost; and can be used in twice or three times weekly regimens. It readily penetrates body tissues as well as the central nervous system. The half-life of INH varies from one to three hours, depending on the acetylation status of the individual. The mechanism of action of INH is to inhibit a cell wall biosynthetic pathway, probably mycolic acid biosynthesis.[9] Therefore, it is only bactericidal for actively growing organisms. The usual daily dose of INH is 300 mg (or 5 mg/kg) while the twice or three times weekly dosage must be increased to 900 mg (or 15 mg/kg).

Toxicity

INH can cause fever, skin rash, hepatitis, and peripheral neuropathy. Fever and skin rash are the most common side-effects and when mild, may not require discontinuation of the drug. Premedication with diphenhydramine (Benadryl) and a nonsteroidal anti-inflammatory agent may provide symptomatic relief. Concomitant use of excess alcohol, acetaminophen or other potentially hepatotoxic drugs (including other TB medications) together with INH has been associated with an increased risk of hepatic toxicity.[10,11] Hepatotoxicity, with symptoms of nausea, vomiting, anorexia, fatigue, or jaundice requires the immediate discontinuation of the drug. Although elevated liver enzymes occur in approximately 10% of patients, only 1% of individuals develop clinical hepatitis.[12,13] The risk of hepatitis from isoniazid increases with age, alcohol consumption, and underlying liver disease such as chronic hepatitis infections.[14] Routine monitoring of liver function tests is not necessary, although patients should be interviewed at least monthly regarding symptoms of hepatitis. Patients should also

Table 6-2. Dosage Recommendations for the Treatment of TB in Children and Adults

Drugs	Daily Dosage		Twice-Weekly Dosage		Thrice-Weekly Dosage	
	Children*	Adults	Children	Adults	Children	Adults
Isoniazid	10–20 mg/kg Max 300 mg	5 mg/kg Max 300 mg	20–40 mg/kg Max 900 mg	15 mg/kg Max 900 mg	15 mg/kg Max 900 mg	15 mg/kg Max 900 mg
Rifampin	10–20 mg/kg Max 600 mg	10 mg/kg Max 600 mg	10–20 mg/kg Max 600 mg	10 mg/kg Max 600 mg	10 mg/kg Max 600 mg	10 mg/kg Max 600 mg
Pyrazinamide	15–30 mg/kg Max 2 gm	Table 2.A	50mg/kg Max 4 gm	Table 2.A	—	Table 2.A
Ethambutol[†]	15–20 mg/kg Max 1 gm	Table 2.B	50 mg/kg Max 4 gm	Table 2.B	—	Table 2.B
Streptomycin	20–40 mg/kg Max 1 gm	15 mg/kg Max 1 gm	25–30 mg/kg Max 1.5 gm	25–30 mg/kg Max 1.5 gm	25–30 mg/kg Max 1.5 gm	25–30 mg/kg Max 1.5 gm
Ofloxacin[‡]		600–800 mg qd		No data		No data
Levofloxacin[‡]		500–1000 mg qd		No data		No data
Moxifloxacin[‡]		400 mg qd		No data		No data
Gatifloxacin±		400 mg qd		No data		No data
Ciprofloxacin[‡]		750–1500 mg qd		No data		No data
Rifabutin		5 mg/kg 300 mg qd		5 mg/kg 300 mg qd	5 mg/kg 300 mg qd	5 mg/kg 300 mg qd

*Children are defined as being 14 years old or less.
[†]Ethambutol is not recommended for children who are too young to be monitored for changes in their vision (less than 8 years old). However, ethambutol should be considered for all children who have TB that is resistant to other drugs but susceptible to ethambutol.
[‡]Quinolones are not recommended for children or during pregnancy. Also, twice weekly dosages have not been defined, although in practice are usually given the same as a daily dose.

be educated about the side-effects of INH so that they can contact the health department immediately if symptoms develop. Peripheral neuritis secondary to vitamin B^6 deficiency has been noted and occurs most often in alcoholics, in persons with poor nutritional intake, and pregnant women. This can usually be prevented by the daily administration of pyridoxine (25 mg orally per day). It is advisable to give pyridoxine to patients with seizure disorders, as INH may precipitate seizures in these patients. INH rarely causes an antibuse effect when taken concurrently with alcohol. Less common side effects include hematological reactions such as agranulocytosis, thrombocytopenia, and anemia. Vasculitis and arthritis may occur, but these side-effects reverse when the drug is discontinued. Dizziness, insomnia, nervousness, mood changes, and stupor occur rarely.

Rifampin

Rifampin (RIF) is bactericidal and metabolized by the liver. RIF is an extremely potent antituberculosis agent and can be given orally or intravenously. The half-life of RIF varies from 1.5–5 hours. RIF inhibits the DNA-dependent RNA polymerase of MTB[15] and is able to interfere with RNA synthesis even when the organism has minimal metabolic activity. This allows it to be effective against the slowly growing or intermittently growing organisms.[3] RIF penetrates tissues and the central nervous system and is extremely effective in killing intracellular organisms. It colors the body fluids orange and may permanently discolor soft contact lens. The usual daily dose of RIF is 600 mg (or 10 mg/kg). Unlike the other first-line agents, RIF requires no adjustment of the dosage when administered twice or three times weekly.

Table 6-3. Adverse Reactions and Recommended Monitoring of Antituberculosis Medication

Drug	Common Adverse Reactions	Recommended Regular Monitoring
Isoniazid	Liver function test (LFT) elevations, usually asymptomatic; clinical hepatitis less common; peripheral neuropathy; headache; mood and sleep disturbances	Liver function tests at baseline, hold INH, and repeat if symptoms occur; Pyridoxine to prevent neuropathy in high risk patients
Rifampin	Orange discoloration of the urine, tears, and other body fluids; many significant drug interactions; hepatitis; flu-like illness occasionally with cytopenias	Liver function as for INH; review all other meds when starting/stopping RIF; discontinue and do not rechallenge if cytopenias develop
Pyrazinamide	Gastrointestinal upset; polyarthralgia; abnormal liver function tests; hepatitis; rash; gout	Liver function tests as for INH; uric acid levels should be checked only in the setting of acute gout symptoms or renal failure
Ethambutol	Optic nerve damage	Monthly testing of visual acuity and color discrimination
Streptomycin	Otovestibular nerve toxicity; nephrotoxicity	Audiograms; renal function tests monthly
Quinolones	GI upset is most common; hypersensitivity and mild central nervous system reactions have been reported; QT-interval prolongation; arthropathy; LFT elevation can occur	Follow EKG for QT-interval in patients at risk
Rifabutin	Uveitis (ocular pain and blurry vision); GI upset, neutropenia, thrombocytopenia, Arthralgia	Visual checks; concomitant use of clarithromycin, azole antifungals increase toxicity risk

Toxicity

Rifampin is usually well tolerated, but as with the other antituberculosis medications, gastrointestinal upset, fever, and rash can occur. Hepatotoxicity can occur rarely and in contrast to INH, when hepatitis occurs, bilirubin elevations with jaundice are more common. When large doses are used intermittently, hypersensitivity reactions may result. Renal failure, hemolytic anemia, thrombocytopenia, and a flu-like syndrome have been described. This is less likely when RIF is used at lower (standard) doses (600 mg). Eosinophilia, light-chain proteinuria, and nervous system symptoms have been seen rarely. RIF interacts with many medications including methadone, protease inhibitors, and non-nucleoside reverse transcriptase inhibitors used to treat HIV infection, cyclosporine, macrolide antibiotics, warfarin, and oral contraceptives. Rifampin profoundly lowers azole antifungal drugs (fluconazole, itraconazole)

making them unreliable to treat serious fungal infections (e.g., cryptococcal meningitis).[16]

The major difficulty associated with rifampin use is the management of these interactions. By upregulating the cytochrome P-450 oxidase system, metabolism of many drugs, and endogenous compounds (e.g., steroids and hormones) is accelerated. This often requires dose adjustment of the other drug, both at the initiation of rifampin therapy as well as upon its completion. When the effect on the other drug is too great, rifabutin may be substituted as it has less effect on P-450 induction.[17,18]

Pyrazinamide

Pyrazinamide (PZA) is bactericidal only to intracellular organisms in an acidic environment.[19] It is uniquely effective in eliminating potential persisters and is used during the first

2 months of chemotherapy to reduce the total length of therapy. Resistance develops rapidly if it is used alone and it should be used with at least one and preferably two other bactericidal agents. Pyrazinamide can be given orally and it is usually well absorbed. Peak concentrations are reached 2 hours after ingestion and the half-life is longer than INH and RIF at 9–10 hours. PZA is cleared through the kidneys. The usual daily dose of PZA is approximately 1.5 g (20 to 30 mg/kg) with a maximum dose of 2 gm. Dosage is increased when PZA is given twice or three times weekly with a maximum dose of 4 gm (Table 6-4.A).

Toxicity

The most important toxic effect of PZA is hepatitis. There is no marked increase in the incidence of hepatotoxicity when PZA is added to INH and RIF in short-course therapy regimens.[20] However, when hepatic toxicity occurs, the liver enzymes are elevated longer after discontinuing the medication than with INH or RIF. In patients with known hepatic dysfunction, the use of PZA should be considered carefully. If hepatotoxicity develops while on therapy, PZA should be discontinued. Gastrointestinal upset is common, particularly with elderly patients as are elevated uric acid levels, although not predictive of development of gout. Acute episodes of gout develop infrequently. Occasionally, patients will complain of arthralgias of peripheral joints, which usually respond to nonsteroidal anti-inflammatory agents without necessitating discontinuation of PZA. Fever and rash also occur rarely.

Ethambutol

Ethambutol (EMB) is only bacteriostatic, but despite this, EMB has been an effective agent in the treatment of TB.[21] Its mechanism of action is not completely understood, but inhibition of glucose incorporation into cell wall components of MTB is suggested by metabolic labeling experiments.[22] Although it is not a good agent to use with PZA alone, it can be coupled with INH and RIF. When used with these other agents, its major function is to prevent emergence of drug resistance. EMB can be given orally, and peak plasma concentrations are achieved two to four hours after ingestion. The half-life is approximately four hours. It is excreted through the kidneys and therefore the dosage must be reduced in patients with renal failure. The usual daily dose of EMB is 15–20 mg/kg. EMB, when given 2 or 3 times a week, requires an increased dosage (Table 6-4.B).

Toxicity

EMB can cause optic neuritis and its use is discouraged in children unable to be monitored for changes in vision. The risk for eye toxicity increases when the daily dose is raised above 15 mg/kg. A risk factor for the development of optic neuritis is renal insufficiency. Symptoms include blurry vision and central scotomata. The earliest effect is usually the loss of the ability to perceive the color green. Under most circumstances, the symptoms reverse when the drug is discontinued. EMB can also cause an increased serum concentration of uric acid.[23]

Streptomycin

Streptomycin (SM), an aminoglycoside, disrupts bacterial protein synthesis, but is bactericidal against only actively growing extracellular organisms. It must be given parenterally and peak concentrations are reached by 1 hour after administration. SM has good tissue penetration, but enters the cerebrospinal fluid only if there is meningeal inflammation. It is cleared through the kidneys and should be used with caution in patients with renal insufficiency. The usual daily dose is 0.75 to 1.0 g (or 10–15 mg/kg). If it is necessary to give SM in elderly patients

Table 6-4.A PZA Table—Suggested Pyrazinamide doses, Using Whole Tablets, for Adults Weighing 40–90 Kilograms

	Weight (kg)*		
	40–55	**56–75**	**76–90**
Daily, mg (mg/kg)	1,000 (18.2–25.0)	1,500 (20.0–26.8)	2,000[†](22.2–26.3)
Thrice weekly, mg (mg/kg)	1,500 (27.3–37.5)	2,500 (33.3–44.6)	3,000[†](33.3–39.5)
Twice weekly, mg (mg/kg)	2,000 (36.4–50.0)	3,000 (40.0–53.6)	4,000[†](44.4–52.6)

*Based on estimated lean body weight.
†Maximum dose regardless of weight.

Table 6-4.B EMB Table—Suggested Ethambutol doses, Using whole Tablets, for Adults Weighing 40–90 Kilograms

	Weight (kg)[*]		
	40–55	**56–75**	**76–90**
Daily, mg (mg/kg)	800 (14.5–20.0)	1,200 (16.0–21.4)	1,600[†](17.8–21.1)
Thrice weekly, mg (mg/kg)	1,200 (21.8–30.0)	2,000 (26.7–35.7)	2,400[†](26.7–31.6)
Twice weekly, mg (mg/kg)	2,000 (36.4–50.0)	2,800 (37.3–50.0)	4,000[†](44.4–52.6)

[*]Based on estimated lean body weight.
[†]Maximum dose regardless of weight.

or those with renal dysfunction, reduce the dose. SM can be given twice or three times weekly, with a maximum single dose of 1.5 g.

Toxicity

Approximately 10% of patients receiving SM will have some toxicity.[24] Hypersensitivity reactions which have been reported include skin rash, eosinophilia, fever, blood dyscrasia, angioedema, exfoliative dermatitis, and anaphylaxis. Eosinophilia may occur in as many as 5% of patients receiving the drug over a long period of time.

The most common toxic effect of SM is damage to the eighth cranial nerve. Usually the vestibular component is involved initially with dizziness or unsteadiness being the first symptom. Nephrotoxicity can also occur, but this is less common than with the other aminoglycosides, amikacin, kanamycin, and capreomycin. The risk is increased in patients with preexisting renal disease or when other nephrotoxic agents are used concurrently. The risks of ototoxicity and nephrototoxicity are related to both cumulative dose and serum concentration. A total dose of more than 120 grams should not be given unless no other therapeutic option is available.

A rare effect of SM is blockade at the neuromuscular junction. This presents a problem especially in patients with myasthenia gravis or in those taking curare-like medications. Dizziness and circumoral paresthesias are not unusual immediately after injection but they cause no harm generally.

Alternate Drugs which may be used in First-Line Regimens

For a complete discussion of alternate drugs used for MDR-TB therapy, see Chap. 7.

Rifabutin

Rifabutin is structurally similar to rifampin, and like rifampin inhibits the DNA-dependent RNA polymerase in bacteria. However, there are important pharmacokinetic differences between the two drugs.[18] Rifabutin is more lipid soluble than rifampin, which results in more extensive tissue uptake and longer half-life (45 hours). Rifabutin and rifampin are equally active against MTB. Rifabutin has less effect on the pharmacokinetics of many antiretroviral drugs, and therefore can be used in conjunction with some protease inhibitors[18] and the non-nucleoside reverse transcriptase inhibitor nevirapine. Similarly, rifabutin's effect on cyclosporine levels is less than that seen in rifampin.[25] Concurrent administration of fluconazole increases the plasma levels of rifabutin and increases the toxicity of rifabutin.[26] The daily dose of rifabutin is 300 mg/day.

Toxicity

Rifabutin may cause polyarthralgias, arthritis, or skin hyperpigmentation. Leukopenia is also common and may be severe. Changing to twice or three times weekly dosing may minimize this risk. When rifabutin is given in conjunction with clarithromycin for treatment of nontuberculous mycobacterial infections, uveitis has been reported.[27]

Aminoglycosides other than Streptomycin

Kanamycin, amikacin, capreomycin, or viomycin may be used in place of streptomycin when necessary. MTB strains that are resistant to SM may be susceptible to these other agents; however, if a strain is resistant to kanamycin, it will also be resistant to amikacin. The aminoglycosides are bactericidal by disrupting bacterial protein synthesis. They are only available in the parenteral form. The toxicities of these agents are similar to those of streptomycin.

Quinolones

The quinolones (moxifloxacin, gatifloxacin, levofloxacin, ofloxacin, and ciprofloxacin) disrupt the bacterial chromosome by inhibiting the supercoiling action of DNA gyrase.[28] These drugs are given orally or intravenously. Several studies using animal models have shown that the 8-methoxy-substituted fluoroquinolones, moxifloxacin and gatifloxacin, to be the most active members of this class against TB,[29,30] although ofloxacin and levofloxacin are also commonly used.[31] Quinolones have been especially valuable in the successful treatment of MDR-TB, and susceptibility to quinolones has been an independent predictor of cure of these patients.[32]

For standard dosing of these agents, see Table 6-2. Side effects include abdominal discomfort, insomnia, photosensitivity, and cardiotoxicity (QT interval prolongation).[33] Their use is discouraged in children and pregnancy because of possible arthropathy. The quinolones should not be ingested with dairy products or antacids since there is binding to calcium/magnesium and they are then not well absorbed.

Long-acting rifamycins

Rifapentine

The role and dosing of Rifapentine in TB therapy today remains unsettled and therefore is not yet widely utilized. Rifapentine is a rifamycin derivative, which has a similar microbiologic profile to rifampin. Rifapentine is taken orally and has a longer half-life than rifampin (approximately 15 hours)[34] and peak concentrations are achieved 8 hours after ingestion. This characteristic prompted investigation into its use in a once weekly regimen together with isoniazid during the continuation phase. This was found to be effective, but the recommendation for use limited to patients who are HIV-negative and without initial cavitary disease on chest radiography. Patient characteristics found to be independently associated with increased risk of failure/relapse were: sputum culture positive at two months; cavitation of chest radiograph; being underweight; bilateral pulmonary involvement; and being a non-Hispanic White person.[35] However among patients without cavitation, failure/relapse rates did not differ between the standard, twice-weekly RIF-INH continuation phase regimen compared with the once-weekly Rifapentine-INH group. Further, relapse, and failure rates were also associated with

being a rapid acetylator of INH (as determined by *NAT*-2 genotype assay) and low serum INH levels.[36] Studies are currently underway to clarify Rifapentine's role, possibly utilizing a higher dose or additional isoniazid.

Concerning HIV-infected TB patients, in a second study arm that was terminated early, acquired rifampin mono-resistant disease was often noted among HIV-seropositive patients treated with the once-weekly (Rifapentine) continuation phase[37]; acquired resistance, however, was not noted among the HIV-negative patients.

Rifapentine is not extensively metabolized and is predominately excreted in the bile intact. Toxicity from rifapentine is similar to that of rifampin.

Drug Regimens

Treatment of TB must be continued for at least 6 months and with some drug regimens, treatment lasts much longer. Tuberculosis must also be treated with at least two drugs to which the organism is susceptible to prevent the emergence of drug resistance. In order to prevent relapse and drug resistance, clinicians must prescribe an adequate regimen and insure that patients adhere to therapy.

Treatment Regimens

The "short course" or 6-month (26 weeks) regimen is preferred for the treatment of newly diagnosed, never-treated TB. This regimen consists of an initial 2-month (8 weeks) phase of treatment with INH, RIF, and PZA followed by a 4-month (18 weeks) continuation phase with INH and RIF. EMB or SM should be included in the initial phase until the results of drug susceptibility studies are available, confirming MTB organism susceptibility to INH and RIF. Normally, EMB is the preferred fourth drug used. All treatment of patients with TB must be done in conjunction with the local public health department. The use of intermittent regimens among HIV-infected is based on the CD4 count as discussed below.

1. INH, RIF, PZA, (EMB or SM) are administered daily (5–7 days per week) for 8 weeks followed by twice weekly doses of INH and RIF for an additional 18 weeks (WHO recommends thrice weekly dosing during the continuation phase);

2. INH, RIF, PZA, (EMB or SM) are administered daily (5–7 days per week) for 2 weeks followed by these four drugs given twice weekly for an additional 6 weeks. INH and RIF are then given twice weekly for the remaining 18 weeks; or

3. INH, RIF, PZA, (EMB or SM) are administered three times a week for 8 weeks (24 doses), followed by INH and RIF three times a week for 18 weeks (54 doses).

4. INH, RIF, EMB daily (5–7 days per week) for 8 weeks, followed by INH and RIF twice weekly for 31 weeks. This regimen is recommended whenever PZA cannot be used or tolerated. EMB is used until drug susceptibility testing confirms INH and RIF susceptibility.

It is important to note that the duration of therapy should be counted as the actual number of doses of medications the patient receives (which will vary depending on the frequency of administration, e.g., daily, twice or thrice-weekly) and not simply the time on therapy. This ensures that any missed doses are completed. Dosages of the medications for daily or intermittent therapy regimens are shown in Table 6-2. Note that twice and thrice-weekly doses are not established for the quinolones. Again, EMB or SM should be added to the regimen initially until the susceptibility of the MTB organism is known. *Extension of the continuation phase by an additional 3 months is now recommended for patients with cavitation and a sputum culture positive at the end of month 2 of therapy.*

Patients resistant or intolerant to INH can be treated with RIF and EMB for 12 months, which can be shortened to 9 months if PZA is used for the first two months. Alternatively, RIF, EMB, and PZA can be used for 6 months total, if PZA can be tolerated for the entire 6 months.[1,38]

Patients found to be resistant to one or more antituberculosis medications should be referred to a specialist in TB therapy for treatment. Treatment of drug-resistant TB will be discussed in Chap. 7.

Drug Interactions

Drugs that increase the microsomal enzyme activity in the liver will prolong the half-life of INH.[39] INH may also inhibit the hepatic metabolism of other drugs (Table 6-5). RIF induces the cytochrome P-450 system and thereby can reduce the effectiveness of many agents

Table 6-5. Drug Interactions

Drugs	Interactions with other Medications and other Cautions
Isoniazid	Decreases clearance of phenytoin, carbamazepine, and anticoagulants.
	Daily ingestion of alcohol or other hepatotoxic drugs may potentiate toxicity i.e., methotrexate, acetaminophen, and cholesterol lowering agents.
Rifampin	Decreases activity of: anticoagulants, methadone, oral hypoglycemics, digoxin, quinidine, disopyramide, dapsone, corticosteroids, cyclosporine, oral contraceptives, narcotics, analgesics, azathioprine, haloperidol, estrogen, most protease inhibitors and non-nucleoside reverse transcriptase inhibitors (NNRTIs), barbiturates, diazepam, verapamil, beta-adrenergic blockers, clofibrate, progestins, disopyramide, mexiletine, theophylline, chloramphenicol, and anticonvulsants.
	Azoles should be avoided when any rifamycins are used. Azoles will increase Rifabutin to toxic levels and rifamycins will lower azole levels. Additionally, Ketoconazole can lower rifampin levels by 40–50%.
Pyrazinamide	Contraindicated during acute episode of gout; caution with liver dysfunction.
	Management of diabetes mellitus may be more difficult. Interferes with Ketostix and Acetest producing a brown color.
Ethambutol	Do not use if patients has optic neuritis.
Streptomycin	Caution should be used in renal dysfunction and/or with use of other nephrotoxic agents.
	Contains metabisulfite, which may cause asthmatic exacerbations.
Quinolones	Ciprofloxacin, but not ofloxacin, prolongs the half-life of theophylline which may lead to theophylline toxicity.
	Antacids containing aluminum hydroxide or magnesium hydroxide or iron supplements substantially reduce absorption.
Rifabutin	Fluconazole and clarithromycin increases rifabutin levels (for other azole interactions, see Rifampin above).
	Effects on protease inhibitors and cyclosporine are less than rifampin.

(Table 6-4).[40] The quinolones may inhibit the cytochrome P-450 system.[41]

Drug Intolerance

Often, specific antituberculosis medications cannot be used, not because the MTB organism is resistant, but because the patient cannot tolerate the drug. Toxicities of these medications can be mild or life-threatening. All patients receiving antituberculosis therapy must be educated as to the symptoms of serious toxicities as well as insignificant changes, such as discoloration of body fluids with the use of rifampin.

If serious side effects occur, such as symptomatic hepatitis (or liver aminotransferases elevations exceeding five times the normal), hematologic derangements, or neuropathy, the antituberculosis medications must be stopped immediately. Hepatotoxicity can result from many drugs and it is often unclear which is causing the liver toxicity. Of the first-line drugs, INH, RIF, and PZA can result in hepatitis with liver enzyme elevations. Liver enzyme tests should be obtained immediately after discontinuing the medications. If the bilirubin is elevated, this may be a clue that RIF is causing the problem. Normally, the liver aminotransferases return to baseline levels within seven days if the toxicity is related to INH[42] while they tend to remain elevated longer with RIF and PZA. Once liver enzymes have returned to baseline levels, a single drug should be given for one to two doses. If this is tolerated, another drug can be added back to the regimen. The most likely offending agent should be held until last. Once the offending drug is identified, it should be substituted with another agent and the duration of therapy should be adjusted as necessary.

Alternate Routes of Drug Administration

Patients with TB who cannot take medication by mouth are limited in the antituberculosis drugs available to treat them. Only INH, RIF, the aminoglycosides and the quinolones (moxifloxacin, gatifloxacin, levofloxacin, ofloxacin, and ciprofloxacin) are available in parenteral form. All the oral forms of antituberculosis medications can be given through nasogastric or other types of feeding tubes. Suspensions can be made up for the medications to make administration easier.

Case Study

L.R. is a 38 year old woman, foreign-born, admitted to the hospital with fever, night sweats, weight loss, and increasing dyspnea of several weeks duration. A CXR reveals extensive bilateral airspace disease without cavitation, and although multiple sputum specimens were smear negative for acid-fast bacilli (AFB), bronchoscopy washings were AFB-positive, with positive cultures for M. tuberculosis. Upon testing, she was found to be HIV-positive with a CD4 count of seven. Multiple drug therapy with INH, rifampin, pyrazinamide, and ethambutol were begun, however her course was complicated by profound watery diarrhea, exacerbated by the administration of TB medications, to the extent that intact tablets appeared in the stool. No specific intestinal pathogen was identified. In view of the immediate life threatening presentation of her TB and total malabsorption of oral medications, she was given an entirely parenteral regimen of moxifloxacin 400 mg IV once daily, rifampin 600 mg IV once daily, isoniazid (Nydrazid) 300 mg IM (intramuscularly) once daily, and streptomycin 1000 mg IV once daily. Over the next 2–3 weeks, her overall condition stabilized, the diarrhea improved, and standard oral TB medications were sequentially introduced without incident.

This case illustrates the use of TB medications in an ICU setting, or when oral administration is difficult due to altered mental status or impaired gastrointestinal function, such as in this case. In these situations, a completely parenteral regimen may be used until the patient can tolerate a standard oral regimen. Aminoglycosides, particularly streptomycin, amikacin, kanamycin as well as the related polypeptide antibiotic capreomycin are all given parenterally. Rifampin is available IV, as are several quinolones used in the treatment of TB (moxifloxacin, gatifloxacin, levofloxacin, ofloxacin, and ciprofloxacin). Isoniazid can also be obtained in an intramuscular (Nydrazid). Pyrazinamide and ethambutol are only available in oral formulations.

Principles governing selection of a parenteral regimen are similar as for an oral regimen, namely, that at least two or more effective drugs are included and that adequate dosing and monitoring of therapy and toxicity are followed. In most instances, the use of parenteral agents will be temporary, and a switch to oral medications can be made when the initial problems improve.

Interruption of Therapy

Occasionally, patients have treatment of their TB interrupted because of illness or patient nonadherence. In general, if it is certain that the patient was taking all the TB medications correctly prior to the interruption (e.g., by DOT), the previous drug regimen can be reinstituted without adding two new drugs. If however, there is any question of improper administration of antituberculosis medications, two new drugs to which the organism is susceptible should be added to the original regimen. As a general rule, if the patient cannot complete the required number of doses for a 6-month regimen within a 9-month period, it is necessary to reevaluate the patient for either treatment extension or re-starting a full course.[1] If the patient remains MTB culture positive after the interruption of therapy, a susceptibility test should be repeated on the MTB organisms and drug therapy adjusted once these results are available.

Monitoring Drug Levels

If adequate blood levels of antituberculosis medications are not achieved, patients are more likely to fail TB therapy or relapse with TB. MTB organisms may acquire drug resistance while a patient is on directly observed therapy (DOT).[43] Obtaining serum levels of antituberculosis drugs at one and two hours after ingestion may prove to be useful for adjusting medication dosing. Situations where drug level monitoring should be considered include coadministration of medications that interfere with the absorption or metabolism of TB drugs, failure to respond to TB drugs as expected, or relapse with TB after adequate therapy.

Patients with TB who fail to convert their sputum culture to negative by the end of month 2 should be evaluated as to their reason(s) for delayed response. Drug resistance and poor adherence to medication can be evaluated by drug susceptibility testing and history of DOT, respectively. If the patient's isolate is pansensitive and DOT is assured, then there is a high likelihood of low serum drug levels, which may be the result of impaired absorption, accelerated metabolism or both. Low levels of rifampin and/or isoniazid may result in an impaired response to treatment, and this can be addressed by increasing the dose of the given drug(s). Effective serum ranges are established for the major TB drugs, and they differ depending on daily versus intermittent therapy (Table 6-6). Although a two hour post-administration peak concentration is usually the most informative, there are occasional patients who peak *early* and will only be accurately assessed by a one hour level.

Samples are drawn and shipped on ice to a reference laboratory equipped to do TB drug levels (e.g., National Jewish Hospital, Denver, CO). The finding of a low level should prompt an increase in dosage and repeat levels to confirm adequate dosing. Our experience has been that most delayed converters who are fully sensitive and are getting DOT have low rifampin levels and may require dosage increments one or more times to achieve target serum concentrations. Excessive dose increments should be cautioned against as rifampin toxicity causing acute renal failure has occurred despite apparently *safe* levels with higher dosages.

SPECIAL SITUATIONS

Drug Resistant Tuberculosis

Drug-resistant organisms have been noted to occur at a greater frequency under the following circumstances:

1. Failure to convert sputum culture within 2 months;
2. History of previous treatment (early relapse or treatment failure as defined by a positive culture after 4 months of therapy);
3. Exposure to known drug-resistant TB; and
4. Tuberculosis exposure in a geographical area where drug-resistant disease is prevalent.

Refer to Chap. 7 for specific recommendations regarding treatment of multidrug resistant TB.

Extrapulmonary Tuberculosis

In general, treatment of extrapulmonary TB is the same as treatment of pulmonary TB. However, infants and children with bone and joint disease or central nervous system disease should receive 9–12 months of therapy.[1] It is often more difficult to obtain tissue specimens for smear and culture from patients with extrapulmonary disease. Surgery may be necessary to obtain diagnostic specimens in some circumstances such as in pericardial or spinal TB.

Corticosteroids

The role of corticosteroids in the treatment of TB is controversial. Inflammation associated with TB may respond to steroid therapy, which may alter outcomes in meningitis or pericarditis.[44,45] The adjunctive use of corticosteroids in disseminated disease has not been studied prospectively. Corticosteroids do not appear to alter stenosis as a result of endobronchial TB.[46] Adrenal insufficiency which may result from adrenal involvement with TB requires corticosteroid supplementation.

Immune Deficiency States

Patients with chronic renal insufficiency, malnutrition, hematologic and reticuloendothelial malignancies, HIV infection,[18] and those taking immunosuppresive agents, including Tumor Necrosis Factor (TNF)-alpha blockers[47,48] are all at increased risk for developing TB if infected.

Table 6-6. Antituberculosis Medications Therapeutic Levels

Medication	Number of Hours Following Dose	Dose	Therapeutic Level
Ethambutol	2–3 hours	15–25 mg/kg (daily)	2–6 mcg/mL
		50 mg/kg (twice weekly)	8–12 ug/mL
Isoniazid	1 and 2 hours (if the sample was drawn at 2 hours post dose, and the concentration is within 1 ug/mL of the daily range or within 3 ug/mL of the twice weekly range, no dosage change is needed)	Daily	3–6 mcg/mL
Isoniazid		Twice weekly	9–15 mcg/mL
Ofloxacin	2 hours	800 mg	8–12 mcg/mL
Rifampin	1 and 2 hours	600 mg	8–24 mcg/mL
p-Aminosalicylic acid	5–7 hours		10–60 mcg/mL
Streptomycin	1 hour		35–45 mcg/mL
Ethionamide	2 and 6 hours		1–5 mcg/mL

If disease develops, these patients with cell-mediated defects have an increased risk of extrapulmonary and disseminated TB.[49,50]

Most patients with AIDS and TB respond to standard antituberculosis chemotherapy although there is a significantly higher mortality risk while on therapy as well as an increased relapse rate after completion, particularly when rifampin is not included in the drug regimen.[51] A higher risk of treatment failure/relapse has been observed in HIV/AIDS patients receiving twice-weekly treatment during the continuation phase, often with acquired rifampin mono-resistant disease.[1,18] Acquired resistance was associated with advanced AIDS and very low CD4 counts, and as a result, *any HIV+ patient being treated for TB should receive either daily or three-times weekly therapy during the entire therapy unless they have a documented recent CD4 count equal to or greater than 100.*

Some experts recommend routine monitoring of drug levels in all HIV-TB patients due to the frequency of enteropathic conditions which may lead to drug malabsorption, but this is not always practical. A history of recurrent or chronic diarrhea is a risk factor for malabsorption of TB drugs. Because rifampin interferes with many of the antiretroviral agents, regimens which do not utilize rifampin are becoming more prevalent in this population. In circumstances where protease inhibitors (PI's) are being used to control the viral load of HIV, rifabutin may be a substitute for rifampin in the treatment regimens. Alternatively, some PI's may be used with rifampin if the PI dose is increased.[18] Alternatively, PI's may be withheld until patients are adequately treated with a rifampin-containing drug regimen. Rifampin may be used together with the nonnucleoside reverse transcriptase inhibitor efavirenz although it is recommended to increase the efavirenz dose from 600–800 mg daily. Nevirapine cannot reliably be used with rifampin, although some have supported coadministration possibly with an increased nevirapine dose.[52,53] Rifabutin use without any dose adjustments is an acceptable alternative. Due to these complex drug interactions and other nuances of TB and HIV coinfection, these patients should be comanaged by specialists in both diseases. See Chap. 19 for additional information.

Patients with TB who are immunosuppressed after receiving an organ transplant also respond to standard anti-tuberculosis chemotherapy. However, cyclosporine, which is often used as an immunosuppressive agent in these patients, also interferes with rifampin metabolism. Rifampin causes cyclosporine levels to be low and thus increases the likelihood of transplant rejection. Twice or thrice weekly regimens are especially difficult when trying to control both the cyclosporine and rifampin levels. As with protease inhibitors, rifabutin has less effect on cyclosporine than rifampin, and a daily regimen containing rifabutin may be optimal in treating TB in this patient population. Monitoring the levels of cyclosporine and rifabutin will help optimize drug therapy.

Treatment in Children (see Chapter 29)

The basic principles of TB treatment apply to children as well as adults. Because it may be difficult to monitor ocular toxicity from ethambutol in very young children, this drug should be avoided if possible. The quinolones may affect cartilage development and should be used in growing children only when necessary. Infants are more likely to have disseminated TB, and vigorous treatment should be started immediately, once the diagnosis is suspected. An asymptomatic neonate born to a mother with active TB should be given a full course of INH. Given the unreliability of the TB skin test below the age of six months, it is very difficult to exclude latent infection. If the chest radiograph shows hilar adenopathy or other abnormalities, the child should be treated for active disease with multiple drugs.[1]

Pregnancy and Lactation

Pregnancy does not preclude the adequate treatment of TB. The initial regimen should include INH and RIF, with EMB added when INH resistance is possible.[54] PZA has been used worldwide without apparent problems in pregnancy, but PZA is not FDA approved for use during pregnancy in the United States. Streptomycin and other aminoglycosides may cause high frequency hearing loss in the fetus and should not be used. The quinolones may interfere with cartilage development. Because of possible nutritional deficiency, pyridoxine is recommended when INH is given. Breast feeding should not be discouraged in mothers receiving antituberculosis medications.

Renal Dysfunction

Patients with renal disease should not be given nephrotoxic drugs, such as the aminoglycosides, unless absolutely necessary. Ethambutol, in reduced dosages, can be used with caution. If these drugs are used, serum levels should be monitored. The dosage and frequency of the quinolones must also be adjusted when renal insufficiency is present (Table 6-7). In patients undergoing hemodialysis, medications may be given after the procedure to avoid removal of the drugs. INH, RIF, and EMB are not appreciably affected by hemodialysis whereas PZA is significantly cleared and should only be given after dialysis. It is generally recommended to treat hemodialysis patients with TB using a thrice-weekly regimen with the drugs given following each dialysis treatment (Table 6-7).[1,55] The clearance of drugs by peritoneal dialysis is unknown.

Liver Dysfunction

If a patient has hepatic failure, they should be treated with drugs that are excreted by the kidneys when possible. INH, RIF (including the rifamycin derivatives), PZA, and the quinolones are all potentially hepatotoxic. Because avoidance of all of these drugs would result in inadequate therapy, a regimen of SM and EMB coupled with one hepatotoxic agent such as INH or RIF should be tried.

Table 6-7. Dosage of Medications Used in Renal Insufficiency

Dosage recommendations for adult* patients with reduced renal function and for adult patients receiving hemodialysis (all dosage is post dialysis treatment)

Drug	Change in Frequency?	Recommended Dose and Frequency for Patients with Creatinine Clearance <30 mL/min or for Patients Receiving Hemodialysis
Isoniazid	No change	300 mg once daily, or 900 mg three times per week
Rifampin	No change	600 mg once daily, or 600 mg three times per week
Pyrazinamide	Yes	25–35 mg/kg per dose three times per week (not daily)
Ethambutol	Yes	15–25 mg/kg per dose three times per week (not daily)
Levofloxacin	Yes	750–1,000 mg per dose three times per week (not daily)
Gatifloxacin	Yes	300–400 mg per dose three times per week (not daily)
Moxifloxacin	Yes	300–400 mg per dose three times per week (not daily)
Ofloxacin	Yes	600–800 mg per dose three times per week (not daily)
Streptomycin	Yes	12–15 mg/kg/dose two or three times per week (not daily)
Capreomycin	Yes	12–15 mg/kg/dose two or three times per week (not daily)
Kanamycin	Yes	12–15 mg/kg/dose two or three times per week (not daily)
Amikacin	Yes	12–15 mg/kg/dose two or three times per week (not daily)

*15 years of age or older

Source: Adapted from American Thoracic Society/Centers for Disease Control and Prevention/Infectious Diseases Society of America. Treatment of tuberculosis. *Am J Respir Crit Care Med.* 2003;167:603–662.[1]

Often mild hepatic dysfunction is present and should not influence the choice of drugs, but will require frequent monitoring of symptoms of hepatotoxicity and levels of liver enzymes throughout therapy.[56]

Malabsorptive States

Patients who have undergone gastrectomy absorb the oral antituberculosis medications well. These medications are absorbed primarily in the small intestine. Rifampin is absorbed in the jejunum; therefore, jejunal resection will interfere with achieving adequate drug levels. Colonic resection does not appear to affect absorption of any of these medications. In patients who have had large portions of their small bowel resected, monitoring drug levels will ensure adequate treatment for TB. A history of recurrent or chronic diarrhea identifies those patients at potential risk of TB drug malabsorption.

REFERENCES

1. American Thoracic Society/Centers for Disease Control and Prevention/Infectious Diseases Society of America. Treatment of tuberculosis. *Am J Respir Crit Care Med.* 2003;167: 603–662.
2. Grosset J. Bacteriologic basis of short-course chemotherapy for tuberculosis. *Clin. Chest Med.* 1980;1:231–243.
3. Mitchison D. Basic Mechanisms of Chemotherapy. *Chest.* 1979;76 Supplement:771–781.
4. Tsukamura M. In vitro antituberculosis activity of a new antibacterial substance ofloxacin (DL8280). *Am J Respir Dis.* 1985;131:349–351.
5. Mitchison D. Drug resistance in mycobacteria. *Br Med Bull.* 1984;40:84–90.
6. Riska P., Jacobs R., Alland D. Molecular determinants of drug resistance in tuberculosis. *Int J Tuberc Lung Dis.* 2000;4:S4–S10.
7. Sbarbaro J. The patient-physician relationship: compliance revisited. *Ann Allergy.* 1990;64:325–332.
8. Komaroff A. The practitioner and the compliant patient. *Am J Public Health.* 1976;66:833–835.
9. Winder F, Collins P. Inhibition by isoniazid of synthesis of mycolic acids in *Mycobacterium tuberculosis. J Gen Microbiol.* 1970;63:41–48.
10. Nolan C, Sandblom R, Thummel K. Hepatotoxicity associated with acetaminophen usage in patients receiving multiple drug therapy for tuberculosis. *Chest.* 1994;105:408–411.
11. Moulding T, Redeker A, Kanel G. Acetaminophen, isoniazid, and hepatic toxicity. *Ann Intern Med.* 1991;114:451.
12. Bailey W, Taylor S, Dascomb W, et al. Disturbed hepatic function during isoniazid chemoprophylaxis. *Am Rev Respir Dis.* 1973;107:523.
13. Byrd R, Horn B, Solomon D, Griggs G. Toxic effects of isoniazid in tuberculosis chemoprophylaxis. *JAMA.* 1979;241: 1239–1241.
14. Turktas H, Unsal M, Tulek N. Hepatotoxicity of antituberculosis therapy (rifampin, isoniazid and pyrazinamide) or viral hepatitis. *Tuber Lung Dis.* 1994;75:58–60.
15. Eng R, Padberg F, Smith S, et al. Bactericidal effects of antibiotics on slowly growing and nongrowing bacteria. *Antimicrob Agents Chemother.* 1991;35:1824–1828.
16. Tucker RM, Denning DW, Hanson LH, et al. Interaction of azoles with rifampin, phenytoin, and carbamazepine: in vitro and clinical observations. *Clin Infect Dis.* 1992;14(1):165–174.
17. Burman WJ, Gallicano K, Peloquin C. Comparative pharmacokinetics and pharmacodynamics of the rifamycin antibacterials. *Clin Pharmacokinet.* 2001;40:327–341.
18. Centers for Disease Control and Prevention. Updated Guidelines for the Use of Rifamycins for the Treatment and Prevention of Tuberculosis Among HIV-Infected Patients Taking Protease Inhibitors or Nonnucleoside Reverse Transcriptase Inhibitors. *Morb Mortal Wkly Rep MMWR.* 2004;53:37.
19. McDermott W, Tompsett R. Activation of pyrazinamide and nicotinamide in acid environment *in vitro. Am Rev Tuberc.* 1954;70:748.
20. Snider D, Graczyk K, Bek E, et al. Supervised 6 month treatment of newly diagnosed pulmonary tuberculosis using isoniazid, rifampin, and pyrazinamide with and without streptomycin. *Am Rev Respir Dis.* 1984;130:1090.
21. Dickinson J, Aber V, Mitchison D. Bactericidal activity of streptomycin, isoniazid, rifampin, ethambutol, and pyrazinamide alone and in combination against *Mycobacterium tuberculosis. Am Rev Respir Dis.* 1977;116:627.
22. Takayama K, Kilburn J. Inhibition of synthesis of arabinogalactan by ethambutol in *Mycobacterium smegatis. Antimicrob Agents Chemother.* 1989;33:1493–1499.
23. Mandell G, Sander M. The Pharmacological Basis of Therapeutics. In: Goodman L, A G, eds. *The Pharmacological Basis of Therapeutics.* New York: MacMillan; 1980: 1199–1218.
24. Feldman W. Streptomycin: Some historical aspects of its development as a chemotherapeutic agent in tuberculosis. *Am Rev Tuberc.* 1954;69:859–868.
25. Vandevelde C, Chang A, Andrews D, et al. Rifampin and ansamycin interactions with cyclosporine after renal transplantation. *Pharmacotherapy.* 1991;11:88–89.
26. Trapnell C, Narang P, Li R, et al. Increased plasma rifabutin levels with concomitant fluconazole therapy in HIV-infected patients. *Ann Intern Med.* 1996;124:573–576.
27. Tseng A, Walmsley S. Rifabutin-associated uveitis. *Ann Pharmacother.* 1995;29:1149–1155.
28. Ji B, Lounis N, Truffot-Pernot C, et al. In vitro and in vivo activities of levofloxacin against Mycobacterium tuberculosis. *Antimicrob Agents Chemother.* 1995;39:1341–1344.
29. Nuermberger EL, Yoshimatsu T, Tyagi S, et al. Moxifloxacin-containing regimen greatly reduces time to culture conversion in murine tuberculosis. *Am J Respir Crit Care Med.* 2004;169:334–335.
30. Pletz MW, De Roux A, Roth A, et al. Early bactericidal activity of moxifloxacin in treatment of pulmonary tuberculosis: a prospective, randomized study. *Antimicrob Agents Chemother.* 2004;48:780–782.

31. Rodriguez JC, Ruiz M, Climent A, et al. In vitro activity of four fluoroquinolones against Mycobacterium tuberculosis. *Int J Antimicrob.* Agents 2001;17:229–231.

32. Tahaoglu K, Torun T, Sevim T, et al. The treatment of multidrug-resistant tuberculosis in Turkey. *N Engl J Med.* 2001;345:170–174.

33. Noel GJ, Natarajan J, Chien S, et al. Effects of three fluororquinolones on QT interval in healthy adults after single doses. *Clin Pharmacol Ther.* 2003;73:292–303.

34. Assandri A, Ratti B, Cristina T. Pharmacikinetics of rafapentine, a new long lasting rifamycin, in the rat, the mouse and the rabbit. *J Antibiot.* 1984;37:1066–1075.

35. Benator D, Bhattacharya M, Bozeman L, et al. Tuberculosis Trials Consortium. Rifapentine and isoniazid once a week versus rifampicin and isoniazid twice a week for treatment of drug-susceptible pulmonary tuberculosis in HIV-negative patients: a randomised clinical trial. *Lancet.* 2002;360: 528–534.

36. Weiner M, Burman W, Vernon A, et al. Tuberculosis Trials Consortium. Low isoniazid concentrations and outcome of tuberculosis treatment with once-weekly isoniazid and rifapentine. *Am J Respir Crit Care Med.* Epub 2003 Jan 16. 2003;167:1341–1347.

37. Vernon A, Burman W, Benator D, et al. Acquired rifamycin monoresistance in patients with HIV-related tuberculosis treated with once-weekly rifapentine and isoniazid. Tuberculosis Trials Consortium. *Lancet.* 1999;353:1843–1847.

38. Hong Kong Chest Service, British Medical Research Council. Five-year follow-up of a controlled trial of five, 6 month regimens of chemotherapy for tuberculosis. *Am Rev Respir Dis.* 1987;136:1339–1342.

39. Weber W, Hein D, Litwin A, et al. Relationship of acetylator status to isoniazid toxicity, lupus erythematosis, and bladder cancer. *Fed Proc.* 1983;42:3080–3097.

40. Miguet J, Mavier P, Soussy C, et al. Induction of hepatic microsomal enzymes after brief administration of rifampicin in man. *Gastroenterology.* 1977;72:924–926.

41. Stork C, Hoffman R. Toxicology of antituberculous drugs. In: Rom W, SM G, eds. *Tuberculosis.* New York: Little, Brown and Company; 1996:829–841.

42. Scharer L, Smith J. Changes in transaminase and liver with isoniazid. *Ann Intern Med.* 1969;71:1113–1120.

43. Kimerling M, Phillips P, Patterson P, et al. Low serum antimycobacterial drug levels in non HIV-infected tuberculosis patients. *Chest.* 1998;113:1178–1183.

44. Girgis N, Farid Z, Kilpatrick M, et al. Dexamethasone adjunctive treatment for tuberculosis meningitis. *Pediatr Infect Dis J.* 1991;10:179–183.

45. Strang J, Gibson D, Nunn A, et al. Controlled trial of prednisolone as adjuvant in treatment of tuberculous constrictive pericarditis. *Lancet.* 1987;2:1418–1422.

46. Chan H, Sun A, Hoheisel G. Endobronchial tuberculosis—is corticosteroid treatment useful?—a report of 8 cases and review of the literature. *Postgrad Med J.* 1990;66: 822–826.

47. Keane J, Gershon S, Wise RP, et al. Tuberculosis associated with infliximab, a tumor necrosis factor alpha-neutralizing agent. *N Engl J Med.* 2001;345:1098–1104.

48. Centers for Disease Control and Prevention (CDC). Tuberculosis associated with blocking agents against tumor necrosis factor-alpha—California, 2002–2003. *Morb Mortal Wkly Rep MMWR.* 2004;53:683–686.

49. Fischl MA, Daikos GL, Uttamchandani RB et al. Clinical presentation and outcome of patients with HIV infection and tuberculosis caused by multiple-drug-resistant bacilli. *Ann Intern Med.* 1992;117:184–190.

50. Dannenberg AM Jr. Immune mechanisms in the pathogenesis of pulmonary tuberculosis. *Rev Infect Dis.* 1989; 11:S369–S378.

51. Murray J, Sonnenberg P, Shearer SC, et al. Human immunodeficiency virus and the outcome of treatment for new and recurrent pulmonary tuberculosis in African patients. *Am J Respir Crit Care Med.* 1999;159:733–740.

52. Oliva J, Moreno S, Sanz J, et al. Co-administration of rifampin and nevirapine in HIV-infected patients with tuberculosis. *AIDS.* 2003;17:637–638.

53. Ribera E, Pou L, Lopez RM, et al. Pharmacokinetic interaction between nevirapine and rifampicin in HIV-infected patients with tuberculosis. *J Acquir Immune Defic Syndr.* 2001;28:450–453.

54. Snider D, Layde R, Johnson M, et al. Treatment of tuberculosis during pregnancy. *Am Rev Respir Dis.* 1980;122:65.

55. Malone RS, Fish DN, Spiegel DM, et al. The effect of hemodialysis on isoniazid, rifampin, pyrazinamide and ethambutol. *Am J Respir Crit Care Med.* 1999;159: 1580–1584.

56. Cross R, Long M, Banner A, et al. Rifampin-isoniazid therapy of alcoholic and nonalcoholic tuberculosis patients in a US Public Health Service Cooperative Therapy Trial. *Am Rev Respir Dis.* 1980;122:349–353.

7

Therapy of Multidrug-Resistant Tuberculosis

Barbara J. Seaworth
Robert Longfield

OVERVIEW

Multidrug-resistant tuberculosis (MDR-TB), strains resistant to at least isoniazid (INH), and rifampin,[1] are difficult to treat and require drugs that are expensive, toxic, and less effective. MDR-TB is a serious threat to global TB control. Inadequately treated patients continue to spread MDR-TB within their families and communities.

Primary and Acquired Drug Resistance

MDR-TB strains are resistant to INH and rifampin,[1] drugs essential for short-course treatment regimens (Table 7-1). Acquired resistance to antituberculosis drugs occurs during selective multiplication of drug-resistant mycobacteria that emerge spontaneously and then flourish as a result of inadequate therapy. Molecular epidemiology indicates that MDR-TB strains arise by sequential accumulation of resistance mutations for individual drugs.[2] Drug resistance which develops during or after a course of treatment was called "acquired drug resistance," but is now referred to as "resistance among previously treated cases" by the WHO. Similarly, drug-resistance with no prior history of TB treatment was categorized as "primary drug resistance" but is now called "resistance among new cases." It is often difficult to obtain an accurate history of treatment, however, "new cases" are defined as persons who have never received antituberculosis drugs or who have received them for less than one month. "Previously treated cases" are persons who have received at least 1 month of therapy.[3]

Errors in Therapy

TB treatment errors resulting in inadequate treatment of drug susceptible disease can lead to MDR-TB. Mahmoudi and Iseman found management errors in 28 of 35 (80%) MDR-TB patients between 1989 and 1990. An average of 3.93 errors per patient was noted. The most frequent errors included inadequate primary treatment regimens, the addition of a single drug to a failing treatment regimen, failure to recognize resistance, failure to recognize or ensure adherence, and inappropriate isoniazid monotherapy of TB disease. Treatment errors have been observed more often in patients cared for by private providers, including respiratory physicians.[4,5] Nearly half the patients cared for outside state or city TB control programs received regimens that deviated from guidelines from the CDC and American Thoracic Society (ATS), i.e., fewer than four initial drugs despite established local isoniazid resistance above 4% of isolates.[6]

Epidemiology

The World Health Organization (WHO) and the International Union Against Tuberculosis and Lung Disease's (IUALT) global projects on drug resistance surveillance identified MDR-TB as an emerging infectious disease on five continents and in 40 of the 44 countries surveyed. The full extent of the MDR-TB problem is unknown. Mathematical models estimate that 3.2% of new TB cases were MDR in 2002, accounting for approximately 273,000 cases world wide (95% CI: 185,000–414,000 cases).[7] The spread of MDR-TB appears to increase considerably as HIV infection is introduced into areas with established MDR-TB[8] HIV patients may actually serve as a sentinel population among whom the earliest cases of MDR-TB may become manifest in a country or region.[9] Hospital or other facility-based outbreaks of MDR-TB have been reported in the United States and elsewhere and have had dramatic impacts on global TB control efforts.[10]

In the U.S., although TB cases in foreign-born and US-born persons are decreasing steadily, the rate of decline is less in the foreign-born. Spread of MDR-TB has been detected to at least 42 states and the District of Columbia.[11] Between 1993 and 1998, approximately 66% of MDR-TB cases occurred in persons born in Mexico, the Philippines, Vietnam, India, China, Haiti, and South Korea, all areas with high rates of TB resistance. The proportion of MDR-TB ranged from 5.4% of those born in India to 14.4% of those born in South Korea.[11] Mexico ranked sixth in MDR-TB incidence among both new and previously treated TB cases.[12] A history of prior treatment significantly increased the likelihood of MDR-TB in both foreign-born (10.6%) and US-born (3.8%).[11]

More than 300 cases of MDR-TB, primarily involving US born persons, were associated with the epidemic of HIV in New York City. Case mortality rates were high in persons with HIV and those infected with the W strain.[13] Cases caused by the MDR-TB W strain, usually resistant to seven antituberculosis agents, have since been documented outside New York, in other US cities and in other countries.[14] Successful containment was achieved following heightened awareness of possible drug resistance, expedited susceptibility testing, extensive infection control measures, expanded use of DOTS, and the use of empiric six- and seven-drug regimens when MDR-TB was suspected. The incidence of MDR-TB has declined significantly in New York in response to these measures, but the full extent of the consequences of these outbreaks is not known. Cases of latent TB infection (LTBI), cannot be specifically identified as having been caused by MDR-TB. Such latent infections with MDR-TB will not respond to isoniazid and will be detected only when disease occurs over the decades to come.[13]

TREATMENT

Second-Line Drugs

Injectable Agents: Kanamycin, Amikacin, and Capreomycin

Streptomycin was the first effective drug for TB. Early patient improvement following mono-therapy with streptomycin was invariably followed by clinical failure. The peril of sequential mono-therapy unfortunately remains a lesson that generations of physicians have had to relearn. Streptomycin has been identified as a second line drug in the latest CDC, ATS, IDSA: Treatment of TB Guidelines, because of the high rate of resistance to Streptomycin especially in foreign-born populations.[15] Aminoglycosides, which act at the 30S ribosome to inhibit protein synthesis, also include amikacin, kanamycin, and the closely related polypeptide, capreomycin. They demonstrate activity against *M. tuberculosis in vitro* and are bactericidal against rapidly growing extra-cellular mycobacteria especially those growing in cavitary lesions.[16] Due to reduced tissue pH and anaerobic conditions, they are not active against slowly growing organisms in caseous lesions or abscesses.[17–19] All aminoglycosides require parenteral administration and, while some patients can tolerate daily IM injections, many prefer IV administration through a long-term venous access device. Serum drug levels are readily available for amikacin and this allows rapid adjustment of the dose as needed. For capreomycin and streptomycin these must be sent to reference laboratories. Adverse events include ototoxicity, nephrotoxicity, and rare neuromuscular blockade. Aminoglycoside and capreomycin use may be complicated by reductions in serum calcium, magnesium, and potassium.[20,21] Primary resistance to streptomycin is significant in isolates from foreign-born persons. Cross resistance is not seen between streptomycin and Amikacin so unless patients have had prior treatment with the agent, these isolates are generally sensitive to amikacin.[22]

Inhaled aminoglycosides may increase local drug concentration and nearly eliminate toxicity. Seven of 12 patients with persistently smear and culture positive MDR-TB had sputum smear conversion to negative, with this as adjunctive therapy. Successful treatment was documented after inhaled streptomycin was added to a previously failing regimen and three other successful uses of this therapy have been reported.[23] Long-term efficacy is unknown and this means of administration will not address bacilli in caseous lesions. Adverse events were limited to airway irritability.[24]

Fluoroquinolones: Ciprofloxacin, Ofloxacin, Levofloxacin, Gatifloxacin, and Moxifloxacin

There has been considerable experience with the long-term efficacy and safety for ciprofloxacin, ofloxacin, and levofloxacin.[25–28] These drugs are bactericidal against both extra-cellular rapidly multiplying bacteria and intracellular nonmultiplying bacteria.[29] The fluoroquinolones penetrate well into tissues (alveolar macrophages), respiratory secretions, and body fluids, with concentrations equal to or higher than in serum.[29–32] The prolonged half-life (5–8 hours for levofloxacin) and significant postantibiotic effect allow once daily dosing.[28,32]

Both ciprofloxacin and ofloxacin have been associated with good outcomes in the treatment of drug susceptible[30,33] and drug-resistant TB.[34–37] Levofloxacin is the active pure L-enantiomer, of which ofloxacin is a racemic mixture.[38] Levofloxacin is highly bactericidal with minimal inhibitory concentrations (MIC) less than those of ciprofloxacin and ofloxacin.[29,39,40] Because of its safety and activity, Levofloxacin has become the fluoroquinolone of choice, despite the absence of clinical trials for TB treatment. The authors have had good experience with advancing the dose of Levofloxin to 750–1000 mg per day as tolerated.

Newer quinolones such as moxifloxacin have increased bactericidal activity and may offer new treatment benefits.[40,41] Moxifloxacin has the highest serum half-life of the currently available fluoroquinolones. Moxifloxacin and levofloxacin have a higher MIC90(1 mg/l) than ciprofloxacin (4 mg/l)and ofloxacin(2 mg/l).[42] Furthermore, moxifloxacin has demonstrated early bactericidal activity in sputum that is equivalent to rifampin at 2 days and to isoniazid at 5 days.[43,44]

Fluoroquinolone resistance develops as a two-step process, and higher serum levels protect against selection of mutants.[45] Resistance to fluoroquinolones develops rapidly when they are used as mono-therapy.[46] These drugs should always be protected by being given in combination with several other active agents.[30]

Rifabutin

Most reports note that 20–30% or more of MDR-TB isolates retain sensitivity to rifabutin.[47–49] Rifabutin is bactericidal with an MIC for TB < or = 2mcg/mL regarded as susceptible. Although peak serum levels are <1mcg/mL., the drug has excellent activity and penetrates into polymorphonuclear leukocytes, lymphocytes, and macrophages. Tissue levels are significantly higher than serum levels. In the lungs, tissue levels are 5–10 times higher than in plasma.[50,51]

Rifabutin is used to replace rifampin in drug regimens for persons with HIV to avoid the drug interactions with HIV protease inhibitors. Outcomes are similar to those patients treated with rifampin. The response to rifabutin in patients with MDR-TB is unclear. A controlled trial to study the effect of rifabutin susceptible isolates in patients with resistance to isoniazid and rifampin has not been done. Most studies have not been able to select a patient group for reliable comparison of results and some studies do not separate outcomes in patients with initial susceptibility to rifabutin from those with resistance.[52,53] A study of 11 patients with MDR-TB treated with rifabutin and other drugs noted: "Two patients had rifabutin-susceptible strains on admission to the study; their temporary responses were among the best and were associated with the emergence of rifabutin resistance, suggesting that rifabutin may have contributed to their response."[54] When laboratory susceptibility to rifabutin is documented, the authors include it at a dose of 450 mg daily and aim for a peak serum level at the higher end of the therapeutic range. Hematological toxicity and uveitis may limit use of rifabutin at this dose in patients with HIV infection, but have been unusual in HIV negative patients in our experience.

Ethionamide

Ethionamide is structurally similar to isoniazid and also appears to inhibit cell wall mycolic acid synthesis. The drug is bactericidal, well absorbed orally and widely distributed. The most frequent adverse effect is gastrointestinal intolerance including nausea, epigastric pain and metallic taste. Significant hepatitis occurs in about 4.3% of patients but transient abnormalities in liver tests are more common. Hypothyroidism develops in a significant number of patients treated with ethionamide. Replacement

of thyroid hormone is required during therapy but can be discontinued when the ethionamide is stopped.[55] A study in healthy volunteers indicated that single doses > or = 500 mg were required to achieve therapeutic serum levels.[56] When susceptibilities permit, ethionamide is used as part of multiagent therapy. To reduce intolerance, ethionamide can be started slowly (250 mg daily) and increased to the total daily dose over the first 7–10 days of treatment. Treatment is usually given in divided doses totaling 500–1000 mg per day.

Cycloserine

Cycloserine is bacteriostatic for mycobacteria, acting to inhibit cell wall synthesis. It is rapidly absorbed after oral administration and is widely distributed. The most common side effects pertain to the central nervous system (CNS): seizures, psychosis, mania, depression, other emotional disturbances, and drowsiness. Neurotoxicity appears dose dependant and is rarely seen if serum drug levels remain below 30 ug/mL. Prior history of neurologic or psychiatric disorder increases the likelihood of CNS adverse events. When susceptibilities permit, cycloserine is used as part of multiagent therapy. The usual adult dose is 750 mg per day, divided into two or three doses. Treatment is usually started at 250 mg twice daily. The authors recommend that serum levels be determined before increasing the dose of cycloserine further.

Para-Aminosalicylic Acid

Para-aminosalicylic acid (PAS) exerts a bacteriostatic effect on *M. tuberculosis* by competitively blocking the conversion of para-aminobenzoic acid (PABA) to folic acid, thereby inhibiting DNA synthesis. PAS is readily absorbed; extensively protein bound (60–70 %), readily diffuses into caseous TB lesions but fails to penetrate non-inflamed meninges. Rapidly metabolized by the liver and excreted by the kidneys, PAS must be administered in large, divided oral doses (8–12 gm/day). Anorexia, nausea, vomiting, and diarrhea are common even with the current formulation of enteric-coated granules. Diarrhea is especially troublesome with the initiation of treatment but often improves after the first weeks of therapy. Many experts recommend starting at a dose of 4 gm daily and increasing over the next 7–10 days to the desired daily dose. Most patients will not tolerate doses >12 gm/day. PAS, especially when given with ethionamide, can cause hypothyroidism. Thyroid hormone replacement should be given until the offending medications are discontinued. The attendant sodium load may cause fluid retention in susceptible patients.

Clofazimine

Clofazimine is a riminophenazine dye compound used to treat *Mycobacterium leprae* with activity against TB. Concentrated in macrophages, clofazimine has proven effective in a murine TB model. Generally well tolerated except for occasional gastrointestinal complaints, the most frequent patient concern is reversible skin darkening due to drug deposition. Clofazimine is now available for MDR-TB treatment only from the manufacturer (Novartis Pharmaceutical Corporation) under an individual patient IND.

Oxazolidinones and Nitroimidazoles: Linezolid and Metronidazole

Linezolid, the first of the new oxazolidinones, is currently marketed for the treatment of resistant gram-positive bacterial infections. Clinical studies in *M. tuberculosis* have not been done, but *in vitro* susceptibility and murine data show some promise.[57,58] Reported adverse events have included hematological, ophthalmologic, and neurologic toxicity.[58a] Serotonin toxicity reactions may occur if patients are not counseled to avoid certain foods and beverages high in tyramine. The long term efficacy and tolerability of linezolid and related agents remains to be established.

The nitroimidazoles are structurally similar to the antibiotic metronidazole, and a new drug in this class has been identified that possesses marked antituberculosis activity. Laboratory and murine studies found it to be highly bactericidal against *M. tuberculosis* and active against growing and stationary phase organisms.[59,60] Murine and guinea pig studies have shown activity similar to isoniazid at 25 mg/kg/day.[61] Although metronidazole has been used for years, clinical trials on these new drugs are still pending, and unsuspected toxicity could occur. Their potential role warrants additional study.

Gamma Interferon

Systemic gamma interferon given to patients with disseminated nontuberculous mycobacteria infections resulted in clinical improvement in seven patients.[62] Interferon likely acts to inhibit mycobacterial growth through activation of alveolar macrophages and the enhanced production of reactive nitrogen species. In an open-label trial, aerosol interferon gamma was given three times weekly for 1 month to five patients with treatment refractory MDR-TB. Interferon was well tolerated, sputum smears became negative, time to a positive culture increased, and cavitary size was reduced in all patients. However, cultures remained positive, and all patients relapsed once interferon was discontinued.[63] Either systemic or inhaled interferon offers some prospect for long-term adjuvant, palliative or salvage therapy. It is likely that other immune-modulating treatments, and potentially therapeutic vaccines, may become available.

High-Dose Isoniazid

Some physicians have recommended the use of high-dose isoniazid, 1200–1500 mg three times weekly or 1000–1500 mg daily in the treatment of MDR-TB. Available studies demonstrated significant improvement in weight, a trend toward improved sputum smear and an acceptable toxicity profile.[64,65] Moulding concluded that high-dose isoniazid may be helpful in patients with low-level isoniazid resistance or who have subpopulations of isoniazid susceptible mycobacteria. Furthermore, patients in developing countries may benefit because isoniazid is inexpensive.[66] Patients with high-level resistance or who have had multiple treatment failures with an isoniazid-containing regimen would not likely benefit from isoniazid, even at high doses.[13,67]

TREATMENT OF PATIENTS WITH DRUG-RESISTANT TUBERCULOSIS (See Table 7-1)

Case Management

The authors concur with Reichmann who asserts that the case management model which is comprised of multidisciplinary teams of health care professionals practicing at TB centers of excellence provides the optimal approach for treating patients with MDR-TB.[68] Intensive case management is provided for the authors' patients both during hospitalization and through partnering with local health department nurse case managers following discharge.

HIV-Negative Patients

To date, no second line regimen has approached the early bactericidal activity and sterilizing ability of isoniazid-rifampin-pyrazinamide in treating sensitive TB.[69] Because of this, treatment for MDR-TB must include more drugs and be given for prolonged periods (18–24 months or longer). Treatment should begin with preferably six but not less than four new drugs with proven susceptibility, two of which should be bactericidal.[70] An aminoglycoside or capreomycin ("injectable") at 15 mg/kg daily or 5 times weekly is recommended during the first 4–6 months of therapy. The authors then continue the injectable 2–3 times weekly for 6–12 months of treatment after cultures convert

Table 7-1. Treatment Regimens for MDR-TB Based on Drug Resistance and Extent of Disease

Resistance	Recommended Regimen	Disease Extent/Duration of Therapy
INH RIF (Rifabutin sensitive)	Rifabutin 450 mg daily EMB 25 mg/kg × 2 months then 15 mg/kg daily PZA 20–25 mg/kg daily LEVO 750–1000 mg daily Amikacin 15 mg/kg 5 ×/week	**Primary or Limited** Amikacin until culture conversion oral drugs 12 months **Extensive** Amikacin × 4–6 months oral drugs 18–24 months
INH RIF RIFABUTIN	Amikacin* 15 mg/kg 5 ×/week LEVO 750–1000 mg daily PZA 20–25 mg/kg daily EMB 25 mg/kg × 2 months then 15 mg/kg daily Ethionamide 500–750 mg daily† B6 100 mg daily	**Primary or Limited** Amikacin 5 ×/week × 4–6 months., 3 ×/week 6–12 months oral drugs 18–24 months **Extensive** Amikacin 5 ×/week × 4–6 months. Then 3 ×/week until culture negative × 12 months Oral drugs × 24 months after culture conversion PAS or cycloserine may be added
INH RIF RIFABUTIN EMB	Amikacin* 15 mg/kg 5 ×/week LEVO 750–1000 mg daily PZA 20–25 mg/kg daily Ethionamide 500–750 mg daily† Cycloserine 500–750 mg Daily† PAS 8–12 gm q. day daily B6 100 mg daily	**Primary or Limited** Amikacin 5 ×/week × 4–6 months then 3 ×/week for 6–12 months PAS or Cycloserine should be included in regimen Oral drugs 18–24 months **Extensive** Amikacin 5 ×/week × 6 months, 3 ×/week until culture negative × 12 months Oral drugs—all five until culture negative × 24 months
INH RIF RIFABUTIN PZA	Amikacin 15 mg/kg 5 ×/week LEVO 750–1000 mg daily EMB 25 mg/kg × 2 months then 15 mg/kg Ethionamide 500–750 mg daily† PAS 8–12 gm daily‡ Cycloserine 500–750 mg daily† B6 100 mg daily	**Primary or Limited** Amikacin 5 ×/week × 4–6 months then 3 ×/week for 6–12 months PAS or cycloserine should be included in regimen Oral drugs 18–24 months **Extensive** Amikacin 5 ×/week × 6 months, 3 ×/week until culture negative × 12 months Oral drugs—all five until culture negative × 24 months
INH RIF RIFABUTIN PZA EMB	Amikacin 15 mg/kg 5 ×/week daily LEVO 750–1000 mg daily Ethionamide 500–750 mg daily† PAS 8–12 gm q. daily Cycloserine 500–750 mg daily† B6 100 mg daily	**Primary or Limited** Amikacin 5 ×/week × 6months, 3 ×/week until culture negative × 12 months Oral drugs × 18–24 months **Extensive** Amikacin 5 ×/week × 6months, 3 ×/week until culture negative × 12 months Oral drugs until culture negative × 24 months Consider 2nd injectable and/or Linezolid 600 mg. daily

(Continued)

Table 7-1. Treatment Regimens for MDR-TB Based on Drug Resistance and Extent of Disease (*Continued*)

Resistance	Recommended Regimen	Disease Extent/Duration of Therapy
Isoniazid (INH) RIF RIFABUTIN PZA EMB ETHIONAMIDE	Amkacin 15 mg/kg 5 ×/week daily LEVO 750–1000 mg daily Cycloserine 500–750 mg daily† PAS 8–12 gm daily‡ Add 2nd injectable and or Linezolid 600 mg. daily for extensive disease	**Primary or Limited** Amikacin 5 ×/week × 6 months, 3 ×/week until culture negative × 12 months Oral drugs × 24 months **Extensive** Amikacin and 2nd injectable 3–5 ×/week × 6–12 months, continue at least one injectable until culture negative × 12 months Linezolid 600 mg.qd should be included. Oral drugs should be continued until culture negative × 24 months
INH RIF RIFABUTIN AMIKACIN CAPREO +/–OTHERS	LEVO 750–1000 mg daily Any 1st line drugs available PAS 8–12 gm daily‡ Cycloserine 500–750 mg daily† Ethionamide 500–750 mg daily† Linezolid 600 mg daily for extensive disease§ B6 100 mg daily	**Primary or Limited** All oral drugs at least 18 months, preferably 18–24 months **Extensive** Linezolid 600 mg daily, and 5–6 oral drugs as available and tolerated Continue for at least 24 months. after cultures convert to negative
INH RIF RIFABUTIN Levofloxacin +/–OTHERS	Test and use any new fluoroquinolone that might be sensitive Amikacin 15 mg/kg 3–5 ×/week Capreomycin 15 mg/kg 3–5 ×/week Linezolid 600 mg daily for extensive disease	**Primary or Limited** Amikacin 5 ×/week × 6 mo., 3 ×/week until culture negative × 12 months at least 4 oral drugs for at least 18 months, preferably 24 months **Extensive** Continue both Amikacin & Capreomycin as long as possible; then Amikacin 3–5 ×/week until cultures convert to negative × 12 months Oral drugs × 24 months after culture conversion

Extensive disease: Extensive infiltrates, cavities, or pulmonary destruction

Levofloxacin and all fluoroquinolones should be given 2 hours before or after calcium or magnesium containing antacid, milk based food supplements, sucralfate, multi-vitamins, and iron

Doses of all injectables, EMB, PZA, Fluoroquinolones, cycloserine, and PAS must be adjusted in patients with chronic renal failure

Treatment should always be in consultation with an expert in management of MDR-TB

* Amikacin may be given IV or IM, capreomycin or streptomycin may be substituted when susceptibility documented

† Ethionamide, cycloserine can be given in a single daily dose or in two divided doses

‡ PAS is usually given in two divided doses—most smaller patients (<70 kg) tolerate 6–8 gm doses per day better than 12 gm

§ 40% incidence myelosuppression noted by 16 weeks Linezolid therapy in patients dosed at 600 mg. b.i.d.

to negative.[71,72] Peak serum drug levels are maintained at amikacin 25 ug/mL. When treatment options are limited or disease is extremely severe, capreomycin can be given along with an aminoglycoside ("dual injectables") as tolerated. Both drugs can be given on the same day 3–5 times a week or on alternate days.

Four to five oral drugs should be given in addition to the injectable agent, and these drugs should be continued for at least 18–24 months after sputum cultures convert to negative. Serum drug levels are obtained after the first several weeks and the doses of medications adjusted to achieve optimal serum levels.

The key oral agent is a once daily fluoroquinolone, which is continued throughout the treatment course.[13,26,72,73] Susceptibility to the fluoroquinolone and all other drugs utilized in the regimen should be documented. Resistance to the quinolones, though uncommon, has been reported within a month of initial therapy.[46] Most clinical experience exists with levofloxacin. For adults a dose of 750–1000 mg is usually well tolerated. Fluoroquinolone levels are often at or over the upper limit of normal but are well tolerated in the authors' experience. Newer fluoroquinolones are now available that have equivalent or improved activity.[42–44,74] The most frequently recommended is moxifloxacin at 400 mg daily. Experience with pushing the dose is limited and at a dose of 400 mg daily, it may not offer much additional benefit over high dose levofloxacin.

When susceptibility to other first-line drugs (pyrazinamide or ethambutol) exists, these should be included. If they have been part of a previously failing regimen, they may be less effective, however, most experts include them especially when limited treatment options remain.[75,76] Ethambutol is initiated at a dose of 25 mg/kg until cultures convert and then decreased to 15 mg/kg. The combination of levofloxacin, ethambutol, and pyrazinamide demonstrated intermediate early bactericidal activity against 12 MDR strains.[69] When PZA is susceptible it should be given throughout the treatment course. Susceptibility to rifabutin will be present in 20 to 30% or more of rifampin-resistant cases.[13,49] Rifabutin appears to be as effective as rifampin in the treatment of drug-susceptible TB,[77,78] but data on its use in MDR-TB are limited. The authors include it whenever susceptibility exists at a dose of 450 mg daily. Tolerance to this dose is excellent in persons without HIV infection. If possible, additional support drugs are included to bring the total number of drugs in the regimen to six. Ethionamide and clofazimine are weakly bactericidal and generally preferred over cycloserine and para-aminosalicylic acid (PAS). Ethionamide, cycloserine, and PAS can all be initiated at low dose and increased over the first 7–10 days of treatment. Patients may tolerate these drugs better when doses are escalated and when they are given twice daily in divided doses.

The patient's underlying medical condition and their ability to tolerate a given drug form the basis for drug selection. For instance, a person with a history of depression, mania or seizures may be unlikely to tolerate cycloserine, so another drug should be chosen. The experience in Peru suggests that depression at the onset of therapy is common and can be managed with the use of an antidepressant.[79] In the authors' experience, when depression develops during therapy with cycloserine it is difficult to manage and medication usually needs to be discontinued. Suicide has been noted in persons suffering from cycloserine associated depression. Careful attention also must be paid during the selection of drug regimens in patients with renal or hepatic dysfunction and drug doses and dosing intervals should be adjusted accordingly. There are no approved intermittent regimens for MDR-TB so treatment must be daily for oral medications.

During a treatment course, the patient may improve clinically and even transiently convert sputum cultures to negative. If the resistant mycobacteria multiply, the patient may have a relapse of symptoms and positive cultures. This phenomenon was recognized in the past and referred to as the "the fall and the rise" of TB.[80] Without a strong regimen, an initial favorable clinical response does not assure a successful outcome nor justify continuing a weak regimen.

Treatment that consists of at least five drugs, includes both a fluoroquinolone[26,72] and an aminoglycoside, and is continued for an adequate duration should have a high degree of success.[13,80–82] Successful MDR-TB treatment has been associated with prolonged inpatient management, particularly in resource poor settings and for patients who are medically complex or who lack social support.[83] Farmer and Yong in Peru report good results using an individually tailored regimen which is based on drug susceptibilities and includes a quinolone and an aminoglycoside as the foundation of the regimen when susceptibility to these agents is documented.[84]

The National Jewish Medical and Research Center reported recent and historical results for patients treated for MDR-TB at their institution. The recent cohort had better long-term success (75 vs. 56%) and a lower death rate (12 vs. 22%). The improvement in outcomes was attributed to the introduction and use of fluoroquinolone therapy, resection surgery, and prolonged hospitalization.[85] A weakness of this approach is that following an intensive period of treatment and ready access to expertise, the patient was then discharged back to communities where expertise and case management services were not available. This diminished the ability to follow patients after discharge and obtain long-term outcome information. Although this approach was successful in a center with extensive surgical and clinical expertise, it is less likely to be successful in other institutions that lack these skills.[86]

Many second line drugs have insufficient data for safety in pregnancy or have been established to be teratogenic. Nonetheless, small case series and the authors' experience have noted favorable maternal and fetal outcomes despite MDR-TB therapy. Women of child bearing potential should be counseled and offered assistance to avoid conception during treatment for MDR-TB.[87]

HIV-Infected Patients

All HIV-infected or otherwise immunocompromised patients with suspected MDR-TB must be recognized quickly, assessed for the most likely susceptibility pattern and started on aggressive combination therapy. Mortality rates have been extraordinarily high in HIV-infected persons with MDR-TB who have delays in therapy. When MDR-TB is diagnosed early and patients receive individualized therapy, they often respond with prolonged survival.[8,13,36]

The authors recommend a six- or seven-drug regimen to prevent the development of any additional drug resistance. Most, if not all of the remaining medications to which the person might be susceptible, should be prescribed. Adverse medication related events are much more common in HIV-infected patients treated for MDR-TB. The empiric regimen should include enough drugs that an adequate regimen will remain even if several need to be stopped.

MONITORING AND MANAGING MEDICATION TOXICITY

Treatment regimens for MDR-TB include drugs with significant toxicity (Table 7-2).[88] Patients should be warned to expect some adverse effects but encouraged that once they complete treatment, they may resume normal lives. In the authors' experience, toxicity nearly always becomes less severe and more tolerable as treatment progresses. One exception is the auditory or vestibular toxicity with injection medications, which is related to the total dose, usually progresses and is irreversible. Increasing the dosing interval can slow hearing loss and allow continued treatment. Vestibular toxicity, however, usually requires prompt discontinuation of the aminoglycoside or capreomycin. Periodic symptom questionnaires, basic audiometric screens and simple bedside vestibular function tests assist in monitoring for ototoxicity.[89,90]

A symptom screen may help identify the onset of drug related hepatitis, behavioral changes including psychosis and depression (cycloserine), tendonitis (fluoroquinolones), and visual problems. Medications should be continued whenever possible as replacements are usually not available, and discontinuation of even a single medication may impact regimen effectiveness. Symptom treatment or a change in dosing schedule may alleviate nausea and anorexia, and should be attempted before discontinuing a medication.[71] Significant elevation of liver enzymes, vestibular toxicity, acute renal failure,[71] vision loss or uveitis, acute tendonitis or evidence of tendon rupture, seizures, psychosis, and serious depression usually require discontinuation of the responsible medication.

Toxicity monitoring should include at least monthly serum creatinine and assessment of glomerular filtration rate (GFR) by MDRD calculation,[106] or, if significant changes are noted, by a timed urine for creatinine clearance. Hepatic enzymes and a complete blood count should be done monthly. A significant percentage of patients on ethionamide or PAS will develop hypothyroidism, after several months of treatment and patients should have a TSH done at least every two to three months. Thyroid hormone replacement should be provided when indicated[55] but can often be discontinued after treatment is completed.[90] Vision exams and visual symptom screens are important for patients on ethambutol or rifabutin (uveitis).[90,97] Rare instances of clofazimine visual toxicity have been noted.[101,102]

Radiology

Computerized tomography (CT) of the chest has proved an invaluable tool in initial and ongoing assessment of MDR-TB cases. Measurable disease, i.e., cavities present on chest CTs serves as an important marker of response to therapy. The CXR should be followed at least yearly during therapy and before any major change in therapy. A film should be obtained prior to the end of treatment to evaluate response and to serve as a reference for following the patient.

LABORATORY

Early Detection of Resistance

Several broth-based automated systems facilitate the early isolation and identification of MDR-TB.[107,108] Luciferase reporter phages offer promise of rapid (54–94 hour) turn around times for initial susceptibilities.[109] Under development are rapid assays that may directly detect the genetic mutations associated with rifampin resistance,

Table 7-2. Characteristics of Second-Line Drugs for Multidrug-Resistant Tuberculosis

Drug	Bactericidal	Minimum Inhibitory Concentration (MIC)(mcg/mL.)	Serum Level	Dosing	Remarks	Side Effects
Streptomycin	Yes	0.25–2.0	25–35	15 mg/kg/day 5–7 days/week 20–25 mg/kg 2–3 days/week	Class Summary: Vestibular screen. Baseline audiogram. Monitor creatinine. Adjust dose and/or interval for renal insufficiency.	Ototoxicity—auditory/vestibular (irreversible), renal toxicity, giddiness, perioral numbness, hypersensitivity, lichenoid eruptions, pain at injection site[57,71,89-91]
Amikacin	Yes	0.5–1.0	25–35	15 mg to 1 kg/day 5–7 days/week 20–25 mg/kg 2–3 days/week		Ototoxicity—auditory/vestibular (irreversible), renal toxicity, pain at injection site
Capreomycin	Yes	1.25–2.5	25–35	15 mg/kg/day 5–7 days/week 20–25 mg/kg 2–3 days/week		Ototoxicity—auditory/vestibular, hypokalemia, hypocalcemia, hypomagnesemia, pain at injection site eosinophilia[71,89,90]
Ciprofloxacin	Yes	0.5–2.0	4–6	750–1000 once daily	Poor central nervous system penetration. Adjust dose for creat cl <50. May increase liver function tests (LFTs).	Class effect: Gastrointestinal (GI) upset, dizziness, hypersensitivity, photosensitivity, headaches, tendonitis, tendon rupture, insomnia, psychosis, agitation, depression, paranoia, seizures, thrush, hepatitis Sucralfate, antacids with Al, Mg, CaSo$_4$ or FeSo$_4$ inhibit absorption as may enteral supplements[25,27,28,32,38,92-96]
Ofloxacin	Yes	0.5–2.0	8–12	800–1200 once daily	L & D isomer (D-inactive) Good central nervous system penetration Adjust dose for creat cl <50	

Table 7-2. Characteristics of Second-Line Drugs for Multidrug-Resistant Tuberculosis (Continued)

Drug	Bactericidal	Minimum Inhibitory Concentration (MIC)(mcg/mL.)	Serum Level	Dosing	Remarks	Side Effects
Levofloxacin	Yes	0.5–1.0	8–12	500–1000 daily (usual 750)	L isomer—All active drug; Good central nervous system penetration; Adjust dose for creat cl <50	Decreased white blood count, decreased platelet count, arthralgias, renal impairment, hyperpigmentation, uveitis, discoloration of body fluids, flushing, erythema of head and trunk, GI upset, hepatitis, agevsia[76,77,97–99]
Moxifloxacin	Yes	0.25	4–6	400 mg daily	Good central nervous system penetration; No dose adjustment with renal failure	
Rifabutin	Yes	0.25–0.5	0.3–0.9	450 mg daily	Extensive drug interactions: P-450 induction (less than rifampin) decrease levels of: protease inhibitors, methadone, oral contraceptives, diabetic medications, fluconazole, and others: see PDR.*; Concentrates in macrophages.	
Ethionamide	Weak	0.3–1.2	1–5	250 mg 2 or 3 times daily or 250 mg am/500 hs	Increase dose gradually, monitor liver function/thyroid function.	Peripheral neuropathy, nausea, vomiting, abdominal pain, hepatitis, hypothyroidism, salivation, metallic taste, giddiness, headache, hypersensitivity, alopecia,

Para-aminosalicylate	No	8.0	20–60 (6 h after dose)	4 gm 2 or 3 times daily	Increases effect of cycloserine	gynecomastia, hypotension, impotence, mental disturbance, menstrual irregularity, hypoglycemia, photosensitivity[55,71,90,93,100]
Clofazimine	Weak	0.12	0.5–2.0	300 mg daily × 2 months then 100 mg daily	Skin problems limited by sunscreen and lubricants	Hyperpigmentation, GI complaints, acne flare, retinopathy, ichthyosis, sunburn[93,101,102]
Cycloserine	No	N/A†	20–35	250 mg 2 times daily or 250 mg am/500 pm	Avoid in patients with seizures/psychotic disease or ethyl alcohol abuse, check level before increasing dose >500 mg. daily. Administer with pyridoxine 100–300 mg daily	Lichenoid eruption, agitation, psychosis, depression, seizures, dizziness, headache, slurred speech, insomnia, Stevens-Johnson syndrome[71,90,91,103,104]
Isoniazid (high-dose)	Yes	<5.0 mcg/mL.	N/A†	1200 mg 3 times weekly	Pyridoxine 150 mg daily, interacts with phenytoin Only useful if MIC <5.0 mcg/mL.	Optic neuritis, positive ANA rash, fever, jaundice, hepatitis, peripheral neuritis, anemia, agranulocytosis, decreased platelets, vasculitis[11,67]

Adapted from References 11, 25, 27, 28, 32, 38, 55, 57, 67, 71, 76, 77, 89–105.
*PDR = Physicians' Desk Reference
†N/A = Not Available.

an essential feature of MDR isolates.[47,110–112] Mutations in the kat-G allele conferring isoniazid resistance can also be identified by PCR.[113] Importantly, current rapid methods under development require initial sputum processing and at least brief cultivation. Useful results may be delayed, particularly with slow growing isolates.

Therapeutic Serum Drug Level Monitoring

The routine use of serum therapeutic drug level monitoring should be considered for all patients with MDR-TB.[10] The therapeutic indexes of second line TB medications are narrow. Serum therapeutic drug level monitoring allows a physician to "push a drug" to exert maximal benefit and still limit toxicity. An attempt should be made to achieve the best ratio of peak serum drug level to MIC. Successful outcomes and prevention of acquired resistance have been achieved by monitoring and adjusting serum fluoroquinolone levels.[34,35,114] Serum levels may avert aminoglycoside renal and auditory toxicity by decreasing the dose or increasing the dosing interval. Levels of cycloserine are important to minimize central nervous system adverse reactions and seizures. Therapeutic monitoring may alert the physician to an unsuspected problem with absorption, patient adherence with treatment, or a drug interaction. Persons with HIV or those at risk for malabsorption should be specifically targeted for therapeutic monitoring.

Surgical Therapy

Persistence of organisms in necrotic lung, poor vascular supply and resultant limited penetration of medications may lead to treatment failure or relapse. Destroyed pulmonary tissue and old cavitary lesions may be sites for recurrent bacterial or fungal infections.[115] Iseman attributes the improved outcomes of patients with MDR-TB treated between 1984 and 1993 to surgical intervention.[26,116] He and others recommended that surgical intervention be considered for patients with destruction of a lobe or entire lung and those with extensive disease including large or persistent cavities. Another surgical indication is life threatening or uncontrolled hemoptysis, although bronchial arterial embolization may facilitate control of bleeding. The optimum timing of surgical intervention is after 3–4 months of therapy and sputum culture conversion to negative. Patients who fail to convert their sputum to negative after 3–4 months of intensive therapy may also benefit from surgical intervention.[26,115,117] Patients should be screened for overall operative risk, likely residual pulmonary function after surgery and risk of devastating broncho-pleural fistula.

Therapy should be continued for at least an additional 18–24 months after surgery.[26,115] The few experienced centers performing lung resection surgery report infrequent morbidity and mortality.[115] However, the reported benefits of resection surgery may be substantially biased by patient selection.[86] Residual lung damage is common and extensive in MDR versus susceptible TB cases. Close follow-up of treated cases is warranted to detect and manage relapses, regardless of previous resection surgery.[118]

INFECTION CONTROL

Patients with MDR-TB are as infectious as any TB patient.[119] Because treatment for LTBI is unproven in this group and has been associated with a high rate of adverse effects,[92] every effort should be employed to prevent transmission of MDR-TB. Improvement of infection control measures in institutions has been credited with decreasing rates of MDR-TB in urban populations with HIV.[13,120] One study demonstrated a rapid decrease in culture positive cough aerosols during the first three weeks of effective therapy for MDR-TB. Culture positive aerosols were associated with interruptions in therapy during the previous week (p = 0.007).[121] Patients with MDR-TB should be placed individually in engineered negative pressure isolation rooms. The CDC recommends continuing respiratory isolation throughout the hospital course, even when cultures are negative.[122] The authors require patients with MDR-TB to remain in respiratory isolation at least until they have three separate final negative sputum cultures while adherent with and responding to an appropriate regimen. After conversion of cultures to negative, patients should continue to be monitored with monthly sputum cultures. Patients may become sputum culture positive, even after months of negative cultures.[71] Decisions about when patients may contact children or immunocompromised individuals are controversial and may need to be individualized following consultation with public health authorities. The issue is often not *if* patients may be discharged but *where* they may be best cared for on an ambulatory basis.[123]

PREVENTION

The WHO recommended directly observed therapy; short course (DOTS) inexpensively treats susceptible TB cases and effectively reduces the emergence of MDR-TB. Directly observed therapy, short course is based on the axiom that "you cannot cure multidrug resistant TB as fast as you can create it.[124,125] The DOTS strategy appears effective for preventing "home grown" but not "imported" cases of MDR-TB.[86] Furthermore, DOTS may serve as a death sentence in countries with a high prevalence of MDR-TB.[126] Following Peru's success with ambulatory treatment regimens for MDR-TB, WHO has since endorsed "DOTS Plus" MDR-TB treatment regimens, but only in countries with well-functioning TB programs.[84,127–132]

TREATMENT OF LATENT INFECTION POSSIBLY DUE TO MULTIDRUG-RESISTANT TUBERCULOSIS

All persons identified as MDR-TB contacts are at risk and should be quickly evaluated for latent infection and active disease. The optimal management of established latent infection (LTBI) is a matter of debate. No regimen has been proved effective, and it is unlikely that a definitive study will be done to guide management. Nevertheless, it is important to follow all persons with presumed latent MDR-TB for at least 2 years following the exposure. Periodic assessments should include clinical exams and chest radiographs every 3 months for persons with HIV or other immune suppressing illness and every 6 months for all others.[133]

Those who are tuberculin skin test-positive, are close contacts of an MDR-TB case and have no prior history of a previously positive tuberculin test can be considered for treatment of latent MDR-TB. After discussion of the risks and benefits of treatment, the patient and physician can make a decision regarding LTBI treatment. Management of tuberculin skin test-negative high-risk contacts, especially infants and persons with HIV, varies. Some recommend empiric therapy after active disease is excluded.[133,134] Most clinicians agree that LTBI treatment should be offered to tuberculin skin test-positive, immunosuppressed individuals with documented exposure to MDR-TB. If assessment indicates the likelihood of exposure to drug-susceptible TB, isoniazid therapy may be preferred.

The selection of agents should be guided by the susceptibility profile of the index case. One possible regimen is a combination of pyrazinamide (25–30 mg daily) and ethambutol (15–25 mg daily). If fluoroquinolone susceptibility is documented, a regimen that combines ciprofloxacin (750 mg), ofloxacin (800 mg), or levofloxacin (750 mg) daily with pyrazinamide might be used. A pyrazinamide-fluoroquinolone combination appears to result in enhanced intramacrophage activity.[135] The authors have seen life-threatening hepatitis reactions with MDR-TB LTBI regimens which contain pyrazinamide. A fluoroquinolone also can be combined with ethambutol. Some have recommended quinolone monotherapy although emergence of resistance is a concern.[134] LTBI treatment is usually prescribed for 6–12 months.

CONCLUSION

MDR-TB is a continuing public health problem. Although control of the MDR-TB epidemic has been achieved in New York City, strains of MDR-TB are found in nearly every state. Much of the world faces a growing problem with no immediate solution. The treatment habits and public health policies that have led to the problem persist. Reichman notes new drug development has been almost nonexistent. The current global interest offers hope that the discovery and development of new antituberculosis drugs will accelerate. However, the mere existence and affordability of new drugs for MDR-TB "will not address the main underlying cause of almost all drug resistance, nonadherence of patients and doctors to recommended regimens."[68] He calls for an equal commitment to improving the knowledge and skills of healthcare workers to use both old and new agents appropriately, so that they may retain their effectiveness for the future.[136]

Each year brings new, at-risk immigrants to the United States from all regions of the globe. They bring all the TB problems of their home countries with them. Foreign-born persons will continue to have a major impact on TB control efforts in the next decade and beyond. In the United States, TB elimination programs will need to strengthen the education of caregivers and improve case finding and treatment for MDR-TB. Developing countries need assistance to develop similar capacity to effectively manage both susceptible and resistant TB. It is estimated that one million persons arrive in the U.S. each week by plane. A cursory review of resistant TB among the foreign-born should convince even skeptics that global TB programs need our urgent and serious support.

ACKNOWLEDGMENTS

The authors acknowledge Araceli Santellanes for assistance with manuscript preparation, Stephanie Ott for developing figures and tables, and the Texas Department of state health service nurses and physicians at the Texas Center for Infectious Disease and across the state for their dedicated care of patients with MDR-TB.

REFERENCES

1. Iseman MD. Treatment of multidrug-resistant tuberculosis. *N Engl J Med.* 1993;329:784–791.
2. Ramaswamy S, Musser JM. Molecular genetic basis of antimicrobial agent resistance in *Mycobacterium tuberculosis: Int J Tuberc Lung Dis.* 1998 update;79(1):3–29.
3. Dye C, Scheele S, Dolin P, et al. Global burden of tuberculosis: Estimated incidence, prevalence, and mortality by country. *JAMA.* 1999;282:677–686.
4. Kopanoff DE, Snider DR, Johnson M. Recurrent tuberculosis. Why do patients develop disease again? A United States Public Health Service Cooperative Survey. *Am J Public Health.* 1998;78:30–33.
5. Byrd RB, Horn BR, Soloman DA, et al. Treatment of tuberculosis by the nonpulmonary physician. *Ann Intern Med.* 1977;86:799–802.
6. Liu A, Shilkret KL, Finelli L. Initial drug regimens for the treatment of tuberculosis: Evaluation of physician prescribing practices in New Jersey, 1994–1995. *Chest.* 1998;113:1446–1451.
7. Espinal MA. The global situation of MDR-TB. *Tuberculosis.* 2003;83:44–51.
8. Salomon N, Perlman DC. Multidrug-resistant tuberculosis—globally with us for the long haul. *Clin Infect Dis.* 1999;29:93–95.
9. Campos PE, Suarez PG, Sanchez J, et al. Multidrug-resistant *Mycobacterium tuberculosis* in HIV-Infected Persons, Peru. *Emerg Infect Dis.* 2003;9(No.2):1571–1578.
10. Braden CR. Multidrug-resistant tuberculosis. *Infect Dis Clin Prac.* 1997;6:437–444.
11. Moore M, Onorato IM, McCray E, et al. Trends in drug-resistant tuberculosis in the United States, 1993–1996. *JAMA.* 1997;278:833–837.
12. Zumla A, Grange JM: multidrug resistant tuberculosis—can the tide be turned. *Lancet Infect Dis.* 2001;1:199–202.
13. Frieden TR, Sherman LF, Maw KL, et al. Epidemiology and clinical outcomes: A multi-institutional outbreak of highly drug-resistant tuberculosis. *JAMA.* 1996;276:1229–1235.
14. Bifani PJ, Pikaytis BB, Kapur V, et al. Origin and interstate spread of New York City multidrug-resistant Mycobacterium tuberculosis clone family. *JAMA.* 1996;275:452–457.
15. Centers for Disease Control and Prevention, American Thoracic Society, Infectious Disease Society of America. Treatment of TB. *MMWR Morb Mortal Wkly Rep.* 2003;52:26–27.
16. Grosset J. Bacteriologic Basis of Short-Course Chemotherapy for Tuberculosis. *Clin Chest Med.* 1980;1:231–241.
17. Mitchison DA, Selkon JB. The Bactericidal Activities of Antituberculous Drugs. Proceedings Symposium on Tuberculosis in Infancy and Childhood. *Am Rev Tuberc.* 1956;2055:109–116.
18. Edson RS, Terrell C. The Aminoglycosides. Symposium on Antimicrobial Agents *Clinical Proc* (Part VIII). 1999;74:519–528.
19. Sanders WE, Hartwig C, Schneider, et al. Activity of Amikacin Against Mycobacteria in vitro and in Murine Tuberculosis. *Tubercule.* 1982;63:201–208.
20. Law KF, Weiden M. *Streptomycin, Other Aminoglycosides, and Capreomycin. Tuberculosis.* Boston, Toronto, and London: Little and Company. 1996:790–792.
21. Shin S, Furin J, Alcantara F, et al. Hypokalemia Among Patients Receiving Treatment for Multidrug-Resistant Tuberculosis. *Chest.* 2004;125(3):974–980.
22. Alangaden GJ, Kreiswirth BN, AQuad A, et al. Mechanism of Resistance to Amikacin and Kanamycin in *Mycobacterium tuberculosis. Antimicrobial Agents Chemother.* 1998;42:1295–1297.
23. Parola P, Brouqui P. Clinical and Microbiological Efficiency of Adjunctive Salvage Therapy with Inhaled Aminoglycos in a Patient with Refractory Cavitary Pulmonary Tuberculosis. *Clin Infect Dis.* 2001;33:1439–?.
24. Sacks LV, Pendle S, Orlovic D, et al. Adjunctive salvage therapy with inhaled aminoglycosides for patients with persistent smear-positive pulmonary tuberculosis. *Clin Infect Dis.* 2001;32:44–49.
25. Berning SE, Madsen L, Iseman MD, et al. Long-term safety of ofloxacin and ciprofloxacin in the treatment of mycobacterial infections. *Am J Respir Crit Care Med.* 1995;151:2006–2009.
26. Iseman MD, Madsen L, Goble M, et al. Surgical intervention in the treatment of pulmonary disease caused by drug-resistant Mycobacterium tuberculosis. *Am Rev Respir Dis.* 1990;141:623–625.
27. Lipsky BA, Baker CA. Fluoroquinolone toxicity profiles: A review focusing on newer agents. *Clin Infect Dis.* 1999;28:352–364.
28. Peloquin CA, Berning SE, Madsen L, et al. Ofloxacin and ciprofloxacin in the treatment of mycobacterial infections: Development of resistance and drug interactions. *J Infect Dis.* 1995;1:45–65.
29. Gillespie SH, Kennedy N. Fluoroquinolones: A new treatment for tuberculosis? *Int J Tuberc Lung Dis.* 1998;2:265–271.
30. Alangaden GJ, Lerner SA: The clinical use of fluoroquinolones for the treatment of mycobacterial diseases. *Clin Infect Dis.* 1997;25:1213–1221.
31. Leysen DC, Haemers A, Pattyn SR. Mycobacteria and the new quinolones (Mini-review). *Antimicrob Agents Chemother.* 1989;33:1–5.
32. Lode H, Borner K, Koeppe P. Pharmacodynamics of fluoroquinolones. *Clin Infect Dis.* 1998;27:33–39.
33. Kohno S, Koga H, Kaku M, et al. Prospective comparative study of ofloxacin or ethambutol for the treatment of pulmonary tuberculosis. *Chest.* 1992;102:1815–1818.
34. Mangunnegoro H, Hudoy A. Efficacy of low-dose ofloxacin in the treatment of multidrug-resistant tuberculosis in Indonesia. *Therapy.* 1999;45(suppl 2):19–25.
35. Maranetra KN. Quinolones and multidrug-resistant tuberculosis. *Therapy.* 1999;45(suppl 2):12–18.

36. Park MM, Davis AL, Schluger NW, et al. Outcome of MDR-TB patients, 1983–1993—prolonged survival with appropriate therapy. *Am J Respir Crit Care Med.* 1996; 153:317–324.

37. Sharma SK, Guleria R, Jain D, et al. Effect of additional oral ofloxacin administration in the treatment of multidrug-resistant tuberculosis. *Indian J Chest Dis Allied Sci.* 1996;38:73–79.

38. Walker RC. The fluoroquinolones. *Mayo Clin Proc.* 1999; 74:1030–1037.

39. Rastogi N, Goh SK, Bryskier A, et al. In vitro activities of levofloxacin used alone and in combination with first- and second-line antituberculosis drugs against *Mycobacterium tuberculosis. Antimicrob Agents Chemother.* 1996;40: 1610–1616.

40. Tomioka H, Sato K, Akaki T, et al. Comparative in vitro antimicrobial activities of the newly synthesized quinolone HSR-903, sitafloxacin (DU-6859a), gatifloxacin (AM-1155), and levofloxacin against *Mycobacterium tuberculosis* and *Mycobacterium avium* complex. *Antimicrob Agents Chemother.* 1999;43:3001–3004.

41. Stein GE: The methoxyfluoroquinolones: Gatifloxacin and moxifloxacin. *Infect med.* 2000;17:564–570.

42. Rodriguez JC, Ruiz M, Climent A, et al. In vitro activity of four fluoroquinolones against *Mycobacterium tuberculosis. Int J Antimicrob Agents.* 2001;17:229–231.

43. Pletz MWR, De Roux A, Roth A, et al. Early Bactericidal Activity of Moxifloxacin in Treatment of Pulmonary Tuberculosis: a Prospective, Randomized Study. *Antimicrob Agents Chemother.* 2004;48 (No.3):780–782.

44. Gosling RD, Uiso LO, Sam NE, et al. The Bactericidal Activity of Moxifloxacin in Patients with Pulmonary Tuberculosis. *Am J Respir Crit Care Med.* 2003;168: 1342–1345.

45. Dong Y, Xu C, Zhao X, et al. Fluoroquinolone action against mycobacteria: Effects of C-8 substitutes on growth, survival, and resistance [abstract]. *Antimicrob Agents Chemother.* 1998;42:2978–2984.

46. Sullivan EA, Kreiswirth BN, Palumbo L, et al. Emergence of fluoroquinolone-resistant tuberculosis in New York City. *Lancet.* 1995;345:1148–1150.

47. Saribas Z, Kocagoz T, Alp A, et al. Rapid Detection of Rifampin Resistance in *Mycobacterium tuberculosis* Isolates by Heteroduplex Analysis and Determination of Rifamycin Cross-Resistance in Rifampin-Resistant Isolates. *J Clin Microbiol.* 2003;41(2):816–818.

48. Grassi C, Peona V. Use of Rifabutin in the Treatment of Pulmonary Tuberculosis. *Clini Infect Dis.* 1996;22 (1):S50–S54.

49. Lee CN, Lin TP, MF Chang, et al. Rifabutin as Salvage Therapy for Cases of Chronic Multidrug-Resistant Pulmonary Tuberculosis in Taiwan. *J Chemother.* 1996;8: 137–143.

50. O'Brien RJ, Lyle MA, Snider DE Jr. Rifabutin (Ansamycin LM 427): A new rifamycin-S derivative for the treatment of mycobacterial diseases. *Rev Infect Dis.* 1987;9:519–530.

51. Kunin C. Antimicrobial Activity of Rifabutin,. *Clin Infect Dis.* 1996;221:S3–S14.

52. Felten MK. Efficacy and safety of rifabutin (Anamycin LM427) in the treatment of rifampin-resistant chronic pulmonary tuberculosis. *Am Rev Respir Dis.* 1988;137:498.

53. Madsen L, Gobel M, Iseman MD. Anasamycin (LM 427) in the retreatment of drug-resistant tuberculosis. *Am Rev Respir Dis.* 1986;133(suppl 4):A206.

54. Hong Kong Chest Service/British Medical Research Council. A controlled study of rifabutin and an uncontrolled study of ofloxacin in the treatment of patients with pulmonary tuberculosis resistant to isoniazid, streptomycin, and rifampicin. *Tuberc Lung Dis.* 1992;73:59–67.

55. Soumakis S, Berg D, Harris W: Hypothyroidism in a patient receiving treatment for tuberculosis. *Clini Infect Dis.* 1998;27:910–911.

56. Zhu M, Namdar R, Stambaugh JJ, et al. Population pharmacokinetics of ethionamide in patients with tuberculosis. *Tuberculosis.* 2002;82(2/3):91–96.

57. Ashtekar DR, Costa-Periera R, Shrinivasan T, et al. Oxazolidinones, a new class of synthetic antituberculosis agent. In vitro and in vivo activities of DuP-721 against *Mycobacterium tuberculosis. Diagn Microbiol Infect Dis.* 1991;14:465–471.

58. Cynamon MH, Klemens SP, Sharpe CA, et al. Activities of several novel oxazolidinones against *Mycobacterium tuberculosis* in a murine model. *Antimicrob Agents Chemother.* 1999;43:1189–1191.

58a. Razonable RR, Osmon DR, Steckelberg JM. Linezolid Therapy for Orthopedic Infections. *Mayo Clin Proc.* 2004;79(6):1137–1144.

59. Ashtekar DR, Costa-Periera R, Nagrajan K, et al. In vitro and in vivo activities of the nitroimidazole CGI 17341 against *Mycobacterium tuberculosis. Antimicrob Agents Chemother.* 1993;37:183–186.

60. Deidda D, Lampis G, Fioravanti R, et al. Bactericidal activities of the pyrrole derivative BM212 against multidrug-resistant and intramacrophagic *Mycobacterium tuberculosis* strains. *Antimicrob Agents Chemother.* 1998; 42:3035–3037.

61. Stover KC, Warrener P, VanDevanter DR, et al. A small-molecule nitroimidazopyran drug candidate for treatment of tuberculosis. *Nature.* 2000;405:22.

62. Holland SM, Eisenstein E, Kuhus DB, et al. Treatment of refractory disseminated nontuberculous mycobacteria infection with interferon gamma. *N Engl J Med.* 1994;330: 1348–1355.

63. Condos R, Rom WN, Schluger NW. Treatment of multidrug-resistant pulmonary tuberculosis with interferon—via aerosol. *Lancet.* 1997;349:1513–1515.

64. Petty TL, Mitchell RS. Successful treatment of advanced isoniazid- and streptomycin-resistant pulmonary tuberculosis with ethionamide, pyrazinamide, and isoniazid. *Am Rev Respir Dis.* 1962;86:503–512.

65. Ramasamy R, Reginald A, Ganesan E. The use of high-dose isoniazid in intermittent regime TB treatment-some preliminary findings. *Trop Doct.* 2000;30:56.

66. Moulding TS. Should isoniazid be used in retreatment of tuberculosis despite acquired isoniazid resistance? *Am Rev Respir Dis.* 1981;123:262–264.

67. Cynamon MH, Zhang Y, Harpster T, et al. High-dose isoniazid therapy for isoniazid-resistant murine *Mycobacterium tuberculosis* infection. *Antimicrob Agents Chemother.* 1999;43: 2922–2924.

68. Tiruviluamala P, Reichman LB. Tuberculosis. *Annu Rev Public Health.* 2002;23:403–426.

69. Wallis RS, Palaci M, Vinhas S, et al. A Whole Blood Bactericidal Assay for Tuberculosis. *J Infect Dis.* 183: 1300–1303.

70. Seung KJ, Joseph K, Hurtado R, et al. Number of Drugs to Treat Multidrug-resistant Tuberculosis. *Am J Respir Crit Care Med.* 2004;(169)1336.

71. Goble M, Iseman MD, Madsen LA, et al. Treatment of 171 patients with pulmonary tuberculosis resistant to isoniazid and rifampin. *N Engl J Med.* 1993;328:527–532.

72. Tahaoglu K, Toron T, Sevim T, et al. The treatment of multidrug-resistant tuberculosis in Turkey. *N Engl J Med.* 2001;345:170–174.

73. Geerligs WA, van Altena R, de Lange WCM, et al. Multidrug-resistant tuberculosis: Long-term treatment outcome in the Netherlands. *Int J Tuberc Lung Dis.* 2000; 4:758–764.

74. Tomioka, H. Prospects for Development of New Antimycobacterial Drugs. J Infect Chemotherpy. 2000;6: 8–20.

75. Hong Kong Chest/British Medical Research Council. Controlled trials of 2, 4, and 6 months of pyrazinamide in 6-month, three times weekly regimens for smear-positive pulmonary tuberculosis, including an assessment of a combined preparation of isoniazid, rifampin, and pyrazinamide: Results at 30 months. *Am Rev Respir Dis.* 1991;143:700–706.

76. Mitchison DA, Nunn AJ. Influence of initial drug resistance on the response to short-course therapy of pulmonary tuberculosis. *Am Rev Respir Dis* Disease. 1986;133:423–430.

77. Gonzalez-Monaner LJ, Natal S, Yongchaiyud P, et al. Rifabutin for the treatment of newly diagnosed pulmonary tuberculosis: A multi-national randomized, comparative study versus rifampicin. *Tuber Lung Dis.* 1994;75:341–347.

78. McGregor NM, Olliaro P, Wolmarans L, et al. Efficacy and safety of rifabutin in the treatment of patients with newly diagnosed pulmonary tuberculosis. *Am J Respir Crit Care Med.* 1996;154:1462–1467.

79. Vega P, Sweetland A, Acha J, et al. Psychiatric Issues in the Management of Patients with Multidrug Resistnt Tuberculosis. *Int J Tuberc Lung Dis.* 2004;8:749–759.

80. Crofton J, Chaulet P, Maher D, et al. *Guidelines for the management of drug-resistant tuberculosis.* Publication # WHO/GTB/96.210. Geneva, Switzerland: World Health Organization; 1997.

81. Chan ED, Laurel V, Chan MI, et al. Retrospective analysis of 208 patients with MDR-TB; comparison to 171 patients

from 1973 to 1983. *Am J Respir Crit Care Med.* 2001; 163:A497.

82. Park SK, Kim CT, Song SD. Outcome of therapy in 107 patients with pulmonary tuberculosis resistant to isoniazid and rifampin. *Int J Tuberc Lung Dis.* 1998;2:877–884.

83. Palmero DJ, Ambroggi M, Brea A, et al. Treatment and Follow-u of HIV-Negative Multidrug-resistant tuberculosis patients in an infectious diseases reference hospital, Buenos Aires, Argentina. *Int J Tuberc Lung Dis.* 2004;8(6)778–784.

84. Farmer P, Yong KJ. Community-based approaches to the control of multidrug-resistant tuberculosis: Introducing "DOTS-plus." *BMJ.* 1998;317:671–674.

85. Chan ED, Laurel V, Strand MJ, et al. Treatment and Outcome Analysis of 205 Patients with Multidrug-resistant Tuberculosis. *Am J Respir Crit Care Med.* 2004;169:1103.

86. Griffith DE. Treatment of Multidrug-Resistant Tuberculosis—Should You Try This at Home? *Am J Respir Crit Care Med.* 2004;169:1082.

87. Shin S, Guerra D, Rich M et al. Treatment of Multidrug-Resistant Tuberculosis during Pregnancy: A Report of 7 cases. *Clin Infect Dis.* 2003;36:996–1013.

88. Seaworth BJ. in Francis J Curry National TB Center and California Department of Health Services, 2004: Drug-Resistant Tuberculosis: A Survival Guide for Clinicians. 149–173.

89. Brummett RE, Fox KE. Aminoglycoside-induced hearing loss in humans. *Antimicrob Agents* Chemother. 1989;33: 797–800.

90. Girling DJ. Adverse effects of antituberculosis drug. *Drugs.* 1982;23:56–74.*****

91. Halevy S, Shai A. Lichenoid drug eruptions. *J Am Acad Dermatol.* 1993;29:249–255.

92. Horn DL, Hewlett D, Alfalla C, et al. Limited tolerance of ofloxacin and pyrazinamide prophylaxis against tuberculosis. *N Engl J Med.* 1994;330:1241.

93. Allen JE, Potter TS, Hashimoto K: Drugs that cause photosensitivity. *Med Lett Drugs Ther.* 1995;37:35–36.

94. Lewis JR, Gums JG, Dickensheets DL: Levofloxacin-induced bilateral achilles tendonitis. *Ann Pharmacother.* 1999;33:792–795.

95. Ridzon R, Meador J, Maxwell R: Asymptomatic hepatitis in persons who received alternative preventive therapy with pyrazinamide and ofloxacin. *Clin Infect Dis.* 1997;24:1264–1265.

96. Traeger SM, Bonfiglio MF, Wilson JA, et al. Seizures associated with ofloxacin therapy. *Clin Infect Dis.* 21: 1504–1506.

97. Havlir D, Torriani F, Dube M. Uveitis associated with rifabutin prophylaxis. Ann Intern Med. 1994;121:510–512.

98. Griffith DE, Brown BA, Wallace RJ Jr. Varying doses of rifabutin affect white blood cell and platelet counts in human immunodeficiency virus-negative patients who are receiving multidrug regimens for pulmonary *Mycobacterium avium* complex disease. *Clin Infect Dis.* 1996;23:1321–1322.

99. Morris JT, Kelly WJ: Rifabutin-induced ageusia. *Ann Intern Med.* 1993;119:171–172.

100. Huang KL, Beutler SM, Wang C. Hypothyroidism in a patient receiving treatment for multidrug-resistant tuberculosis. *Clinical Infectious Disease.* 1998;27:910–911.

101. Craythorn JM, Swartz M, Creel DJ. Clofazimine-induced bull's-eye retinopathy. *Retina.* 1986;6:50–52.

102. Cunningham CA, Friedberg DN, Carr RE. Clofazimine-induced generalized retinal degeneration. *Retina.* 1990;10:131–134.

103. Akula SK, Aruna AS, Johnson JE, et al. Case study. Cycloserine-induced Stevens-Johnson syndrome in an AIDS patient with multidrug-resistant tuberculosis. *Int J Tuberc Lung Dis.* 1997;1:187–190.

104. Shim JH, Kim TY, Kim HO, et al. Cycloserine-induced lichenoid drug eruption: Case report. *Dermatology.* 1995;191:142–144.

105. Naik HR, Siddique N, Chandrasekar PH. Unusual pigmentation in patients with AIDS who are receiving rifabutin for bacteremia due to *Mycobacterium avium/Mycobacterium intracellulare* complex. *Clin Infect Dis.* 1995;21:1515–1516.

106. Levey AS, Bosch JP, Breyer LJ, et al. A More Accurate Method to Estimate Glomerular Filtration Rate from serum Creatinine: A New Prediction Equation. *Ann Intern Med.* 1999;130:461–470.

107. Scarparo C, Ricordi P, Ruggiero Giuliana, et al. Evaluation of the Fully Automated BACTEC MGIT 960 System for Testing Susceptibility, Isoniazid, Rifampin, and Ethambutol and Comparison with the Radiometric BACTEC 460TB Method. *J Clinical Microbiology.* 2004;42(No. 3):1109–1114.

108. Bemer P, Bodmer T, Munzinger J, et al. Multicenter Evaluation of the MB/BACT System for Susceptibility Testing of *Mycobacterium tuberculosis*. *J Clinical Microbiology.* 2004;42(No.3):1030–1034.

109. Hazbon MH, Guarin N, Ferro BE, et al. Photographic and Luminometric Detection of Luciferase Reporter Phages for Drug Susceptibility Testing of Clinical *Mycobacterium tuberculosis* Isolates. *Eur J Clin Microbial.* 2003;41(No.10):4865–4869.

110. Johansen IS, Lundgren B, Sosnovskaja, et al. Early Detection of Multidrug-Resistant *Mycobacterium tuberculosis* in Clinical Specimens in Low- and High-Incidence Countries by Line Probe Assay. *Eur J Clin Microbiol.* 2003:4454–4456.

111. Ruiz M, Torres MJ, Llanos AC, et al. Direct Detection of Rifampin- and Isoniazid-Resistant *Mycobacterium tuberculosis* in Auramine-Rhodamine-Positive Sputum Specimens by Real-Time PCR. *Eur J Clin Microbiol.* 2004;42(4):1585–1589.

112. Mayta H, Gilman RH, Arenas F, et al. Evaluation of a PCR-Based Universal Heteroduplex Generator as a Tool for Rapid Detection of Multidrug-Resistant Myco in Peru. *Eur J Clin Microbiol.* 2003;41(12):5774–5777.

113. Van Doorn RH, Claas ECJ, Templeton KE, et al. Detection of a Point Mutation Associated with High-Level Isoniazid Resistance in *Mycobacterium tuberculosis* by Using Real-Time PCR Technology with 3'-Minor Groove Binder-DNA Probes. *Eur J Clin Microbiol.* 2003;41(10):4630–4635.

114. Yew WW, Kwan SY, Ma WK, et al. In vitro activity of ofloxacin against Mycobacterium tuberculosis and its clinical efficacy in multiply resistant pulmonary tuberculosis. *J Antimicrob Chemother.* 1990;26:227–236.

115. Treasure RL, Seaworth BJ. Current role of surgery in *Mycobacterium tuberculosis*. *Ann Thorac Surg.* 1995;59:1405–1407.

116. Iseman MD. Treatment and implications of multidrug-resistant tuberculosis for the 21st century. Therapy 1999;45(suppl 2):34–40.

117. Van Leuven M, De Groot M, Shean KP, et al. Pulmonary resection as an adjunct in the treatment of multiple drug-resistant tuberculosis. *Ann Thorac Surg.* 1997;63:1368–1363.

118. de Valliere S, Barker RD: Residual Lung Damage after Completion of Treatment. *Int J Tuberc Lung Dis.* 2004;8(6):767–771.

119. Snider DE Jr, Kelly GD, Cauthen GM, et al. Infection and disease among contacts of tuberculosis cases with drug-resistant and drug-susceptible bacilli. *Am Rev Resp Dis.* 1985;132:125–132.

120. Wenger PN, Otten J, Breeden A, et al. Control of nosocomial transmission of MDR-TB among health care workers and HIV-infected patients. *Lancet.* 1995;345:235–240.

121. Fennelly KP, Martyny JW, Fulton KE, et al. Cough-generated Aerosols of *Mycobacterium tuberculosis*—A New Method to Study Infectiousness. *Am J Respir Crit Care Med.* 2004;169:604:609.

122. Centers for Disease Control and Prevention. *Core Curriculum on Tuberculosis—What the Clinician Should Know,* 4th ed. Atlanta, GA: Centers for Disease Control and Prevention; 2000.

123. Sepkowitz KA. Tuberculosis control in the 21st century. *Emerg Infect Dis.* 2001;7:2.

124. Enarson DA. Resistance to antituberculosis medication. Hard lessons to learn. *Arch Intern Med.* 2000;160:581–582.

125. Hopewell C. Global tuberculosis control: An optimist's perspective. *Int J Tuberc Lung Dis.* 1999;3:270–272.

126. Heldal E, Arnadottir T, Cruz JR, et al. Low failure rate in standardized retreatment of tuberculosis in Nicaragua: Patient category, drug resistance, and survival of "chronic" patients. *Int J Tuberc Lung Dis.* 2001;5:129–136.

127. Grange JM, Zumla A. Tuberculosis progress report: Paradox of the global emergency of tuberculosis. *Lancet.* 1999;353:996.

128. Iseman MD. TB elimination in the 21st century, a quixotic dream? *Int J Tuberc Lung Dis.* 2000;4:S109–S110.

129. Nolan CM. The fruits of the labor: Reinvesting the savings from good tuberculosis control in the United States. *Int J Tuberc Lung Dis.* 2000;4:191–192.

130. Snider DE Jr, Castro KG. The global threat of drug-resistant tuberculosis. *N Engl J Med.* 1998;338:1689–1690.
131. World Health Organization Tuberculosis Programme. The WHO/IUATLD global project on antituberculosis drug resistance surveillance. Antituberculosis drug resistance in the world. WHO Report 2, Geneva, Switzerland: WHO; 2000.
132. Lambregts-van Weezenbeek KSB, Reichman LB. DOTS and DOTS-plus: What's in a name? *Int J Tuberc Lung Dis.* 2000;4:995–996.
133. Centers for Disease Control and Prevention. Management of persons exposed to multidrug-resistant tuberculosis. *MMWR Morb Mortal Wkly Rep.* 1992;41:59–71.
134. Shuter J, Bellin E. Multidrug-resistant tuberculosis. *Infect Dis Clin Prac.* 1997;6:430–437.
135. Chan ED, Iseman MD. Current medical treatment for tuberculosis. *BMJ.* 2002;325:1282–1286.
136. Reichman LB, Fanning A. Drug development for tuberculosis: The missing ingredient. *Lancet.* 2001;357:9251.

8

Role of Surgery in the Diagnosis and Management of Pulmonary Tuberculosis

Wing Wai Yew
Shui Wah Chiu

INDICATIONS FOR SURGICAL MANAGEMENT IN PULMONARY TUBERCULOSIS

Before the availability of antituberculosis chemotherapy, various surgical procedures were used to collapse tuberculous cavities in the lungs in an attempt to cure the disease. These included artificial pneumothorax, phrenic nerve crush, extrapleural pneumonolysis (plombage), and thoracoplasty.[1] Apart from thoracoplasty, these surgical treatment methods have become obsolete.[2,3] Newer procedures such as lung resection have been incorporated into the surgical armamentarium. The global resurgence of tuberculosis (TB), the concomitant human immunodeficiency virus (HIV) epidemic, and the emergence of multidrug-resistant tuberculosis (MDR-TB) since the mid-1980s underscore the renewed interest of surgical management of pleuro-pulmonary TB.[4] Broadly speaking, the role of surgery therein resides in three major areas. These are (1) establishment of definitive diagnosis of TB after failed attempts with noninvasive or less invasive investigative procedures, (2) treatment of MDR-TB, tuberculous empyema, and other complications of active TB, and (3) treatment of complications that represent the sequelae of previous TB.

DIAGNOSIS OF TB BY SURGICAL METHODS

Mediastinal Lymphadenopathy

The heterogeneous appearance of the lymph nodes on chest computed tomography (CT) may suggest tuberculous adenopathy, especially when the enlarged nodes have low-attenuation centers and enhancing rims or calcification.[5] These findings are of greatest relevance in a young person in whom Mantoux test results are positive.

However, histological confirmation is often still necessary. This is particularly true for the immunocompromised hosts. Although transbronchial needle biopsy via the fiberoptic bronchoscope has yielded encouraging results,[6–8] more experience is required to delineate the efficiency of such investigative procedures. Therefore, the standard procedure for biopsy of mediastinal lymph nodes remains conventional mediastinoscopy or mediastinotomy.[9,10] The choice of the operation reflects the location of the lymph nodes. Since about a decade ago, video-assisted thoracoscopic surgery (VATS) has been used effectively in the assessment of mediastinal pathology in thoracic oncology,[11] and it is hoped that this technique will be applicable for the diagnosis of tuberculous mediastinal lymphadenopathy, though such experience is still rather limited.[12,13]

Lung Parenchymal Lesion

Histologic examination of transbronchial lung biopsy obtained via the fiberoptic bronchoscope was shown to give a diagnostic yield of smear-negative pulmonary TB in only 30–58% of cases.[14–17] This can provide the sole means of diagnosis in HIV-infected subjects and elderly patients.[18,19] Percutaneous transthoracic needle biopsy of benign lung lesions was reported in 1980s to give rather disappointing results, with a diagnostic yield of less than 20%.[20] In the decade that followed, data from several series have however provided more favorable yields of 60–90%.[15,21–25] These reported series mainly included patients with tuberculomas. Notwithstanding these encouraging results, lung resection might still be needed to furnish a definitive diagnosis in selected cases, especially when lung malignancy is a consideration.[9,26,27] The advent of VATS in the last decade has provided a new avenue for resection of solitary lung nodules of indeterminate origin.[28–31] Compared with formal thoracotomy, a reduction of duration of chest tube drainage, hospital stay, and postoperative analgesic requirement have been documented[30,31]; however, thoracoscopic wedge resection of lung has to meet the following selection criteria.[31] The nodule destined for resection should be (1) smaller than 3 cm in its maximum diameter, and (2) located in the peripheral third of the lung or close to a major fissure.

Pleural Effusion

Closed-needle biopsy of the pleura has been widely accepted as the single most useful procedure for rapid diagnosis of tuberculous pleuritis. Despite this view, the diagnostic yield still ranges from 50–80% only.[32]

VATS has provided a relatively new and also safe method for diagnosis of tuberculous pleural effusion in virtually all cases.[31,33] The low morbidity was illustrated by a mean duration of postoperative chest tube drainage of only 2 days in one study.[31] In experienced hands, medical thoracoscopy using local anesthesia and sedation can be rewarding in the diagnosis of tuberculous effusion.[11]

SURGICAL TREATMENT OF PLEUROPULMONARY TUBERCULOSIS

Preoperative Assessment and Management

Surgical treatment of pulmonary TB is usually performed on an elective rather than emergency basis.[26] Preoperative investigations, including lung function study, CT of chest, and lung ventilation-perfusion scan, have been found useful in estimating the risk, feasibility, and extent of required surgery.[2,9,26,34] Nutritional status of the patient should be optimized because this favorably influences patient outcome.[9,26] Chemotherapy has to be administered to patients prior to and after surgery.

Treatment of Active Pleuropulmonary Tuberculosis

Multidrug-Resistant Tuberculosis

There are three basic selection criteria for surgical treatment of patients with MDR-TB (Table 8-1).[34] Figure 8-1 depicts the chest radiograph of a candidate suitable for adjunctive surgical treatment. Other patient groups that could also be considered for surgical treatment include

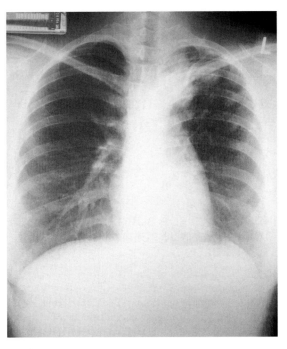

Fig. 8-1. Localized Multidrug-resistant TB for Surgical Treatment. A 24-year-old lady had MDR-TB with disease predominantly localized to the left upper lobe. The lesion harbored bacilli resistant to all first-line drugs, viz isoniazid, rifampin, streptomycin, ethambutol, and pyrazinamide, as well as some second-line drugs, viz kanamycin, ethionamide, and ofloxacin. Thus, she was offered adjunctive surgical resection with favorable outcome eventually.

Table 8-1. Selection Criteria for Surgical Treatment of Multidrug-Resistant Tuberculosis

1. Drug resistance as revealed by *in vitro* susceptibility is so severe or extensive that there is a high probability of failure or relapse with medical therapy alone.
2. Disease is sufficiently localized that the great preponderance of radiographically discernible disease could be resected with expectation of adequate cardiopulmonary capacity after surgery.
3. Drug activity is adequate to diminish the mycobacterial burden enough to facilitate healing of the bronchial stump.

Source: Adapted with permission from Iseman MD, Madsen L, Goble M, et al. Surgical intervention in the treatment of pulmonary disease caused by drug-resistant tuberculosis. *Am Rev Respir Dis.* 1990;141:623–625.

the followings[9,26,27] (1) patients with thick-walled tuberculous abscess harboring drug-susceptible bacilli initially but exhibiting poor response to medical therapy, presumably because of suboptimal drug penetration and activity in the diseased area, and (2) patients with very poor adherence who are likely to develop MDR-TB.

Patients must receive chemotherapy prior to surgery.[9,26,27,34,35] A minimum duration of 3 months has been suggested.[35] If possible, patients should preferably be rendered sputum culture-negative preoperatively.[34,35] In experienced hands, lung resection in form of lobectomy, bilobectomy, or pneumonectomy is a viable option of therapy for selected patients with MDR-TB. Table 8-2 depicts some important worldwide examples.[27,35–40] The number of patients studied in these series ranged from 19–172. The treatment success rate (with continuation of

Table 8-2. Some Experience of Surgical Treatment of Multidrug-resistant Tuberculosis Worldwide

Investigator	Patient Number	Success Rate	Operative Mortality Rate	Postoperative Complication Rate	Reference Number
Treasure et al.	19	89%	0%	9%	27
van Leuven et al.	62	75%	2%	23%	36
Kir et al.	27	96%	0%	26%	37
Sung et al.	27	96%	0%	26%	38
Pomerantz et al.	172	98%	3%	12%	35
Chiang et al.	27	92%	4%	11%	39
Park et al.	49	94%	0%	16%	40

postoperative chemotherapy) reached ≥90% in the majority of series. Operative mortality rate ranged from 0–4%, and postoperative complication rate ranged from 9–26%. Furthermore, adjunctive surgical procedures are often required. These might include (1) application of a muscle pedicle to the bronchial stump to promote healing and prevent leakage, and (2) tailored thoracoplasty to eliminate a persistent pleural space after lung resection or to close a bronchopleural fistula.[9,26,27,34,35]

The feasibility of therapeutic lung resection using the VATS approach for MDR-TB and other indications has not yet been fully established.[31] This is probably because of the anticipated difficulty during the procedure as a result of chronic inflammatory changes and distorted anatomy.[41] For patients who are frail, clinically debilitated, and harboring persistent apical cavities, and who have failed medical treatment, thoracoplasty as a definitive therapy can be considered when lung resection cannot be tolerated.[2] Other methods of collapse therapy such as plombage are also worthy of exploration.[42]

Tuberculous empyema

Tuberculous empyema generally results from the development of a bronchopleural fistula spreading the infection directly from the lung into the pleural space. Because of the presence of thick pus and encapsulation by chronic inflammatory tissue, poor drug penetration poses a genuine problem. Subtherapeutic drug levels resulting in failure of medical treatment and development of acquired drug resistance are constant threats.[43,44] Adjunctive surgical treatment has therefore proved most valuable.

Tube thoracostomy has a limited place except in patients who are not fit for surgery.[27,45] In one center, however, the experience supported the method of surgical treatment of tuberculous empyema to be guided by its stage and state of

the underlying lung.[46] Decortication has been, most of the time, the first-choice operation[9,45,47] for empyema including that following collapse therapy. This procedure can also be performed via the VATS approach.[31] Although the latter technique can result in lower morbidity, this is feasible only for an early empyema. When the decorticated lung cannot fill the pleural space subsequently, the modified Eloesser technique (window thoracostomy) has been recommended.[45,47] Then, cleaning of the empyema sac is followed by tailored thoracoplasty and myoplasty.[2,45,47] This approach of open drainage followed by the adjunctive procedures noted could be highly successful in closure of a bronchopleural fistula and elimination of any residual space; however, there is an inevitable associated loss of lung function.[47,48] A radical procedure devised by Iioka and associates[47] that involves decortication of the visceral peel and obliteration of the dead space by collapsing the parietal wall without rib resection can also be recommended for selected patients. This procedure has the advantage of being cosmetically more appealing and allows better preservation of lung function after decortication.[47] Pleuropneumonectomy or empyemectomy together with lung lesions is also an appropriate radical procedure for complicated empyema,[9,26,46,47] but cannot be performed in the elderly because of high morbidity and mortality. The success rate of surgical treatment of empyema is in general lower for tuberculous etiology compared with that of non-specific etiology.[49]

Massive Hemoptysis

Massive hemoptysis in the setting of active pulmonary TB is less common than in inactive pulmonary TB.[9] The type of surgical intervention recommended is the same and is discussed in the following part of the chapter.

Other Indications

Mediastinal lymphadenopathy is a hallmark of intrathoracic TB in children. Successful decompression of lymph nodes that are acutely or chronically compromising the tracheo-bronchial tree constitutes an important role of surgery for childhood TB.[50] In centers with expertise in thoracoscopy, emptying caseous nodes in certain sites via the said approach is feasible.[51]

Cold abscesses of chest wall are rare tuberculous locations. The general opinion is in favor of their origin from tuberculous lymph nodes in the vicinity. Adequate surgical debridement and antituberculosis drugs are required for optimal treatment and prevention of recurrence.[52]

In addition to the standard approach via thoracotomy in management of primary and secondary spontaneous pneumothorax, VATS has been found to be effective in the surgical treatment of spontaneous pneumothorax associated with TB,[53] although the technical difficulty, morbidity rate, hospital stay, and incidence of persistence and recurrence are generally greater than those associated with such method of treatment for primary spontaneous pneumothorax.

Treatment of Sequelae of Previous Pleuropulmonary Tuberculosis

Bronchostenosis

Endobronchial TB is a serious complication of pulmonary TB. The efficacy of corticosteroids in preventing stricture formation in the cicatricial phase is controversial.[54,55] Once stricture formation sets in, significant morbidity follows subsequent lobar or total lung collapse in the form of recurrent infection and deterioration of lung function. The efficacy of simple bronchial dilation by bougienage is limited.[56] Lung resection can help to control lung infection, but postoperative complications, such as bronchopleural fistula and possible loss of functioning lung parenchyma, can be problematic.[57] Bronchoplastic procedures for tuberculous bronchial stenosis[57-59] though technically demanding, have been shown to provide the best permanent solution. The reported improvement in lung function was most satisfactory.[57-59] However, anastomotic stenosis was also found to be a real problem and necessitated reoperation or bronchial dilational procedures in some patients.[57-59] In older patients and patients with substantial operative risks, alternative procedures such as balloon dilation,[60,61] insertion of silicone/expandable metallic tracheobronchial stents,[62-65] and laser photoresection therapy[66,67] can be considered. Use of cryotherapy might merit further exploration as well.[68] Balloon dilation can offer immediate symptom

relief alongside patient safety, operator familiarity, and avoidance of general anesthesia.[61] Till date, experience with these afore-mentioned techniques on treating tuberculous stricture still remains limited.

Bronchiectasis and Mycetoma

Recurrent infection and hemoptysis are the two main clinical problems pertaining to post-tuberculous bronchiectasis and mycetoma formation in the destroyed lung. Post-tuberculous lung destruction has a left-sided preponderance.[69] One example is shown in Fig. 8-2. Hemoptysis can be massive and life-threatening. When bleeding is due to active pulmonary TB, treatment by bronchial artery embolization proves effective even in severe settings.[70-73] Surgery is required rather infrequently.[72,74] However, lung resection still remains the most reliable modality of treatment of selected patients with severe or recurrent hemoptysis, despite higher associated morbidity and mortality in comparison with bronchial artery embolization.[72,74] Furthermore, treatment of posttuberculous bronchiectasis (due to inactive pulmonary TB), with or without concomitant mycetoma by lung resection on an elective basis has offered a good chance of cure.[75-77] As in

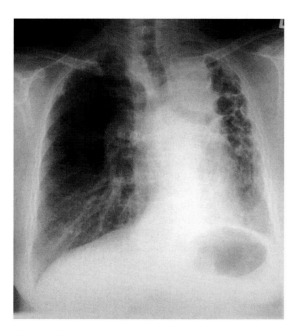

Fig. 8-2. Chest radiograph of a 79-year-old lady with extensive posttuberculous bronchiectasis affecting the left lung.

treatment of MDR-TB, ancillary procedures such as thoracoplasty might need to follow therapeutic lung resection; however, removal of a calcified broncholith representing a fistularized mediastinal lymph node via thoracotomy is followed by minimal or no lung resection.[9] It is still controversial whether antituberculosis drug "cover" is required for surgery on the diseased sites with no clinical activity. Empirical chemotherapy has been advised on the premise that manipulation and trauma might reactivate disease.[9] Longer duration of treatment had been used in patients whose resected lung yielded *Mycobacterium tuberculosis* on culture or in those in whom chemotherapy for TB was inadequately documented prior to surgery.[9] Bronchial artery embolization has the advantages of repeatability and fewer major complication rates.[70,71] Another procedure, namely intracavitary instillation of amphotericin B, can also be applied for treatment of mycetoma-related hemoptysis,[78–80] though its success rate is lower and its recurrence rate is higher, when compared with bronchial artery embolization or surgical resection.

Calcified Pyothorax

Calcified pyothorax usually refers to an old empyema resulting from previous artificial pneumothorax for treatment of TB in the predrug era.[9,47] Surgery is usually prompted by recurrent infections and the possibility of subsequent development of lymphoma.[81] The surgical approach is virtually identical to that for an active tuberculous empyema.

Postoperative Complications of Surgery

The mortality and morbidity of surgical management of pleuropulmonary TB vary somewhat among different series.[9,26,27,35–40] Some series reported minimal mortality.[27,37,38,40] Different confounding variables, such as severity of illness, and extent and nature of intervention, might be partially responsible. Mortality could be related to surgery or to the TB disease itself.[27] The former type of mortality includes complications such as bleeding, acute respiratory distress syndrome, and pulmonary embolism. The latter type includes complications such as hematogenous spread of tubercle bacilli to vital organs.

The reported morbidity is given in Table 8-3.[9,26,27,35–40] Some complications occur earlier and others later in the postoperative period. Reoperation such as reexploration for bleeding and adjunctive thoracoplasty for empyema might be required.[26,27,35–40] The comparatively favorable

Table 8-3. Complications of Surgical Treatment of Pleuropulmonary Tuberculosis

Severity	Complication
Major	Bronchopleural fistula
	Residual space problem
	Empyema
	Pneumonia
	Wound breakdown
	Bleeding
	Pulmonary hypertension
	Respiratory failure
	Recurrent laryngeal nerve palsy
	Disseminated intravascular coagulation
Minor	Pleural effusion
	Superficial wound infection
	Atelectasis
	Mental confusion
	Superficial thrombophlebitis

morbidity of VATS in selected clinical settings has been alluded to earlier.[31]

CONCLUSION

The changing status and behavior of pulmonary TB in the 1990s have generated challenges in both diagnosis and therapy. As part of the response to these challenges, new indications for surgical approaches to diagnosis and therapy are being devised to complement older, time-honored techniques. These approaches merit a thorough, ongoing assessment of their role in combating this ancient scourge of humanity.

REFERENCES

1. Shepherd MP. Plombage in the 1980s. *Thorax.* 1985;40: 328–340.
2. Hopkins RA, Ungerleider RM, Staub EW, et al. The modern use of thoracoplasty. *Ann Thorac Surg.* 1985;40:181–187.
3. Dewan RK, Singh S, Kumar A, et al. Thoracoplasty: an obsolete procedure? *Indian J Chest Dis Allied Sci.* 1999; 41:83–88.
4. Weissberg D, Refaely Y. The place of surgery in the treatment of re-emerging pulmonary tuberculosis. *Ann Ital Chir.* 2000;71:649–652.
5. Kim WS, Moon WK, Kim IO, et al. Pulmonary tuberculosis in children: evaluation with CT. *AJR Am J Roentgenol.* 1997;168:1005–1009.

6. Serda GJ, Rodriguez de Castro F, Sanchez-Alarcos JMF. Transcarinal needle aspiration in the diagnosis of mediastinal adenitis in a patient infected with the human immunodeficiency virus. *Thorax.* 1990;45:414–415.

7. Cetinkaya E, Yildiz P, Kadakal F, et al. Transbronchial needle aspiration in the diagnosis of intrathoracic lymphadenopathy. *Respiration.* 2002;69:335–338.

8. Win T, Stewart S, Groves AM, et al. The role of transbronchial needle aspiration in the diagnosis of bronchogenic carcinoma. *Respir Care.* 2003;48:602–605.

9. Mouroux J, Maalouf J, Padovani B, et al. Surgical management of pleuropulmonary tuberculosis. *J Thorac Cardiovasc Surg.* 1996;111:662–670.

10. Langdale LA, Meissner M, Nolan C, et al. Tuberculosis and the surgeon. *Am J Surg.* 1992;163:505–509.

11. Mathur PN, Loddenkemper R. Medical thoracoscopy: Role in pleural and lung diseases. *Clin Chest Med.*1995;16: 487–496.

12. De Montpreville VT, Dulmet EM, Nashashibi N. Frozen section diagnosis and surgical biopsy of lymph nodes, tumors and pseudotumors of the mediastinum. *Eur J Cardiothorac Surg.* 1998;13:190–195.

13. Chen JS, Chang YL, Cheng HL, et al. Video-assisted thoracoscopic surgery for the diagnosis of patients with hilar and mediastinal lymphadenopathy. *J Formos Med Assoc.* 2001; 100:213–216.

14. So SY, Lam WK, Yu DY. Rapid diagnosis of suspected pulmonary tuberculosis by fiberoptic bronchoscopy. *Tubercle.* 1982;63:195–200.

15. Yew WW, Kwan SY, Wong PC, et al. Percutaneous transthoracic needle biopsies in the rapid diagnosis of pulmonary tuberculosis. *Lung.* 1991;169:285–289.

16. Fujii H, Ishihara J, Fukaura A, et al. Early diagnosis of tuberculosis by fiberoptic bronchoscopy. *Tuber Lung Dis.* 1992;73:167–169.

17. Charoenratanakul S, Dejsomritrutai W, Chaiprasert A. Diagnostic role of fiberoptic bronchoscopy in suspected smear negative pulmonary tuberculosis. *Respir Med.* 1995; 89:621–623.

18. Salzman SH, Schindel ML, Aranda CP, et al. The role of bronchoscopy in the diagnosis of pulmonary tuberculosis in patients at risk for HIV infection. *Chest.* 1992;102:143–146.

19. Patel YR, Mehta JB, Harvill L, et al. Flexible bronchoscopy as a diagnostic tool in the evaluation of pulmonary tuberculosis in an elderly population. *J Am Geriatr Soc.* 1993; 41:629–632.

20. Calhoun P, Feldman PS, Armstrong P, et al. The clinical outcome of needle aspirations of the lung when cancer is not diagnosed. *Ann Thorac Surg.* 1986;41:592–596.

21. Gomes I, Trindade E, Vidal O, et al. Diagnosis of sputum smear-negative forms of pulmonary tuberculosis by transthoracic fine-needle aspiration. *Tubercle.* 1991;72: 210–213.

22. Yuan A, Yang P-C, Chang D-B, et al. Ultrasound guided aspiration biopsy for pulmonary tuberculosis with unusual radiographic appearances. *Thorax.* 1993;48:167–170.

23. Yew WW, Wong PC, Lee J, et al. Rapid diagnosis of smear-negative pulmonary tuberculosis (Letter). *Chest.* 1994;106: 326–327.

24. Das DK, Pant CS, Pant JN, et al. Transthoracic (percutaneous) fine needle aspiration cytology diagnosis of pulmonary tuberculosis. *Tuber Lung Dis.* 1995;76:84–89.

25. Ferreiros J, Bustos A, Merino S, et al. Transthoracic needle aspiration biopsy: value in the diagnosis of mycobacterial lung opacities. *J Thorac Imaging.* 1999;14:194–200.

26. Rizzi A, Rocco G, Robustellini M, et al. Results of surgical management of tuberculosis: experience in 206 patients undergoing operation. *Ann Thorac Surg.* 1995;59:896–900.

27. Treasure RL, Seaworth BJ. Current role of surgery in Mycobacterium tuberculosis. *Ann Thorac Surg.* 1995;59: 1405–1407.

28. Daniel TM, Kern JA, Tribble CG, et al. Thoracoscopic surgery for diseases of the lung and pleura: effectiveness, changing indications and limitations. *Ann Surg.* 1993;217: 566–574.

29. Rieger R, Woisetschlager R, Schinko H, et al. Thoracoscopic wedge resection of peripheral lung lesions. *Thorac Cardiovasc Surg.* 1993;41:152–155.

30. Yim AP, Ko KM, Chau WS, et al. Video-assisted thoracoscopic anatomic lung resections: The initial Hong Kong experience. *Chest.* 1996;109:13–17.

31. Yim AP. The role of video-assisted thoracoscopic surgery in the management of pulmonary tuberculosis. *Chest.* 1996; 110:829–832.

32. Yew WW, Chan CY, Kwan SY, et al. Diagnosis of tuberculous pleural effusion by the detection of tuberculostearic acid in pleural aspirates. *Chest.* 1991;100: 1261–1263.

33. Yim AP, Ho JK, Lee TW, et al. Thoracoscopic management of pleural effusions revisited. *Aust N Z J Surg.* 1995;65: 308–311.

34. Iseman MD, Madsen L, Goble M, et al. Surgical intervention in the treatment of pulmonary disease caused by drug-resistant Mycobacterium tuberculosis. *Am Rev Respir Dis.* 1990;141:623–625.

35. Pomerantz BJ, Cleveland JC Jr, Olson HK, et al. Pulmonary resection for multidrug-resistant tuberculosis. *J Thorac Cardiovasc Surg.* 2001;121:448–453.

36. van Leuven M, De Groot M, Shean KP, et al. Pulmonary resection as an adjunct in the treatment of multiple drug-resistant tuberculosis. *Ann Thorac Surg.* 1997;63: 1368–1372.

37. Kir A, Tahaoglu K, Okur E, et al. Role of surgery in multidrug-resistant tuberculosis: results of 27 cases. *Eur J Cardiothorac Surg.* 1997;12:531–534.

38. Sung SW, Kang CH, Kim YT, et al. Surgery increased the chance of cure in multidrug resistant pulmonary tuberculosis. *Eur J Cardiothorac Surg.* 1999;16:187–193.

39. Chiang CY, Yu MC, Bai KJ, et al. Pulmonary resection in the treatment of patients with pulmonary multidrug-resistant tuberculosis in Taiwan. *Int J Tuberc Lung Dis.* 2001;5:272–277.

40. Park SK, Lee CM, Heu JP, et al. A retrospective study for the outcome of pulmonary resection in 49 patients with multidrug-resistant tuberculosis. *Int J Tuberc Lung Dis.* 2002;6:143–149.

41. Massard G, Dabbagh A, Wihlm JM, et al. Pneumonectomy for chronic infection is a high-risk procedure. *Ann Thorac Surg.* 1996;62:1033–1037.

42. Jouveshomme S, Dautzenberg B, Bakdach H, et al. Preliminary results of collapse therapy with plombage for pulmonary disease caused by multidrug-resistant mycobacteria. *Am J Respir Crit Care Med.* 1998;157:1609–1615.

43. Iseman MD, Madsen LA. Chronic tuberculous empyema with bronchopleural fistula resulting in treatment failure and progressive drug resistance. *Chest.* 1991;100:124–127.

44. Elliott AM, Berning SE, Iseman MD, et al. Failure of drug penetration and acquisition of drug resistance in chronic tuberculous empyema. *Tuber Lung Dis.* 1995;76:463–467.

45. Pairolero PC, Trastek VF. Surgical management of chronic empyema: the role of thoracoplasty. *Ann Thorac Surg.* 1990;50:689–690.

46. Al-Kattan KM. Management of tuberculous empyema. *Eur J Cardiothorac Surg.* 2000;17:251–254.

47. Iioka S, Sawamura K, Mori T, et al. Surgical treatment of chronic empyema: a new one-stage operation. *J Thorac Cardiovasc Surg.* 1985;90:179–185.

48. Beard GA, Chapman CM, Sznajder JI. Late complications of thoracoplasty and plombage for tuberculosis. *Clinical Pulmonary Medicine.* 1996;3:9–14.

49. Soysal O, Topcu S, Tastepe I, et al. Childhood chronic pleural empyema: a continuing surgical challenge in developing countries. *Thorac Cardiovasc Surg.* 1998;46:357–360.

50. Hewitson JP, Von Oppell UO. Role of thoracic surgery for childhood tuberculosis. *World J Surg.* 1997;21:468–474.

51. Balquet P, Larroquet M, Philippe-Chomette P, et al. The role of surgery in tuberculosis in children. *Rev Mal Respir.* 1997;14(Suppl 5):S121–S123.

52. Faure E, Souilamas R, Riquet M, et al. Cold abscess of the chest wall: a surgical entity? *Ann Thorac Surg.* 1998;66:1174–1178.

53. Andres B, Lujan J, Robles R, et al. Treatment of primary and secondary spontaneous pneumothorax using videothoracoscopy. *Surg Laparosc Endosc.* 1998;8:108–112.

54. Ip MS, So SY, Lam WK, et al. Endobronchial tuberculosis revisited. *Chest.* 1986;89:727–730.

55. Lee JH, Park SS, Lee DH, et al. Endobronchial tuberculosis: clinical and bronchoscopic features in 121 cases. *Chest.* 1992;102:990–994.

56. Iles PB. Multiple bronchial stenoses: treatment by mechanical dilatation. *Thorax.* 1981;36:784–786.

57. Hsu HS, Hsu WH, Huang BS, et al. Surgical treatment of endobronchial tuberculosis. *Scand Cardiovasc J.* 1997;31:79–82.

58. Kato R, Kakizaki T, Hangai N, et al. Bronchoplastic procedures for tuberculous bronchial stenosis. *J Thorac Cardiovasc Surg.* 1993;106:1118–1121.

59. Nakajima Y, Shiraishi Y. Surgical treatment and endobronchial stent placement for tuberculous tracheobronchial strictures. *Kekkaku.* 1999;74:897–905.

60. Nakamura K, Terada N, Ohi M, et al. Tuberculous bronchial stenosis: treatment with balloon bronchoplasty. *AJR Am J Roentgenol.* 1991;157:1187–1188.

61. Sheski FD, Mathur PN. Long-term results of fiberoptic bronchoscopic balloon dilation in the management of benign tracheobronchial stenosis. *Chest.* 1998;114:796–800.

62. Dumon J-F. A dedicated tracheobronchial stent. *Chest.* 1990;97:328–332.

63. Tsang V, Williams AM, Goldstraw P. Sequential silastic and expandable metal stenting for tracheobronchial strictures. *Ann Thorac Surg.* 1992;53:856–860.

64. Nomori H, Kobayashi R, Kodera K, et al. Indications for an expandable metallic stent for tracheobronchial stenosis. *Ann Thorac Surg.* 1993;56:1324–1328.

65. Filler RM, Forte V, Chait P. Tracheobronchial stenting for the treatment of airway obstruction. *J Pediatr Surg.* 1998;33:304–311.

66. Dumon J-F, Reboud E, Garbe L, et al. Treatment of tracheobronchial lesions by laser photoresection. *Chest.* 1982;81:278–284.

67. Tong MC, van Hasselt CA. Tuberculous tracheobronchial strictures: clinicopathological features and management with the bronchoscopic carbon dioxide laser. *Eur Arch Otorhinolaryngol.* 1993;250:110–114.

68. Mathur PN, Wolf KM, Busk MF, et al. Fiberoptic bronchoscopic cryotherapy in the management of tracheobronchial obstruction. *Chest.* 1996;110:718–723.

69. Ashour M, Pandya L, Mezraqji A, et al. Unilateral posttuberculous lung destruction: the left bronchus syndrome. *Thorax.* 1990;45:210–212.

70. Ramakantan R, Bandekar VG, Gandhi MS, et al. Massive hemoptysis due to pulmonary tuberculosis: control with bronchial artery embolization. *Radiology.* 1996;200:691–694.

71. Mal H, Rullon I, Mellot F, et al. Immediate and long-term results of bronchial artery embolization for life-threatening hemoptysis. *Chest.* 1999;115:996–1001.

72. Lee TW, Wan S, Choy DK, et al. Management of massive hemoptysis: a single institution experience. *Ann Thorac Cardiovasc Surg.* 2000;6:232–235.

73. Yu-Tang Goh P, Lin M, Teo N, et al. Embolization for hemoptysis: a six-year review. *Cardiovasc Intervent Radiol.* 2002;25:17–25.

74. Ong TH, Eng P. Massive hemoptysis requiring intensive care. *Intensive Care Med.* 2003;29:317–320.

75. Chen JC, Chang YL, Luh SP, et al. Surgical treatment for pulmonary aspergilloma: a 28 year experience. *Thorax.* 1997;52:810–813.

76. Babatasi G, Massetti M, Chapelier A, et al. Surgical treatment of pulmonary aspergilloma: current outcome. *J Thorac Cardiovasc Surg.* 2000;119:906–912.

77. Al-Kattan K, Ashour M, Hajjar W, et al. Surgery for pulmonary aspergilloma in post-tuberculous vs

immuno-compromized patients. *Eur J Cardiothorac Surg.* 2001;20:728–733.

78. Jackson M, Flower CD, Shneerson JM. Treatment of symptomatic pulmonary aspergillomas with intracavitary instillation of amphotericin B through an indwelling catheter. *Thorax.* 1993;48:928–930.

79. Munk PL, Vellet AD, Rankin RN, et al. Intracavitary aspergilloma: Transthoracic percutaneous injection of amphotericin gelatin solution. *Radiology.* 1993;188: 821–823.

80. Ortiz de Saracho J, Perez-Rodriguez E, Zapatero J, et al. Therapeutic alternatives in complicated nonsurgical pulmonary aspergillomas. *Arch Bronconeumol.* 1995;31:83–85.

81. Nakatsuka S, Yao M, Hoshida Y, et al. Pyothorax-associated lymphoma: a review of 106 cases. *J Clin Oncol.* 2002;20: 4255–4260.

9

BCG and New Vaccines Against Tuberculosis

Jerome M. Larkin
C. Fordham von Reyn

INTRODUCTION

It has long been recognized that an effective immunization strategy would provide the optimal approach to global control of tuberculosis (TB). Several types of vaccines have been shown to reduce the risk of disease and death due to TB in humans, but only one is currently used in global immunization programs:

Mycobacterium bovis, Bacille Calmette-Guérin (BCG). BCG is an attenuated live vaccine administered at birth to children in most countries where TB is endemic. It is the most widely administered vaccine in the world, and it is estimated that more than 3 billion doses have been administered.[1] BCG has likely reduced the burden of TB in many areas, but it has numerous limitations. These limitations, together with the continuation of the global TB epidemic have made the development of a more effective vaccine against TB a major international public health priority.[2,3] Development of new vaccines has been informed by evolving data on the natural history and immunology of infection with *M. tuberculosis*, by reanalysis of the role of nontuberculous mycobacteria in protection against TB, by a clearer understanding of the limitations of BCG, by new data on prime-boost immunization strategies, and by molecular techniques that have permitted identification of immunodominant antigens of *M. tuberculosis* and new methods of antigen delivery.

GLOBAL TUBERCULOSIS IN THE BCG ERA

Approximately one third of the world's population is infected with *M. tuberculosis* and the annual incidence of new infections in the developing world is 1–5%. In 2002, there were a total of 8,797,000 new cases of active disease and 1,823,000 deaths. This compares with 8,768,000 new cases and 2,977,000 deaths in 1995. Most of these cases occur in areas of the world where BCG is now administered routinely at birth with coverage levels >80% and where 50% of more of adults have BCG scars. While the largest numbers of both cases and deaths occur in

southeast Asia, the incidence per 100,000 population for both cases (350) and deaths (83) is highest in Africa. This is attributed to the concurrent epidemic of HIV infection with an estimated 500,000 new cases of HIV-associated TB annually. The increase in new infections in Africa is also thought to be influenced by the impact of war and its attendant economic and social displacements.[4] The incidence of TB in the United States and many developed countries is low and falling, but high risk subgroups have been identified including immigrants from high prevalence countries, homeless persons, and persons in lower socioeconomic strata.[5–7]

It is estimated that each person with active disease will infect between 10 and 15 people per year. Only 20% of persons infected receive adequate treatment. Worldwide, TB is the most common cause of death from HIV. Tuberculosis accounts for 7% of all deaths annually and it is estimated by the World Bank that 26% of preventable mortality is attributable to TB. The rate of multidrug resistant TB, defined as resistance to at least both INH and rifampin, is estimated at 1–2% of all infections and is likely rising.[8]

INFECTION AND DISEASE DUE TO *M. TUBERCULOSIS*: IMPLICATIONS FOR PREVENTIVE IMMUNIZATION

Initial infection and the immune response

Humans are infected with *Mycobacterium tuberculosis* when droplet nuclei containing viable organisms are inhaled and reach the alveoli of a nonimmune host. An initial bacteremia distributes organisms to other organ sites and to other areas of the lung. A humoral and cellular host immune response ensues, which successfully contains infection for a lifetime in over 90% of infected persons (latent infection) and results in cutaneous delayed-type hypersensitivity to tuberculin. Approximately 10% of infected persons subsequently develop active disease: 5% who develop progressive primary disease within the first 2 years of infection and 5% who develop reactivation disease in the lung, or another organ site, years later.

Cellular immune responses are considered to be essential in the control of latent infection. At the time of initial infection *M. tuberculosis* is ingested by host macrophages. Subsequent activation of CD4+ T cells and secretion of interferon-γ (IFN-γ) results in macrophage activation, phagolysosomal acidification and release of reactive oxygen intermediates. Th1 cytokine responses are important as demonstrated by the fact that individuals with genetic deficiencies in IFN-γ and IL-12 receptors have enhanced susceptibility to disseminated mycobacterial disease. CD8+ cells also play an important role in containing infection through both cytokine activation and cytolytic activity and may be important in preventing reactivation disease.[3]

Tuberculosis in Children

Most new infections and approximately 25% of all cases of disease due to *M. tuberculosis* worldwide occur in children under the age of five. Among two million new cases of active disease in the world annually, approximately 650,000 occur in children.[9,10]

Congenital disease due to *M. tuberculosis* is rare owing at least in part to the fact that infection in the female genital tract often leads to infertility. When congenital disease does occur it is often the result of a primary infection in the mother just prior to or during the pregnancy. Infection occurs transplacentally. The primary focus is usually in the fetal liver with secondary dissemination.[11–14]

Most infections in neonates result from exposure of the infant to an adult with active pulmonary disease soon after delivery.[15] Both congenital and early neonatal disease are likely to present in the second or third week of life. There is often a miliary pattern on chest x-ray. Meningitis occurs in 30–50%. Mortality is very high as a result of delay in diagnosis.[16,17]

Primary infection in children is often asymptomatic. However, approximately 40% of infants and 15% of children under the age of five will develop active disease within one to two years of infection. Primary disease in young children is most likely to occur in the lung. The most common form of extrapulmonary disease in children is superficial lymphadenitis, usually developing within 6–9 months after infection. The most serious complication of TB in young children is meningitis and is usually fatal without effective therapy. It is a complication of approximately 0.3% of primary infections and usually occurs between six months and four years of age. The course of illness may be gradual or rapidly catastrophic.

The protean manifestations of childhood TB, the difficulty in diagnosis, and the high mortality are all arguments for a more effective vaccination strategy to prevent TB in children.

Tuberculosis in Older Children and Adults

After infancy and early childhood, progression of latent infection to active disease is most common in early adulthood (15–25 years of age) and in the elderly. While infection in children from age five to fourteen years may occur, this age group is relatively resistant to disease progression. Active disease, when it occurs, tends to resemble the pulmonary disease of earlier childhood.

Infection after the age of 15, progresses to active disease in 5% in the first two years and then 5% over the remainder of life. Infection after age 35 is less likely to progress to active disease[18] and has a better prognosis. New or reinfection in the elderly tends to progress to active disease in a manner similar to adolescents, and has a high mortality.[19] As in children, extrapulmonary TB may involve the gastrointestinal, genitourinary, cardiovascular, musculoskeletal, reticuloendothelial, and central nervous systems. The high rate of disease and high mortality in the elderly emphasize the importance of a vaccine strategy that produces durable immunity.

Tuberculosis in HIV Infection

The risk of progression from latent TB infection to active TB disease is altered by various interventions or underlying diseases (e.g., steroid therapy, TNF blockers, silicosis). The most significant of these is untreated HIV infection and its associated impairment of CD4 cellular immunity, which increases the likelihood of active TB to 10% per year. In most areas of the world where TB is endemic, it is the most common cause of death in persons with HIV infection.[20] In HIV-endemic countries more than 50% of new cases of TB occur in HIV-positives, and this figure reaches 70% in some regions of sub-Saharan Africa.[20] Although most of the TB risk in HIV-positives is thought to be due to an increased risk of reactivation disease, patients with HIV infection also have a substantial risk of reinfection with *M. tuberculosis*.[21] This implies that diminished CD4 function in HIV infection impairs the relative protection against reinfection that has been observed in healthy subjects. A special feature of HIV-associated TB is the high rate of bacteremia and disseminated disease, manifestations which may serve as sensitive endpoints for assessing the efficacy of new vaccines against TB.[22] Therapy with antiretroviral therapy and consequent improvement in CD4 numbers and function has been shown to reduce the risk of TB by 80%.[23] HIV infection plays a critical role in the global TB epidemic. Thus, improved immunization strategies against TB should be designed for safety and efficacy in persons with HIV infection.

IMMUNOLOGIC PROTECTION AGAINST TUBERCULOSIS

Virtually any prior mycobacterial infection that has been investigated, whether naturally-acquired or vaccine-induced, appears to produce some level of protection against subsequent disease due to TB (Table 9-1).

Table 9-1. Immunologic Protection Against Tuberculosis in Humans

---

Prior mycobacterial infection
M. tuberculosis
Nontuberculous mycobacteria

Immunization
BCG (live)
M. microti (live)
Whole cell mycobacterial vaccines (inactivated)

This suggests that protection is conferred by immune responses to common mycobacterial antigens. The magnitude of this protection is often not quantified but is not likely to be absolute. Natural infections, which confer protection against TB, include prior infection with *M. tuberculosis* itself or prior infection with nontuberculous mycobacteria. Vaccines, which have been shown to confer protection against TB in humans, include BCG, *Mycobacterium microti* and inactivated whole cell vaccines.

Natural Infection or Disease due to *M. tuberculosis*

Epidemiologic and experimental animal studies indicate that prior infection with TB confers relative protection against subsequent disease due to re-exposure.[24,25] Such protection seems to be diminished in the face of cellular immunodeficiency, exemplified by reports of reinfection with new strains of *M. tuberculosis* among patients with untreated HIV infection.[21] The fact that reinfection has now been demonstrated in some persons does not contradict the prevailing view that most healthy persons with TB have some level of protection against reinfection. Nor does it suggest that protective immunization against TB is not possible. Population based studies will be required to assess the magnitude of the protective effect of prior infection and its implications for TB vaccine development.

Natural Infection with Nontuberculous Mycobacteria

Skin test studies in humans suggest that prior infection with nontuberculous mycobacteria (NTM), acquired naturally from exposure to colonized water or soil, confers protection against TB.[26,27] Experimental data in animals demonstrate that infection with NTM protects against TB.[27,28] Infection with NTM is common in most regions of

the world,[29] and infections are usually acquired in childhood.[30] In the United States approximately 40% of adults have positive skin test reactions to NTM organisms of the *Mycobacterium avium* complex (MAC) and most of these adults have negative tuberculin skin tests.[31] Naturally acquired NTM infection may produce levels of protection against TB equal to BCG, and high rates of background infection with NTM in older children and adults have been proposed as an explanation for the lack of efficacy of BCG in some areas of the world.[27] Prior mycobacterial infection may also reduce the efficacy of BCG by limiting its replication. Recent data indicate that infection of mice with environmental mycobacteria inhibits BCG replication and induction of a BCG-mediated immune response and abrogates the protective effect of BCG after challenge with *M. tuberculosis*.[32]

Immunization with Live *Mycobacterium microti*

The Medical Research Council conducted a controlled clinical trial of another live mycobacterial vaccine, *M. microti* or the vole bacillus in 1950. A single dose of *M. microti* was found to have a 5 year efficacy of 84%, equivalent to BCG, in a trial involving 54,239 tuberculin-negative British adolescents.[33] These data indicate that antigens other than those derived from *Mycobacterium tuberculosis* or *Mycobacterium bovis*, may protect humans against TB. Immunologic techniques were not available to assess mycobacteria-specific cellular immune responses, thus the in vitro correlates of protection with this vaccine have not been identified.

Immunization with Inactivated Whole Cell Mycobacterial Vaccines

Inactivated whole cell mycobacterial vaccines were tested before the widespread acceptance of BCG and were shown to be effective in preventing TB in humans. Multiple doses were required and animal studies indicated that the inoculum had to be higher than BCG since replication did not occur after immunization.[34] Dr. Jules Freund demonstrated that a multiple dose series of heat-killed *M. tuberculosis* had an efficacy of 42% against TB in a controlled clinical trial in the 1930s.[35] More than 100,000 Italian children were immunized with inactivated whole cell mycobacterial vaccines (including a vaccine that combined *Mycobacterium tuberculosis*, *Mycobacterium bovis*, and *Mycobacterium avium*) and a study in more than 18,000 of these children showed a reduction in TB mortality from 5% in unimmunized children to 0% in immunized children.[34]

BCG VACCINE

History

Mycobacterium bovis, Bacille Calmette-Guérin (BCG) was developed by Leon Calmette and Camille Guérin, the former a physician, the latter a veterinarian. Beginning in 1902 they passed a strain of *M. bovis* isolated from a cow with tuberculous mastitis in culture every three weeks for a total of 230 passages. Beginning in 1913 they inoculated calves and then guinea pigs with the attenuated *M. bovis* strain with no evidence of infection. They subsequently challenged immunized cows with a wild-type, virulent strain of *M. bovis*, without any resulting evidence of infection. Protection was then demonstrated in pigs, rabbits and horses. In 1921 the vaccine was first administered orally to humans. The first recipient was a three-day-old infant whose mother had died of TB a few hours after giving birth. The grandmother also had advanced TB and was the child's guardian. In these circumstances, which mimic the current recommendation for use of BCG in the United States by the American Academy of Pediatrics, the infant's risk of developing infection with disseminated disease and/or meningitis was deemed to outweigh the risk of the new vaccine. The child had no ill effects from the vaccine and was raised by the grandmother without developing TB. Between 1921 and 1924 the vaccine was given to an additional 600 children without serious complications. Production and vaccination efforts were increased so that approximately 100,000 doses had been administered by 1928, including to Calmette's own grandchildren.[36] In 1928 the vaccine was certified as safe by the League of Nations. Soon thereafter, 251 children were vaccinated in Lubeck, Germany with a lot contaminated with virulent *M. tuberculosis*. This resulted in 172 deaths and at least 108 cases of active disease.[37]

BCG Strain Variation

Although all strains of BCG originated from the parent BCG strain developed by Calmette and Guérin, this strain was distributed and maintained by different laboratories and subsequently evolved into several genetically distinct strains.[38] The first randomized, controlled trial of vaccine efficacy was undertaken by Aronson et al. between 1935 and 1938.[39] In 1947 the World Health Organization (WHO) initiated a TB control program that included widespread use of BCG. From the mid-1950s until 1997 seed lots of vaccine were established under the direction of the WHO and administered by the Danish State Serum Institute in Copenhagen. Responsibility for vaccine manufacture and quality control now rests with the individual manufacturer and with regulatory agencies in the country of production. Four strains (Glaxo, Danish, Pasteur, and Tokyo) account for over 90% of vaccine currently administered.[38]

Immune Response to BCG Immunization

In Vitro Responses

Immunization with BCG induces a mild systemic infection in healthy hosts. Autopsy studies of recently immunized children who died from diverse causes indicate widespread granuloma formation.[40] The immune response to this attenuated mycobacterial infection provides cross-protection against subsequent disease due to other mycobacteria including *Mycobacterium tuberculosis, Mycobacterium leprae, Mycobacterium ulcerans,* and *Mycobacterium avium* complex.

Both humoral and cellular immune responses to mycobacteria can be detected in vaccine recipients. Antibody responses are induced to *M. tuberculosis* whole cell lysates and are of the dominant type including IgG subtypes 1, 2, and 3.[41] Cellular immune responses have been characterized both by lymphocyte proliferation assays (LPA) and by induction of interferon-gamma. LPA responses occur to both secreted antigens (e.g., Ag 85 or MTB culture filtrate) and whole cell (e.g., MTB whole cell lysate) or cell wall antigens.[42–44] IFN-γ responses are stimulated to both whole cell and secreted antigens.[42–44] BCG vaccination at birth results in a strong Th1 type immune response to mycobacterial antigens.[45] Intradermal immunization is more immunogenic than subcutaneous immunization[42] and normal or high dose BCG is more immunogenic than low dose BCG.[44] A trial underway in Cape Town, South Africa is comparing the efficacy of percutaneous and intradermal immunization with Tokyo BCG in newborns (Geiter L, personal communication). Published studies have produced conflicting results on whether BCG induces cytotoxic responses to mycobacteria-infected cells.[46,47] Cellular immune responses to *M. tuberculosis* whole cell lysate in BCG-immunized humans correlate with post immunization tuberculin skin test results.[42] Vaccine site reactions to BCG also correlate with *in vitro* cellular immune responses raising the possibility that local reactogenicity may be a necessary consequence of successful immunization against TB.[42] Although the studies cited above have characterized the human immune responses considered most relevant to protection against TB, these methods were not available during BCG efficacy trials and so we remain without a proven *in vitro* or *in vivo* surrogate for vaccine-induced protection against TB.[2]

Tuberculin Skin Test Responses

Most tuberculin negative subjects who are immunized with BCG develop a positive tuberculin skin test several weeks later. This effect wanes with time and thus it is recommended that tuberculin reactions >10 mm several years after immunization be interpreted as latent infection with *M. tuberculosis* rather than the persistent effect of BCG. However, BCG induced tuberculin reactions are often larger than 10 mm and can be boosted with repeated tuberculin skin tests. Although it is generally stated the development of BCG induced tuberculin sensitivity is not a surrogate for protective immunity against TB this issue has not been rigorously studied in a BCG efficacy trial. Further, a recent volunteer study in the United States showed a correlation between BCG-induced tuberculin sensitivity and contemporary *in vitro* markers of immune response to BCG.[48]

Efficacy of BCG against Tuberculosis

Overview

Although most countries and international bodies have concluded that childhood BCG immunization is effective in the prevention of TB, this view was never widely accepted in the United States. The controversy is based largely on the variable results of BCG efficacy trials and on different interpretations of these trials. Reexamination of the major trials in the light of contemporary knowledge of mycobacterial immunity and an improved understanding of critical trial design issues supports the view that childhood immunization is effective.

Because prior infection with either *M. tuberculosis* or NTM confers protection against TB comparable to BCG, vaccine efficacy for childhood immunization programs can only be assessed adequately by results of BCG immunization in mycobacteria-naïve hosts, i.e., newborns. Numerous older trials attempted to screen out older children and adults with pre-existing mycobacterial

immunity by using intradermal skin tests. However, contemporary *in vitro* studies demonstrate that many skin test negative subjects have demonstrable cellular and humoral immune responses to mycobacteria and are therefore not mycobacteria-naïve.[41,43,49,50] Thus, efficacy trials should be separated into those conducted in mycobacteria-naïve newborns and those conducted in mycobacteria-experienced older children and adults.

Trials in Mycobacteria-Naïve Subjects

Four prospective trials have assessed the efficacy of BCG immunization against TB in newborns and infants (Table 9-2).[39,51–54] Collectively these trials demonstrate an efficacy of 73% against disease and 87% against death. An exemplary trial in this group was the randomized, placebo controlled study conducted in Chicago in the 1930s by Rosenthal et al.[53] Participants were infants < three months of age and BCG was given by the multiple puncture technique. Approximately 1700 subjects were enrolled in each arm and followed for 12–23 years to demonstrate a vaccine efficacy of 74%. Trials in children have demonstrated that BCG is 86% effective in the prevention of bacteremic disease including disseminated TB and tuberculous meningitis.[55]

Trials in Mycobacteria-Experienced Subjects

Numerous BCG trials have been conducted in older children and adults. Each of these trials is subject to the potential bias of including subjects who have already been infected with *M. tuberculosis* (in tuberculosis-endemic regions) or nontuberculous mycobacteria (in most areas of the world). As noted above contemporary in vitro immunologic techniques suggest that the tuberculin skin tests used to screen out mycobacteria-experienced subjects may not have been sufficiently sensitive to identify pre-existing mycobacterial immunity. Thus, negative trials in

Table 9-2. Efficacy of BCG Against Tuberculosis: Trials in Newborns

Author	Year	Location	Subjects	No.	Efficacy (disease)	Efficacy (death)	Reference
Aronson	1948	Western US	Newborns (native Americans)	232	59%	100%	39
Ferguson and Simes	1949	Montreal	Newborns	609	80%	78%	51
Rosenthal et al.	1960	Chicago	Newborns	451	74%	100%	52
Rosenthal et al.	1961	Chicago	Newborns	3381	72%	84%	53
TOTAL				4673	73%	87%	

this category may simply have been an attempt to immunize persons with naturally acquired immunity.

However, some studies in older children and adults have been able to demonstrate protective efficacy. One example is the large trial conducted between 1935 and 1938 in Native Americans by Aronson and colleagues.[39] This was a randomized, placebo controlled study of persons ages 0–20 years (28% < age 5) with baseline single and extra strength tuberculin screening to exclude those with prior mycobacterial exposure. The original study enrolled 3287 participants. Evaluation at 11 years demonstrated a 75% reduction in radiographically diagnosed TB and evaluation at 20 years demonstrated an 82% reduction in mortality. Overall vaccine efficacy was 70%. A recent report provided the longest term follow-up of any BCG trial: data on 1998 of 2963 original participants showed vaccine efficacy of 52% against disease after 50–60 years.[56]

Another well-designed prospective study conducted among 14–15 year old British school children in the 1950s enrolled over 25,000 subjects in the vaccine and control groups. Baseline screening excluded children with reactions to standard or extra strength tuberculin. Vaccine efficacy was determined to be 76% over a follow up period of 15 years.[33]

Chingleput South India Trial

The South India trial deserves special consideration since it was designed as the ultimate randomized, controlled trial to investigate the protective efficacy of BCG against TB,[57,58] and is often cited to show that BCG is not effective. The study had the objectives of comparing the efficacy of different BCG strains and doses and assessing the efficacy of BCG in those with and without prior infection (determined by baseline tuberculin skin testing). In fact, the trial was principally a study of the effect of BCG in older children and adults, many of whom were already tuberculin positive, and all of whom lived in an area of high leprosy prevalence. The trial was initiated in 1968 and enrolled over 270,000 subjects, but only enrolled 1500 (0.6%) aged 0–1 month for randomization to vaccine or placebo. Surveillance for TB was based on a positive chest x-ray and these were only performed at age 5 or above; those with positive x-rays had sputum microbiology. Tuberculosis endpoints were only said to be positive if the subject had a positive sputum culture or positive AFB stain, and there were no methods for detecting extrapulmonary TB. Collectively these endpoint definitions would be very insensitive for detecting TB in children. Further, surveillance in the overall study was not uniform in all subject groups and the rate of TB endpoints was only half the predicted rate. The most reasonable interpretation of this large trial is that BCG vaccination of mycobacteria-experienced older children and adults in India did not lead to reduction in sputum culture positive pulmonary TB.

Trials in HIV Infection

No prospective trials have been conducted to assess the efficacy of childhood BCG immunization against TB in persons with HIV infection. Retrospective and case control studies have provided conflicting results with one study suggesting protection against disseminated TB[59] and another showing no protection.[60]

Interpretation of Trials

Two meta-analyses have evaluated the major prospective trials of BCG efficacy. A review by Feinstein and colleagues evaluated the methodology of eight community trials with specific reference to susceptibility bias, surveillance bias, and diagnostic testing bias; confidence intervals for reported efficacy were also calculated. The three trials judged to meet strict methodologic criteria were the North American Indian, Chicago and British trials: all showed protective efficacy (Table 9-3).[61] These three were also the only three with narrow confidence intervals; the remaining five, including those that purported to show negative efficacy, had broad confidence intervals including negative and positive efficacy. The South India trial was not interpreted to have adequate protection against surveillance bias and diagnostic testing bias.

A review by Colditz and colleagues analyzed 14 prospective trials and 12 case-control studies, including several that were considered to have inadequate methods by the Feinstein analysis.[63,64] Based on both prospective and case-control studies the Colditz reviewers concluded that the overall protective efficacy of BCG was 50% for TB disease, 71% for TB mortality and 64% for tuberculous meningitis.

Other possible explanations for observed variations in the efficacy of BCG have included differences in potency of various strains, genetic or age differences in target populations, variations in efficacy against different forms of disease, and reduced virulence of some strains of *M. tuberculosis*.[63] None of these hypotheses explain the observed variations as well as methodologic differences in the trials and/or differences in pre-existing mycobacterial immunity.

Table 9-3. Efficacy of BCG Against Tuberculosis: Trials Meeting Strict Methodologic Criteria

Author	Year	Location	Subjects	Efficacy No.	Efficacy (disease)	(death)	Reference
Stein and Aronson	1953	Western U.S.	Age 0–20 (native Americans)	3,008	67%	82%	62
Hart and Sutherland	1977	England	Newborns	26,465	76%	NA	33
Rosenthal et al.	1961	Chicago	Newborns	3,381	72%	84%	53
TOTAL				32,854	71%	82%	

Source: Studies selected based on analysis by Clemens JD, Chuong JJ and Feinstein AR. The BCG controversy: a methodological and statistical reappraisal. *JAMA* 1983;249:2362–2369.

BCG Revaccination

Although a few countries still administer booster doses of BCG to tuberculin negative children, there is no evidence that revaccination is effective. A large trial conducted in Malawi showed that BCG boosters provided additional protection against leprosy but had no protective efficacy against TB.[65] Another trial,[66] recently completed in Brazil, also failed to show benefit from a second dose of BCG (L Rodrigues, personal communication). Similar data are available from Hong Kong.[67] Since BCG must replicate to induce immunity[32] it may be that the initial dose of BCG confers a sufficient immune response against the organism to prevent replication of the subsequent dose.

Efficacy of BCG against Other Diseases

Mycobacterium leprae

Several studies have demonstrated efficacy of 50–80% against *M. leprae* and this effect may be increased with booster doses of BCG.[65]

Mycobacterium ulcerans

BCG is also approximately 50% effective in preventing Buruli ulcer disease due to *M. ulcerans*.[68] This includes protection against osteomyelitis, a major complication of *M. ulcerans* infection.[69]

Mycobacterium avium Complex (MAC)

BCG also provides cross protection against childhood lymphadenitis due to MAC.[70] Cessation of childhood BCG immunization has been associated with a marked increase in the rate of childhood adenitis due to NTM.[71]

Childhood mortality

In addition, BCG immunization of children in developing countries has been associated with reduced all cause mortality.[72,73] This effect is not specifically attributable to reduction in mortality from TB and is not fully understood.

Administration of BCG

Two BCG vaccines are licensed in the United States: Tice BCG (Organon) and Aventis Pasteur BCG. Reconstituted vaccine contains a mixture of killed and live bacilli with a range of 37,500–3,000,000 CFU (colony forming units) per dose.[74] For the Tice vaccine the manufacturer recommends that 0.2–0.3 ml of vaccine reconstituted in 1.0 ml of sterile water be administered in the lower deltoid area by the multiple puncture technique (0.2–0.3 ml reconstituted in 2 ml sterile water for infants < one year of age). For the Aventis Pasteur vaccine the manufacturer recommends intradermal administration of 0.1 ml (0.05 ml for infants < one year of age). Individual manufacturer's instructions should be consulted. Reconstituted vaccine should be refrigerated and should be protected from exposure to light. Unused vaccine should be discarded after 2–4 hours and should be treated as infectious waste as should all equipment used in vaccine preparation and manufacture. Tuberculin skin test conversion usually occurs 6–12 weeks after immunization.

Side Effects of BCG

General

Side effects of BCG immunization have been shown to be dependent on the BCG strain, dose, method of administration and recipient.[75] Neonates are more likely to experience complications than older children and adults.

Small clusters of increased complication rates have been associated with a change in the strain or method of vaccination. Among strains currently in use, the Pasteur and Danish have been associated with the highest rate of side effects. For example, lymphadenitis is more common with the Pasteur strain than with Tokyo or Brazil strains.[76] The average CFU of viable bacilli varies by vaccine strain and most products also include nonviable bacilli. Intradermal inoculation is associated with a higher rate of local reactions. The multiple puncture technique has a lower rate of local reactions but is more costly, less precise, time consuming and technically involved.[76] Adverse effects of BCG immunization are summarized in Table 9-4.

Common and Local Reactions

The most common side effect of BCG is a local reaction at the site of inoculation characterized by pain, swelling and erythema. This is seen in 95% of vaccine recipients, typically lasts several weeks and usually resolves by three months without any complication other than scar formation.[77] Approximately 75% of vaccinees will also experience some myalgia. Seventy percent will have ulceration with drainage at the vaccine site. Vaccine site abscess has been reported in 2% of recipients and regional lymphadenitis in 1–2%.[79,82]

Among those who develop adenitis, ulceration with drainage is more likely if the lesion develops rapidly and within two months after vaccination. Surgery is usually required if fistulas and drainage develop. The role of adjunctive antimycobacterial therapy remains controversial. More indolent and later developing lesions are best managed with observation alone.[83,84]

Osteomyelitis

Osteitis has been reported at a rate of between 0.01 per million vaccinees in Japan (multipuncture technique), to 300 per million in Finland (intradermal technique).[79] Treatment of osteomyelitis is with isoniazid and rifampin (BCG is resistant to pyrazinamide).

Disseminated Disease

Disseminated disease, including fatal outcome, is reported at between 0.19 and 1.56 per million vaccinees. Disseminated disease is usually associated with cellular immunodeficiency such as HIV or Severe Combined Immune Deficiency (SCID). Treatment is with isoniazid and rifampin.[85]

Current Use of BCG

Developing Countries

BCG is administered routinely to newborns in TB-endemic countries.[86] Vaccine is typically administered over the deltoid or on the forearm. Current coverage is >80% because BCG is included in list of recommended childhood immunizations by the World Health Organization.

Developed Countries

BCG is still administered universally at birth in some developed countries (to tuberculin negative adolescents in the UK), and is administered selectively in other developed countries such as Sweden where the incidence of TB is falling.[86,87] Selective immunization can strike a

Table 9-4. Adverse Effects of Parenteral BCG Immunization

Reaction Type	Incidence	Comment	Reference
Local Reaction			
-Induration, pain, erythema	95%	Essentially all vaccines	77
-Ulceration at inoculation site	70%		75,78
-Local ulceration/ adenopathy	1–2%	Varies with strain Increased in neonates	76,78
Osteomyelitis	.01–300/million	Varies with strain	78,79
Disseminated Infection	.19–1.56/million	Associated with immuno- compromised state (CGD, SCID, HIV, etc)	78,80,81

CGD = chronic granulomatous disease, SCID = severe combined immune deficiency.

reasonable balance between protection and vaccine side effects in countries where the general incidence of TB is falling but high risk groups can be identified at birth.[88]

BCG has never been administered routinely in the United States but was used more widely before the incidence of TB reached its current low levels. For example, health care workers were often immunized in the last century and many physicians and nurses who practiced in that era still have BCG scars.[89] Because US policy for the prevention of TB places a strong emphasis on tuberculin skin testing and treatment of latent infection, and because BCG may interfere with the tuberculin skin test there has been a strong reluctance to endorse BCG for all potential high risk groups. Current guidelines from American Academy of Pediatrics and from the CDC Advisory Committee on Immunization Practices are listed in Table 9-5. The guidelines recommend BCG for a child who is continually exposed to a person with untreated or ineffectively treated TB and cannot be given antituberculous therapy. Additionally, BCG is recommended for a child exposed to a person with multidrug resistant TB when the child cannot be removed from contact with the index case. These guidelines are sufficiently restrictive that BCG manufacturers have been reluctant to distribute vaccine in the US. The guidelines do not include other important other high risk groups such as homeless persons in the United States,[7] medical relief personnel from low incidence countries working in TB-endemic areas[90] and US children moving to TB endemic countries. Most current use of BCG in the United States is topical installation in the bladder for treatment of bladder cancer.[91]

NEW VACCINES AGAINST TUBERCULOSIS
Rationale

The favorable and unfavorable characteristics of BCG are summarized in Table 9-6. Based on these features there is universal agreement that an improved vaccine strategy against TB is a major international health priority. A critical shortcoming is judged to be the inconsistent efficacy of BCG and its inadequate standardization; however, as noted above, the efficacy of BCG against TB

Table 9-5. Recommendations for BCG use in the United States

Advisory Group Recommendations
1. Children with continuous exposure to a person with contagious MDR TB (and cannot be removed from contact with the person).*
2. Children with continuous exposure to a person with untreated or ineffectively treated pulmonary TB (and cannot be removed from contact with the person).*
3. Health care workers exposed to contagious MDR in settings where infection control programs have failed to prevent transmission.†

Additional Recommendations
1. Tuberculin negative homeless persons.[7]
2. Infants or tuberculin negative adults moving to TB endemic countries.
3. Health care workers (medical students, physicians, nurses etc), medical relief workers, missionaries and others traveling to conduct direct patient care activities in TB endemic countries.[90]

Contraindications
1. HIV infection or other immunodeficiency (e.g., SCID, DiGeorge Syndrome).
2. Hematologic or generalized malignancy.
3. Immune suppression (e.g., TNF blocking agents, chronic steroid therapy, alkylating agents, antimetabolites, radiation).
4. Positive tuberculin skin test or prior TB.

MDR = multiple drug resistant, SCID = Severe Combined Immune Deficiency, TNF = tumor necrosis factor
*American Academy of Pediatrics, 2003 Report of the Committee on Infectious Diseases, Elk Grove Village, IL, 2003
†Centers for Disease Control and Prevention. The role of BCG vaccine in the prevention and control of TB in the United States: a joint statement by the Advisory Committee for the Elimination of Tuberculosis and the Advisory Committee on Immunization Practices. *MMWR Morb Mortal Wkly Rep.* 1996;45:1–18.

Table 9-6. Characteristics of BCG

Favorable Characteristics

Newborn immunization reduces risk of disease and
death due to childhood TB

Newborn immunization reduces risk of miliary and
meningeal TB

Newborn immunization reduces risk of childhood
nontuberculous lymphadenitis, leprosy,
Mycobacterium ulcerans

Low cost

Unfavorable Characteristics

Limited efficacy against reactivation disease

Limited efficacy in mycobacteria-experienced children
and adults

Uncertain efficacy in HIV infection

Limited duration of efficacy

Genetic variation in licensed vaccine strains

Frequency and duration of local vaccine site reactions

Risk of BCG adenitis or osteomyelitis in healthy
recipients

Risk of disseminated BCG in HIV-infected recipients

Absence of booster effect

Requirement for parenteral immunization

Effect on skin test reaction to tuberculin

is high when administered to newborns, but its duration of protection has been found to be limited to 15 years or less in most studies and it appears to provide minimal if any protection against reactivation TB in adults. Thus, although enhanced potency is cited as one goal, a more important goal may be improving the duration of protection. For this reason many investigators are now focused on development of novel booster vaccines for BCG or on the development of prime-boost strategies using two novel vaccines. Because HIV-associated TB may now account for more than 50% of global cases of TB, another important goal is the development of a safe, effective and durable vaccine strategy for the prevention of HIV-associated TB.[92] New vaccines should be economical and single dose vaccines would be preferable to those that require multiple doses. It would also be advantageous to have a vaccine that does not require parenteral immunization.[93] Another goal has been development of a vaccine that does not interfere with the tuberculin skin test. However, newer and more specific in vitro diagnostic tests for latent TB are likely to eliminate this problem in the near future.[94]

Identification of Antigens

Many candidate antigens have been selected from extensive screening of *M. tuberculosis* antigens in animal models. Because secreted and surface-exposed antigens seem to be the first antigens encountered by the immune system, these antigens have been widely screened for immunogenicity and protection.[3] Other antigens have been selected from those to which healthy PPD positive donors (i.e., persons who have successfully contained latent infection) respond.[95] Other vaccine antigens have been selected based on older vaccines showing protective efficacy in humans, including whole cell inactivated vaccines[96] and live *M. microti*.[97] Leading subunit antigens include *M. tuberculosis* Ag85, ESAT, CFP 10 and Mtb72f.

Animal Testing

Candidate vaccines are typically screened for immunogenicity and protective efficacy in the mouse model. BCG vaccine is used as a gold standard and generally produces a 0.7 log reduction in CFU in the lung after virulent *M. tuberculosis* challenge.[98] Although this model is useful, it is not always predictive. For example, *M. microti* is effective in humans but was found to have only marginal activity in the standard mouse model.[98] The guinea pig is more sensitive than the mouse to *M. tuberculosis* infection and demonstrates higher CFUs after challenge and progressive lung pathology. In this model protection can be assessed using the endpoints of survival time and degree of lung pathology.[98] Macaques can also be used for preclinical evaluation of vaccine candidates and have several advantages over rodent models (disease more closely mimics human TB, antigen presentation and T cell receptor repertoire similar to humans, more relevant safety evaluation) but testing in primates is expensive.[99]

Human Trials

Candidate vaccines are first tested for safety in small numbers of healthy adults, subsequently in children and then in immunocompromised subjects, particularly persons with HIV infection. Safety trials are conducted in both mycobacteria-naïve and mycobacteria-experienced populations including subjects with and without prior BCG, and subjects from TB endemic regions. Safe vaccines then proceed to human immunogenicity (Phase II) testing in the same populations. Relevant immune responses are those identified above and include antibody responses, lymphocyte proliferative responses, interferon-γ responses and cytotoxic responses to mycobacterial antigens. Further Phase II studies are designed to determine optimal doses and schedules. Controlled efficacy trials (Phase III) then follow. Trials in adult subjects can be targeted to high-risk subjects to reduce sample sizes and follow up periods.[100] Household contacts of TB cases and persons with early HIV infection would both be suitable. In pediatric and HIV-positive subjects both pulmonary and bacteremic TB should be used as endpoints.[22]

Vaccine Strategies

An emerging consensus is that successful and durable immunization against TB will be best achieved with a prime boost strategy: an initial mycobacterial vaccine to prime a Th-1 response against *M. tuberculosis* and a second vaccine to boost this response.[2,101–103] Because most TB-endemic regions of the world administer BCG at birth, many investigators favor first testing new candidate vaccines as booster vaccines to those who received BCG at birth. Another strategy under development is mucosal immunization against TB. Oral, intranasal or aerosol delivery may be capable of eliciting stronger cellular immune responses against TB at the site of initial infection in the pulmonary alveolus.[93,104–106]

Candidate Vaccines

Numerous new vaccines against TB are in various stages of development and testing.[92] These include enhanced potency BCG, live-attenuated mycobacterial vaccines, live *Mycobacterium microti*, viral vaccines expressing mycobacterial antigens, subunit vaccines, DNA vaccines and inactivated vaccines. Each approach has theoretical advantages and disadvantages: enhanced potency BCG may be more immunogenic but may have high rates of reactogenicity; live mycobacterial vaccines present diverse antigens but might not replicate in patients with prior BCG; subunit vaccines may have a low rate of reactogenicity but may not contain a sufficiently diverse number of protective epitopes; live vaccines may pose safety risks in HIV infection, inactivated vaccines may be safe in HIV but require 3 or more injections. Selected vaccines with current or imminent testing in humans are listed in Table 9-7 and are described below.

Table 9-7. Selected New Candidate Vaccines Against Tuberculosis

Vaccine (Type)	Rationale/Description	Comment	Human Studies	References
rBCG30 (live)	Recombinant BCG enhanced by overexpression of Ag 85	Live vaccine with protection and survival superior to BCG alone in guinea pig model	Phase I beginning in 2004	107,108
Mycobacterium vaccae (inactivated)	NTM infection protects against TB	Protective in mouse model. Safe, immunogenic, boosts BCG responses in HIV positives	Phase II complete Phase III started 2001	96,109
ESAT/Ag 85B (subunit)	Combination of immunodominant secreted antigens	Subunit vaccine which shows protection in mouse and guinea pig models	Pending	110
Mtb 72f (fusion protein)	Combination of Mtb 39 cell membrane-associated protein and Mtb 32 modified serine protease	Fusion protein which shows protection in mouse, guinea pig and monkey models	Phase I in 2004	111
BCG > MVA-Ag 85 (live)	BCG followed by modified vaccinia virus Ankara expressing Ag 85	More effective than BCG alone in mouse model, effective in primates, induces IFN-γ response	Phase I in 2003	112

Ag = antigen, MVA = modified vaccinia virus Ankara, NTM = nontuberculous mycobacteria.

Enhanced Potency BCG

Modified BCG has been produced by introducing a plasmid coding for the 30-kDa major secretory or extracellular protein, also known as antigen 85 B. Extracellular proteins of *M. tuberculosis* are encountered by the host early in infection and are thought to be key immunoprotective molecules. Lymphocyte proliferative responses to this antigen, for example, are more common in healthy PPD positive family contacts than in household members with active TB.[113] In a guinea pig model the recombinant BCG vaccine expressing Ag 85 is associated with reduced CFUs in liver and lung and prolonged survival compared to the parent BCG strain.[108,114]

Inactivated Whole Cell Vaccines

An inactivated whole cell vaccine derived from a nontuberculous mycobacterium, *Mycobacterium vaccae*, is protective against TB in animal models and generates mycobacteria-specific cytotoxic responses.[115,116] Multiple dose controlled human studies have shown that *M. vaccae* is safe and stimulates mycobacteria-specific antibody, lymphocyte proliferative, and interferon-γ responses in both healthy and HIV-positive BCG-primed subjects.[96,109] A prime-boost efficacy trial for the prevention of bacteremic and pulmonary TB in HIV positives with childhood BCG immunization was initiated with this vaccine in Tanzania in 2001. Whole cell inactivated BCG has also been studied using intranasal administration with an adjuvant.[117]

Subunit Vaccines

Many *M. tuberculosis* derived antigens have been screened, for subunit vaccines and there have been mainly surface-exposed or secreted proteins. Promising antigens include the secreted proteins ESAT 6 and Ag 85 and the fusion protein Mtb72f. The antigens in subunit vaccines are delivered in one or more forms: protein or peptides (usually accompanied with adjuvant), DNA, or live vector. Because single protein antigens may not provide a protective immune response, multiple proteins are often combined.[3]

Prime-Boost Vaccines

The approach termed prime-boost is based on the concept of successive administration of the same mycobacterial antigen expressed by two different vaccine vectors: e.g., intramuscular immunization with naked DNA expressing the antigen followed by intradermal immunization with modified vaccinia virus expressing the same antigen.[103] This is considered *heterologous boosting* in contrast with conventional *homologous boosting* in which the antigens are delivered by the same delivery system with each dose. Phase I studies in human volunteers have confirmed the safety and immunogenicity of a prime-boost approach using BCG followed by a recombinant modified vaccinia virus Ankara expressing Ag 85A.[112]

REFERENCES

1. Fine PE, Carneiro IA, Milstien JB, et al. Issues relating to the use of BCG in immunization programs: a discussion document. Geneva, Switzerland: Department of Vaccines and Biologicals, World Health Organization; 1999:1–45.
2. Brennan MJ, Fruth U. Global forum on TB vaccine research and development. World Health Organization, June 7–8, 2001, Geneva. *Tuberculosis*. 2002;81:365–368.
3. Andersen P. TB vaccines: progress and problems. *Trends Immunol.* 2001;22:160–168.
4. Organization WH. Global Tuberculosis Control: WHO Report 2001. Geneva, Switzerland: World Health Organization; 2001.
5. Dye C, Sheele S, Doli P, et al. Global burden of tuberculosis: estimated incidence, prevalence, and mortality by country. *JAMA*. 1999;282:677–686.
6. Talbot EA, Moore M, McCray E, et al. Tuberculosis among foreign-born persons in the United States, 1993–1998. *JAMA*. 2000;284:2894–2900.
7. Brewer TF, Heymann SJ, Krumplitsh SM, et al. Strategies to decrease tuberculosis in US homeless populations. *JAMA*. 2001;286:834–842.
8. Dye C, Espinal MA, Watt CJ, et al. Worldwide incidence of multidrug-resistant tuberculosis. *J Infect Dis*. 2002; 185:1197–1202.
9. Organization WH. Global Tuberculosis Control: WHO Report 2001. Geneva, Switzerland: World Health Organization; 2001.
10. Walls T, Shingadia D. Global epidemiology of pediatric tuberculosis. *J Infect*. 2004;48:13–22.
11. Shingadia D, Novelli V. Diagnosis and treatment of tuberculosis in children. *Lancet Infect Dis*. 2003;3:624–632.
12. Nemir RL, O'Hare D. Congenital tuberculosis. Review and diagnostic guidelines. *Am J Dis Child*. 1985;139:284–287.
13. Cantwell MF, Shehab ZM, Costello AM, et al. Brief report: congenital tuberculosis. *N Engl J Med*. 1994;330:1051–1054.
14. Loeffler AM. Pediatric tuberculosis. *Semin Respir Infect*. 2003;18:272–291.
15. Starke JR. Transmission of *Mycobacterium tuberculosis* to and from children and adolescents. *Sem Ped Inf Dis*. 2001;12:115.
16. Schaaf HS, Gie RP, Beyers N, et al. Tuberculosis in infants less than 3 months of age. *Arch Dis Child*. 1993;69:371–374.

17. Jaffe IP. Tuberculous meningitis in childhood. *Lancet.* 1982;1:738.

18. Horsburgh CR, Jr. Priorities for the treatment of latent tuberculosis infection in the United States. *N Engl J Med.* 2004;350:2060–2067.

19. Stead WW, Lofgren JP, Warren E et al. Tuberculosis as an endemic and nosocomial infection among the elderly in nursing homes. *N Engl J Med.* 1985;312:1483–1487.

20. Harries AD, Hargreaves NJ, Kemp J, et al. Deaths from tuberculosis in sub-Saharan African countries with a high prevalence of HIV-1. *Lancet.* 2001;357:1519–1523.

21. Sonnenberg P, Murray J, Glynn JR et al. HIV-1 and recurrence, relapse, and reinfection of tuberculosis after cure: a cohort study in South African mineworkers. *Lancet.* 2001;358:1687–1693.

22. von Reyn CF. The significance of bacteremic tuberculosis among persons with HIV infection in developing countries. *AIDS.* 1999;13:2193–2195.

23. Badri M, Wilson W and Wood R. Effect of highly active antiretroviral therapy on incidence of tuberculosis in South Africa: a cohort study. *Lancet.* 2002;359:2059–2064.

24. Flahiff EW. The occurrence of tuberculosis in persons who failed to react to tuberculin, and in persons with positive tuberculin reactions. *Am Jour Hyg.* 1939;30:69–74.

25. Ziegler JE, Edwards ML and Smith DW. Exogenous reinfection in experimental airborne tuberculosis. *Tubercle* 1985;66:121–128.

26. Edwards LB, Palmer CE. Identification of the tuberculous-infected by skin tests. *Ann NY Acad Sci.* 1968;154:140–148.

27. Fine PEM. Variation in protection by BCG: implications of and for heterologous immunity. *Lancet.* 1995;346:1339–1345.

28. Edwards ML, Goodrich JM, Muller D, et al. Infection with *Mycobacterium avium-intracellulare* and the protective effects of Bacille Calmette-Guérin. *J Infect Dis.* 1982;145:733–741.

29. von Reyn CF, Barber TW, Arbeit RD, et al. Evidence of previous infection with *M. avium* among healthy subjects: An international study of dominant mycobacterial skin test reactions. *J Infect Dis.* 1993;168:1553–1558.

30. Fairchok MP, Rouse JH and Morris SL. Age-dependent humoral responses of children to mycobacterial antigens. *Clin Diagn Lab Immunol.* 1995;2:443–447.

31. von Reyn CF, Horsburgh CR, Olivier KN, et al. Skin test reactions to *Mycobacterium tuberculosis* purified protein derivative and *Mycobacterium avium* sensitin among health care workers and medical students in the United States. *Int J Tuber Lung Dis.* 2001;5:1122–1128.

32. Brandt L, Cunha JF, Olsen AW, et al. Failure of the *Mycobacterium bovis* BCG vaccine: some species of environmental mycobacteria block multiplication of BCG and induction of protective immunity to tuberculosis. *Infect Immun.* 2002;70:672–678.

33. Hart PD, Sutherland I. BCG and vole bacillus vaccines in the prevention of tuberculosis in adolescence and early adult life. *Brit Med J.* 1977;2:293–295.

34. Weiss DW. Vaccination against tuberculosis with non-living vaccines. I. The problem and its historical background. *Am Rev Respir Dis.* 1959;80:676–688.

35. Opie EL, Flahiff EW and Smith HH. Protective inoculation against human tuberculosis with heat-killed tubercle bacilli. *Am J Hyg.* 1939;29:155–164.

36. Sakula A. BCG: who were Calmette and Guérin? *Thorax.* 1983;38:806–812.

37. Bendiner E. Albert Calmette: a vaccine and its vindication. *Hosp Pract* (Off Ed). 1992;27:113–6, 119–122, 125 passim.

38. Behr MA. Correlation between BCG genomics and protective efficacy. *Scand J Infect Dis.* 2001;33:249–252.

39. Aronson JD. Protective vaccination against tuberculosis with special reference to BCG vaccination. *Am Rev Tuberc.* 1948;58:255–281.

40. Trevenen CL, Pagtakhan RD. Disseminated tuberculoid lesions in infants following BCG vaccination. *Can Med Assoc J.* 1982;127:502–504.

41. Hoft DF, Kemp EB, Marinaro O, et al. A double-blind, placebo-controlled study of *Mycobacterium*-specific human immune responses induced by intradermal Bacille Calmette-Guérin vaccination. *J Lab Clin Med.* 1999;134:244–252.

42. Kemp EB, Belshe RB and Hoft DF. Immune responses stimulated by percutaneous and intradermal Bacille Calmette-Guérin. *J Infect Dis.* 1996;174:113–119.

43. Ravn P, Boesen H and Pedersen BK. Human T cell responses induced by vaccination with *Mycobacterium bovis* Bacillus Calmette-Guérin. *J Immunol.* 1997;158:1949–1955.

44. Lowry PW, Ludwig TS, Adams JA, et al. Cellular immune responses to four doses of percutaneous Bacille Calmette-Guérin in healthy adults. *J Infect Dis.* 1998;178:138–146.

45. Marchant A, Goetghebuer T, Ota MO, et al. Newborns develop a Th1-type immune response to *Mycobacterium bovis* Bacillus Calmette-Guérin vaccination. *J Immunol.* 1999;163:2249–2255.

46. Hoft DF, Brown RM and Roodman ST. Bacille Calmette-Guérin vaccination induces human $\gamma\delta$ T cell responsiveness suggestive of a memory-like phenotype. *J Immunol.* 1998;161:1045–1054.

47. Ravn P, Demissie A, Eguale T, et al. Human T cell responses to the ESAT-6 antigen from *Mycobacterium tuberculosis*. *J Infect Dis.* 1999;179:637–645.

48. Hoft DF, Tennant JM. Persistence and boosting of Bacille Calmette-Guérin-induced delayed-type hypersensitivity. *Ann Intern Med.* 1999;131:32–36.

49. von Reyn CF, Williams P, Lederman H, et al. Skin test reactivity and cellular immune responses to *Mycobacterium avium* sensitin in AIDS patients at risk for disseminated *M. avium* infection. *Clin Diag Lab Immun.* 2001;8:1277–1278.

50. Vuola J, Cole B, Matee M, et al. Baseline mycobacterial immunity in HIV-positive adults entering the DARDAR TB booster vaccine trial in Tanzania [abstract 882]. In: 42nd Annual Meeting of the Infectious Disease Society of America, 2004.

51. Ferguson RG, Simes AB. BCG vaccination of infant Indians in Saskatchewan. *Tubercle.* 1949;30:5–11.

52. Rosenthal SR, Loewinsohn E, Graham ML, et al. BCG vaccination in tuberculous households. *Am Rev Respir Dis.* 1960;84:690–704.

53. Rosenthal SR, Loewinsohn E, Graham ML, et al. BCG vaccination against tuberculosis in Chicago: a twenty year study statistically analyzed. *Pediatrics.* 1961;28:622–641.

54. Levine MI, Sackett MF. Results of BCG immunization in New York City. *Am Rev Tuberc.* 1948;53:517–532.

55. Rodrigues LC, Diwan VK and Wheeler JG. Protective effect of BCG against tuberculosis meningitis and miliary tuberculosis: a meta-analysis. *Int J Epidemiol.* 1993;22: 1154–1158.

56. Aronson NE, Santosham M, Comstock GW, et al. Long-term efficacy of BCG vaccine in American Indians and Alaska Natives: A 60-year follow-up study. *JAMA.* 2004; 291:2086–2091.

57. Tuberculosis MTP. Trial of BCG vaccines in South India for tuberculosis prevention. *Indian J Med Res.* 1980;72 (Suppl):1–74.

58. Tripathy SP. Fifteen year follow-up of the Indian BCG prevention trial. In: *International Union Against Tuberculosis.* Singapore: Professional Postgraduate Services KK, 1986.

59. Marsh BJ, von Reyn CF, Edwards J, et al. The risks and benefits of childhood Bacille Calmette-Guérin immunization among adults with AIDS. *AIDS.* 1997;11:669–672.

60. Waddell RD, Lishimpi K, von Reyn CF, et al. Bacteremia due to *Mycobacterium tuberculosis* or *M. bovis*, Bacille Calmette-Guérin (BCG) among HIV-positive children and adults in children. *AIDS* 2001;15:55–60.

61. Clemens JD, Chuong JJ and Feinstein AR. The BCG controversy: a methodological and statistical reappraisal. *JAMA.* 1983;249:2362–2369.

62. Stein SC, Aronson JD. The occurrence of pulmonary lesions in BCG vaccinated and unvacccinated persons. *Am Rev Tuberc.* 1953;68:692–712.

63. Colditz GA, Berkey CS, Mosteller F, et al. The efficacy of Bacille Calmette-Guérin vaccination of newborns and infants in the prevention of tuberculosis: meta-analyses of the published literature. *Pediatrics* 1995;96:29–35.

64. Colditz GA, Brewer TF, Berkey CS, et al. Efficacy of BCG vaccine in the prevention of tuberculosis: meta-analysis of the published literature. *JAMA.* 1994;271:698–702.

65. Karonga Trial Prevention Group. Randomised controlled trial of single BCG, repeated BCG, or combined BCG and killed *Mycobacterium leprae* vaccine for prevention of leprosy and tuberculosis in Malawi. *Lancet.* 1996;348:17–24.

66. Barreto ML, Rodrigues LC, Cunha SS, et al. Design of the Brazilian BCG-REVAC trial against tuberculosis: a large, simple randomized community trial to evaluate the impact on tuberculosis of BCG revaccination at school age. *Control Clin Trials.* 2002;23:540–553.

67. Leung CC, Tam CM, Chan SL, et al. Efficacy of the BCG revaccination programme in a cohort given BCG vaccination at birth in Hong Kong. *Int J Tuberc Lung Dis.* 2001;5:717–723.

68. Smith PG, Revill WD, Lukwago E, et al. The protective effect of BCG against *Mycobacterium ulcerans* disease: a controlled trial in an endemic area of Uganda. *Trans R Soc Trop Med Hyg.* 1977;70:449–457.

69. Portaels F, Aguiar J, Debacker M, et al. *Mycobacterium bovis* BCG vaccination as prophylaxis against *Mycobacterium ulcerans* osteomyelitis in Buruli ulcer disease. *Infect Immun.* 2004;72:62–65.

70. Katila ML, Brander E and Backman A. Neonatal BCG vaccination and mycobacterial cervical adenitis in childhood. *Tubercle.* 1987;68:291–296.

71. Romanus V, Hallander HH, Wahlen P, et al. Atypical mycobacteria in extrapulmonary disease among children. Incidence in Sweden from 1969 to 1990, related to changing BCG-vaccination coverage. *Tubercle and Lung Disease.* 1995;76:300–310.

72. Roth A, Jensen H, Garly ML, et al. Low birth weight infants and Calmette-Guérin bacillus vaccination at birth: community study from Guinea-Bissau. *Pediatr Infect Dis J.* 2004;23:544–550.

73. Kristensen I, Aaby P and Jensen H. Routine vaccinations and child survival: follow up study in Guinea-Bissau, West Africa. *BMJ* 2000;321:1435–1438.

74. Smith KC, Starke JR. Bacille Calmette-Guérin Vaccine. In: Plotkin SA, Orenstein WA, eds. *Vaccines.* Philadelphia, PA: W.B. Saunders; 1999:121.

75. Lotte A, Wasz-Hockert O, Poisson N, et al. BCG complications. Estimates of the risks among vaccinated subjects and statistical analysis of their main characteristics. *Adv Tuberc Res.* 1984;21:107–193.

76. Praveen KN, Smikle MF, Prabhakar P, et al. Outbreak of Bacillus Calmette-Guérin-associated lymphadenitis and abscesses in Jamaican children. *Pediatr Infect Dis J.* 1990;9:890–893.

77. Brewer MA, Edwards KM, Palmer PS, et al. Bacille Calmette-Guérin immunization in normal healthy adults. *J Infect Dis.* 1994;170:476–479.

78. Lotte A, Wasz-Hockert O, Poisson N, et al. Second IUATLD study on complications induced by intradermal BCG-vaccination. *Bull Int Union Tuberc Lung Dis.* 1988; 63:47–59.

79. Kröger L, Korppi M, Brander E, et al. Osteitis caused by Bacille Calmette-Guérin vaccination: a retrospective analysis of 222 cases. *J Infect Dis.* 1995;172:574–576.

80. Ninane J, Grymonprez A, Burtonboy G, et al. Disseminated BCG in HIV infection. *Arch Dis Child.* 1988;63:1268–1269.

81. Besnard M, Sauvion S, Offredo C, et al. Bacillus Calmette-Guérin infection after vaccination of human immunodeficiency virus-infected children. *Pediatr Infect Dis J.* 1993;12:993–997.

82. Turnbull FM, McIntyre PB, Achat HM, et al. National study of adverse reactions after vaccination with Bacille Calmette-Guérin. *Clin Infect Dis.* 2002;34:447–453.

83. Caglayan S, Yegin O, Kayran K, et al. Is medical therapy effective for regional lymphadenitis following BCG vaccination? *Am J Dis Child.* 1987;141:1213–1214.

84. Goraya JS, Virdi VS. Treatment of Calmette-Guérin bacillus adenitis: a metaanalysis. *Pediatr Infect Dis J.* 2001;20:632–634.

85. Talbot EA, Perkins MD, Silva SFM, et al. Disseminated Bacille Calmette-Guérin disease after vaccination: case report and review. *Clin Infect Dis.* 1997;24:1139–1146.

86. Tala E, Romanus V, Tala-Heikkilä M. Bacille Calmette-Guérin vaccination in the 21st century. *Eur Respir Mon.* 1997;4:327–353.

87. Romanus V, Svensson A and Hallander HO. The impact of changing BCG coverage on tuberculosis incidence in Swedish born children between 1969 and 1989. *Tubercle.* 1992;73:150–161.

88. Hersh AL, Tala-HeikkilÑ M, Tala E, et al. A cost-effectiveness analysis of universal versus selective immunization with *Mycobacterium bovis* Bacille Calmette-Guérin in Finland. *Int J Tuberc Lung Dis.* 2002;7:22–29.

89. Abruzzi WA, Jr., Hummel RJ. Tuberculosis: incidence among American medical students, prevention and control and the use of BCG. *N Engl J Med.* 1953;248:722–729.

90. Cobelens FG, van Deutekom H, Draayer-Jansen I, et al. Risk of infection with *Mycobacterium tuberculosis* in travellers to areas of high tuberculosis endemicity. *Lancet.* 2000;356:461–465.

91. Shelley MD, Wilt TJ, Court J, et al. Intravesical Bacillus Calmette-Guérin is superior to mitomycin C in reducing tumour recurrence in high-risk superficial bladder cancer: a meta-analysis of randomized trials. *BJU Int.* 2004;93: 485–490.

92. von Reyn CF, Vuola J. New vaccines for the prevention of tuberculosis. *Clin Infect Dis.* 2002;35:465–474.

93. Hoft DF, Brown RM and Belshe RB. Mucosal Bacille Calmette-Guérin vaccination of humans inhibits delayed type hypersensitivity to purified protein derivative but induces mycobacteria-specific interferon-gamma responses. *Clin Infect Dis.* 2000;30 (Suppl 3):S217–S222.

94. Doherty TM, Demissie A, Olobo J, et al. Immune responses to the *Mycobacterium tuberculosis*-specific antigen ESAT-6 signal subclinical infection among contacts of tuberculosis patients. *J Clin Microbiol.* 2002; 40:704–706.

95. Alderson MR, Bement T, Day CH, et al. Expression cloning of an immunodominant family of *Mycobacterium tuberculosis* antigens using human CD4+ T cells. *J Exp Med.* 2000;191:551–559.

96. Waddell RD, Chintu C, Lein D, et al. Safety and immunogenicity of a 5 dose series of inactivated *Mycobacterium vaccae* vaccination for the prevention of HIV-associated tuberculosis. *Clin Infect Dis.* 2000;30 (Suppl 3): S309–S315.

97. Manabe YC, Scott CP and Bishai WR. Naturally attenuated, orally administered *Mycobacterium microti* as a tuberculosis vaccine is better than subcutaneous *Mycobacterium bovis* BCG. *Infect Immun.* 2002;70:1566–1570.

98. Orme IM, McMurray DN and Belisle JT. Tuberculosis vaccine development: recent progress. *Trends Microb.* 2001;9:115–118.

99. Langermans JA, Andersen P, van Soolingen D, et al. Divergent effect of Bacillus Calmette-Guérin (BCG) vaccination on *Mycobacterium tuberculosis* infection in highly related macaque species: implications for primate models in tuberculosis vaccine research. *Proc Natl Acad Sci U. S. A.* 2001;98:11497–11502.

100. Horsburgh CR. A large, simple trial of a tuberculosis vaccine. *Clin Infect Dis.* 2000;30 (Suppl 3):S213–S216.

101. Barker LF, Geiter L, Rayner RE, et al. TB vaccine products and regimens—can boosting improve protection? In: Fourth World Congress on Tuberculosis; 2002; Washington, D.C. Abstract 48.

102. Goonetilleke NP, McShane H, Hannan CM, et al. Enhanced immunogenicity and protective efficacy against *Mycobacterium tuberculosis* of Bacille Calmette-Guérin vaccine using mucosal administration and boosting with a recombinant modified vaccinia virus Ankara. *J Immunol.* 2003;171:1602–1609.

103. McShane H, Brookes R, Gilbert SC, et al. Enhanced immunogenicity of CD4+ T-cell responses and protective efficacy of a DNA-modified vaccinia virus Ankara prime-boost vaccination regimen for murine tuberculosis. *Infect Immun.* 2001;69:681–686.

104. Chen L, Wang J, Zganiacz A, et al. Single intranasal mucosal *Mycobacterium bovis* BCG vaccination confers improved protection compared to subcutaneous vaccination against pulmonary tuberculosis. *Infect Immun.* 2004;72:238–246.

105. Lagranderie M, Balazuc AM, Abolhassani M, et al. Development of mixed Th1/Th2 type immune response and protection against *Mycobacterium tuberculosis* after rectal or subcutaneous immunization of newborn and adult mice with *Mycobacterium bovis* BCG. *Scand J Immunol.* 2002;55:293–303.

106. Barclay WR, Busey WM, Dalgard DW, et al. Protection of monkeys against airborne tuberculosis by aerosol vaccination with Bacillus Calmette-Guérin. *Am Rev Resp Dis.* 1973;107:351–358.

107. Horwitz MA. New vaccines against tuberculosis more potent than BCG. In: Infectious Diseases Society of America 39th Annual Meeting. San Francisco; CA. 2001. Abstract S113.

108. Horwitz MA, Harth G, Dillon BJ, et al. Recombinant Bacillus Calmette-Guérin (BCG) vaccines expressing the major secretory protein induce greater protective immunity against tuberculosis than conventional BCG vaccines in a highly susceptible animal model. *PNAS.* 2000;97:13853–13858.

109. Vuola J, Ristola M, Cole B, et al. Immunogenicity of an inactivated mycobacterial vaccine for the prevention of HIV-associated tuberculosis: a randomized, controlled trial. *AIDS.* 2003;17:2351–2355.

110. Olsen AW, Pinxteren LA, Okkels LM, et al. Protection of mice with a tuberculosis subunit vaccine based on a fusion protein of Ag85B and ESAT-6. *Infect Immun.* 2001;69: 2773–2778.

111. Skeiky YA, Alderson MR, Ovendale PJ, et al. Differential immune responses and protective efficacy induced by components of a tuberculosis polyprotein vaccine, Mtb72F, delivered as naked DNA or recombinant protein. *J Immunol.* 2004;172:7618–7628.

112. McShane H, Pathan AA, Sander CR, et al. Recombinant modified vaccinia virus Ankara expressing antigen 85A boosts BCG-primed and naturally acquired anti-mycobacterial immunity in humans. *Nature Medicine 2004*. In press.

113. Torres M, Mendez-Sampeiro P, Jimenez-Zamudio L, et al. Comparison of the immune response against *Mycobacterium tuberculosis* antigens between a group of patients with active pulmonary tuberculosis and healthy household contacts. *Clin Exp Immun.* 1994;96:75–78.

114. Horwitz MA, Lee BE, Dillon BJ, et al. Protective immunity against tuberculosis induced by vaccination with major extracellular proteins of *Mycobacterium tuberculosis. Proc Nat Acad Sci USA.* 1995;92:1530–1534.

115. Abou-Zeid C, Gares M-P, Inwalrd J, et al. Induction of a type 1 immune response to a recombinant antigen from *Mycobacterium tuberculosis* expressed in *Mycobacterium vaccae. Infect Immun.* 1997;65:1856–1862.

116. Skinner MA, Yuan S, Prestidge R, et al. Immunization with heat-killed *Mycobacterium vaccae* stimulates CD8+ cytotoxic T cells specific for macrophages infected with *Mycobacterium tuberculosis. Infect Immun.* 1997;65: 4525–4530.

117. Haile M, Schroder U, Hamasur B, et al. Immunization with heat-killed *Mycobacterium bovis* Bacille Calmette-Guérin (BCG) in Eurocrine™ L3 adjuvant protects against tuberculosis. *Vaccine.* 2004;22:1498–1508.

10

Tuberculosis—A WHO Perspective

Dermot Maher
Mario C. Raviglione

INTRODUCTION

Tuberculosis (TB) was the first disease for which WHO declared a global emergency.[1] Subsequently in 2003, WHO also declared the failure to deliver antiretroviral treatment for AIDS to the millions of people who need it as a global health emergency.[2] The declaration of TB as a global emergency served to focus attention on a disease that many people thought belonged to a previous era (see Preface). In response to this emergency, WHO has promoted the strategy known as DOTS (a brand name derived from "Directly Observed Treatment, Short-course") to control TB by the interruption of transmission through the rapid identification and cure infectious cases. While the development of new tools for TB control (e.g., a more effective vaccine, better diagnostic tests, and improved preventive and therapeutic approaches) holds out the prospect of dramatic progress in TB control in the future (see Chap. 9), the DOTS strategy relies on the currently available methods of diagnosis and treatment. The strategy is effective, affordable, and adaptable in different settings; however, one of the main themes of this chapter is the importance of new approaches to improving the extent and effectiveness of implementation of the DOTS strategy. The chapter first reviews the global burden of TB, with particular focus on the epidemic in developing countries and on the increasingly important issues of human immunodeficiency virus (HIV) infection and multidrug-resistant (MDR) TB. A brief description of the DOTS strategy for TB control is followed by an update on the current status of TB control achievements worldwide. There is an account of new approaches to improving the extent and effectiveness of implementation of the DOTS strategy, with an emphasis on strengthened delivery through the full range of primary care providers, including the many nongovernmental health providers that are often not linked to national TB control programs, e.g., private practitioners, academic institutions, nongovernmental organization (NGO) services, and traditional healers. The new approaches also include a strategy of

expanded scope to counter HIV-related TB and the DOTS-Plus strategy against MDR-tuberculosis. The conclusion reviews the factors likely to determine the future prospects for global TB control.

REVIEW OF THE GLOBAL TUBERCULOSIS EPIDEMIC

Tuberculosis ranks among the top three infectious diseases as a cause of disease burden, expressed as disability-adjusted life years (DALYs).[3] The unprecedented scale of the TB epidemic and the human rights approach to TB demand effective and urgent action.[4] This section summarizes the current status of the global TB epidemic in terms of morbidity, mortality, and the economic burden of TB.

Burden of Tuberculosis Morbidity and Mortality

Tuberculosis Case Notifications

Case notification data are important because in practice it is difficult to obtain the real incidence of TB. In fact, case notifications in countries with effective TB control programmes closely approximate to the true incidence of TB. Case notifications, however, often represent only a fraction of the true incident cases, particularly in those developing countries where only a minority of the population has access to effective TB care. Alternatives to case notifications are therefore necessary for estimating incidence and the size of the TB disease burden.

Tuberculosis case notification data reflect health service coverage and the efficiency of case-finding and reporting activities of national TB control programs. Often, poor performance of these programs results in considerable under-detection and under-reporting of cases. In addition, case definitions vary among countries and case notification data often include all cases, both new and retreatment cases. Despite limitations, case notifications under stable program conditions in any country may provide useful data on the trend of incidence and for obtaining rates by age, sex, and risk group.

WHO publishes TB notifications worldwide that are provided by its member states.[5] Overall, 4.1 million cases of TB were reported in 2002. Table 10-1 shows TB case notifications and rates by WHO region.[5] Figure 10-1 shows the worldwide distribution of notified cases: 36% in the South-East Asian region, 20% in the Western Pacific region, 24% in the African region, 6% in the American region, 5% in the Eastern Mediterranean

Table 10-1. Tuberculosis Case Notifications and Rates by WHO Region, 2002

WHO Region	No. of Cases Notified (All Forms)	Rate (Per 100,000) Population
Africa	992,054	148
Americas	233,648	27
Eastern Mediterranean	188,458	37
Europe	373,497	43
South-East Asia	1,487,985	94
Western Pacific	806,112	47
Global	4,081,754	66

region, and 9% in the European region.[5] Figure 10-2 shows TB case notification rates by country in 2002.[5]

Estimated Tuberculosis Incidence and Mortality

WHO estimates of TB incidence are based on a variety of inputs, including surveys of prevalence of TB infection and disease, vital registration data, and independent assessments of quality of surveillance systems.[6,7] The global incidence rate of TB is growing at approximately 1.1% per year.[5] This overall global trend hides much faster increases in sub-Saharan Africa and in countries of the former Soviet Union, although the increase has been decelerating in both these regions since the mid 1990s.[5]

Worldwide in 2002 there were an estimated 8.8 million new cases of TB, with an incidence rate of 141/100,000.[5] Figure 10-3 shows estimated TB incidence rates by country.[5] The few countries which routinely report TB mortality are mostly in the industrialized world.[8] Global mortality must therefore be estimated, as with incidence. Table 10-2 shows a summary of TB incidence and mortality estimates in 2002 by WHO regions.[5,6] Developing countries suffer the brunt of the TB epidemic. Overall, it is estimated that 95% of the world's TB cases and 98% of the TB deaths occur in the developing world,[9] and that TB causes over 25% of avoidable adult deaths in the developing world.[10]

The global TB burden remains serious for several reasons, including the following: a) poverty and the widening gap between rich and poor in various populations (e.g., developing countries, inner city populations in developed countries); b) previous neglect of TB control (inadequate case detection, diagnosis, and cure); c) changing demography (increasing world population and changing age structure); d) the impact of the HIV pandemic.[11]

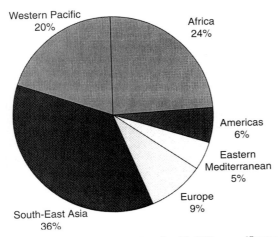

Fig. 10-1. Worldwide distribution of notified TB cases. (*Source:* Data from World Health Organization. Global Tuberculosis Control, Surveillance, Planning, Financing. WHO Report 2004 (WHO/HTM/TB/2004.331). Geneva; World Health Organization; 2004.) *Arch Intern Med.* 2003;163:2775–83. Copyright 2003, AMA. All right reserved.

HIV-Related Tuberculosis

Untreated HIV infection leads to progressive immunodeficiency and increased susceptibility to infections, including TB. Persons infected with HIV who subsequently become infected with *M. tuberculosis* have an extraordinarily high risk of developing active TB within a short period of time.[12,13] Therefore HIV infection can

TB notification rates, 2002

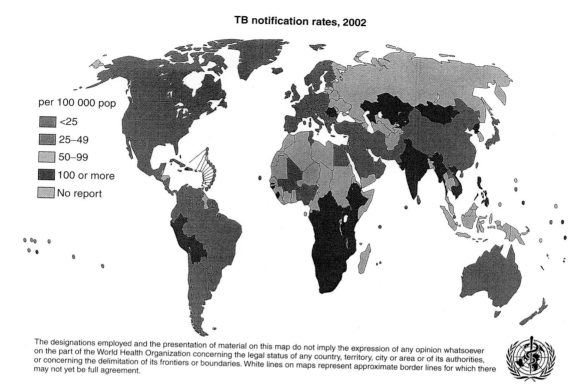

per 100 000 pop

- <25
- 25–49
- 50–99
- 100 or more
- No report

The designations employed and the presentation of material on this map do not imply the expression of any opinion whatsoever on the part of the World Health Organization concerning the legal status of any country, territory, city or area or of its authorities, or concerning the delimitation of its frontiers or boundaries. White lines on maps represent approximate border lines for which there may not yet be full agreement.

Fig. 10-2. Tuberculosis case notification rates by country in 2002.

"telescope" a TB epidemic of both susceptible and drug-resistant strains, shortening the time to generate the epidemic from years to months. The HIV pandemic has fuelled TB in populations in which there is overlap between those infected with HIV and those infected with *Mycobacterium tuberculosis.* The increased number of TB cases[6] and increased case fatality[14] pose a challenge to health services, TB control programmes, and clinicians.[15] In estimating the global burden of TB, WHO has reviewed interactions with HIV.[6] Table 10-2 shows the breakdown of global estimates in 2002 of the burden of HIV-related TB by WHO region. Thirteen percent of all new TB cases in adults aged between 15 and 49 years were attributable to HIV infection. In 2002, of the global total of 1.82 million deaths from TB, 237,000 (13%) were attributable to HIV.[6,7] Sub-Saharan Africa bears the brunt of the burden of HIV-related TB, with 506,000 incident TB cases attributable to HIV and 208,000 deaths from TB in HIV-positive individuals in 2002. In 2002 the estimated proportion of

TB cases in adults attributable to HIV infection was 11% worldwide but 31% in sub-Saharan Africa.

Multidrug-Resistant Tuberculosis

MDR-tuberculosis is a serious threat, since it arises wherever there has been, or is currently, inadequate application of antituberculosis chemotherapy. WHO and the International Union Against Tuberculosis and Lung Disease launched the Global project on Antituberculosis Drug Resistance Surveillance in 1994 to measure the prevalence and monitor the trend of antituberculosis drug resistance worldwide using a standardized methodology.[16] During the last few years, surveys in over 60 countries have identified a high prevalence of MDR-tuberculosis in specific regions of the world, e.g., Estonia, Latvia, the Oblasts of Ivanovo and Tomsk in Russia, and the provinces of Henan and Zhejiang in China.[17] More representative geographical coverage of global antituberculosis drug

Estimated TB incidence rates, 2002

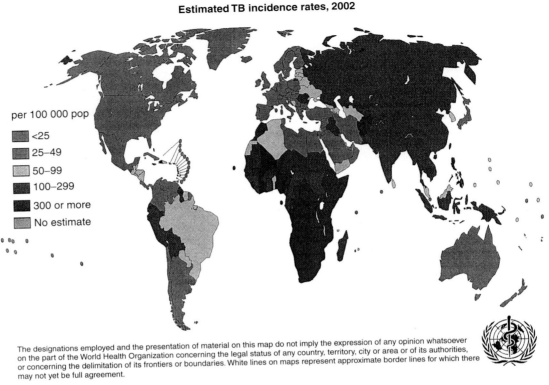

per 100 000 pop

- <25
- 25–49
- 50–99
- 100–299
- 300 or more
- No estimate

The designations employed and the presentation of material on this map do not imply the expression of any opinion whatsoever on the part of the World Health Organization concerning the legal status of any country, territory, city or area or of its authorities, or concerning the delimitation of its frontiers or boundaries. White lines on maps represent approximate border lines for which there may not yet be full agreement.

Fig. 10-3. Estimated TB incidence rates by country.

resistance surveillance, with further data from longitudinal studies, will enable more accurate and comprehensive monitoring of global trends in the spread of MDR-tuberculosis.

Economic Burden of Tuberculosis

As a fundamental human right, health deserves investment for its own sake. Tuberculosis patients and their families pay the cost of TB in suffering, pain, and grief. Tuberculosis also causes psychological and social costs. Tuberculosis patients may be rejected by family and friends or lose their jobs. In some societies, TB patients are seen as damaged for life or unmarriageable. Such discrimination can result in anxiety, depression, and reduction in the quality of life.

In addition to alleviation of these human costs, alleviation of the global economic burden of TB also represents a justification for investment in TB control from the health economics perspective.[18] The economic costs of TB fall into two categories: a) indirect costs to society, the community, and the patient's family through lost production; and b) direct costs to the health services and to

the patient and the patient's family. The largest indirect cost of TB for a patient is income lost by being too sick to work. Studies suggest that on average 3–4 months of work time are lost, resulting in average lost potential earnings of 20–30% of annual household income. For the families of those who die from the disease, there is the further loss of about 15 years of income because of the premature death of the TB sufferer. Regarding direct costs, the substantial nontreatment costs borne by TB patients and their families are often greater than the costs of treatment borne by the health sector. The case study of India provides an example of the enormous potential economic benefits of investing in TB control.[19]

Households have developed strategies for coping with the costs of illness and death that result in actual losses being less than the potential losses. However, some of these short-term strategies can have significant long-term costs. In particular, selling assets can reduce a household's economic prospects. Reducing children's food intake or removing them from school can seriously undermine their health, education, and future prospects.

Table 10-2. Summary of Tuberculosis Estimates in 2002 by WHO Region

WHO region	AFR	AMR	EMR	EUR	SEAR	WPR	Global
Population (millions)	672	857	507	877	1,591	1,718	6,222
New Cases of TB, All forms							
Number of incident cases (thousands)	2,354	370	622	472	2,890	2,090	8,798
Incidence rate (per 100,000)	350	43	123	54	182	122	141
Change in incidence rate 97–00 (% per year)	5.9	−3.6	0.7	1.9	−2.1	0.2	1.1
HIV prevalence in new adult cases (%)	37	5.5	2.8	3.6	3.5	1.2	12
Attributable to HIV (thousands)	506	11	9.8	10.0	56	14	656
Attributable to HIV (% of adult cases)	31	5.0	2.5	3.3	2.9	1.1	11
New Smear-Positive Cases of TB							
Number of incident cases (thousands)	1,000	165	279	211	1,294	939	3,888
Prevalence rate SS+ TB (per 100,000)	224	25	102	34	166	104	112
% of prevalent SS+ cases HIV+ve	6.9	1.0	0.4	0.7	0.5	0.2	1.8
Deaths from TB							
Deaths from TB (thousands)	556	53	143	73	625	373	1,823
Deaths from TB (per 100,000)	83	6.2	28	8.3	39	22	29
Deaths from TB in HIV+ve adults (thousands)	208	3.7	4.8	3.0	26	5.5	251
% of adult AIDS deaths due to TB	15	5.4	20	13	7.6	14	13
TB deaths attributable to HIV (%)	34	6.5	3.2	3.9	3.8	1.4	13

AFR = Africa, AMR = Americas, EMR = Eastern Mediterranean, EUR = Europe, SEAR = South-East Asia, WPR = Western Pacific, TB = tuberculosis, SS+ = sputum smear-positive, HIV+ve = HIV-positive, adult = 15–49 years old.
WHO African Region comprises sub-Saharan Africa and Algeria. The remaining North African countries are included in the WHO Eastern Mediterranean Region.

Source: Data from World Health Organization. Global Tuberculosis Control. Surveillance, Planning, Financing. WHO Report 2004. (WHO/HTM/TB/2004.331). Geneva: World Health Organization; 2004. Corbett EL, Watt CJ, Walker N. et al. The growing burden of tuberculosis: global trends and interactions with the HIV epidemic. *Arch Intern Med.* 2003;163:1009–1021. Copyright 2003, AMA. All right reserved.

THE DOTS STRATEGY FOR TUBERCULOSIS CONTROL AND GLOBAL TARGETS

Development of the DOTS Strategy

The overall objectives of TB control are to reduce mortality, morbidity and disease transmission, while preventing the development of antituberculosis drug resistance.[20] Tuberculosis control programs in many developing countries have failed to meet these objectives, because they have not cured enough TB patients, particularly the infectious (sputum smear-positive) patients. The main reasons for this failure are the following: 1) reliance on special TB care facilities which have failed to ensure directly observed treatment and which have not been accessible for many patients; 2) use of inadequate chemotherapy and failure to use standardized treatment regimens; 3) lack of an information management system for the rigorous evaluation of treatment outcomes of TB patients. In 1974 the WHO Expert Committee on Tuberculosis formulated four principles which are still applicable to any developing country national TB program (NTP). The NTP must be: integrated into general health services, within the Ministry of Health; country-wide; permanent, because of the nature and chronicity of the disease; adapted to the needs of the people, with TB services being as close to the community as possible.[21]

In response to the global TB emergency declared in 1993, WHO adopted the DOTS strategy for effective TB control. The organizational principles of the DOTS strategy are the following: 1) availability of a decentralized diagnostic and treatment network based on existing health facilities and integrated with Primary Health Care; 2) good program management based on accountability and supervision of health care workers; 3) an in-built system for programme evaluation. The DOTS strategy provides for the treatment of all TB patients with standardized short-course chemotherapy under proper case management conditions. Regarding smear-positive pulmonary TB cases (the source of infection), the aim is to achieve a cure rate of at least 85%. NTPs that achieve this cure rate have the following impact on TB: tuberculosis prevalence and the rate of TB transmission both decrease rapidly; TB incidence decreases gradually; there is less drug resistance (which makes future treatment of TB easier and more affordable).

The five elements of the DOTS strategy represent the policy package for delivering the essential basics of TB case finding and cure: 1) government commitment to TB control; 2) case detection through case-finding by sputum smear examination of TB suspects in general health services; 3) standardized short-course chemotherapy for, at least, all smear-positive cases, under proper case management conditions; 4) regular, uninterrupted supply of all essential drugs; 5) standardized recording and reporting system for program supervision and evaluation.[22]

Global Targets for Tuberculosis Control

World Health Assembly Targets for Tuberculosis Control

In 1991, all countries adopted a World Health Assembly (WHA) resolution setting two TB control targets for the year 2000: to detect at least 70% of all new infectious cases and to cure at least 85% of those detected.[23] These targets are based on the observation that in the absence of TB control measures (case-finding and chemotherapy), each infectious TB case causes on average about 20 new infections, out of which two new cases will arise (one infectious and one noninfectious).[24,25] The reproduction number (the number of new cases arising from a single infectious case) is therefore one for infectious cases, and the TB epidemic is in a steady state. Achievement of 85% cure rate and 70% case detection eventually reduces both the prevalence of infectious TB cases and the number of infected contacts by about 40%.[24] Since the assumption is that in the absence of control measures the prevalence of sputum smear-positive TB cases is twice the incidence of sputum smear-positive TB cases,[24] achievement of these targets will reduce the incidence of infectious cases by 20%.

The choice of these global targets in 1991 reflected the need to achieve a significant epidemiologic impact through reaching targets that field experience had demonstrated were feasible in high TB incidence countries. Reaching the 70% case detection and an 85% cure rate targets leads to an expected decline in annual TB incidence rate of 6–7% per year.[26] The NTP in Peru, for example, achieved these targets during the 1990s (and has now reached more than 90% case detection and 93% cure rate), and has seen an average annual rate of decline in TB incidence of 6.5% per year.[27] The NTP in China has reported a 32% reduction between 1991 and 2000 in the prevalence of smear-positive TB in the areas of China comprising the half of the country implementing the DOTS strategy and achieving high cure rates.[28]

It became apparent by 1998 that the year 2000 targets would not be met on time. This realization served to galvanize international activities. WHO convened an *ad hoc* Committee to review barriers to progress and make recommendations to strengthen implementation of the DOTS strategy and accelerate impact.[29] Most of those recommendations have materialized today, including the establishment of a global alliance named the Stop TB Partnership,[30] the creation of a Global Drug Facility providing quality antituberculosis drugs to countries in need,[31] a Ministerial Conference in Amsterdam in 2000 to call for renewed political commitment,[32] and a strategic focus on the 22 highest-burden countries (HBCs), responsible for 80% of estimated global TB incidence. In 2000, the WHA decided to postpone the date to achieve the targets to 2005.[33]

Millennium Development Goals

The United Nations (UN) Millennium Development Goals (MDGs) provide an unprecedented framework and opportunity for international cooperation in redressing the global injustice of poverty, including improving the health of the poor. The framework recognizes health as both a human right and a contributing factor in poverty reduction. As a disease of poverty, TB is one of the priority communicable diseases (along with HIV/AIDS and malaria) to which the MDGs apply. The MDG relevant to TB (Goal 6, Target 8) is "to have halted and begun to reverse incidence by 2015."[34] The MDG indicators 23 and 24 for measuring achievement of this goal are TB prevalence and deaths, and the proportion of cases detected and successfully treated under the DOTS strategy for TB control.[34] The epidemiologic interpretation of these goals set by politicians is to decrease TB prevalence and deaths by half by 2015, through sustained achievement of the WHA global targets of detecting 70% of new infectious cases and successfully treating 85% of those detected.

CURRENT STATUS OF TUBERCULOSIS CONTROL ACHIEVEMENTS WORLDWIDE

WHO coordinates a global TB monitoring and evaluation project in which countries report annual progress in implementing the DOTS strategy.[35] The main indicators of progress include the number of countries implementing the strategy, population coverage by the DOTS strategy, case detection, and cure rate. This section summarizes the most recent assessment of the status of global TB control as set out in the 2004 WHO Report, which reports on the cases detected in 2002 and the outcomes of treatment of patients detected in 2001.[5]

Number of Countries Implementing the DOTS Strategy

By 2002 the number of countries implementing the DOTS strategy was 180 (out of 210). Figure 10-4 shows the increasing number of countries implementing the DOTS strategy since 1992.

Population Coverage by the DOTS Strategy

Measuring population coverage by the DOTS strategy is not easy. Countries currently report DOTS coverage as the proportion of the population residing in administrative areas with in-principle access to TB care consistent with the DOTS strategy; however, in practice, the

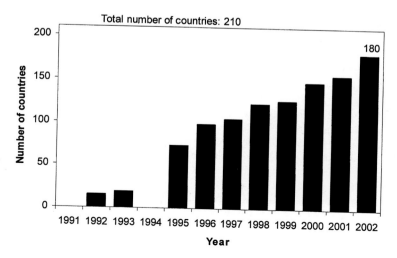

Fig. 10-4. The number of countries implementing the DOTS strategy (1992–2002). (*Source:* From World Health Organization. Global Tuberculosis Control. Surveillance, Planning, Financing, WHO Report 2004, (WHO/HTM/TB/2004.331). Geneva, Switzerland: WHO; 2004.)

proportion of the population with access to the DOTS strategy is less than this administrative figure, on account of several possible barriers to access, including geographic, financial, and cultural, within the administrative area. By the end of year 2002, 69% of the world's population lived in administrative areas of countries where the DOTS strategy was being implemented.

Cases Detected under Programs Implementing the DOTS Strategy

Through a global TB monitoring and evaluation project, countries report annually the number, and type of TB cases detected and treated, under DOTS and non-DOTS programs. In 2002 approximately 3 million patients with newly-diagnosed TB, 1.4 million of whom were smear-positive, were notified in DOTS programs. A total of 13.3 million TB patients, and 6.8 million smear-positive patients, were treated in DOTS programs between 1995 and 2002.

Regarding new cases of sputum smear-positive pulmonary TB, for the calculation of case detection rate in each country, the numerator is the number of annual cases reported under DOTS and the denominator is the estimated annual incidence of cases in that country. The numerator is derived annually from country reports of registered cases and the denominator is an estimate based on a variety of inputs, as outlined earlier. The 1.4 million smear-positive cases notified globally by DOTS programs in 2002 represent 37% of the estimated incidence, just over half way to the 70% target. The increment in smear-positive cases notified under DOTS between 2001 and 2002 (214,656) was greater than the average from 1995–2000 (134,157). Nevertheless, to reach 70% global case detection by the end of 2005, DOTS programs must detect an additional 433,000 smear-positive cases in each of the years 2003–2005.

Treatment Success

The cure rate is reported by each country through cohort analysis of treatment outcomes of registered patients. Since practice varies considerably between countries in documenting negative sputum smears on completion of treatment, for practical purposes we consider the treatment success rate (cure + treatment completion) as a proxy for cure rate. Treatment success under DOTS for the 2001 cohort was 82% on average. As in previous years, treatment success was substantially below average in the WHO African region (71%) and in Eastern Europe (70%). Low treatment success in these two regions is attributable, in part, to NTPs failing to cope with the

increased case load fuelled by HIV, and the problem of drug resistance, respectively. All indicators of treatment outcome were much worse in non-DOTS areas.

Figure 10-5 shows treatment outcomes for those patients not successfully treated in DOTS and non-DOTS areas, by WHO region, for the 2001 cohort. Note that the true outcome of treatment is unknown for a high proportion of patients in non-DOTS areas due to lack of systematic reporting when programme are weak. Regarding patients treated in DOTS areas, fatal outcomes were most common in Africa (7.2%), where a higher fraction of cases are HIV-positive, and Europe (5.9%), where a higher fraction of cases occur among the elderly. Treatment interruption (default) was most frequent in the African (10.3%), Eastern Mediterranean (7.2%), and South-East Asian (6.7%) regions. Transfer without follow-up was also especially high in Africa (6.6%). Treatment failure was conspicuously high in the European region (8.1%), mainly because of high failure rates in former Soviet countries, most likely due to high MDR-TB prevalence.

Countries Achieving the WHO Targets

Eighteen countries had reached targets for case detection and cure by the end of 2002, but Vietnam was the only HBC among them (following the departure of Peru from the list of HBCs in 2001).

NEW APPROACHES TO ACCELERATING GLOBAL TUBERCULOSIS CONTROL

Setting the Strategic Direction for Global Tuberculosis Control

The development of new tools for TB control, e.g., a more effective vaccine,[36] better diagnostic tests,[37] and improved preventive[38] and therapeutic[39] approaches, holds out the prospect of rapid progress in TB control in the future (see Chap. 20). In the meantime, the challenge in maximizing the impact of currently available methods of diagnosis and treatment lies in implementing the DOTS strategy as effectively and as widely as possible. The above assessment of progress towards the WHA 2005 targets for case detection (70%) and treatment success (85%) indicates a considerable achievement. Since the publication of the first WHO annual report on global TB control in 1995, for sputum smear-positive cases under DOTS programs the case detection rate has increased from 11–37% and the treatment success has increased from 77% to 82%[5]; however, NTPs face not only the immediate challenge of speeding up progress towards the

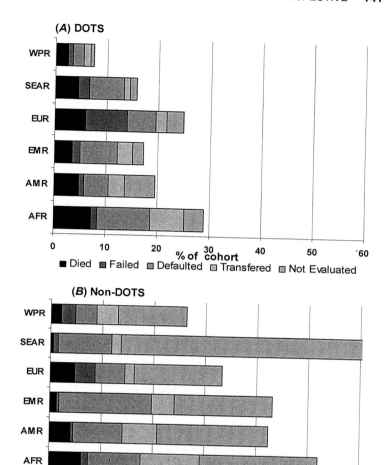

Fig. 10-5. Treatment outcomes for those patients not successfully treated in (*A*) DOTS and (*B*) non-DOTS areas, by WHO region, 2001 cohort. *Note:* That the true outcome of treatment is unknown for a high proportion of patients in non-DOTS areas.

WHA 2005 targets but also the long term challenge of sustaining achievement of those targets in order to reach the 2015 targets and thereby have an impact on the global TB burden.

In 2003 the Stop TB Partnership convened a second *ad hoc* Committee on the TB epidemic to seek solutions to constraints to more rapid progress in global TB control and to make recommendations to overcome those constraints.[40,41] The Committee reviewed the key constraints and corresponding challenges in overcoming them identified by the NTP managers of the 22 HBCs (Table 10-3).[42]

The Committee recognized that progress in TB control can contribute to improved health and poverty reduction, and depends on actions which are beyond the specifics of

TB control. In setting the mid-term strategic direction towards the 2015 targets for global TB control, the committee made recommendations under the following seven headings (many of which cut across the different aspects of TB control): 1) consolidate, sustain, and advance achievements; 2) enhance political commitment (and its translation into policy and action); 3) address the health workforce crisis; 4) strengthen health systems, particularly primary care delivery; 5) accelerate the response to the TB/HIV emergency; 6) mobilize communities and the corporate sector; 7) invest in research and development to shape the future.[41] The following section addresses three priority needs, firstly, to strengthen health systems, particularly primary care

Table 10-3. Key Constraints and Corresponding Challenges in Overcoming them

Constraints	Corresponding Challenges in Overcoming Constraints
1. Insufficient funding	How to convince governments of developing countries and development partners to mobilize more funds for TB control?
2. Lack of involvement of full range of health care providers in delivery of the DOTS strategy	How to equip national TB programmes for stewardship of TB control activities involving the full range of health providers?
3. Insufficient political commitment	How to advocate and lobby for improved political commitment?
4. Inadequate human resource capacity	How to develop increased human resource capacity?
5. Inadequate quality of implementation of the DOTS strategy	How to provide technical assistance for improved quality of implementation of the DOTS strategy?
6. Aligning TB control with health system reforms	How to maximize opportunities and minimize threats for TB control arising from health system reforms?
7. Weak primary care infrastructure	How to develop and strengthen primary care infrastructure?
8. TB epidemic exacerbated by HIV	How to improve collaboration between TB and HIV programmes in tackling HIV-related TB?
9. High prevalence of MDR-TB	How to extend the provision of better management of MDR-TB?

delivery, by engaging the full range of primary care providers in TB case finding and treatment, and secondly, to improve the response to HIV and to drug-resistant TB.

Engaging the Full Range of Primary Care Providers in Tuberculosis Control

For several reasons patients obtain TB care from health providers whose delivery of TB care is not consistent with the DOTS strategy.[43] Firstly, some countries have not adopted the DOTS strategy and most have not achieved full geographical DOTS strategy coverage.[5] Secondly, not all TB care provision through government health facilities is linked to the NTP and follows its standards. Depending on the setting, this is true for different branches of health facilities under the Ministry of Health,[44] or for other government health facilities not under the Ministry of Health, e.g., urban administrations,[45] social security schemes, prisons[46] and army health facilities. Thirdly, many nongovernmental health providers are often not linked to the NTP, e.g., private practitioners,[47] academic institutions, nongovernmental organization (NGO) services, and traditional healers.

There is increasing experience of engaging different health providers under NTP stewardship: government services, whether Ministry of Health (nationally and locally administered services) or non-Ministry of Health services (e.g., social security schemes, prisons, military), and nongovernmental services, e.g., NGOs, community groups,[48] private practitioners,[49] and employers.[50]

In practice, all health providers should either refer patients to public health facilities delivering TB care under the DOTS strategy or deliver TB care consistent with the DOTS strategy in collaboration with the NTP. In order to engage the full range of health providers, many countries will need to undertake legislative and policy reform and invest in developing human resource capacity (for strengthened NTP stewardship and service delivery). The following sections on the contributions of community groups and private practitioners provide examples of success in harnessing these primary care providers.

Community Contribution to Tuberculosis Care

Communities have played an important role in TB control in developed countries.[51] They are also essential to demand and deliver TB care under the DOTS strategy in developing countries. Two key roles include, firstly, supporting patients in adhering to and completing treatment[52] and secondly, voicing demand for quality TB-care under the DOTS strategy. There is a particular need for expansion of community contribution to TB care in sub-Saharan Africa, where pilot projects in several different settings have shown this to be feasible, effective, affordable and cost-effective in maintaining a satisfactory cure rate.[53] Local nongovernmental organizations are crucial to mobilize people and organize action.[54] In collaboration with financial and technical partners, NTPs should intensify efforts to scale up community contribution to TB care consistent with the DOTS strategy.

Private Practitioners' Contribution to Tuberculosis Care

Private practitioners are the most common first contact for a large proportion of people with TB in many countries.[55] Since private practitioners are often not linked to the NTP, they often do not follow the standard of TB care set by the NTP in line with the DOTS strategy.[55] Engaging private practitioners in the provision of TB care in line with the DOTS strategy is therefore crucial to achieving the global targets for case detection and cure.[56] WHO has promoted the contribution of private practitioners to TB care through the public-private mix (PPM) approach to implementing the DOTS strategy, reflecting the collaboration necessary between the public institution responsible for overall stewardship of national TB control programs and the private health care providers.[56] Treatment outcome has been evaluated for over 20,000 TB patients in a series of 15 PPM DOTS projects reviewed by WHO since 1999, with treatment success rates close to or above the global target of 85% in most projects that provided drugs free of charge to patients (personal communication, Mukund Uplekar).

The success factors for PPM DOTS include the following: government commitment to NTP stewardship functions, financing of PPM operations (including drug costs and cost for staff for supervision) and monitoring and evaluation activities; involvement of public sector providers, requiring coordination on government level, and collaboration between different ministries; a dialogue between all stakeholders to build trust; use of a nongovernmental organization or a medical association as a "neutral ground" to facilitate dialogue and collaboration; training of NTP staff and the private providers; improved referral and information systems; provision of drugs free of charge to patients.[57] Following the demonstration of the feasibility and effectiveness of the PPM approach in pilot projects, the main challenge is to scale up the approach so that all patients receive TB care from private practitioners in line with the DOTS strategy.

Response to HIV and to Drug-resistant Tuberculosis

Two particular challenges in TB control are the impact of HIV in fuelling the TB epidemic and drug-resistant TB. Control of HIV-related TB depends on collaboration between TB and HIV programmes in implementing the strategy of expanded scope,[58] consisting of interventions against TB and interventions against HIV (and therefore indirectly against TB), adapted in relation to a country's HIV prevalence.[59] Although progress in widespread implementation of the DOTS strategy will help to prevent the further emergence of drug-resistant TB, the adaptation of the DOTS strategy known as DOTS-Plus is necessary to control the current contribution of drug-resistant cases to the overall TB epidemic.

Strategy of Expanded Scope to Control HIV-related Tuberculosis

The interaction between TB and HIV has implications for the public health approach to TB control among HIV-infected people. Tuberculosis in high HIV prevalence populations is a leading cause of morbidity and mortality, and HIV is driving the TB epidemic in many countries (especially in sub-Saharan Africa). Tuberculosis programs and HIV programs therefore share mutual concerns: prevention of HIV should be a priority for TB control; TB care and prevention should be priority concerns of HIV/AIDS programs. The public health approach to decreasing the burden of TB/HIV requires more effective delivery of the available interventions by health service providers, with increased population coverage. Whereas previously TB programs and HIV/AIDS programs have largely pursued separate courses, they need to exploit synergies in supporting health service providers to deliver these interventions. WHO has developed a new strategic framework to decrease the burden of the intersecting epidemics of TB and HIV (TB/HIV).[58] Instead of the previous "dual strategy for a dual epidemic", the new framework represents a strengthened unified health sector strategy to control HIV-related TB as an integral part of the strategy for HIV/AIDS. The strategic goal is to reduce TB transmission, morbidity, and mortality (while minimizing the risk of antituberculosis drug resistance), as part of overall efforts to reduce HIV-related morbidity and mortality in high HIV prevalence populations.

Up to now, the efforts to control TB among HIV-infected people have mainly focused on implementing the DOTS strategy for TB control, i.e., identifying and curing infectious TB cases (among patients presenting to general health services). This targets the final step in the sequence of events by which HIV fuels TB, namely the transmission of *Mycobacterium tuberculosis* infection by infectious TB cases. The expanded scope of the new strategy for TB control in high HIV prevalence populations comprises interventions against TB (intensified case-finding and cure and TB preventive treatment) and interventions against HIV (and therefore indirectly against TB), e.g., condoms, treatment of sexually transmitted infections, safe injecting drug use, and highly active antiretroviral treatment (HAART).[58]

Several requirements are necessary for countries to strengthen general health service providers in implementing the interventions to control TB as part of the overall health service response to HIV/AIDS. These include: increased funding (by national governments and the donor community); changes in international and national policy away from specific HIV/AIDS activities towards responding to the care needs of high HIV prevalence populations through strengthened general health services; improved general health service capacity to deliver interventions (human resources, infrastructure, and commodities); operational research to find out how best HIV/AIDS and TB programs can work together to help general health services deliver an effective response; effective coordination of activities on the part of the many role players often involved.

DOTS-Plus

The management of MDR-tuberculosis is generally more complex and requires more resources than the management of drug-susceptible TB.[60,61] DOTS-Plus refers to the programmatic approach to the diagnosis and treatment of MDR-tuberculosis within the context of DOTS-programmes. Management involves the diagnosis of MDR-tuberculosis through quality-assured culture and drug susceptibility testing and treatment with second-line drugs under proper case management conditions. In response to the seriousness of MDR-tuberculosis as a global public health problem, the DOTS-Plus Working Group was established in 1999 to promote improved management of MDR-TB in resource-limited countries. The working group aims to assess the feasibility and cost-effectiveness of the use of second-line antituberculosis drugs DOTS in DOTS-Plus projects. Since 2000, the Working Group's Green Light Committee has successfully negotiated with the pharmaceutical industry substantial concessionary prices for second-line drugs that otherwise were unaffordable in poor settings. As a result, prices of the most expensive regimens have dropped by 95%.[62]

CONCLUSION—THE FUTURE

The global progress in implementation of the DOTS strategy and progress in the development of new and improved TB control tools (drugs, diagnostics and vaccines) indicate some cause for optimism regarding future prospects for controlling the global TB epidemic; however, several factors mitigate prospects for improved TB control, including the spread of HIV, war, natural disasters, demographic changes, and increasing antituberculosis drug resistance. The extent of future expansion of the HIV pandemic is uncertain, especially in South-East Asia, the WHO region of the world with the biggest share of the TB burden. If unchecked, the further spread of HIV has the potential to dramatically undermine TB control efforts in regions other than sub-Saharan Africa. As a result of war, famine and drought, large populations of displaced, malnourished people in crowded living conditions will continue to contribute to high TB case rates in particular areas.[63] Demographic changes will contribute to an increasing global TB burden. In regions with high population growth rates, children born in recent decades are now reaching the high-incidence ages for TB morbidity and mortality. Even without changes in age-specific TB incidence rates, the increasing numbers of people entering the high TB incidence age groups will result in an increase in the number of new TB cases and deaths.

Continued progress in global TB control depends on continued and increased investment in research for the development of new TB control tools and in widespread and effective implementation of the DOTS strategy, including the new approaches described above. In many developing countries, government per capita expenditure on health is falling, and expenditure on national TB control programs is often not protected. Despite a substantial increase in external aid flows for TB control to developing countries over the past decade, TB control globally is still under-funded. Through two slightly different estimation methods, both the Global DOTS Expansion Plan[64] and the Global Plan to Stop TB[65] estimated that a total of 6 billion US$ would be needed over the 5 years from 2000 to 2005 to achieve the WHA 2005 global targets. The governments of the high TB incidence countries are expected to cover an estimated 69% of the financial need. Thus the current global financial gap stands at around 300 million US$ annually. Closing this financial gap is paramount to enable universal access to effective TB care in line with the DOTS strategy and the above new approaches and thereby decrease the global burden of TB on humanity. All concerned with TB control and poverty reduction must help mobilize the political will necessary to ensure adequate funds to implement effective programs that can be sustained for several decades.

REFERENCES

1. World Health Organization. 47th World Health Assembly: Provisional agenda item 19. Tuberculosis programme - Progress report by the Director-General, (WHA47/1994/A47/12). Geneva: WHO; 1994.

2. World Health Organization. 57th World Health Assembly: Provisional agenda item 12.1. HIV/AIDS—Report by the Secretariat, (WHA57/2004/A57/4). Geneva: WHO; 2004.

3. World Health Report 2002. Reducing risks, promoting healthy life. ISBN 9241562072. Geneva: WHO; 2002.

4. World Health Organization. Guidelines for social mobilization: a human rights approach to tuberculosis, (WHO/CDS/TB/2001.9). Geneva, Switzerland: WHO; 2001.

5. World Health Organization. Global Tuberculosis Control. Surveillance, Planning, Financing, WHO Report 2004, (WHO/HTM/TB/2004.331). Geneva, Switzerland: WHO; 2004.

6. Corbett EL, Watt CJ, Walker N, et al. The growing burden of tuberculosis: global trends and interactions with the HIV epidemic. *Arch Intern Med.* 2003;163:1009–1021.

7. Dye C, Scheele S, Dolin P, et al. for the WHO Global Surveillance and Monitoring Project. Global burden of tuberculosis: estimated incidence, prevalence and mortality by country. *JAMA.* 1999;282:677–686.

8. World Health Organization. World Health Statistics Annual 1995. Geneva, Switzerland: WHO; 1996.

9. Raviglione MC, Snider D, Kochi A. Global epidemiology of tuberculosis: morbidity and mortality of a worldwide epidemic. *JAMA.* 1995;273(3):220–226.

10. Murray CJL, Styblo K, Rouillon A. Tuberculosis in developing countries: burden, intervention and cost. *Bull Int Union Tuberc Lung Dis.* 1990;65:6–24.

11. Raviglione MC, Luelmo F. Update on the global epidemiology of tuberculosis. *Curr Issues Public Health.* 1996; 2: 192–197.

12. Di Perri G, Cruciani M, Danzi MC, et al. Nosocomial epidemic of active tuberculosis among HIV-infected patients. *Lancet.* 1989;2:1502–1504.

13. Daley C, Small P, Schecter G, et al. An outbreak of tuberculosis with accelerated progression among persons with the human immunodeficiency virus: an analysis using restriction-fragment-length polymorphism. *N Engl J Med.* 1992;326:231–235.

14. Mukadi YD, Maher D, Harries A. Tuberculosis case fatality rates in high HIV prevalence populations in sub-Saharan Africa. *AIDS.* 2001;15:143–152.

15. Harries AD, Maher D. TB/HIV: A Clinical Manual, Second edition, (WHO/HTM/TB/2004.329). Geneva, Switzerland: WHO; 2004.

16. World Health Organization. Guidelines for surveillance of drug resistance in tuberculosis, (WHO/CDS/CSR/RMD/2003.3). Geneva, Switzerland:.WHO; 2003.

17. World Health Organization. Antituberculosis drug resistance in the world, Report number 2: prevalence and trends, (WHO/CDS/TB/2000.278). Geneva, Switzerland: WHO; 2000.

18. World Health Organization. The economic impacts of tuberculosis. The Stop TB Initiative 2000 Series, (WHO/CDS/STB/2000.5). Geneva, Switzerland: WHO; 2000.

19. Dholakia R. The potential economic benefits of the DOTS strategy against TB in India, (WHO/TB/96.218). Geneva, Switzerland: WHO; 1996.

20. World Health Organization: Treatment of tuberculosis. Guidelines for national programmes. Third edition, (WHO/CDS/TB/2003.313). Geneva, Switzerland: WHO; 2003.

21. WHO Expert Committee on Tuberculosis: Ninth Report: Technical report Series 552. Geneva,Switzerland: WHO; 1974.

22. World Health Organization: An expanded DOTS framework for effective tuberculosis control,(WHO/CDS/TB/2002.297). Geneva, Switzerland: WHO; 2002.

23. World Health Organization. Forty-fourth World Health Assembly. Resolutions and Decisions. Resolution WHA 44.8, (WHA44/1991/REC/1). Geneva, Switzerland: WHO; 1991.

24. Styblo K, Bumgarner JR. Tuberculosis can be controlled with existing technologies: evidence. Tuberculosis Surveillance Research Unit Progress Report. 1991;2:60–72.

25. Styblo K. Epidemiology of tuberculosis. Selected papers, vol. 24, KNCV, 1991.

26. Dye C, Williams BG. Criteria for the control of drug-resistant tuberculosis. *Proc Natl Acad Science.* 2000;97:8180–8185.

27. Suarez PG, Watt CJ, Alarcon E, et al. The dynamics of tuberculosis in response to 10 years of intensive control effort in Peru. *J Infect Dis.* 2001;184:473–478.

28. China Tuberculosis Control Collaboration. The effect of tuberculosis control in China. *Lancet.* 2004;364:417–422.

29. World Health Organization. Global Tuberculosis Programme. Report of the ad hoc Committee on the Tuberculosis Epidemic, (WHO/TB/98.245). London, 17–19 March 1998. Geneva, Switzerland: WHO;1998.

30. Stop TB Partnership. Annual Report 2001, (WHO/CDS/STB/2002.17). Geneva, Switzerland: WHO; 2001.

31. Stop TB Initiative. Global TB Drug Facility-Prospectus. (WHO/CDS/STB/2001.10a.). Geneva, Switzerland: WHO; 2001.

32. Stop TB Initiative—"Tuberculosis and Sustainable Development". Report of a Conference, Amsterdam 22–24 March 2000, (Document WHO/CDS/STB/2000.6.). Geneva, Switzerland: WHO; 2000.

33. World Health Organization. Fifty-third World Health Assembly. Resolutions and Decisions. Resolution WHA 53.1. Geneva, Switzerland: WHO; 2000.

34. United Nations Statistics Division. Millennium Indicators Database. Avaiable at: http://unstats.un.org/unsd/mi/mi_goals.asp. Accessed August 4, 2004.

35. Raviglione MC, Dye C, Schmidt S, et al. Assessment of worldwide tuberculosis control. *Lancet.* 1997;350:624–629.

36. Young DB. Current tuberculosis vaccine development. *Clin Infect Dis.* 2000;30(Suppl. 3):S254–S256.

37. Perkins MD. New diagnostics for tuberculosis. *Int J Tuberc Lung Dis.* 2000;4(12):S182–S188.

38. Centers for Disease Control and Prevention. Prevention and treatment of tuberculosis among patients infected with human immunodeficiency virus: principles of therapy and revised recommendations. *MMWR Morb Mortal Wkly Rep.* 1998;47(No. RR-20):1–58.

39. Barry CE III, Slayden RA, Sampson AE, et al. Use of genomics and combinatorial chemistry in the development of new antimycobacterial drugs. *Biochem Pharmacol.* 2000; 59:221–231.

40. World Health Organization. Background document prepared for the meeting of the second ad hoc Committee on the TB epidemic, (WHO/HTM/STB/2004.27). Geneva, Switzerland: WHO; 2004.

41. World Health Organization. Report on the meeting of the second ad hoc Committee on the TB epidemic, (WHO/HTM/STB/2004.28.). Montreux, Switzerland: 18–19 September 2003. Recommendations to Stop TB partners. Geneva, Switzerland: WHO; 2004.

42. World Health Organization. Report on DOTS Expansion Working Group meeting, (Internal document). Montreal, Canada: WHO: October 2002.

43. Elzinga G, Raviglione MC, Maher D. Scale up: meeting targets in global tuberculosis control. *Lancet.* 2004;363: 814–819.

44. Chen X, Zhao F, Duanmu H et al. The DOTS strategy in China: results and lessons after 10 years. *Bull World Health Organ.* 2002;80:430–436.

45. Chakraborty AK, Rangan S, Uplekar M, eds. *Urban tuberculosis control: problems and prospects.* Bombay, India: The Foundation for Research in Community Health; 1995.

46. Coninx R, Maher D, Reyes H, et al. Tuberculosis in prisons in countries with high prevalence. *Br Med J.* 2000;320: 440–442.

47. Uplekar M, Pathania V, Raviglione M. Private practitioners and public health: weak links in tuberculosis control. *Lancet.* 2001;358:912–916.

48. Maher D. The role of the community in the control of tuberculosis. *Tuberculosis.* 2003;83:177–182.

49. Murthy KJR, Frieden TR, Yazdani A, et al. Public-private partnership in tuberculosis control: experience in Hyderabad, India. *Int J Tuberc Lung Dis.* 2001;5:354–359.

50. World Health Organization and International Labour Office. Guidelines for workplace TB control activities, (WHO/CDS/TB/2003.323). Geneva, Switzerland: WHO; 2003.

51. Broekmans JF, Migliori GB, Rieder HL et al. European framework for tuberculosis control and elimination in countries with a low incidence. *Eur Respir J.* 2002;19: 765–775.

52. Maher D, Gorkom JLC van, et al. Community contribution to tuberculosis care in high tuberculosis prevalence countries:

past, present and future. *Int J Tuberc Lung Dis.* 1999;3: 762–768.

53. World Health Organization. Community contribution to TB care: practice and policy, (WHO/CDS/TB/2003.312). Geneva, Switzerland: WHO; 2003.

54. World Health Organization, Regional Office for South-East Asia. NGOs and TB control. Principles and examples for organizations joining the fight against TB, (SEA/TB/213)., New Delhi, India: World Health Organization Regional Office for South-East Asia; 1999.

55. Uplekar M, Juvekar S, Morankar S, et al. Tuberculosis patients and practitioners in private clinics in India. *Int T Tuberc Lung Dis.* 1998;2(4):324–329.

56. Uplekar M. Involving private health care providers in delivery of TB care. *Tuberculosis.* 2003;83:156–164.

57. Lönnroth K, Uplekar M, Arora VK, et al. Public-Private Mix for Improved TB Control—what makes it work? *Bull. World Health Organization.* In press.

58. World Health Organization. A strategic framework to decrease the burden of TB/HIV, (WHO/CDS/TB/2002.296). Geneva, Switzerland: WHO; 2002.

59. World Health Organization. Interim policy on collaborative TB/HIV activities, (WHO/HTM/TB/2004.330). Geneva, Switzerland: WHO; 2004.

60. World Health Organization. Guidelines for the management of drug-resistant tuberculosis, (WHO/TB/96.201). Geneva, Switzerland: WHO; 1996.

61. World Health Organization. Guidelines for establishing DOTS-Plus pilot projects for the management of multidrug-resistant tuberculosis, (WHO/CDS/TB/2000.279) Geneva, Switzerland: WHO; 2000.

62. Gupta R, Kim JY, Espinal MA et al. Responding to market failure in tuberculosis control. *Science.* 2001;293:1049–1051.

63. World Health Organization and the Office of the United Nations High Commissioner for Refugees. Tuberculosis control in refugee situations: an inter-agency field manual, (WHO/TB/97.221). Geneva, Switzerland: WHO; 1997.

64. World Health Organization. Global DOTS Expansion Plan - Progress in TB control in high burden countries 2001, 1 year after the Amsterdam Ministerial Conference, (WHO/CDS/STB/2001.11). Geneva, Switzerland: WHO; 2001.

65. Stop TB Partnership. The Global Plan to Stop Tuberculosis, (WHO/CDS/STB/2001.16). Geneva, Switzerland: WHO; 2002.

11

Tuberculosis in Enclosed Populations

Sorana Segal-Maurer

INTRODUCTION

The past two decades saw a dramatic resurgence in cases of tuberculosis (TB), especially among those of nosocomial and multidrug-resistant tuberculosis (MDR-TB). Numerous reports from congregate settings emphasized the increased transmission of TB in closed or indoor environments, particularly among high-risk hosts. Factors that contributed to outbreaks of TB in hospitals, prisons, shelters, and nursing homes in the early 1990s included: the decay in public health infrastructure, the rise of human immunodeficiency virus (HIV) coinfection, the increase in the number of homeless and destitute persons, health care workers' decreased vigilance, and few existing adequate isolation facilities. The resulting major public health efforts to upgrade facilities in hospitals and jails, provide directly observed treatment, and educate healthcare workers (HCWs) and the public all led to a dramatic decrease in new TB cases (especially MDR-TB) from 10.5 cases per 100,000 in 1992 to 5.8 cases per 100,000 in 2000.[1,2] Over the last several years we have seen a decrease in nosocomial transmission of TB and MDR-TB but an increase in reactivation with transmission among immigrants and residents of homeless shelters.[3–5] This chapter reviews the factors involved in the transmission of TB in congregate facilities and the methods employed for curtailment and prevention. Focus is on implementation of infection-control practices for the safety of residents, patients, and health care workers.

EPIDEMIOLOGY OF TRANSMISSION

The probability of transmission of *Mycobacterium tuberculosis* (MTB) depends on the concentration of infectious droplet nuclei in the air, the duration of exposure to these particles, and the closeness of contact with infectious persons.[6] Infection is best transmitted in overcrowded environments and confined spaces where poor ventilation or air recirculation permits the accumulation of infectious particles.[6,7] Numerous non-health-care, community-based outbreaks of TB have been described in schools, offices and work places, neighborhood bars, ships, and airplanes.[8] All outbreaks were characterized by highly infectious persons in proximity to susceptible persons in enclosed, poorly ventilated environments.

OUTBREAKS OF THE 1990s—"THE PROBLEM"

Nosocomial outbreaks of TB in the United States before 1990 were relatively few, propagated slowly among patients, and rarely involved MDR-TB strains.[9] Healthcare personnel who were infected as a result of these exposures demonstrated close and prolonged contact with patients with either unrecognized TB or TB in the initial phases of treatment. In many reports, specific aerosol-producing medical procedures, such as bronchoscopy, endotracheal intubation, wound manipulation, respiratory tract manipulation, or autopsy, were associated with transmission.[9] Patient-to-patient transmission of TB was uncommon. By contrast, nosocomial spread of TB in the 1990s occurred as multiple institutional outbreaks that propagated rapidly and involved MDR-TB strains. In New York alone, 57 medical facilities (including the Medical Examiner's office) and 2 correctional facilities reported outbreaks with MDR-TB.[10,11]

Many outbreaks involved strain W, a strain of MTB multiply resistant to more than six antituberculosis medications. It accounted for one-third of New York City's MDR-TB cases and one-fourth of all US MDR-TB cases during 1990-1993.[11] Attack rates were highest among US-born, HIV coinfected patients, and among the HCWs caring for them. Molecular epidemiology of TB in New York City and San Francisco indicated that over 40% of TB cases were a result of recent transmission rather than reactivation of latent disease.[12,13] Although there have been no further institutional outbreaks involving strain W, its presence is still detected in the community among a number of patients whose exposure risk is frequently traced to contacts with a prior infected patient.[11] Spread of strain W outside New York City and across the United States has been attributed to relocation of prior patients, released inmates, and HCWs with prior infection or contact with infected patients during 1990 to 1993.[11,14]

HIV infection dramatically increases the risk of progression from latent TB infection to active TB disease, explaining in part the increased prevalence of nosocomial outbreaks in areas where patients with acquired immunodeficiency syndrome (AIDS) work, receive care, or reside.[15–28] In spite of an overall dramatic reduction in cases of TB in HIV coinfected persons in the US, HIV infection is still found in over 25% of adults with newly diagnosed TB.[27,28] In addition, symptoms of TB disease can be altered and clinical progression may occur more rapidly in the face of HIV-related immunosuppression, leading to delays in diagnosis.[27]

Acute Care Facilities

Numerous descriptions exist of nosocomial spread of TB in the early 1990s.[15–22,24–26,29–33] These outbreaks were characterized by HIV coinfection prevalence greater than 80%, median of 8 weeks from the time of diagnosis to death (average 4–16 weeks), and a mortality rate in excess of 70%. Temporal clustering of clinical cases and distinct antituberculosis medication susceptibility patterns led to the eventual recognition of distinct outbreaks. In most instances, patients were housed in dedicated HIV wards, or attended HIV clinics.[17–19,25,26] Numerous HCWs were infected, and a number developed active disease.

Factors that contributed to patient and HCW infection are listed in Table 11-1. Common to each outbreak was the failure to isolate patients early and to maintain isolation pending clinical improvement or diagnosis. Laboratory delays, infection control lapses, and facility shortcomings all contributed to spread of MDR-TB among patients and staff. The period between specimen collection and the identification of MTB (6 weeks) and completion of susceptibility testing (up to 12 weeks) frequently occurred after the patient's death.[16] Since the presence of resistant organisms was not recognized quickly, patients remained on inadequate antituberculosis regimens for prolonged periods, and many persons were removed from isolation while still infectious.[17,22,25,26]

Nosocomial transmission of TB declined sharply following the issuance and widespread implementation of the Center for Disease Control (CDC) guidelines in 1994.[34] Advances in HIV antiretroviral therapy improved patients' health and decreased hospitalizations, thereby reducing a highly susceptible population. In addition, the concern over bioterrorism, new strains of influenza, and severe acute respiratory syndrome (SARS), increased our awareness regarding airborne infections.[35] In spite of this, isolated outbreaks still occur due to breaches in infection control and HCWs' low-index of suspicion.[36] HCWs with active TB have even been identified during SARS screening efforts in Taiwan.[37]

Correctional Facilities

The risk of developing TB increases significantly following the first year of incarceration.[38] By 1992, the

Table 11-1. Factors Contributing to Nosocomial Outbreaks of Multidrug-Resistant Tuberculosis During 1990s

Source or Patient Factors
Increased homelessness
Human immunodeficiency virus (HIV)
    Advanced disease (i.e., end-stage AIDS)
    Atypical presentation of MTB
    Attendance in a dedicated HIV clinic
    Housing in HIV congregate setting
Previous hospitalization, especially prior exposure
    (on the same ward) to infectious MDR-TB patient
Aerosolized pentamidine treatment

Infection Control Factors
Low clinical suspicion (leading to delayed recognition)
Cohorting of patients
Problems with isolation of infectious patients
    Delayed institution of isolation
    Premature discontinuation of isolation
    Inadequate isolation facilities
    Lack of enforcement of strict isolation policies
Slow laboratory turnaround time for AFB smears,
    culture, and susceptibility results
Delayed initiation of effective treatment regimens
    (undiagnosed MDR-TB) resulting in prolonged
    period of infectiousness

Source: From references 15, 17–20, and 27.

incidence of TB among prisoners was ten-fold greater than that in the general US population.[39,40] This was, in great part, the result of 11 outbreaks of TB (most with MDR-TB) occurring in prisons in eight states during 1985–1992.[23,41–44] Over 171 inmates with TB were diagnosed in the New York State prison system alone during 1990–1991. Approximately one-third of them had MDR-TB and 97% were HIV coinfected.[23] Infectious inmates were transferred through a number of correctional facilities and local hospitals for medical care prior to diagnosis of TB. One-third of inmates who were exposed converted their tuberculin skin test (TST) (one-half after close contact with index patients) as well as a number of HCWs and patients at local hospitals.[23,41,44] Federal and state systems reported 25% prevalence of TB infection, increased TST conversions, and over 10% HIV coinfection rate among inmates incarcerated during 1990–1995.[45,46] Factors that contributed to correctional-facility TB outbreaks included the rise in HIV coinfection and rapid progression of disease, low-index of suspicion

Table 11-2. Factors Contributing to the Rise of Tuberculosis in Correctional Facilities

---

National drug control strategy with incarceration of illegal substance-using persons

Increase in HIV-positive or HIV-at-risk inmates (primarily due to intravenous substance use)

Overcrowding of facilities

Security (not health care) as prime objective in policy and edifice design

Increasing rates in communities

Nosocomial spread in acute care facilities to and from transferred inmates

Diagnostic failures (clinical and laboratory delays)

Inter-correctional facility transfer of infectious inmates

Inadequate tuberculin skin test screening and loss to follow-up

Noncompliance with therapy and prophylactic therapy

Long or multiple incarcerations

Source: Data adapted from references 16, 23, 38, 40–42, 44, and 46.

for TB, the increase in MDR-TB with extensive resistance to empiric antituberculosis regimens, as well as inadequate isolation facilities (Table 11-2).

TB in correctional facilities remains endemic. Overcrowding with inadequate isolation facilities has been described as a cause of continued failure of TB infection control in spite of recent facility improvements and CDC guidelines.[40,47–50] Average time spent in pre-screening areas may be anywhere from 3–24 hours (from admission to symptom screening), increasing risk of spreading TB. The most recent CDC-investigated outbreak occurred throughout two states and included a homeless shelter, three jails and a state prison with over three hundred contacts (including inmates and staff).[51] Although the index patient had symptoms consistent with a diagnosis of pulmonary TB, his TST was negative and no screening chest radiograph was performed until he reached the state prison system, approximately one year later. The greatest rate of TST conversions occurred in the two jails (15.6–22.2%) and the least in the state prison (1.7%).[51] The jails had an open-cell design with multiple inmates per cell while the state prison had single-occupancy cells with solid walls and doors.

Facility design and lapses in early identification of TB cases continue to promulgate outbreaks with rapid spread among inmates and staff, as well as visitors and the nearby community.[52–54] A recent study in Tennessee reported that 43% of persons identified with TB in the city of Memphis had previous contact with a single urban jail and no other identified common exposure.[48]

Homeless Shelters, SROs, and Other Facilities

Two and a half percent of adult Americans, or about five million people, reported being homeless during 1995–2000.[55] TB infection occurs in over 30%, and clinically active TB in 10% of homeless persons.[55–63] The incidence of TB among substance users on welfare in New York City is 14.8 times greater than that of the age-matched general population in New York City and 70 times greater than the incidence in the United States.[64] Social risk factors for TB infection such as poverty, crowded living conditions, stress, malnutrition, alcoholism, drug addiction, mental illness, and prior incarceration, are all common among the homeless.[7,56,57,65–68] In addition, the degree of "homelessness" has been linked to risk of acquisition of TB, with persons sleeping in a shelter or on the street being less likely to acquire TB than those sleeping in a single-resident occupancy (SRO) hotel or a rehabilitation program.[69] A decade ago, a significant proportion of homeless persons with active TB residing in large urban centers were HIV-coinfected.[56–58,60] Although there has been a decrease in the number of HIV and MTB coinfected homeless, it is still double that found among the nonhomeless.[3] A summary of risk factors for acquisition of TB among the homeless appears in Table 11-3.

TST screening, initiating, and completing treatment for latent TB infection (LTBI) in individuals with unstable housing prove to be difficult tasks. Homeless persons are frequently reluctant to answer screening questions related to symptoms or past TB infection for fear they may be denied a benefit (such as a shelter bed or substance use treatment) or be compelled to enter coercive treatment.[70] Although numerous persons are potentially exposed in shelter outbreaks, their transient and migratory lifestyles hinder the ability to identify and follow-up contacts.[71–73] Even when contacts are identified, less than half of those who begin LTBI treatment actually complete a full course.[72]

Use of restriction fragment length polymorphism (RFLP) pattern indicates most cases identified are due to recent acquisition (or primary TB) and not reactivation of prior infection.[55,56,59,60,66,69,71–74] In the early 1990s, over 90% of a New York City homeless cohorts with newly diagnosed TB was lost to follow-up or failed to complete therapy.[56] One-quarter were readmitted within the first year after discharge with continued active TB; and, of

Table 11-3. Risk Factors for Spread of *Mycobacterium tuberculosis* in Shelters and Single Resident Occupancy (SRO) Hotels

Human Factors

Increasing age of occupants
Socioeconomic factors (poverty, stress, malnutrition)
Substance use (intravenous drug use, alcoholism)
HIV coinfection
Mental illness
Transient nature of homeless persons
History of prior incarceration, hospitalization,
    or contact with others with such history

Facility Factors

Close living quarters in open areas
Increasing length of stay (>24 months)
Inadequate ventilation

Infection Control Factors

Inability to identify contacts due to nature of transient
    status or fear of incarceration
Poor medical screening and health care

Source: Data adapted from references 22, 56–60, and 65.

Table 11-4. Risk Factors for Spread of *Mycobacterium tuberculosis* in Nursing Homes and Long-term Care Facilities

Source or Patient Factors

Elderly age
High prevalence of TST positivity (and increased
    risk of recrudescence)
Comorbid medical conditions increasing the risk
    of reactivation or of exogenous reinfection
Waning of immunity to prior infection
Unsuspected disease (confused with carcinoma
    or bacterial infection)
Prolonged exposure
Atypical chest radiograph appearance of TB

Facilities and Infection Control Factors

Congregate surroundings/close contact
Few or no isolation facilities
Variable compliance with annual TST programs
Inadequate education concerning infection and
    transmission
Inadequate use of prophylactic therapy

Source: Data adapted from references 75, 76, and 79.

these, the majority was lost to follow-up on the second discharge. In 2003, the New York City Department of Health reported that only 6.6% of new cases with TB among homeless persons were lost to follow-up prior to completing treatment courses.[71] Increases in rates of TB among the homeless are now due to isolated outbreaks in shelters or SRO hotels.[5]

Nursing Homes and Long-term Care Facilities

In spite of increased incidence among younger persons, the elderly continue to experience a large proportion of TB cases, most due to recrudescence of past infection.[75–77] Many persons older than 64 years of age with active TB live in a long-term care facility (LTCF) or nursing home at the time of diagnosis.[78] Although the majority of TB in older persons presents as pulmonary reactivation, a quarter of persons will present with atypical symptoms of extrapulmonary or disseminated disease.[77] TST results are positive in a third of persons entering LTCFs and only a minority of elderly persons fail to react to two-step testing.[75,79,80] Nonetheless, 20% of LTCF residents develop active TB as a result of a recent exposure.[76] Factors contributing to transmission of TB in nursing homes and LTCFs appear in Table 11-4.

Long-term care facilities caring for the handicapped have also reported TB outbreaks.[81] These were facilitated by prolonged contagiousness due to delay in diagnosis of the source, difficulty in medical examination or communication with impaired or psychotic patients, crowded or communal living conditions, and lack of isolation facilities.[81]

IMPACT ON HEALTHCARE WORKERS

Baseline prevalence of TST positivity among HCWs is reported to be 1.4% to 3.9%.[82–86] While HCW ethnicity, socio-economic status, and location of residence may play a role in community transmission of TB to HCWs, TST reaction prevalence rates among HCWs are 10 to 100 times greater than those in the general population and are explained by occupational exposure.[83,84,87] Although, frequent and prolonged exposure is necessary to produce disease in HCWs, recent studies have demonstrated relatively short but close contact with an infectious patient or involvement with aerosol-producing procedures to be a source of widespread infection.[82,84,87–89]

During nosocomial outbreaks of the 1990s, conversion rates occurred in over three-quarters of exposed HCWs, with a risk eight-fold greater for exposed than nonexposed HCWs.[29,89,90] Higher disease rates and increased mortality has been described among HIV coinfected HCWs following occupational exposure to TB.[29,91,92] Spread of TB from HCWs to others (coworkers and patients) is unusual but has been described.[92,93] Exogenous re-infection in spite of prior TB infection is possible in the HIV coinfected or in those with other immunosuppressive medical conditions.[85,90] Although the prevalence of TST conversions among HCWs decreased after the peak of the TB epidemic in the early 1990s (26.4–3.9%), the conversion rate among HCWs in high-risk occupational settings for TB exposure continues to be greater than that among HCWs in low-risk settings.[94]

CURTAILMENT AND PREVENTION—"THE SOLUTION"

TB reemerged in the United States at a time when compliance with existing guidelines for prevention of nosocomial spread of TB was not strictly enforced.[26,30,33,86,95–97] In most cases, outbreaks were curtailed with implementation of established infection control practices, increased diagnostic and therapeutic aggressiveness, and establishment of an active TST surveillance program, prior to any environmental or personal protective equipment changes (i.e., masks or respirators).[30,32,96] Administrative measures alone at one hospital in New York City led to a marked decrease in TST conversion rates among HCWs from 17–5%, a decrease to the same rate of conversion as seen among controls.[31]

The direct contribution of personal protective equipment (PPE) use to outbreak curtailment is unclear since neither use nor model chosen were uniform among facilities.[30,32,96] Many facilities implemented a number of changes simultaneously, and individual contributions could not be assessed.[31,32] A survey conducted by the Occupational Safety and Health Administration (OSHA) of 272 health care facilities found greater compliance with administrative than respiratory protection equipment guidelines.[98] This is consistent with most health care practitioners' belief that adherence to basic infection control tenets is paramount in controlling nosocomial transmission of TB.[98]

The CDC has published TB control guidelines for acute care facilities, correctional facilities, homeless persons, and long-term care facilities.[34,40,47,62,76,95,99] A comparison among these different policies appears in Table 11-5. In December 2004, the CDC submitted the draft of its "Guidelines for preventing the transmission of *Mycobacterium tuberculosis* in health-care settings, 2005"

to the Federal Register for public comment.[99] The guidelines are designed for broad application in various settings and facilities (both in- and out-patient) where health care is delivered. Emphasis is placed on developing and instituting a local TB infection control program based on annual institutional TB risk assessment (determination of prevalence, incidence, and risk of acquisition of TB infection to ascertain risk of nosocomial spread of TB). The CDC facilitated this process with numerous detailed worksheets and tables found throughout the document. The hierarchy of TB controls remains: (1) administrative controls with guidelines for programs in patient care (education, diagnosis, isolation, treatment) and HCW safety (education, TST, LTBI treatment), (2) environmental controls (improvement in ventilation, decontamination of air and equipment), (3) use of PPE (selection, education, fit-testing). Specific needs for each facility type are addressed below within each hierarchy category.

Administrative Controls

Surveillance (gathering and timely analysis of data) and education remain the cornerstones for nosocomial TB control. The most important steps in limiting exposure are isolation of the patient when TB is suspected on clinical grounds and compliance with isolation procedures until laboratory and clinical data can eliminate the possibility of TB or the risk of contagion. Rapid diagnosis and empiric (and appropriate) antituberculosis therapy (after adequate samples are obtained for culture) are additional factors in decreasing the potential for spread. TST screening of patients, inmates, residents, and HCWs, and the use of LTBI treatment add to an effective TB infection control program.

TST Screening

Guidelines for TST screening are published and are discussed in Chapter 4.[34,80,99] During the outbreaks of the 1990s, many facilities performed TST of their HCWs based upon perceived risk and, as a result, did not always have a reliable baseline to document conversions following exposures.[17,18,86] Frequency of TST depends on the results of baseline testing and risk classification for exposure.[34,99] The CDC encourages use of a two-step TST program for all new HCWs (especially for those from areas where Bacille Calmette-Guérin, or BCG, vaccination is administered and/or infections with mycobacteria are endemic). The newer QuantiFERON-TB test can be used in place of the traditional TST, when deemed appropriate.[99] Although the cost of implementing and maintaining a TST program

Table 11-5. Comparison of Recommendations from CDC Guidelines for Acute Care, Correctional, Long-Term Care Facilities and Facilities Housing Homeless Persons

Type of Facility	Administrative Controls				Environmental Controls			
	Facility Risk Analysis	Infection Control program (ICP)	HCW Program[x]	Source or Patient Management[y]	Ventilation[z]	HEPA filters	UVGI	PPE
Acute Care*	1	1	1	1	1	1	1	1
Correctional[†]	1	1	1	1, 5	1	2	2	4
Long-term care[‡]	1	1	1	1, 5	1	4	4	4
Homeless[§]	1	1	1	1, 5	1	4	1	4

Recommendations and grade importance:

1 Recommendation in official guidelines.

2 Recommendation in official guidelines but questions remain regarding exact utilization of modality.

3 Information from other CDC data or studies; modality of probable utility.

4 No recommendation provided in official guidelines.

5 Isolation requires transfer to on-site or off-site medical or acute care facility.

Program components:

[x]HCW Program: Education, TST Screening

[y]Source or Patient Management: Symptom and TST screening, Isolation, LTBI treatment, Treatment

[z]Ventilation: Air changes, negative pressure, exhaust

CDC Guidelines for Tuberculosis Program priorities:

*Administrative (risk analysis, ICP, TST program, effective work practices, education, source screening), environmental (isolation, ventilation, exhaust, negative pressure, HEPA filtration, UVGI), PPE

[†]Screening of inmates and HCWs, containment of infectious persons (treatment and LTBI treatment), analysis of data. Correctional medical facilities are included under guidelines for "acute care facilities."

[‡]Surveillance (screening and reporting), containment (treatment and LTBI treatment), analysis of data, education. Environmental and respiratory control programs based on individual risk assessment.

[§]Surveillance activities (case finding, reporting, and treatment), TST screening and preventive therapy (priority for HIV-seropositive/high-risk persons, recent converters, persons with medical conditions and/or abnormal chest radiographs), evaluation of inadequate treatment.

CDC = Centers for Disease Control; HCW = healthcare workers; HEPA = high-efficiency particulate air; ICP = Infection Control Program; PPE = personal protection equipment; UVGI = ultraviolet germicidal irradiation.

Source: Data adapted from references 34, 40, 47, 62, 76, 95, and 99.

in hospitals and health departments can be significant (estimated at $41–$362/HCW), the benefit of monitoring conversions and early intervention well outweighs the cost.[100]

Although all HCWs who experience conversion of their TST status should receive LTBI treatment, many refuse or do not complete a full course. At one medical center, only one-third of physicians eligible for LTBI treatment completed at least 6 months of therapy.[85] It is illegal to compel workers to accept preventive therapy as a condition of continued employment in a health care institution. Unfortunately, some infected employees who would not or could not comply with preventive therapy have gone on to develop active TB and to expose others.[26,30,31,89,92]

Acute Care Facilities

Key elements in reducing nosocomial outbreaks are case recognition and a high index of suspicion for the myriad clinical presentations of TB. Special considerations should be made for the unusual manifestations of TB in the elderly (frequently mistaken for aspiration pneumonia or carcinoma) and in HIV coinfected persons.[20,25,26,56,76,101] In one facility; an outbreak was curtailed with isolation of all HIV-infected patients with abnormal chest radiograph results.[96]

Not every (non-HIV) person with pulmonary complaints or symptoms can or should be isolated (especially during seasonal increases in viral and bacterial respiratory infections). Recent focus on bioterrorism and epidemics of

SARS has increased HCWs' awareness of patients with pulmonary complaints and increased the use of airborne isolation, especially in emergency departments.[37] Awareness of TB prevalence rates in the community and other facilities, as well as active surveillance of all patients, determines an institution's threshold for isolation of patients.

Unfortunately, some degree of over-isolation will continue to occur. Multidisciplinary triage teams have been implemented successfully in busy emergency rooms in endemic areas to limit the use of airborne isolation.[30–32,96,102] In patients unlikely to have infectious TB disease, isolation may be discontinued after an alternative diagnosis has been made or three negative AFB sputum smears are obtained (8–24 hours apart).[99] Recent studies analyzed the value of three AFB smears prior to discontinuation of respiratory isolation for patients suspected of TB disease.[103,104] Fewer than three AFB specimens may be sufficient to discontinue isolation in low-prevalence areas and in nonoutbreak situations.[103,104] However, further data are needed prior to changing current recommendations.

The length of time required for a TB patient to become noninfectious after initiating TB therapy varies considerably. Isolation should be discontinued only when the patient is receiving effective therapy, is improving clinically, and has had three consecutive negative AFB smears from specimens collected on different days. Although smear-negative TB patients are less likely to transmit TB, the rate is not low enough to discontinue isolation and place patients in the general hospital population.[99,105] Isolation is continued for hospitalized patients in whom the suspicion of TB remains in spite of negative AFB sputum smears until the patients are on standard multidrug anti-TB treatment and are clinically improving (or an alternative diagnosis is made).[99] Table 11-6 lists

Table 11-6. Criteria for MTB Airborne Isolation

Criteria for Initiation of Isolation

Persons with HIV coinfection with respiratory or constitutional symptoms and/or abnormal chest radiograph

Persons with:

Unexplained systemic symptoms

Respiratory illness without response to adequate/broad antimicrobial therapy within 72 hours

Prior history of TB or tuberculin skin test-positive with respiratory symptoms and/or abnormal chest radiograph

Prior history of contact with institution with prior outbreak of multidrug-resistant TB and respiratory symptoms and/or abnormal radiograph

Undergoing treatment for TB with unknown compliance or with documented persistent sputum AFB positive

Criteria for Continuation of Isolation

Sputum smear AFB-negative without alternative diagnosis and persistent symptoms while undergoing further work-up

Empiric antituberculous therapy begun without evidence clinical and/or radiographic improvement

Persistent AFB smear-positive in spite of clinical improvement and unable to discharge to appropriate home setting (i.e., presence in the home of children, immunocompromised persons, or home healthcare personnel)

Criteria for Discontinuation of Isolation

Clinical, AFB smear, and radiographic improvement on empiric antituberculous therapy

Verification of compliance and documented improvement from Directly Observed Therapy/Department of Health sources

Alternative diagnosis made or improvement with institution of non-anti TB treatment (i.e., improvement with antibacterial agents, or diagnosis of non-infectious etiology of radiographic or clinical symptoms)

HIV = human immunodeficiency virus; AFB = acid-fast bacillus
Source: Data adapted from references 96, 99, 103–105.

some criteria for establishing as well as discontinuing airborne isolation for potentially infectious patients.

New York City Department of Health (NYCDOH) implemented a number of administrative controls in their chest clinics to reduce the risk of exposure from potentially infectious patients in 1992.[94] These included earlier morning appointments scheduled at times when the clinic would be empty; immediate triage with reduced waiting time; the use of PPE by patients and staff; and physical separation from other patients through the use of a separate waiting area.[94] A summary of these measures appears in Table 11-7.

Correctional Facilities

Initial TB screening of inmates includes a detailed history regarding active symptoms, TST and HIV status, and chest radiographs.[40,45,105] Using both TST and chest radiographs is superior to screening with TST alone among short-term incarcerated persons and among HIV-infected persons exhibiting cutaneous anergy.[40,106–108] High-speed radiographic screening (100-mm mini chest radiographs) is cost-effective in large correctional facilities with a high prevalence of TB.[106] Although policies require annual TST and symptom screening of all inmates and correctional staff, LTBI treatment is not mandatory.[99,109]

Table 11-7. NYCDOH Modalities for Improvement of MTB Control in Chest Clinics

Administrative
Separate waiting areas
Appointments for infectious patients at times of least
  clinic activity
Immediate triage without waiting in congregate spaces

Environmental
Installation of ultraviolet germicidal irradiation
  (UVGI) in all moderate to high-risk areas (waiting
  areas, examination rooms, and sputum induction areas)
Specific handling for sputum induction areas:
  Sputum induction booths fitted with HEPA filtration
    systems for external air exhaust
  Negative pressure with a minimum of 50 AC/hr
Use of PPE by patients and staff

Source: Data adapted from Cook S, Maw KL, Munsiff SS, et al. Prevalence of tuberculin skin test positivity and conversions among healthcare workers in New York City during 1994 to 2001. *Infect Control Hosp Epidemiol.* 2003;24:807–813.

To date, state and federal systems report high rates of TST screening of inmates at intake following incarceration and annually thereafter (over 90%), higher than city and county systems (40–60%).[45] Since 1992, over three quarters of correctional facilities reported isolating inmates until three negative sputa were collected on consecutive days and the number of inmates enrolled in directly observed therapy (DOT) programs while receiving treatment for active TB exceeded 90%.[45] In the past, compliance with isoniazid therapy was variable (approximately 60% among state and federal inmates and 35% among city and county inmates). Compliance levels rose significantly recently when the majority of inmates less than 35 years old, of new converters, and of those coinfected with HIV, received isoniazid therapy while enrolled in directly observed preventive therapy (DOPT) programs.[45] Local departments of health continue to provide DOT and DOPT for a majority of inmates after institutional discharge.

CDC guidelines for TB control in correctional facilities emphasize three major factors in a TB infection control program: screening, containment, and assessment.[40] Medical settings within correctional facilities are required to conform to TB infection control program components similar to those applicable to acute care facilities.[99] Inmates must be transferred to other facilities or hospitals if appropriate isolation facilities are not available. Isolation can be discontinued only if the diagnosis of TB has been excluded or if the patient is determined not to be infectious.[40] Table 11-8 lists some modalities for improved TB control in correctional facilities. Increased vigilance, cooperation among correctional facilities, and communication with local departments of health significantly decreased numbers of TB cases and new conversions among inmates.[45] When isolated outbreaks occur, they do so due to decreased vigilance, lack of communication, and lack of organized follow-up of patients/inmates.

Homeless Shelters, SROs, and Other Facilities

Because of the transient nature of homeless persons, the highest priority of TB control is surveillance (detection, evaluation, and reporting) of active TB and completion of an appropriate course of treatment.[62] The second priority is screening for latent infection, especially among high-risk groups (i.e., HIV coinfected persons, those with chronic medical conditions, or active substance users). Incentives such as food, housing, vouchers, and financial rewards have been used with some success to aid compliance.[60,62,110,111] Specialized housing programs based on infectivity have been locally successful with compliance

Table 11-8. Modalities for Improvement of MTB Control in Correctional Facilities

Information Systems (Tracking inmates within and across correctional facilities)
Improve completeness of medical records
    HIV testing, screening of symptoms, history of TB risk (prior incarceration, homelessness, drug use, contact with above), TST, chest radiograph, therapy
Develop aggregate record-keeping systems for MTB-related data
Periodic review of TB trend data and radiographic results
Close working relationship with DOH for prior MTB diagnosis and treatment history as well as follow-up after release

Infection Control
Isolate quickly (minimize time in prescreening and other congregate areas)
Maintain isolation until diagnosis and/or response to therapy
Use negative pressure rooms that are monitored frequently (preferably smoke tube)
Separate air handling for intake areas (use HEPA filters if possible)
Use of UVGI for communal areas

Source: Data adapted from CDC. Prevention and control of TB in correctional facilities: recommendations of the Advisory Council for the Elimination of Tuberculosis. *MMWR Morb Mortal Wkly Rep.* 1996;45(NoRR-8).

with treatment regimens.[112] Short-term incarceration (less than 30 days) can be used for those where DOT alone is not successful and is sometimes continued for the whole duration of the TB treatment course.[113]

Mass TST and chest radiograph screening has not proven to be effective in identifying all cases among contacts of such a transient and migratory population.[71] An additional tool implemented by the New York City Department of Health to identify contacts has been to search the TB registry which identifies patient clusters by address of residence.[71] Applying a calculated "homelessness score" to focus contact identification efforts on locations frequented by homeless patients and the average amount of time spent at these locations during the infectious period may increase success in contact tracing.[69] Some modalities employed by the NYCDOH for improved TB control among these persons appear in Table 11-9.[71]

Nursing Homes and Long-term Care Facilities

Guidelines for nursing homes and other long-term care facilities (LTCFs) include the same components of surveillance and record-keeping (TST of residents and employees at baseline, intervals, and following exposures), containment of active cases, LTBI treatment of exposed persons (residents and employees, regardless of age), and education of residents and employees.[76,77] Unusual or atypical presentation of TB may occur, and emphasis is placed on identification of active cases and referral to

a setting where they can be evaluated and managed (if deemed infectious and the LTCF does not have the appropriate TB environmental and respiratory protection controls in place).[99,101]

Environmental Controls

Environmental control of TB refers to engineering modalities for removal or disinfection of air containing MTB.

Table 11-9. NYCDOH Modalities for Improvement of MTB Control among the Homeless

Enhanced case management
Review of all Department of AIDS Services referrals for history of TB by cross-matching to the TB registry and a brief questionnaire
Provision of directly observed treatment for TB patients on site in particular Division of AIDS Services (DAS) hotels
Offering of incentives and peer counseling to ensure treatment completion
Creation of a shelter specifically to house homeless persons with TB until treatment completion
Use of short- or long-term incarceration for completion of treatment

Source: Data adapted from Li J, Driver CR, Munsiff SS, Fujiwara PI. Finding contacts of homeless TB patients in New York City. *Int J Tuberc Lung Dis.* 2003;7:S397.

These include ventilation of a given space measured in air changes per hour (AC/hour), directional airflow and pressurization (laminar and negative or positive pressure), air mixing, air filtration, and air disinfection.[114–116] Conditions which increase the spread of TB include poorly ventilated environments (or those using recirculated air), overcrowding, or clinical procedures that effectively aerosolize MTB particles.[6–8,34,95,114–116]

In 2003, CDC and the Healthcare Infection Control Practices Advisory Committee (HICPAC) released updated guidelines for environmental infection control in healthcare facilities.[47] The following items are required to meet standards for airborne isolation of patients infected with organisms spread via droplet nuclei (<5 μm diameter, i.e., MTB): 12 or more AC/hr for new construction after 2001 and 6 or more AC/hr for construction before 2001; negative pressure; external exhaust preferred (25 feet or more from air intake vents, 6 feet above ground, or 3 feet above roof levels) but recirculation permitted if air is first passed through high particulate air (HEPA) filter.[47] In addition, anterooms should be installed whenever possible and negative pressure maintained.[47,99] Although mechanical ventilation is universally available in modern buildings and generally adaptable to current needs, it is most effective in smaller areas, such as individual patient rooms. Attempting to retrofit older buildings to comply with the appropriate AC/hour with direct outdoor exhaust and negative pressure differential could be a daunting experience requiring significant investment of capital and resources. As a result, the new CDC guidelines offer the ability to increase the airflow to 12 AC/hr either by adjusting the existing ventilation system or by using air-cleaning methods (i.e., portable HEPA filter-containing units or ultraviolet germicidal irradiation systems) to increase the equivalent AC/hr.[99]

Ultraviolet germicidal irradiation (UVGI) is the least well understood of the three approaches to air disinfection despite its use for over 70 years. Although there are good laboratory data supporting the germicidal activity against a number of virulent bacteria, viruses and mycobacteria (including MTB), there are few recent field trials showing it can prevent TB transmission in populations.[6,34,114–116] UVGI has been implemented successfully in large areas where ventilation is insufficient to cleanse stagnant air pockets.[6,114–116] Upper air UVGI may minimize the spread of MTB, especially from unsuspected patient sources.[116–118] Additional recent studies performed with mannequins "aerosolizing" mycobacteria in isolation rooms found a linear relationship between UV irradiation and germicidal efficacy.[119] However, efficacy dropped drastically (89% to 9%) when air humidity was raised above 75% and when ventilation mixing fans were turned off and wintertime

ventilation conditions were established.[119] More recently, UVGI has been studied as a possible adjuvant to diminish airborne infections associated with bioterrorism.[35]

Milwaukee County Hospital documented a decrease in TST conversions among HCWs working on wards with installed UVGI.[117] Nonetheless, HCWs' apprehension of eye and skin toxicity has been a major obstacle to increasing the use of UVGI. UVGI placed in enclosed ducts, in wall-mounted metal boxes with fans, or in wall-mounted devices with upward-directed louvers can address this concern.[34,108,114] Guidelines exist for care and low maintenance of UVGI devices and emphasis is placed on close monitoring of air flow resistance indicators as markers for the need to change filters that are full.[115] CDC guidelines for use and placement of UVGI fixtures in healthcare facilities appeared recently.[47,99] UVGI fixtures should be placed on the wall near the ceiling, suspended from the ceiling, in the air-return duct of an isolation room, or in areas specially designated for sputum induction.[47,99] UVGI should not be used in place of high efficiency particulate air (HEPA) filters when discharging air from isolation booths or enclosures directly into the surrounding room or area, or when discharging air into the general ventilation system.[99]

Air filtration has been a long-practiced modality in industry for removal of airborne contaminants.[114] HEPA filters have pore sizes <1 μm and are able to remove 99.97–99.99% of particles >1 μm (e.g., droplet nuclei). Although there exist few data concerning MTB, experience with *Aspergillus* outbreaks on oncology wards has affirmed HEPA filtration capacity and efficiency.[34] The efficacy of HEPA filters is closely related to having a well-functioning ventilation system that is able to move air past them, and to the adequacy of prefilters which, when placed upstream, significantly extend the life of HEPA filters by removing larger debris. HEPA filters incorporated into the ventilation systems: (1) must be used when discharging air back into the general ventilation system when direct outside discharge is impossible; (2) can be used when recirculating air within a room (when the existing system is incapable of adjustments) or discharging to the outside (as an added safety measure).[99]

HEPA filters can also be used for air recirculation when contained in portable air cleaners (many of which also contain UVGI).[47,99] Use of these units is considered when a room has either no general ventilation system or when the existing system cannot provide adequate AC/hr.[99] As with placement of HEPA filters in ventilation ducts, the effectiveness of portable HEPA filter units depends on the ability to circulate as much of the air in the room as possible through the HEPA filter. This is dependent on the room's configuration (including location of furniture, position of air supply diffusers and exhaust grilles, and the persons in the room). Furthermore, patients and HCWs sometimes turn off these units due to their perception that the noise and heat generated by the fans interfere with healthcare delivery. As a result, special attention must be paid to ensure their proper and continuous functioning. Filters must be monitored for quality and cleanliness with scheduled changes as designated by manufacturers.[47,99]

In 1992, the NYCDOH implemented a number of environmental changes in its chest clinics to minimize exposure to potentially infectious patients.[94] These are listed in Table 11-7 and include installation of UVGI in all moderate to high-risk areas, such as patient waiting areas, examination rooms, and areas where sputum induction was performed. In addition, sputum induction booths were fitted with HEPA filtration systems for external air exhaust.[94] The rooms in which the sputum induction booths were located were maintained under negative pressure and had a minimum of 50 AC/hr.[94] As demonstrated by the NYCDOH environmental interventions, ventilation was maximized in smaller areas where control of airflow is easier to manage, and HEPA filters were installed for cleansing of exhaust air. UVGI was used in large congregate spaces, such as waiting rooms, where control of airflow is not easily accomplished and in high-risk areas, such as examination rooms, as an adjuvant to ventilation.

Acute Care Facilities

Hospital MDR-TB outbreaks of the early 1990s occurred in spite of the 1990 CDC guidelines recommendations for minimum 6 AC/hour, negative pressure, and supplemental use of air filtration and UVGI.[82,95] In facilities with more than six TB patients, respiratory isolation rooms in compliance with 1990 CDC guidelines were associated with significantly lower rates of TST conversions among HCWs than those not employing such measures.[86] The New York State Department of Health reported varied compliance with ventilation and negative pressure in a number of facilities during 1992 to 1998.[120] Over a quarter of facilities that performed daily smoke testing of isolation rooms reported a discrepancy with measurements of automated monitoring devices.[121] The CDC, however, reported marked nationwide improvement in appropriate airborne isolation (from 63–100% of the facilities), appropriate mask use (60–90% of facilities), and overall decreased HCW TST conversion rates.[122] In spite of such tremendous improvements, human error can still play a significant factor when failing to identify at-risk patients and isolate them.[123,124]

The effort to reduce both energy expenditure and cost has forced many facilities to recirculate air, to seal windows to prevent heat loss, and to operate the ventilation system in cycles rather than continuously. Air pressure relationships within a large facility such as a hospital are contingent on the local ventilation patterns and may be disrupted even with the opening of a door or window. Retrofitting existing rooms requires a change in ventilation volume and pattern as well as creating provisions for safe discharge of contaminated air. Anterooms serve as buffers to airflow disruptions and insulate isolation rooms from corridor and patient traffic. Regularly scheduled maintenance is more cost-effective than the installation of intricate alarm systems.

Several other hospital areas pose environmental problems, such as special procedure areas (i.e., bronchoscopy suites), emergency and ambulatory care areas, mycobacterial laboratories, and morgues. Improved ventilation of bronchoscopy suites, and the addition of UVGI (contained in either louvered or enclosed metallic boxes with fans) and/or portable HEPA filters are reasonable modalities to interrupt TB transmission during these aerosol-generating procedures.[99,125] In addition, the utility of PPE cannot be stressed enough in areas with high MTB aerosol concentrations.[99,126] The large spaces of emergency and ambulatory care areas with increased patient and HCW traffic can overwhelm ventilation systems and additional UVGI (and/or portable HEPA filters) should be considered after a risk assessment is performed. Signs for patients to cover their mouths while coughing along with providing tissues and surgical masks can significantly decrease the spread of droplet nuclei.

Inadequate ventilation and creation of aerosols during post-mortem examinations, and processing of tissue or mycobacteriology samples have led to transmission of TB to susceptible HCWs.[87,127] Better education, increased ventilation, use of UVGI, and strict use of PPE have all helped to reduce TB exposures among pathologists. Frequent testing of ventilation and hood operation are crucial in mycobacteriology and pathology areas.[128] Specific recommendations for ventilation systems for various facility areas have appeared recently.[99]

Correctional Facilities

Some jails still recirculate air from intake areas to other parts of the facilities. When direct outdoor exhaust is not possible, then use of HEPA filters in ventilation ducts is recommended. UVGI is best used to supplement ventilation in high-risk, over-crowded areas such as holding and communal areas and can be installed as ceiling or wall fixtures or within ventilation ducts.[40] Inmates suspected of having TB should wear surgical masks covering mouth and nose whenever they need to be transported outside their isolation rooms for medically essential procedures. All HCWs and corrections staff that care for or transport these inmates must wear PPE. [40]

Specialized facilities for housing inmates with TB can supplement comprehensive TB surveillance programs within correctional facilities.[108] A recent National Institute of Justice and CDC joint survey of correctional facilities' use of negative pressure in infirmaries reported an increase from 30% in 1992 to 65% in 1994.[45] A follow-up survey in 1997 found a further increase to 98% for Federal and state facilities and 85% for local jail systems.[70] Recent guidelines mandate medical settings in correctional facilities to conform to the same environmental and respiratory program recommendations that apply to acute care facilities.[99]

Homeless Shelters, SROs, and Other Facilities

Installation of UVGI can reduce the risk of transmission of TB in shelters where large and open communal areas exist to serve transient residents who may not adhere to accepted TB surveillance programs.[6,62,74,116] Financial support for shelters is meager and does not support retrofitting of ventilation systems in older buildings. Installation of UVGI in ceiling fixtures led to decreased TB transmission in a Boston shelter.[129]

Nursing Homes and Long-term Care Facilities

LTCFs were not designed with infection control as a primary objective. Few or no isolation rooms exist, and ventilation systems are for occupant comfort rather than disease transmission control. Implementation of administrative controls, including symptom screening, is of primary importance. The decision to implement environmental and respiratory protection programs (i.e., creation of isolation rooms, changes in ventilation, exhaust, implementation of HEPA and/or UVGI, PPE, and etc.) is based upon individual facility TB risk assessment.[99] Residents with suspected or confirmed TB should not stay in LTCF unless adequate environmental and respiratory programs are in place.[99]

Personal Protective Equipment

Respirators are distinct from ordinary surgical masks. Respirators are designed to prevent inhalation of particulate air contaminants, including infectious droplet nuclei, whereas surgical masks protect the operating field from the wearer. Unlike environmental control, PPE use requires active implementation and the foresight that there is a risk at hand. Unfortunately, contact with unsuspected infectious cases still accounts for most TB transmission. In 1994, the CDC mandated PPE use for all HCWs caring for patients with identified or suspected TB disease and OSHA enforced the directive.[34,130] At the time, healthcare facilities were attempting to implement long-needed engineering changes and perceived the PPE mandate as an added hardship requiring diversion of limited healthcare dollars.

While workers in industry use PPE for protection from inhalation of particles in defined work settings, the role of respiratory protective devices in healthcare areas remains secondary to other measures in the prevention of the spread of TB.[114] PPE is a modality for added HCW protection in situations of probable high MTB-aerosol content as found when entering isolation rooms, during bronchoscopy procedures, and during autopsies.[34,99,131,132] Masking of patients with infectious TB is still considered an effective source of control by all experts. It is important to reiterate that nosocomial outbreaks were frequently curtailed through rigorous implementation of established infection control practices. In the instances where several modalities were employed simultaneously, the value of individual components in curtailing the outbreak could not be ascertained.[133]

In 1995, the National Institute for Occupational Safety and Health (NIOSH) revised categories of particulate filter respirators.[134] There are two essential components of respirator function: filtration media and face seal. Among the many choices available, the healthcare industry selected the N95 particulate filter respirator (Technol, Fort Worth, TX) as a compromise of efficacy, comfort, and cost.[99,134] It has an efficiency of 95% for filtering particles smaller than 1 μm but is less costly and far more comfortable than the portable HEPA respirator. Re-aerosolization of MTB droplet nuclei is unlikely once they have been trapped by the N95 respirator.[135] A summary of applicable respirators and their uses appears in recent CDC guidelines and options provided for HCWs whose facial features, especially facial hair, make it impractical to wear the N95 respirator.[99]

Following the initial hotly debated implementation of the N95 respirator by the medical community, the CDC and the Healthcare Infection Control Practices Advisory Committee (HICPAC) have made it mandatory for all HCWs to wear it whenever entering airborne isolation.[47,99] In addition, as of early 2004, healthcare facilities became subject to the same standards for annual fit-testing of N95 respirators as is currently recommended in industrial settings.[70,99,136]

Other Methods for Healthcare Worker Protection

Bacille Calmette-Guérin (BCG) vaccination (see Chap. 9) is a potential protective modality for HCWs caring for patients with MDR-TB when transmission of infection is likely and comprehensive TB infection control precautions have failed to curtail spread of infection.[137] Cohort studies suggest that rates of TB may be substantially lower among HCWs who receive BCG vaccine than among those who remain unvaccinated, and efficacy appears to increase with risk of exposure (69%–85%).[138,139] A recent decision analysis comparing BCG vaccination with LTBI treatment for MDR-TB demonstrated a slight benefit for the use of BCG vaccination in healthy, non-HIV-infected North American HCWs exposed to MDR-TB.[140]

A national policy on use of BCG has not been endorsed in this country for multiple reasons including: (1) overall low risk of acquiring TB; (2) difficulty interpreting TST in light of BCG vaccination; (3) incomplete vaccine protection; and (4) inability to administer vaccine to HIV-infected or immunosuppressed persons. In a recent outbreak of TB in a facility for the mentally handicapped, investigators found all patients and staff to have TST induration of ≤10 mm at the time of initial exposure investigation. They attributed the reaction to a prior history of BCG administration, and did not administer isoniazid therapy. Follow-up TST performed 8–12 weeks later found no change in induration. Six patients and HCWs developed TB following exposure in spite of the history of prior vaccination (molecular fingerprinting confirmed clonality among cases).[81]

CONCLUSIONS

Recent nosocomial spread of TB serves as a reminder of the importance of adequate clinical, diagnostic, and infection control practices. Clinicians must maintain a high index of suspicion for TB. The least expensive and most cost-effective intervention is an institutional administrative TB control program. Even those institutions with limited resources for implementation of all environmental changes can implement surveillance, isolation, empiric therapy, and rapid diagnostic plans. Adjuvant environmental control programs can reduce transmission of TB from unsuspected sources. Complete elimination of transmission to HCWs and among patients may not be possible.[87] More realistic is the reduction of risk to the level of that found in the local general population.

Airborne isolation policies must be enforced. Persons entering airborne isolation rooms should wear PPE (i.e., N95 particulate filter respirator). Transfer of patients with TB from acute care facilities can occur when they are no longer infectious or when appropriate isolation is arranged. Guidelines exist for discharging these patients into the general community.[99] Facilities providing care for persons with TB must develop relationships with local, state, and federal programs for the control of this disease. Local and state departments of health have made a significant impact on the control of TB with DOT and a decrease in hospitalization rates.[2]

In late 2003, OSHA withdrew its 1997 proposed standard on occupational exposure to TB due to the already dramatic decrease in TB rates (and HCW exposures) as a result of Federal and state, and local initiatives.[70] Only overall reduction of TB in the general population could decrease the residual risk posed to HCWs from source patients with unsuspected or undiagnosed TB.[70] Current CDC guidelines offer specific TB infection control program recommendations but emphasize basing components on individual and local risk assessment.[47,99]

The remaining challenge is the reintegration of discharged inmates, homeless persons, or hospitalized patients with recently identified TB and to continue to follow them in a systematic fashion. Although the purpose of SROs was to temporarily house homeless persons, many residents remain in such facilities for prolonged periods and are lost to follow-up. These persons become integrated into their local community and continue to expose others. Cooperation with local and state departments of health continues to remain of paramount importance.

Following a decade of decline in numbers of TB cases, 2003 data marked the smallest annual decline in new TB cases since 1992. These data raise concerns that increased efforts might be required to maintain the progress made in controlling TB.[4] There are a number of questions the answers to which can guide future approaches to TB control: the nature of TB "infectivity" and end-points for contagion; the role of HIV coinfected HCWs in the care of patients with TB; the role of special facilities for the care of patients with TB; and the role of newer techniques for immediate clinical diagnosis, susceptibility testing, epidemiological analyses, and quality control, among others. In addition, we are witnessing an increase in the number of TB cases among those infected during recent outbreaks (i.e., HCWs) as well as persistent pockets of infection among high-risk groups. Close cooperation at the federal, state, city, and facility level is required to meet future challenges. Tuberculosis is a disease not yet eradicated.

ACKNOWLEDGMENTS

I wish to thank Sonal S. Munsiff MD and Cynthia R. Driver RN MPH at New York City Department of Health and Rachel L. Stricof MPH at the New York State Department of Health for recent data and critical review.

REFERENCES

1. Geng E, Kreiswirth BA, Driver C, et al. Changes in the transmission of tuberculosis in New York City from 1990 to 1999. *N Engl J Med.* 2002;346:1453.
2. Terry MB, Desvarieux M, Short M. Temporal trends in tuberculosis hospitalization rates before and after implementation of directly observed therapy: New York City, 1988–1995. *Infect Control Hosp Epidemiol.* 2002;23:221.
3. Li JH, Driver CR, Munsiff SS, et al. Differential decline in tuberculosis incidence among US- and non-US-born persons in New York City. *Int J Tuberc Lung Dis.* 2003; 7:451.
4. CDC. Trends in tuberculosis—United States, 1998–2003. *MMWR Morb Mortal Wkly Rep.* 2004;53:209.
5. Tuberculosis in New York City, 2003: Information Summary. New York: New York City Department of Health and Mental Hygiene; 2004.
6. Nardell EA. Environmental infection control of tuberculosis. *Semin Respir Infect.* 2003;18:307.
7. Beggs CB, Noakes CJ, Sleigh PA, et al. The transmission of tuberculosis in confined spaces: an analytical review of alternative epidemiological models. *Int J Tuberc Lung Dis.* 2003;7:1015.
8. Raffalli J, Sepkowitz KA, Armstrong D. Community-based outbreaks of tuberculosis. *Arch Intern Med.* 1996;156: 1053.
9. Huttom MD, Dooley SW, Cauthen GM. Nosocomial TB transmission: Characteristics of source-patients in reported outbreaks, 1970–1991. *First World Congress on Tuberculosis,* November 15–18, 1992, Rockville, MD.
10. Moss AR, Alland D, Telzak E, et al. A city-wide outbreak of a multiple-drug-resistant strain of Mycobacterium tuberculosis in New York. *Int J Tuberc Lung Dis.* 1997;1:115.
11. Munsiff SS, Nivin B, Sacajiu G, et al. Persistence of a highly resistant strain of tuberculosis in New York City during 1990–1999. *J Infect Dis.* 2003;188:356.
12. Alland D, Kalkut GE, Moss AR, et al. Transmission of tuberculosis in New York City: An analysis by DNA fingerprinting and conventional epidemiologic methods. *N Engl J Med.* 1994;330:1710.
13. Small PM, Hopewell PC, Singh SP, et al. The epidemiology of tuberculosis in San Francisco: A population-based study using conventional and molecular methods. *N Engl J Med.* 1994;330:1703.
14. Agerton TB, Valway SE, Blinkhorn RJ, et al. Spread of strain W, a highly drug-resistant strain of Mycobacterium tuberculosis, across the United States. *Clin Infect Dis.* 1999;29:85.
15. Pitchenik AE, Burr J. Laufer M, et al. Outbreaks of drug-resistant tuberculosis at AIDS center. *Lancet.* 1990;336:440.
16. Centers for Disease Control. Nosocomial transmission of multidrug-resistant tuberculosis among HIV-infected persons-Florida and New York, 1988–1991. *MMWR Morb Mortal Wkly Rep.* 1991;40:585.
17. Edlin BR, Tokars JI, Grieco MH, et al. An outbreak of multidrug-resistant tuberculosis among hospitalized patients with the acquired immunodeficiency syndrome. *N Engl J Med.* 1992;326:1514.
18. Pearson ML, Jereb JA, Frieden TR, et al. Nosocomial transmission of multidrug-resistant Mycobacterium tuberculosis: A risk to patients and health care workers. *Ann Intern Med.* 1992;117:191.
19. Beck-Sagué C, Dooley SW, Hutton MD, et al. Hospital outbreak of multidrug-resistant *Mycobacterium tuberculosis* infections: Factors in transmission to staff and HIV-infected patients. *JAMA.* 1992;268:1280.
20. Fischl MA, Daikos GL, Uttamchandani RB, et al. Clinical presentation and outcome of patients with HIV infection and tuberculosis caused by multiple-drug-resistant bacilli. *Ann Intern Med.* 1992;117:184.
21. Centers for disease Control and Prevention. Outbreak of multidrug-resistant tuberculosis at a hospital-New York City, 1991. *MMWR Morb Mortal Wkly Rep.* 1993;42:427.
22. Small PM, Shafer RW, Hopewell PC, et al. Exogenous reinfection with multidrug-resistant *Mycobacterium tuberculosis* in patients with advanced HIV infection. *N Engl J Med.* 1993;328:1137.
23. Valway SE, Greifinger RB, Papania M, et al. Multidrug-resistant tuberculosis in the New York State prison system, 1990–1991. *J Infect Dis.* 1994;170:151.
24. Ikeda RM, Birkhead GS, DiFerdinando GT Jr, et al. Nosocomial tuberculosis: an outbreak of a strain resistant to seven drugs. *Infect Control Hosp Epidemiol.* 1995;16:152.
25. Castro KG. Tuberculosis as an opportunistic disease in persons infected with human immunodeficiency virus. *Clin Infect Dis.* 1995;21(suppl 1):S66.
26. Frieden TR, Sherman LF, Maw KL, et al. A multi-institutional outbreak of highly drug-resistant tuberculosis: Epidemiology and clinical outcomes. *JAMA.* 1996;276:1229.
27. Bock N, Reichman LB. Tuberculosis and HIV/AIDS: Epidemiological and clinical aspects (world perspective). *Semin Respir Crit Care Med.* 2004;25:337.
28. Reichler MR, Bur S, Reves R, et al. Results of testing for human immunodeficiency virus infection among recent contacts of infectious tuberculosis cases in the United States. *Int J Tuberc Lung Dis.* 2003;7:S471.
29. Jereb JA, Klevens RM, Privett TD, et al. Tuberculosis in health care workers at a hospital with an outbreak of multidrug-resistant *Mycobacterium tuberculosis. Arch Intern Med.* 1995;16:141.
30. Stroud LA, Tokars JI, Grieco MH, et al. Evaluation of infection control measures in preventing the nosocomial transmission of multidrug-resistant *Mycobacterium tuberculosis* in a New York City hospital. *Infect Control Hosp Epidemiol.* 1995;16:141.

31. Maloney SA, Pearson ML, Gordon MT, et al. Efficacy of control measures in preventing nosocomial transmission of multidrug-resistant tuberculosis to patients and health care workers. *Ann Intern Med.* 1995;122:90.

32. Wenger PN, Otten J, Breeden A, et al. Control of nosocomial transmission of multidrug-resistant Mycobacterium tuberculosis among healthcare workers and HIV-infected patients. *Lancet.* 1995;345:235.

33. Jarvis WR. Nosocomial transmission of multidrug-resistant *Mycobacterium tuberculosis. Am J Infect Control.* 1995;23:146.

34. Centers for Disease Control and Prevention. Guidelines for preventing the transmission of Mycobacterium tuberculosis in health-care facilities, 1994. *MMWR Morb Mortal Wkly Rep.* 1994;43(RR-13):1.

35. Brickner PW, Vincent RL, First M, et al. The application of ultraviolet germicidal irradiation to control transmission of airborne disease: bioterrorism countermeasure. *Public Health Rep.* 2003;118:99.

36. CDC. Tuberculosis outbreak in a community hospital—District of Columbia, 2002. *MMWR Morb Mortal Wkly Rep.* 2004;53:214.

37. CDC. Nosocomial transmission of Mycobacterium tuberculosis found through screening for Severe Acute Respiratory Syndrome—Taipei, Taiwan, 2003. *MMWR Morb Mortal Wkly Rep.* 2004;53:321.

38. Bellin EY, Fletcher DD, Safyer SM. Association of tuberculosis infection with increased time in or admission to the New York City jail system. *JAMA.* 1993;269:2228.

39. Takashima HT, Cruess DF, McDonald KR, et al. Tuberculosis and HIV infection in new inmates in Federal Bureau of Prison facilities. *Mil Med.* 1996;161:265.

40. CDC. Prevention and control of tuberculosis in correctional facilities: recommendations of the Advisory Council for the Elimination of Tuberculosis. *MMWR Morb Mortal Wkly Rep.* 1996;45(No. RR-8):1.

41. Centers for Disease Control. Transmission of multidrug-resistant tuberculosis among immunocompromised persons in a correctional system-New York, 1991. *MMWR Morb Mortal Wkly Rep.* 1992;41:507.

42. Centers for Disease Control. Tuberculosis transmission in a state correctional institution-California, 1990–1991. *MMWR Morb Mortal Wkly Rep.* 1992;41:927.

43. Centers for Disease Control and Prevention. Probable transmission of multidrug-resistant tuberculosis in correctional facility-California. *MMWR Morb Mortal Wkly Rep.* 1993;42:48.

44. Valway SE, Richards SB, Kovacovich J, et al. Outbreak of multi-drug-resistant tuberculosis in a New York State Prison, 1991. *Am J Epidemiol.* 1994;140:113.

45. Wilcock K, Hammett TM, Widom R, et al. Tuberculosis in correctional facilities 1994–1995. National Institute of Justice, Research in Brief, July 1996, p 1.

46. Centers for Disease Control and Prevention. Tuberculosis prevention in drug-treatment centers and correctional facilities-selected US sites, 1990–1991. *MMWR Morb Mortal Wkly Rep.* 1993;42:211.

47. CDC. Guidelines for environmental infection control in health-care facilities: recommendations of CDC and the Healthcare Infection Control Practices Advisory Committee (HICPAC). *MMWR Morb Mortal Wkly Rep.* 2003;52 (No. RR-10):1.

48. Jones TF, Craig AS, Valway SE, et al. Transmission of tuberculosis in a jail. Ann *Intern Med.* 1999;131:557–563.

49. Brock NN, Reeves M, LaMarre M, et al. Tuberculosis case detection in a state prison system. *Public Health Rep.* 1998;113:359.

50. Cone JE, Harrison R, Katz E, et al. Tuberculosis transmission to prison employees during an outbreak among prisoners at two California prisons. *J Healthcare Safety* 2000;4:75.

51. CDC. Tuberculosis transmission in multiple correctional facilities—Kansas, 2003–2003. *MMWR Morb Mortal Wkly Rep.* 2004;53:734.

52. McLaughlin SI, Spradling P, Drocluk D, et al. Extensive transmission of Mycobacterium tuberculosis among congregated, HIV-infected prison inmates in South Carolina, United States. *Int J Tuberc Lung Dis.* 2003;7:665.

53. CDC. Tuberculosis outbreaks in prison housing units for HIV-infected inmates—California, 1995-1996. *MMWR Morb Mortal Wkly Rep.* 1999;48:79.

54. Ijaz K, Yang Z, Templeton G, et al. Persistence of a strain of *Mycobacterium tuberculosis* in a prison system. *Int J Tuberc Lung Dis.* 2004;8:994.

55. Moss AR, Hahn JA, Tulsky JP, et al. Tuberculosis in the homeless: a prospective study. *Am J Respir Crit Care Med.* 2000;162:460.

56. Brudney K, Dobkin J. Resurgent tuberculosis in New York City: Human immunodeficiency virus, homelessness, and the decline of tuberculosis control programs. *Am Rev Respir Dis.* 1991;144:745.

57. Brickner PW, Scharer LL, McAdam JM. Tuberculosis in homeless populations. In: Reichman LB, Hershfield ES, eds. *Tuberculosis: A Comprehensive International Approach.* New York, NY: Marcel Dekker; 1993:433.

58. Torres RA, Mani S, Altholz, et al. Human immunodeficiency virus infection among homeless men in a New York City shelter: association with *Mycobacterium tuberculosis* infection. *Arch Intern Med.* 1990;150:2030.

59. Nolan CM, Elarth AM, Barr H, et al. An outbreak of tuberculosis in a shelter for homeless men: a description of its evolution and control. *Am Rev Respir Dis.* 1991;143:257.

60. Zolopa AR, Hahn JA, Gorter R, et al. HIV and tuberculosis infection in San Francisco's homeless adults: Prevalence and risk factors in a representative sample. *JAMA.* 1994;272:455.

61. Pablos-Mendez A, Raviglione MC, Battan R, et al. Drug resistant tuberculosis among the homeless in New York City. *N Y State J Med.* 1990;90:351.

62. Centers for Disease Control. Prevention and control of tuberculosis among homeless persons: Recommendations

of the Advisory Council for the Elimination of Tuberculosis. *MMWR Morb Mortal Wkly Rep.* 1992;41(RR-5):1.

63. Bureau of Tuberculosis Control. *Information summary 1995.* New York, NY: New York City Department of Health; 1995:1.

64. Friedman LN, Williams MT, Singh TP, et al. Tuberculosis, AIDS, and death among substance abusers on welfare in New York City. *N Engl J Med.* 1996;334:828.

65. Perlman DC, Salomon N, Perkins MP, et al. Tuberculosis in drug users. *Clin Infect Dis.* 1995;21:1253.

66. CDC. Tuberculosis outbreak in a homeless population— Portland, Maine, 2002–2003. *MMWR Morb Mortal Wkly Rep.* 2003;52:1184.

67. Cantwell MF, McKenna MT, McCray E, et al. Tuberculosis and race/ethnicity in the United States: impact of socioeconomic status. *Am J Respir Crit Care Med.* 1998;157:1016.

68. Barr RG, Diez-Roux AV, Knirsch CA, et al. Neighborhood poverty and the resurgence of tuberculosis in New York City, 1984–1992. *Am J Public Health.* 2001;91:1487.

69. Barnes PF, Yang Z, Preston-Martin S, et al. Patterns of tuberculosis transmission in central Los Angeles. *JAMA.* 1997;278:1159.

70. Department of Labor Occupational Safety and Health Administration. 29 CFR Part 1910 Occupational Exposure to Tuberculosis; Proposed rule; Termination of rulemaking respiratory protection for M tuberculosis; Final rule; Revocation. *Federal Regist.* 2003(December 31);68 (250):75768–75775.

71. Li J, Driver CR, Munsiff SS, Fujiwara PI. Finding contacts of homeless tuberculosis patients in New York City. *Int J Tuberc Lung Dis.* 2003;7:S397.

72. Yun LWH, Reves RR, Reichler MR, et al. Outcomes of contact investigation among homeless persons with infectious tuberculosis. *Int J Tuberc Lung Dis.* 2003;7:S405.

73. CDC. Tuberculosis outbreak among homeless persons – King County, Washington, 2002–2003. *MMWR Morb Mortal Wkly Rep.* 2003:52:1209.

74. Nardell E, McInnis B, Thomas B, et al. Exogenous reinfection with tuberculosis in a shelter for the homeless. *N Engl J Med.* 1986;315:1570.

75. Stead WW: Special problems in tuberculosis: Tuberculosis in the elderly and in residents of nursing homes, correctional facilities, long-term care hospitals, mental hospitals, shelters for the homeless, and jails. *Clin Chest Med.* 1989;10:397.

76. Centers for Disease Control. Prevention and control of tuberculosis in facilities providing long-term care to the elderly: Recommendations of the Advisory Committee for the Elimination of Tuberculosis. *MMWR Morb Mortal Wkly Rep.* 1990;39(RR-10):1.

77. Rajagopalan S, Yoshikawa TT. Tuberculosis in long-term-care facilities. *Infect Control Hosp Epidemiol.* 2000;21: 611.

78. Hutton MD, Cauthen GM, Bloch AB. Results of a 29-state survey of tuberculosis in nursing homes and correctional facilities. *Public Health Rep.* 1993;108:305.

79. Naglie G, McArthur M, Simor A, et al. Tuberculosis surveillance practices in long-term care institutions. *Infect Control Hosp Epidemiol.* 1995;16:148.

80. Centers for Disease Control and Prevention. Screening for tuberculosis and tuberculosis infection in high-risk populations: Recommendations of the Advisory Council for the Elimination of Tuberculosis. *MMWR Morb Mortal Wkly Rep.* 1995;44(RR-11):11.

81. Lemaitre N, Sougakoff W, Coetmeur D, et al. Nosocomial transmission of tuberculosis among mentally-handicapped patients in a long-term care facility. *Tubercle Lung Dis.* 1996;77:531.

82. Markowitz SB. Epidemiology of tuberculosis among health care workers. *Occup Med.* 1994;9:589.

83. Bowden KM, McDiarmid MA. Occupationally acquired tuberculosis: What's known. *J Occup Med.* 1994;36:320.

84. Sepkowitz KA. AIDS, tuberculosis, and the health care worker. *Clin Infect Dis.* 1995;20:232.

85. Fraser VJ, Kilo CM, Bailey TC, et al. Screening physicians for tuberculosis. *Infect Control Hosp Epidemiol.* 1994;15:95.

86. Fridkin SK, Manangan L, Bolyard E, et al. SHEA-CDC TB survey, part I: Status of TB infection control programs at member hospitals, 1989–1992. *Infect Control Hosp Epidemiol.* 1995;16:129.

87. Menzies D, Fanning A, Yuan L, et al. Tuberculosis among health care workers. *N Engl J Med.* 1995;332:92.

88. Hutton M, Stead WW, Cauthen G. et al. Nosocomial transmission of tuberculosis associated with a draining abscess. *J Infect Dis.* 1990;161:286.

89. Griffith DE, Hardeman JL, Zhang Y, et al. Tuberculosis outbreak among healthcare workers in a community hospital. *Am J Respir Crit Care Med.* 1995;152:808.

90. Sepkowitz KA. Tuberculin skin testing and the health care worker: lessons of the Profit Survey. *Tuber Lung Dis.* 1996;77:81.

91. Sepkowitz KA, Friedman CR, Hafner A, et al. Tuberculosis among urban health care workers: A study using restriction fragment length polymorphism typing. *Clin Infect Dis.* 1995;172:1542.

92. Zaza S, Blumberg HM, Beck-Sagué C, et al. Nosocomial transmission of *Mycobacterium tuberculosis:* role of health care workers in outbreak propagation. *J Infect Dis.* 1995;172:1542.

93. Bock NN, Sotir MJ, Parrott PL, et al. Nosocomial tuberculosis exposure in an outpatient setting: evaluation of patients exposed to healthcare providers with tuberculosis. *Infect Control Hosp Epidemiol.* 1999;20:421.

94. Cook S, Maw KL, Munsiff SS, et al. Prevalence of tuberculin skin test positivity and conversions among healthcare workers in New York City during 1994 to 2001. *Infect Control Hosp Epidemiol.* 2003;24:807.

95. Centers for Disease Control. Guidelines for preventing the transmission of tuberculosis in health-care settings, with special focus on HIV-related issues. *MMWR Morb Mortal Wkly Rep.* 1990;39(RR-17):1.

96. Blumberg HM, Watkins DL, Berschling JD, et al. Preventing the nosocomial transmission of tuberculosis. *Ann Intern Med.* 1995;122:658.

97. Fridkin SK, Manangan L, Bolyard E, et al. SHEA-CDC TB survey, part II: Efficacy of TB infection control programs at member hospitals, 1992. *Infect Control Hosp Epidemiol.* 1995;16:135.

98. McDiarmid M, Gamponia MJ, Ryan MAK, et al. Tuberculosis in the workplace: OSHA's compliance experience. *Infect Control Hosp Epidemiol.* 1996;17:159.

99. CDCP. Draft: Guidelines for Preventing the Transmission of *Mycobacterium tuberculosis* in Health-Care settings. Available at: http://www.cdc.gov/nchstp/TB/FederalRegister/default/htm. Accessed 2005.

100. Lambert L, Rajbhandary S, Qualls, et al. Costs of implementing and maintaining a tuberculin skin test program in hospitals and health departments. *Infect Control Hosp Epidemiol.* 2003;24:814.

101. Steimke EH, Tenholder MF, McCormick MI, et al. Tuberculosis surveillance: Lessons from a cluster of skin test conversions. *Am J Infect Control.* 1993;21:236.

102. Fazal BA, Telzak EE, Blum S, et al. Impact of a coordinated tuberculosis team in an inner-city hospital in New York City. *Infect Control Hosp Epidemiol.* 1995;16:340.

103. Craft DW, Jones MC, Blanchet CN, et al. Value of examining three acid-fast bacillus sputum smears for removal of patients suspected of having tuberculosis from the "Airborne Precautions" category. *J Clin Microbiol.* 2000;38:4285.

104. Siddiqui AH, Perl TM, Conlon M, et al. Preventing nosocomial transmission of pulmonary tuberculosis: when may isolation be discontinued for patients with suspected tuberculosis? *Infect Control and Hosp Epidemiol.* 2002;23:141.

105. Hernandez-Garduno E, Cook V, Kunimoto D, et al. Transmission of tuberculosis from smear negative patients: a molecular epidemiology study. *Thorax.* 2004;59:286–290.

106. Puisis M, Feinglass J, Lidow E, et al. Radiographic screening for tuberculosis in a large urban county jail. *Public Health Rep.* 1996;111:330.

107. Zoloth SR, Safyer S, Roen J, et al. Anergy compromises screening for tuberculosis in high-risk populations. *Am J Public Health.* 1993;83:719.

108. Safyer SM, Richmond L, Bellin E, et al. Tuberculosis in correctional facilities: The tuberculosis control program of the Montefiore Medical Center Rikers Island Health Services. *J Law Med Ethics.* 1993;21:342.

109. Greifinger RB, Heywood NJ, Glaser JB. Tuberculosis in prison: balancing justice and public health. *J Law Med Ethics.* 1993;21:332.

110. Tulsky JP, Pilote L, Hahn JA, et al. Adherence to isoniazid prophylaxis in the homeless: a randomized controlled trial. *Arch Intern Med.* 2000;160:697.

111. Tulsky JP, Hahn JA, Long HL, et al. Can the poor adhere? Incentives for adherence to TB prevention in homeless adults. *Int J Tuberc Lung Dis.* 2004;8:83.

112. LoBue P, Cass R, Lobo D, et al. Development of housing programs to aid in the treatment of tuberculosis in homeless individuals: a pilot study. *Chest.* 1999;115:218.

113. Burman WJ, Cohn DL, Rietmeijer CA, et al. Short-term incarceration for the management of noncompliance with tuberculosis treatment. *Chest.* 1997;112:57.

114. Segal-Maurer S, Kalkut GE. Environmental control of tuberculosis: Continuing controversy. *Clin Infect Dis.* 1994;19:299.

115. Nagin D, Pavelchak N, London M, et al. Control of tuberculosis in the workplace: Engineering controls. *Occup Med.* 1994;9:609.

116. Nardell EA. Interrupting transmission from patients with unsuspected tuberculosis: A unique role for upper-room ultraviolet air disinfection. *Am J Infect Control.* 1995;23:156.

117. Stead WW, Yeung C, Hartnett C. Probable role of ultraviolet irradiation in preventing transmission of tuberculosis: A case study. *Infect Control Hosp Epidemiol.* 1996;17:11.

118. Ko G, Burge HA, Nardell EA, et al. Estimation of tuberculosis risk and incidence under upper room ultraviolet germicidal irradiation in a waiting room in a hypothetical scenario. *Risk Anal.* 2001;21:657.

119. Xu P, Pecciaa J, Fabiana P, et al. Efficacy of ultraviolet germicidal irradiation of upper-room air in inactivating airborne bacterial spores and Mycobacteria in full scale studies. *Atmos Environ.* 2003;37:405.

120. Pavelchak N, DePersis RP, London M, et al. Identification of factors that disrupt negative pressurization of respiratory isolation rooms. *Infect Control Hosp Epidemiol.* 2000;21:191.

121. Pavelchak N, Cummings K, Stricof R, et al. Negative-pressure monitoring of tuberculosis isolation rooms within New York State Hospitals. *Infect Control Hosp Epidemiol.* 2001;22:518.

122. Manangan LP, Bennett CL, Tablan N, et al. Nosocomial tuberculosis prevention measures among two groups of US hospitals, 1992 to 1996. *Chest.* 2000;117:380.

123. Tokars JI, McKinley GF, Otten J, et al. Use and efficacy of tuberculosis infection control practices at hospitals with previous outbreaks of multidrug-resistant tuberculosis. *Infect Control Hosp Epidemiol.* 2001;22:449.

124. Iwata K, Smith BA, Santos E, et al. Failure to implement respiratory isolation: why does it happen? *Infect Control Hosp Epidemiol.* 2002;23:595–599.

125. Mehta AC, Minai OA. Infection control in the bronchoscopy suite. *Clin Chest Med.* 1999;20:19.

126. Menzies D, Adhikari N, Arietta M, et al. Efficacy of environmental measures in reducing potentially infectious bioaerosols during sputum induction. *Infect Control Hosp Epidemiol.* 2003;24:483.

127. Ussery XT, Bierman JA, Valway SE, et al. Transmission of multidrug-resistant Mycobacterium tuberculosis among persons exposed in a medical examiner's office, New York. *Infect Control Hosp Epidemiol.* 1995;16:160.

128. Segal-Maurer S, Kreiswirth BN, Burns JM, et al. *Mycobacterium tuberculosis* specimen contamination

revisited: The role of laboratory environmental control in a pseudo-outbreak. *Infect Control Hosp Epidemiol.* 1998;19:101.

129. Nardell EA. Ultraviolet air disinfection to control tuberculosis in a shelter for the homeless. In: Kundsin RB, ed. *Architectural design and indoor microbial pollution.* Oxford : Oxford University Press; 1988:296.

130. Clark RA. OSHA enforcement policy and procedures for occupational exposure to tuberculosis. *Infect Control Hosp Epidemiol.* 1993;14:694.

131. Hodous TK, Coffey CC. The role of respiratory protective devices in the control of tuberculosis. *Occup Med.* 1994;9:631.

132. Jarvis WR, Bolyard EA, Bozzi CJ, et al. Respirators, recommendations, and regulations: The controversy surrounding protection of health care workers from tuberculosis. *Ann Intern Med.* 1995;122:142.

133. Fella P, Rivera P, Hale M, et al. Dramatic decrease in tuberculin skin test conversion rate among employees at a hospital in New York City. *Am J Infect Control.* 1995;23:352.

134. Rosenstock L. 42 *CFR* Part 84: Respiratory protective devices implications for tuberculosis control. *Infect Control Hosp Epidemiol.* 1995;16:529.

135. Reponen TA, Wang Z, Willeke K, et al. Survival of mycobacteria on N95 personal respirators. *Infect Control Hosp Epidemiol.* 1999;20:237.

136. Department of Labor Occupational Safety and Health Administration 29 *CFR* Part 1910 Occupational Exposure to Tuberculosis; Proposed rule; Termination of rulemaking respiratory protection for *M tuberculosis*; Final rule; Revocation. *Federal Register.* December 31, 2003;68 (250):75776–75780.

137. Centers for Disease Control and Prevention. The role of BCG vaccine in the prevention and control of tuberculosis in the United States: A joint statement by the Advisory Council for the Elimination of Tuberculosis and the Advisory Committee on Immunization Practices. *MMWR Morb Mortal Wkly Rep.* 1996;45(RR-4):1.

138. Sepkowitz KA. Tuberculosis and the health care worker: A historical perspective. *Ann Intern Med.* 1994;120:71.

139. Brewer TF, Colditz GA. Bacille Calmette-Guérin vaccination for the prevention of tuberculosis in HCWs. *Clin Infect Dis.* 1995;20:136.

140. Stevens JP, Daniel TM. Bacille Calmette-Guérin immunization of health care workers exposed to multidrug-resistant tuberculosis: A decision analysis. *Tuber Lung Dis.* 1996;77:315.

12

Role of the Health Department—Legal and Public Health Considerations

Philip LoBue
Zachary Taylor

Tuberculosis (TB) is an archetypical public health disease. Tuberculosis is caused by an infectious organism, it is spread through a common vehicle, the air, and public health measures are essential for control of the disease. There are three priority strategies for TB prevention and control in the United States: 1) identifying and treating persons who have TB disease; 2) finding persons exposed to infectious TB patients, evaluating them for *M. tuberculosis* infection and disease, and providing subsequent treatment, if appropriate; and 3) screening populations at high risk for latent tuberculosis infection (LTBI) and progression to TB disease to detect infected persons and provide treatment to prevent progression to disease.[1]

Although prevention and control of TB in the United States is primarily the responsibility of state and local TB control programs, rarely are these activities implemented solely by the health department. Patients with TB disease are usually diagnosed and often treated by private providers. Contacts to infectious cases may also be evaluated and treated by their private physicians or other community providers. Private providers, as well as nonhealth department community or governmental entities, also screen and treat individuals at high risk for LTBI. However, the health department is responsible for coordination and oversight of these activities to ensure that objectives related to TB prevention and control are achieved.

The Advisory Council for the Elimination of Tuberculosis identified seven core components of public health TB control programs[1]:

1. Conducting overall planning and development of policy
2. Identifying persons who have clinically active TB
3. Managing persons who have or who are suspected of having disease
4. Identifying and managing persons infected with *M. tuberculosis*
5. Providing laboratory and diagnostic services
6. Collecting and analyzing data
7. Providing training and education

This chapter will describe the role of the health department in the context of these core components. This discussion is primarily limited to TB prevention and control programs in the United States.

HISTORICAL AND EPIDEMIOLOGIC CONTEXT OF TUBERCULOSIS CONTROL

Public health control measures for TB have mirrored the knowledge and availability of treatment options. Prior to the discovery of the tubercle bacillus by Koch, there were few public health measures to control TB, although morbidity and mortality data were collected by some jurisdictions. Following the discovery of the tubercle bacillus and the advent of the sanatorium movement, the primary public health measure became the isolation of infectious persons in sanatoria. Hospitalization in sanatoria was intended for treatment initially, but soon evolved into a control measure as well with the forced hospitalization of some patients;[2] however, the availability of beds never met the demand. In 1945, the United States had 450 TB hospitals with 79,000 beds, despite having many more reported incident cases. With the advent of effective chemotherapy, hospitalization duration declined as the adoption of outpatient treatment of TB became the standard. In the 1960s and early 1970s, the situation in 1945 was reversed with many beds in TB hospitals remaining empty and the eventual closure of the TB hospitals. Hospitalization is now reserved for acute care, although forced confinement continues for a small number of recalcitrant patients.[3–6]

Tuberculosis incidence and mortality from TB began declining in the United States prior to the widespread use of sanatoria and well before the advent of effective chemotherapy.[7] National statistics, which have been kept since 1953, demonstrate a steady decline in disease from 1953 to 1985. In 1953, there were 83,304 incident cases reported, and in 1985, 22,201 incident cases were reported.[8] As cases of TB declined to historical lows in the United States, the public health infrastructure for control also declined, as categorical federal funding ended and local funding was shifted to other priorities.[1] Reported incident TB cases increased from 22,768 cases in 1986 to 26,673 cases in 1992. This increase coincided with the onset of the human immunodeficiency virus (HIV) epidemic, and TB in HIV infected persons contributed to the increase.[1] Other factors associated with the increase in TB included nosocomial and institutional transmission of *M. tuberculosis* and increased cases occurring in foreign-born persons who immigrated from countries with high rates of TB.[1] Following the resurgence of TB, federal resources for TB prevention and control were substantially increased. These resources were directed to improve surveillance, increase the capacity of public health laboratories, and increase the number of TB patients treated with directly observed therapy.[9] As a result, the incidence of TB steadily declined from 1993 through 2003; in 2003, a historical low of 14,874 incident cases of TB were reported in the United States.[10]

The complexity of TB control and the challenges facing elimination of TB have, however, not diminished. In 2003, greater than 50% of cases reported in the United States occured in persons born in other countries.[10] A local TB control program may now have individuals from several different countries with TB disease in their jurisdiction. Therefore, the program must provide interpreter services, be responsive to the cultural issues of their patients, and provide patient education to persons who may have different perceptions regarding TB disease and treatment than health department staff and providers. Along the US/Mexico border, persons with TB travel back and forth, complicating treatment of their TB and the identification and follow-up of contacts.[11] Persons diagnosed and beginning treatment in Mexico, may travel to the United States to continue and complete treatment, a burden of prevalent cases not included in incident case reports. Coinfection with HIV occurs in 9% of patients reported with TB.[10] This complicates treatment options because of drug-drug interactions between highly active antiretroviral therapy (HAART) and antituberculous medications.[12,13] Outbreaks in low incidence areas often overwhelm local TB control program staff, resulting in increased transmission of and morbidity from TB. Although rates of drug resistant TB, particularly multi-drug resistant TB, have declined since 1993, these cases continue to complicate treatment and prevention efforts.[10] All of these factors complicate efforts to control and eventually eliminate TB in the United States.

ORGANIZATION OF PUBLIC HEALTH TUBERCULOSIS CONTROL PROGRAMS

Tuberculosis control in the United States is the legal responsibility of the state and local governments.[1] Most of the activities of TB control, such as surveillance, case management, and contact investigation, are conducted by the local (city, county, or district) health departments with oversight by the state TB control program. Medical care for patients with TB disease or LTBI is often provided by the health department; however, in many areas of the United States, medical care is provided by private, community physicians who may have an established relationship with the local TB control program. Regardless of where the medical care is provided, local TB control programs continue to have responsibility for supervision of care and ensuring that the patient completes treatment for their disease.

State TB control programs generally provide funding and technical support to local programs. State programs also compile and report surveillance data, as do large local programs. State programs may assist local programs with investigations of outbreaks. Some state programs also conduct operational and epidemiologic research related to TB control. Public health laboratories are generally part of the state program, although large cities or counties may also have public health laboratories. State programs are responsible for interactions with other state government entities that may have a role in TB control, such as correctional facilities.

The U.S. Centers for Disease Control and Prevention (CDC) is primarily responsible for the federal public health response to TB control. This includes providing funding for state and local TB programs, providing technical assistance to programs, compiling and reporting surveillance data, providing support for and investigating outbreaks of TB, and funding and conducting operational, epidemiologic, clinical, and basic and applied laboratory studies related to TB control.

LEGAL BASIS FOR PUBLIC HEALTH AUTHORITY

In the United States, "police power," i.e., the authority to protect the health and safety of citizens, lies primarily with the individual states. The state public health department generally assumes the executive function with regard to protecting the public from infectious diseases, although frequently certain duties are delegated to municipal or county health departments, especially in large or populous states. The individual state health department's powers, including the ability to limit individual freedom, have been broadly defined and upheld by the U.S. Supreme Court.[14,15] While involuntary confinement is permitted under these powers, the court has found that individuals are entitled to due process protections when such actions are initiated.[14,16] To facilitate

TB control, health departments are invested with a number of legal powers. These include the abilities to require disease reporting; isolate contagious patients; order medical examinations; mandate therapy, including directly observed therapy (DOT); and, if necessary, detain or incarcerate nonadherent patients (Table 12-1).

Reporting of active TB by medical providers and facilities is required by all states, although the time allowed between knowledge or suspicion of disease and reporting varies.[17] Some states have additional reporting or approval requirements. In Missouri, LTBI must also be reported, while in California, patients with suspected or confirmed TB may not be discharged from a medical facility without prior approval of the discharge plan by the local health department.[18,19]

Similarly, there is significant state-to-state variation in laws related to isolation of contagious patients. Many states use long-standing quarantine regulations to "quarantine" contagious patients in their homes or in the hospital. Technically, quarantine consists of segregating persons

Table 12-1. Types of Regulatory Action*

Description	Evidence Required	Basis for Rescinding Order
Order for examination for suspected TB as outpatient or in detention	Clinical symptoms or history of TB and refusal by patient to come to clinic or submit to examination in hospital	After minimal time required, TB can be either diagnosed or ruled out. No forcible examination allowed.
Order to complete treatment	History of leaving hospital against medical advice or noncompliance early in course of treatment	Patient completes treatment or is given another order.
Order for directly observed therapy	Noncompliance with voluntary directly observed therapy or history of leaving hospital against medical advice or previous order for detention while infectious	Patient completes treatment, self-administration of medication is allowed, or patient is detained.
Written warning of possible detention	Failure to adhere to order for directly observed therapy without plausible excuse or <80 percent compliance for more than 2 weeks	Patient completes treatment or is detained.
Order for detention while infectious	Proof of suspected infectiousness, either by smears or clinical symptoms, plus failure to abide by infection-control guidelines or inability to be separated from others as outpatient	Patient has three negative smears or clinical evidence of noninfectiousness.
Order for detention while noninfectious	Proof of substantial likelihood that patient cannot complete treatment as outpatient (e.g., documented noncompliance with directly observed therapy, denial of diagnosis of TB, history of inability to be located)	Patient is discharged early to court-ordered directly observed therapy or patient completes therapy. Order must be periodically reviewed by court.
Discharge from detention before cure (for noninfectious patient)	Change in circumstances so that compliance with outpatient, directly observed therapy is likely (e.g., new insight, substance-abuse treatment, new home environment, or family support)	Patient completes treatment or is detained again if patient fails to comply with outpatient treatment.

*None of the orders permit the forcible administration of medication.

Source: Reproduced with permission from Gasner MR, Law Maw K, Feldman GE, et al. The use of legal action in New York City to ensure treatment of TB. *N Engl J Med.* 1999;340:359–366. Copyright 1999 Massachusetts Medical Society. All right reserved. Reproduced by permission.

recently exposed to an infectious disease who are not yet manifesting symptoms. In its narrowest definition, this intervention is not really applicable to TB control, where the goal is to isolate contagious patients until they are no longer able to transmit TB, thereby preventing others from being exposed and infected. Nevertheless, the "quarantine" power has been used by some states to enforce respiratory isolation. The lack of uniformity and, in some cases, antiquated nature of state public health laws related to isolation and quarantine poses potential problems in the face of new bioterrorism threats. This has led to development of model public health law proposals which may have applicability to TB, especially in outbreak situations.[20]

The most controversial public health powers are those that allow the state to detain or confine TB patients who do not adhere to treatment. Confining an individual should only be done as a last resort after all less restrictive measures have been exhausted.[2] Voluntary DOT is the initial intervention used to facilitate adherence to treatment. All reasonable additional steps should be taken to remove barriers for patients to adhere to voluntary DOT before instituting more restrictive measures. Such steps include attempting to accommodate the patients work or school schedule, arranging a convenient site for administering DOT, and providing incentives and enablers including transportation tokens, food vouchers, and housing if needed.[21,22] If these interventions fail, usually the next action is to serve the patient with a legal order for DOT. If there is continued nonadherence with legally ordered DOT, detention may be necessary.

Because of the restrictions on personal liberty, attempts to detain an individual must allow for due process. This includes the ability to challenge a detention order in court and the right to an attorney to assist with the challenge.[2,21] If detention is ordered, it should be carried out in the least restrictive environment possible, a locked hospital ward being preferred over a correctional facility. Detention orders are usually subject to periodic judicial review (e.g., every 90 days), with the health department required to provide evidence that continued detention is necessary. All legal orders should be immediately rescinded when they are no longer needed for public health protection.

A recent review of the use of legal action for TB control in New York City found that the issuing of regulatory orders was uncommon, with less than 4% of 8000 patients receiving such orders.[21] Legal orders tended to be reserved for patients who were repeatedly nonadherent or who left the hospital against medical advice. Even among patients with significant social problems (e.g., substance abuse, homelessness), only a minority required legal action to complete treatment.

CONDUCTING OVERALL PLANNING AND DEVELOPMENT OF POLICY

Rational planning for TB program activities begins with an analysis of current data with close attention to recent trends. Morbidity trends (total cases and case rates) provide a general indication of future resource requirements. Not only do they provide insight into the amount of resources necessary for the management of TB patients, but they also help to predict resources needed for contact investigation and tuberculin testing and LTBI treatment since the numbers of contact investigations conducted and persons with LTBI tend to be proportional to TB morbidity.

The next level of analysis should focus on epidemiologic trends, specifically the distribution of TB morbidity in the population served by the health department. Although general associations between TB and certain risk groups have been well documented (e.g., HIV-infected, homeless, foreign-born, and racial and ethnic minorities), the relative importance of these risk groups varies based on location. Therefore analysis of morbidity trends among these groups at the state and local level is crucial to planning activities and interventions. This type of analysis also informs the TB program with respect to the needs for outreach to specific communities and hiring employees with suitable cultural and linguistic competencies.

Formal program evaluation is a critical process that contributes to both planning and accountability. In program evaluation, measurable indicators of program performance are created, and objectives are set for each indicator. This allows the program to determine if it is achieving its goals. CDC has developed a framework for program evaluation of public health practices.[23] The CDC framework is based on four principles: utility—ensuring that the user's information needs are satisfied; feasibility—ensuring that the evaluation is viable and pragmatic; propriety—ensuring that the evaluation is ethical; and accuracy—ensuring that the evaluation produces findings that are considered correct. The framework includes six steps:

1. Engage stakeholders
2. Describe the program
3. Focus the evaluation design
4. Gather credible evidence
5. Justify conclusions
6. Ensure use and share lessons learned

Use of this methodology allows detailed examination of various aspects of a TB program. The program can determine which aspects are successful and which are in need of improvement. For those that need improvement, action steps can be designed and implemented to address shortcomings. Program evaluation should be a continual, iterative process.

Some TB programs have created sets of indicators to provide an overall assessment of performance.[24] A good example of TB program evaluation using the CDC framework has been reported by the Massachusetts Department of Public Health.[25] Massachusetts applied the CDC framework to TB contact investigation in five city health departments. Stakeholders of the evaluation were engaged. Models describing the components of contact investigation at the state and local level were created, and self-evaluation tools were developed. Based on this experience, Massachusetts plans to apply the evaluation process statewide and use the findings to target areas that need improvement.

IDENTIFYING PERSONS WHO HAVE CLINICALLY ACTIVE TUBERCULOSIS

The first priority of TB control in the United States is detection and treatment of patients with active TB. Discovery of a previously undiagnosed TB patient triggers several interventions that interrupt transmission. These include placing the patient in respiratory isolation if contagious, starting the patient on TB treatment, and conducting a contact investigation. Health departments seek to be notified of patients with TB as early as possible, and use active and passive methods of case finding to achieve this goal.

Active case finding occurs through contact and outbreak investigations and screening of high-risk populations. The purpose of contact investigation is to find persons recently infected with TB. Although most recently infected individuals will have LTBI, approximately 1–2% of contacts evaluated will be diagnosed with active TB.[26] When several TB cases are linked through traditional or molecular epidemiological methods, this may constitute an outbreak. Because an outbreak indicates significant ongoing transmission, more intensive methods may be used to ensure all cases in the outbreak have been discovered. This may include screening with chest radiographs (CXRs) and sputum sampling regardless of tuberculin skin test (TST) results or symptoms. Because these tests incur considerable additional cost, their use in the initial phase of screening has usually been restricted to large outbreaks or those involving congregate settings or very high-risk populations (e.g., homeless shelters, prisons, HIV-infected persons).[27]

Screening of high-risk populations generally begins with targeted tuberculin testing. As with contact investigation, most persons found to be infected with TB have LTBI, but occasionally individuals with active TB are also identified.[28] The health department may also work with congregate facilities with high rates of active disease to conduct active case finding using chest radiographic screening. Several of these screening programs have been successful in early case detection.[29,30]

Passive case finding consists of accepting reports of TB suspects and patients from community medical providers. In all U.S. states, reporting of TB patients is required by law.[17] While patients found through the passive reporting system frequently have advanced disease, this passive case-finding mechanism remains important because it allows mobilization of health department services, including monitoring of respiratory isolation, case management, directly observed therapy, and contact investigation, that help to prevent further transmission. In addition, this surveillance activity makes possible the collection of epidemiological data, facilitating the examination of TB trends at the local, state, and national levels. By examining these trends, TB programs are able to utilize resources more effectively.

EVALUATION OF IMMIGRANTS

All persons attempting to enter the United States as refugees or through application for an immigrant visa must undergo a medical examination that includes screening for active TB. The TB screening process occurs in two phases: it is initiated by panel physicians (selected by the U.S. Department of State) in the country of departure and completed in the United States by state and local health departments.[31]

Overseas, all immigrants and refugees at least 15 years of age are required to have a CXR. Based on the CXR results, the panel physician determines if the immigrant should submit three sputum specimens for acid-fast bacilli (AFB) smear staining. Using the CXR and sputum results, the immigrant is classified as Class A—active TB, infectious (AFB smear positive); Class B1—active TB, noninfectious (AFB smear negative); Class B2—inactive TB; or no TB infection. Individuals with active or inactive TB are required to report to the local or state health department for further evaluation after arriving in the United States. Those with infectious TB cannot enter the United States until they have received sufficient treatment to render them noninfectious. Immigrants younger than 15 years of age are not required to have a CXR routinely. If such individuals have had contact with a known TB case or are suspected of having TB for other reasons, they must have a TST. If there is induration or erythema of any size, a CXR is required. Additional evaluation is conducted as it is for persons older than 15 years of age.

Initial testing for TB at a U.S. local or state health department usually includes a medical examination, CXR, and TST.[32] Additional testing, such as sputum examination, is performed at the discretion of the evaluating medical provider. Several studies have demonstrated that Class B immigrant screening by U.S. health departments has a high rate of case detection with on average about 7% of immigrants discovered to have active TB.[32–34] Many of the immigrants who do not have active TB have LTBI (as high as 70%), providing an excellent opportunity for prevention through LTBI treatment.[32] Because of this high yield for finding TB cases (higher than for contact investigation) and LTBI, evaluation of Class B immigrants should be considered a high priority activity for health departments.

MANAGING PERSONS WHO HAVE OR ARE SUSPECTED OF HAVING DISEASE

After a patient with TB has been reported to the health department, it is the responsibility of the health department, in conjunction with the patient's medical provider (if the provider is not the health department), to ensure the patient completes an adequate treatment regimen.[35] In this context, case management involves accessing and employing the medical and social resources needed to shepherd a patient through completion of treatment.

The first task of the case manager is to make certain that the patient has a medical provider who will assume responsibility for the patient's TB treatment. The case manager should also oversee the administration of directly observed therapy, making it as convenient as possible for the patient, while closely monitoring adherence. Monitoring for adverse effects and response to treatment (e.g., collection of follow-up sputum samples) should be performed, with any problems being promptly reported to the patient's medical provider.

In addition to oversight of medical care, it is also important to assist the patient to overcome social barriers that may impede adherence to treatment.[36] Being ill with TB can impose significant financial hardship due to costs of medical care that may not be covered by the health department (e.g., hospitalization), and inability to work. Patients may be eligible for medical and financial benefits such as Medicaid, Medicare, or disability insurance. The case manager should help the patient access social services to obtain these benefits and direct the patient to other governmental or nongovernmental community-based programs that can assist with housing, food, and transportation if needed (Table 12-2).[22,35]

Culture and language present other potential barriers to adherence. It is preferable that culturally and linguistically competent staff be used to provide medical care and education.[36] If not available, it is essential to have ready access to interpreters. In addition, all education materials should be appropriate for the culture, language, and reading level of the patient.

The final responsibility of the case manager is to review the treatment record before the case is closed to the health department. The case manager should ensure that an adequate number of doses of medication have been taken within the recommended duration and that the patient has had a good response to therapy indicative of cure. If these criteria have not been met, the case manager should confer with the TB controller and the patient's medical provider to determine the appropriate course of action.

MEDICAL CONSULTATION

As TB cases have decreased in the United States, so have the number of medical providers with experience in treating TB patients.[37] For this reason, the only local or statewide clinical expertise may reside within the public health department. Therefore it is often necessary that health department physicians and nurses be available to provide medical consultation on diagnostic and treatment issues. Frequently this service can be provided via telephone or e-mail. In some areas, medical providers can refer patients to a health department TB clinic for a more formal consultation. However, even health departments may no longer possess expertise in treating TB if they are in low incidence areas. To address this need and increase access to expert medical consultation, CDC is funding regional training and medical consultation centers to provide coverage throughout the United States.

INTERJURISDICTIONAL REFERRALS

Ensuring completion of treatment for all patients is critical in achieving and maintaining TB control. When patients move from one health department jurisdiction to another, making certain they complete treatment becomes more difficult. According to one study, patients who move are five times more likely to default.[38] This underscores the necessity of close cooperation and coordination between TB control programs when caring for mobile patients if optimal outcomes are to be attained.

Table 12-2. Possible Components of a Multifaceted, Patient-centered Treatment Strategy

Enablers: Interventions to Assist the Patient in Completing Therapy

Transportation vouchers

Child care

Convenient clinic hours and locations

Clinic personnel who speak the languages of the populations served

Reminder systems and follow-up of missed appointments

Social service assistance (referrals for substance abuse treatment and counseling, housing, and other services)

Outreach workers (bilingual/bicultural as needed; can provide many services related to maintaining patient adherence, including provision of DOT, follow-up on missed appointments, monthly monitoring, transportation, sputum collection, social service assistance, and educational reinforcement)

Integration of care for TB with care for other conditions

Incentives: Interventions to Motivate the Patient, Tailored to Individual Patient Wishes and Needs and, thus, Meaningful to the Patient

Food stamps or snacks and meals

Restaurant coupons

Assistance in finding or provision of housing

Clothing or other personal products

Books

Stipends

Patient contract

Source: Reproduced from American Thoracic Society, Centers for Disease Control and Prevention and Infectious Disease Society of America. Treatment of TB. *MMWR Morb Mortal Wkly Rep.* 2003;52(No. RR-11):1–80.

To deal with the complexities of managing TB patients relocating while on therapy, the National Tuberculosis Controllers Association (NTCA) has developed a system for interjurisdictional referrals. A brief protocol can be downloaded from their website (http://www.ntca-tb.org). A form for transferring pertinent information about TB patients from the discharging health department to the receiving health department can also be found on the website. Information collected on the form includes identifying, demographic, clinical, laboratory, and treatment data. In addition, the form allows for exchange of information related to contact investigation and patients being treated for LTBI. When the discharging jurisdiction has reported the patient as a case to CDC, it is also responsible for reporting the treatment outcome. Therefore, the receiving jurisdiction should provide follow-up information on transferred patients to the discharging jurisdiction. A form and instructions for providing interjurisdictional follow-up are available on the NTCA website.

The NTCA system is primarily meant for interstate referrals. For intrastate referrals, it is best for local health departments to contact their state TB control program. Some states, such as California, have existing intrastate interjurisdictional referral systems that are similar to the one implemented by NTCA.

Occasionally TB programs may need to exchange information regarding TB patients with TB programs in other countries. The Cure-TB binational referral program, which is managed by the County of San Diego's Tuberculosis Control Program (website: www.sandiegotb-control.org), assists with managing TB patients moving to or from Mexico. For assistance in exchanging information about patients moving to or from countries other then Mexico, it is recommended that health departments contact the International Research and Programs Branch of CDC's Division of Tuberculosis Elimination.

IDENTIFYING AND MANAGING PERSONS INFECTED WITH *M. TUBERCULOSIS*

Investigation of Contacts to Infectious Tuberculosis Cases

Contact investigations are an essential function of TB control in the United States and have been identified as a priority strategy for prevention and control of TB.[1]

Among close contacts, approximately 1–2% will have TB disease and 31–36% will have LTBI.[39,40] Approximately 5% of contacts with newly acquired LTBI will develop TB within two years of infection.[41] Contact investigations are therefore an effective method for active case finding and identifying persons with LTBI who are also at a high risk of developing TB disease. State and local public health agencies are responsible for ensuring that contact investigations are effectively conducted and that all exposed contacts are identified, evaluated for TB infection and disease, and appropriately treated. Consequently, 90% of contact investigations in the United States are performed by public health departments.[37]

Targeted Testing and Treatment of LTBI

The number of persons in the United States with LTBI is currently estimated at 9.5–14.7 million.[42] To continue progress toward the elimination of TB in the United States, public health programs must devise effective strategies to address the challenge of preventing TB in this population of infected persons. Guidelines on targeted testing and treatment of LTBI have been published and revised.[43–44] Those guidelines include recommendations for diagnosis and treatment of LTBI, as well as recommendations for identifying persons and groups to target for testing.

The health department has several potential roles in testing for, and treatment of, persons with LTBI. Health departments may evaluate and treat persons who have been referred to the health department following diagnosis of LTBI by community providers. The health department may also test persons who are required to document that they are free from TB because of existing state and local regulations. This group may include food handlers, teachers, or students. Since these two activities are not necessarily targeted towards populations at risk for TB infection, their impact and effectiveness tend to be limited.

Potentially greater impact can be achieved by targeting populations at greater risk for LTBI and at greater risk for progression to TB if infected. The health department can do this by providing technical assistance and collaborating with persons, facilities, or agencies providing health care services to populations at risk; or by implementing targeted testing and treatment programs in high-risk populations. Health departments must regularly evaluate the effectiveness and impact of their targeted testing activities to ensure resources are appropriately allocated. Ineffective practices, such as testing low-risk populations, should be discontinued.

PROVIDING LABORATORY AND DIAGNOSTIC SERVICES

Public health TB control programs are responsible for ensuring that suitable laboratory and diagnostic services are available for TB suspects and patients. The most important component is the availability of mycobacteriology laboratory services. The TB control program and community providers should have access to accurate and rapid laboratory tests to isolate and identify *M. tuberculosis*. Rapid methods should also be available for testing of *M. tuberculosis* isolates for susceptibility to first-line drugs used for treatment. The TB control program should work with the laboratory to ensure prompt reporting of all results to treating clinicians and to the health department.

The health department should also ensure that outpatient and inpatient facilities involved in the diagnosis and treatment of TB have access to chest radiology services, including interpretation. Prompt reporting of CXR findings is essential to providing care to TB suspects and patients. HIV counseling, testing, and referral must be readily available also. Finally, facilities providing TB treatments should provide adequate laboratory and diagnostic services to monitor patients for adverse reactions to treatment.

COLLECTING AND ANALYZING DATA

Public health programs cannot function effectively without rapid and accurate disease surveillance systems. The critical first step in maintaining effective surveillance is prompt TB case reporting. A vital element of this process is reporting of positive test results from laboratories to the health department. Reporting from physicians, hospitals, and other community health care providers also plays a crucial role. The health department should institute both passive and active case findings to facilitate case reporting. Active case finding includes routine communication with infection control practitioners in hospitals, correctional facilities, and other facilities that diagnose TB. The health department should create a TB registry and have the capacity for the electronic storage of records with updated information on all current and suspect TB cases. Data collection should include all information necessary to ensure the appropriate follow-up of TB suspects and patients and for compiling local, state, and national surveillance reports. All clinically relevant information, including diagnostic laboratory results, drug susceptibility results, and treatment regimens, should be included in the registry. Ideally, the health department should also collect and store data on contacts and persons tested for LTBI.

Sufficient safeguards to ensure the quality of the data and to protect the confidentiality of the records should be instituted.

Tuberculosis control programs should analyze the data collected to monitor morbidity trends, determine the demographic characteristics of their patient population, monitor drug resistance rates, and determine the outcomes of treatment. Additional analyses should be done on the effectiveness and outcomes of contact investigations and LTBI targeted testing and treatment programs. These analyses should be used to assess program performance and progress towards achieving locally and nationally established program objectives. Planning for use of resources and implementation of interventions should be based on the results of the analysis of surveillance and program data. Annual reports of local TB morbidity rates and trends should be prepared and distributed to community providers and organizations, professional societies, and leaders.

An important component of data collection by the local health department is the prompt and complete reporting of TB cases to state TB control programs, with the states forwarding the reports to CDC. These data are essential for state and national planning, assessment, and resource allocation.

PROVIDING TRAINING AND EDUCATION

The primary training responsibility of state and local health departments is training the health department staff directly involved in TB prevention and control activities. Health department staff need ongoing training and education to remain current on treatment, patient management, and programmatic issues. As new guidelines for TB treatment, prevention, and control are published, staff need updates and related training. New staff members need intensive training to become adept in their job and gain general knowledge regarding TB transmission, infection, and disease, and develop proficiency in infection control procedures.

A secondary responsibility is education of the external community to ensure that community providers and clinicians have the knowledge and skills to appropriately diagnose and treat TB. Health care planners and policy makers should be educated on the continuing need to control and eliminate TB in their jurisdictions. Institutions, such as hospitals, correctional facilities, nursing homes, and homeless shelters, should be instructed on the need to maintain vigilance and adequate infection control practices to prevent the transmission of TB within their facilities. Tuberculosis control programs must work diligently with community groups, minority organizations, professional societies, and medical and nursing schools to meet the training and education needs of the community.

CONCLUSION

With the continued decline in TB incidence, programs must confront the decline in resources available for TB control and the decline in knowledge and skills among community providers and their own staff regarding the diagnosis, treatment, and control of TB. At the same time, outbreaks of TB resulting from delayed diagnosis of persons with infectious TB will continue to occur and can easily overwhelm the capacity of small public health programs to respond. New paradigms of public health response to TB, such as strengthening laboratory networks and regionalization of programs, will be necessary to meet the needs of low incidence areas.

If current trends in the epidemiology of TB persist, TB in the United States will eventually be a disease of persons born in other countries. This will continue to challenge public health programs as they struggle to control TB in patient populations with diverse languages, cultures, and understanding of and beliefs about TB. Many programs have already adapted to this changing epidemiology of TB. Ultimately, control and elimination of TB in the United States will depend not only on the efforts of the state and local health departments and community providers, but also on the success of international efforts.

In *Ending Neglect: The Elimination of Tuberculosis in the United States*, the Institute of Medicine recommended that the United States should maintain control of TB while adjusting control measures to declining incidence of disease and while also accelerating the rate of decline of TB.[37] This fundamental challenge for TB public health programs will define their efforts and activities in the coming years.

REFERENCES

1. Centers for Disease Control and Prevention. Essential components of a tuberculosis prevention and control program: recommendations of the Advisory Council for the Elimination of Tuberculosis. *MMWR Morb Mortal Wkly Rep.* 1995;44(No. RR-11):1–17.
2. Lerner BH. Catching patients: tuberculosis and detention in the 1990s. *Chest.* 1999;115:236–241.
3. Burman WJ, Cohn DL, Rietmeijer CA, et al. Short-term incarceration for the management of noncompliance with tuberculosis treatment. *Chest.* 1997;112:57–62.
4. Singleton L, Turner M, Haskal R, et al. Long-term hospitalization for tuberculosis control. *JAMA.* 1997;278:838–842.

5. Oscherwitz T, Tulsky JP, Roger S, et al. Detention of persistently nonadherent patients with tuberculosis. *JAMA.* 1997;278:843–846.

6. Feldman G, Srivastava P, Eden E, et al. Detention until cure as a last resort: New York City's experience with involuntary in-hospital civil detention of persistently nonadherent tuberculosis patients. *Semin Respir Crit Care Med.* 1997;18:493–501.

7. Horsburgh RC, Moore M, Castro KG. Epidemiology of tuberculosis in the United States. In: Rom WN, Garay SM, eds. *Tuberculosis.* Philadelphia, PA: Lippincott Williams & Wilkins; 2004:31–45.

8. Centers for Disease Control. *Reported Tuberculosis in the United States, 2002.* Atlanta, GA: U.S. Department of Health and Human Services, September 2003.

9. Centers for Disease Control and Prevention. Tuberculosis elimination revisited: obstacles, opportunities, and a renewed commitment. Advisory Council for the Elimination of Tuberculosis (ACET). *MMWR Morb Mortal Wkly Rep.* 1999;48(No. RR-9):1–13.

10. Centers for Disease Control. *Reported Tuberculosis in the United States, 2003.* Atlanta, GA: U.S. Department of Health and Human Services, September 2004.

11. Centers for Disease Control and Prevention. Preventing and controlling tuberculosis along the U.S.-Mexico border: work group report. *MMWR Morb Mortal Wkly Rep.* 2001;50 (No. RR-1):1–27.

12. Centers for Disease Control and Prevention. Prevention and treatment of tuberculosis among patients infected with human immunodeficieincy virus: principles of therapy and revised recommendations. *MMWR Morb Mortal Wkly Rep.* 1998;47(No. RR-20):2–58.

13. Centers for Disease Control and Prevention. Updated Guidelines for the use of Rifabutin or Rifampin for the treatment and prevention of tuberculosis among HIV-infected patients taking protease inhibitors or non-nucleoside reverse transceiptase inhibitors. *MMWR Morb Mortal Wkly Rep.* 2000;49:185–187.

14. Annas GJ. Control of tuberculosis-the law and the public's health. *N Engl J Med.* 1993;328:585–588.

15. *Jacobson v. Massachusetts*, 197 U.S. 11 (1904).

16. *Addington v. Texas*, 441 U.S. 418 (1979).

17. Centers for Disease Control and Prevention: Tuberculosis control laws-United States, 1993: recommendations of the Advisory Council for the Elimination of Tuberculosis (ACET). *MMWR Morb Mortal Wkly Rep.* 1993;42(RR-15):1–28.

18. Missouri Department of Health and Senior Services. Communicable disease investigation manual. Section 4.0, Subsection latent tuberculosis infection. (www.dhss.state. MO.US/CDmanual/CDmanual.htm). Accessed July 5, 2005.

19. California Health and Safety Code. Section 121361. (www.leginfo.ca.gov/calaw.html). Accessed July 5, 2005.

20. Gostin LO, Sapsin JW, Teret SP, et al. The Model State Emergency Health Powers Act: planning for and response to bioterrorism and naturally occurring infectious disease. *JAMA.* 2002;288:622–628.

21. Gasner MR, Law Maw K, Feldman GE, et al. The use of legal action in New York City to ensure treatment of tuberculosis. *N Engl J Med.* 1999;340:359–366.

22. LoBue PA, Cass R, Lobo D, et al. Development of housing programs to aid in the treatment of tuberculosis in homeless individuals: a pilot study. *Chest.* 1999:115:218–223.

23. Centers for Disease Control and Prevention. Framework for program evaluation in public health. *MMWR Morb Mortal Wkly Rep.* 1999;48(RR-11):1–40.

24. Rodrigo T, Cayla JA, Galdos-Tanguis H et al. Proposing indicators for evaluation of tuberculosis control programmes in large cities based on the experience of Barcelona. *Int J Tuberc Lung Dis.* 2001;5:432–440.

25. Logan S, Boutotte J, Wilce M, Etkind S. Using the CDC framework for program evaluation in public health to assess tuberculosis contact investigations programs. *Int J Tuberc Lung Dis.* 2003;7:s375–s383.

26. Jereb J, Etkind SC, Joglar OT et al. Tuberculosis contact investigations: outcomes in selected areas of the United States, 1999. *Int J Tuberc Lung Dis.* 2003;7:S384–S390.

27. Narita M, Lofy K, Lake L et al. An intensive screening strategy utilized in a TB outbreak involving the homeless community in Seattle-King County. *Am J Respir Crit Care Med.* 2004;169:A235.

28. Saunders DL, Olive DM, Wallace SB et al. Tuberculosis screening in the federal prison system: an opportunity to treat and prevent tuberculosis in foreign-born populations. *Public Health Rep.* 2001;116:210–213.

29. Barry MA, Wall C, Shirley L et al. Tuberculosis screening in Boston's homeless shelters. *Public Health Rep.* 1986;101:487–494.

30. Puisis M, Feinglass J, Lidow E et al. Radiographic screening for tuberculosis in a large urban county jail. *Public Health Rep.* 1996;111:330–334.

31. Binkin NJ, Zuber PL, Wells CD et al. 1996. Overseas screening for tuberculosis in immigrants and refugees to the United States: current status. *Clin Infect Dis.* 23:1226–1232.

32. DeRiemer K, Chin DP, Schecter GF et al. Tuberculosis among immigrants and refugees. *Arch Intern Med.* 1998;158:753–760.

33. Sciortino S, Mohle-Boetani J, Royce SE et al. B notifications and the detection of tuberculosis among foreign-born recent arrivals in California. *Int J Tuberc Lung Dis.* 1999;3:778–785.

34. Zuber PL, Binkin NJ, Ignacio AC et al. Tuberculosis screening for immigrants and refugees. Diagnostic outcomes in the state of Hawaii. *Am J Respir Crit Care Med.* 1996;154:151–155.

35. American Thoracic Society, Centers for Disease Control and Prevention and Infectious Disease Society of America. Treatment of tuberculosis. *MMWR Morb Mortal Wkly Rep.* 2003;52(No. RR-11):1–80.

36. Chaulk CP, Kazandjian VA. Directly observed therapy for treatment completion of pulmonary tuberculosis: consensus statement of the public health tuberculosis guidelines panel. *JAMA.* 1998;279:943–948.

37. Institute of Medicine. *Ending neglect: the elimination of tuberculosis in the United States*. Washington, DC:, National Academy Press; 2000.

38. Cummings KC, Mohle-Boetani J, Royce SE, et al. Movement of tuberculosis patients and the failure to complete antituberculosis treatment. *Am J Respir Crit Care Med*. 1998;157:1249–1252.

39. Marks SM, Taylor Z, Qualls NL, et al. Outcomes of contact investigations of infectious tuberculosis patients. *Am J Respir Crit Care Med*. 2000;162:2033–2038.

40. Reichler MR, Reves R, Bur S, et al. Evaluation of investigations conducted to detect and prevent transmission of tuberculosis. *JAMA*. 2002;287:991–995.

41. Ferebee SH. Controlled chemoprophylaxis trials in tuberculosis. A general review. *Bibl Tuberc*. 1970;26:28–106.

42. Bennett DE, Courval JM, Onorato IM, et al. Prevalence of TB infection in the U.S. population, 1999–2000 [abstract]. *Program and Abstracts, the Annual Meeting of the American Public Health Association 2003*. San Francisco, CA. November 15–19, 2003. Abstract 67921.

43. American Thoracic Society/Centers for Disease Control and Prevention. Targeted tuberculin testing and treatment of latent tuberculosis infection. *Am J Respir Crit Care Med*. 2000;161(4 Pt 2):S221–S247.

44. Centers for Disease Control and Prevention. Updated: fatal and severe liver injuries associated with rifampin and pyrazinamide for latent tuberculosis infection, and revisions in American Thoracic Society/CDC recommendations-United States, 2001. *MMWR Morb Mortal Wkly Rep*. 2001;50: 733–735.

13

Pulmonary Tuberculosis

Mary Elizabeth Kreider
Milton D. Rossman

INTRODUCTION

The lung is the most commonly affected organ in tuberculosis (TB) infection in the immunocompetent host, with estimates of lung involvement in subjects with active TB of 80–87%.[1,2] Estimates of lung involvement are similar in the immunocompromised hosts such as those with human immunodeficiency virus (HIV) infection, with studies from the 1980–1990s suggesting that the rates of pulmonary involvement were on the order of 70–92%.[3–5] However, these individuals are also more likely to have extrapulmonary disease as well.[6]

The lung is the portal of entry in the majority of cases of TB.[7,8] The first contact with the organism results in few or no clinical symptoms or signs. Ordinarily, the tubercle bacillus sets up a localized infection in the periphery of the lung where it has been deposited by inhalation. Body defenses appear to have little effect on the organism until the time of development of tuberculin hypersensitivity (4–6 weeks). At this time, mild fever and malaise develop, and occasionally other hypersensitivity manifestations are noted.

In the majority of patients, no additional evidence of TB develops, and the process is contained by local and systemic defenses. Since the primary pulmonary focus is usually subpleural, rupture into the pleural space may result, with the development of a tuberculous pleurisy with effusion. This is usually accompanied by the classic but nonspecific symptoms of pleurisy. Local spread to the hilar lymph nodes is a common occurrence, and from there the disease spreads to other areas of the body. It is this hematogenous dissemination of the organism that results in the pulmonary and extrapulmonary foci that are responsible for the major clinical manifestations of TB. Radiographically, spread is manifested by enlargement of the lymph nodes, with later calcification of both the lymph nodes and the parenchymal lesion. This is the classic Ghon's complex and is suggestive not only of an old tuberculous infection but also of diseases such as histoplasmosis. Progressive (reactivation) TB usually develops after a period of dormancy and arises from the sites of hematogenous dissemination.[9]

Thus, the first infection with TB frequently is clinically insignificant and unrecognized. In the majority of patients, the disease stays dormant either indefinitely or for many years and when a breakdown occurs, it may be secondary to a decrease in body immunity (Table 13-1).

CLINICAL PRESENTATION

Symptoms and Signs

Pulmonary TB frequently develops without any striking clinical evidence of disease; however, since the disease has a wide spectrum of manifestations ranging from skin positivity with negative x-rays to far advanced TB, a variety of clinical presentations may also occur. Ordinarily, until the disease is moderately or far advanced, as shown by changes on the roentgenogram, symptoms are minimal and often attributable to other causes, such as excessive smoking, hard work, pregnancy, or other debilitating conditions.

Symptoms may be divided into two categories, constitutional and pulmonary. The frequency of these symptoms differs according to whether the patient has primary TB or reactivation TB. Subjects with primary TB are much more likely to be asymptomatic or minimally symptomatic. See Table 13-2 for a list of the most common symptoms and their relative frequency in representative case series of both primary and reactivation TB. The constitutional symptom most frequently seen is fever, low-grade at the onset but becoming quite marked if the disease progresses. Characteristically, the fever develops in the late afternoon and may not be accompanied by pronounced symptoms. With defervescence, usually during sleep, sweating occurs—the classic "night sweats." Other signs of toxemia, such as malaise, irritability, weakness, unusual fatigue, headache, and weight loss, may be present. With the development of caseation necrosis and concomitant liquefaction of the caseation, the patient will usually notice

Table 13-1. Increased Susceptibility to TB

Nonspecific Decrease in Resistance
Adolescence
Senescence
Malnutrition
Postgastrectomy state
Diabetes mellitus

Decrease in Resistance Due to Hormonal Effects
Pregnancy
Therapy with adrenocortical steroids

Decrease in Local Resistance
Silicosis
Decrease in specific immunity
Lymphomas
Uremia
Immunosuppressive therapy
Sarcoidosis
Live virus vaccination
HIV infection

cough and sputum, often associated with mild hemoptysis. Chest pain may be localized and pleuritic. Shortness of breath usually indicates extensive disease with widespread involvement of the lung and parenchyma or some form of tracheobronchial obstruction and therefore usually occurs late in the course of the disease.

Physical examination of the chest is ordinarily of minimal help early in the disease. At this stage, the principal finding over areas of infiltration is one of fine rales detected on deep inspiration followed by full expiration and a hard, terminal cough—the so-called posttussive rales. This sign is found particularly in the apexes of the lungs, where reactivation disease has its onset in a large majority of patients.

Table 13-2. Clinical Symptoms of Patients Presenting with Active Tuberculosis

	% of Patients Affected	
Symptoms	Primary	Reactivation
Cough	23–37	42
Fever	18–42	37–79
Weight loss	NR	7–24
Hemoptysis	8	9

Estimates based on several studies (References 2, 10–13).
NR = not reported.

As the disease progresses, more extensive findings are present, corresponding to the areas of involvement and type of pathology. Allergic manifestations may occur, usually developing at the time of onset of infection. These include erythema nodosum and the phlyctenular conjunctivitis. Erythema induratum, involvement of the lower leg and foot with redness, swelling, and necrosis, probably represents a combination of local subcutaneous bacterial infection with an allergic response and should not be confused with erythema nodosum, the latter considered to be due to circulating immune complexes with resultant localized vascular damage. Initially, erythema nodosum occurs in the dependent portion of the body and, if the reaction is severe, may be followed by a more disseminated process.

Laboratory Examination

Routine laboratory examinations are rarely helpful in establishing or suggesting the diagnosis.[14] A mild normochromic normocytic anemia may be present in chronic TB. The WBC count is often normal, and counts over 20,000/μL would suggest another infectious process; however, a leukemoid reaction may occasionally occur in miliary TB, but not in TB confined to the chest. Although a "left shift" in the differential WBC count can occur in advanced disease, these changes are neither specific nor useful. Other nonspecific tests that may be elevated in active TB include the sedimentation rate, α_2-globulins, and γ-globulin. The finding of pyuria without bacteria by Gram's stain is suggestive of renal involvement. Liver enzymes (transaminases and alkaline phosphatase) may occasionally be elevated prior to treatment; however, this finding is usually due to concomitant liver disease secondary to other problems such as alcoholism, rather than to tuberculous involvement. Since the drugs used in the treatment of TB are often associated with hepatotoxicity, it is important to quantitate any hepatic abnormalities prior to treatment.[15] On rare occasions, the serum sodium may be depressed owing to inappropriate secretion of antidiuretic hormone. This only occurs in advanced pulmonary TB.

A positive delayed hypersensitivity reaction to tuberculin (as discussed in Chapter 4) indicates only the occurrence of a prior primary infection.[16]

CHEST RADIOGRAPHY

The chest radiograph is the single most useful study for suggesting the diagnosis of TB. The appearance of the radiograph differs in primary (Figs. 13-1, 13-2, and 13-3) and reactivation TB.[17]

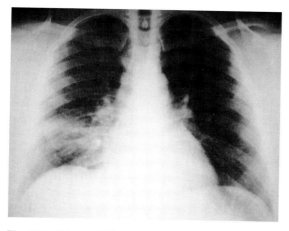

Fig. 13-1. Primary TB in an adult. Right lower lobe infiltrate with bilateral hilar adenopathy.

Primary Tuberculosis

As opposed to reactivation TB, which usually involves the superior and dorsal segments, in primary TB parenchymal involvement can happen in any segment of the lung.[18] In the primary infection there is only a slight predilection for the upper lobes; also, anterior as well as posterior segments can be involved. The air-space consolidation appears as a homogeneous density with ill-defined borders (Fig. 13-1), and cavitation is rare except in malnourished or other immunocompromised patients. Miliary involvement at the onset is seen in less than 3% of cases, most commonly in children under 2–3 years of age, but can also be seen in adults (Fig. 13-2).

Hilar or paratracheal lymph node enlargement is a characteristic finding in primary TB. In 15% of the cases, bilateral hilar adenopathy may be present. More commonly, the adenopathy is unilateral. Unilateral hilar adenopathy and unilateral hilar and paratracheal adenopathy are equally common. Massive hilar adenopathy may herald a complicated course.

Atelectasis with an obstructive pneumonia may result from bronchial compression by inflamed lymph nodes or from a caseous lymph node that ruptures into a bronchus. Obstructive "emphysema" or a localized hyperinflated segment at times precede atelectasis. The most common segments involved are the anterior segment of the right upper lobe or the medial segment of the right middle lobe. Right-sided collapse is twice as common as left-sided collapse. Residual bronchiectatic changes may persist after the obstruction has cleared.

An isolated pleural effusion of mild-to-moderate degree may be the only manifestation of primary TB; however, the most common radiographic appearance of primary TB is a normal radiograph.

Reactivation Tuberculosis

Although reactivation TB may involve any lung segment, the characteristic distribution usually suggests the disease. In 95% of localized pulmonary TB, the lesions will be present in the apical or posterior segment of the upper lobes or the superior segment of the lower lobes (Figs. 13-3 and 13-4). The anterior segment of the upper lobe is almost never the only manifest area of involvement.[19] Although some radiologists attempt to describe the activity of a lesion on the basis of its radiographic appearance, the documentation of activity is best left to bacteriologic and clinical evaluation (Table 13-3). Too often a lesion described as inactive or stable by radiography will progress to symptomatic TB.

The typical parenchymal pattern of reactivation TB is of an air-space consolidation in a patchy or confluent nature. Frequently there are increased linear densities to the ipsilateral hilum (Fig. 13-3). Cavitation is not uncommon, and lymph node enlargement is rarely seen. As the lesions become more chronic, they become more sharply circumscribed and irregular in contour. Fibrosis will lead to volume loss in the involved lung.

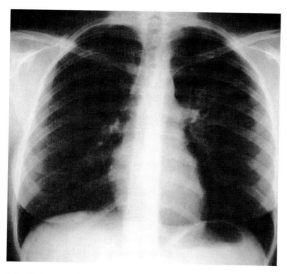

Fig. 13-2. Left upper lobe TB. A typical fibronodular pattern of reactivation TB with linear densities extending to the left hilum.

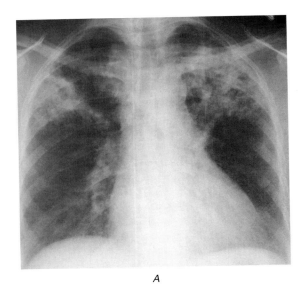

A

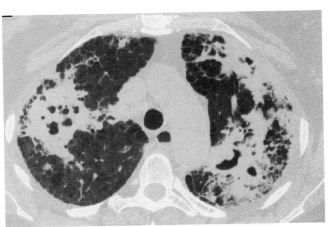

B

Fig. 13-3. Late changes of upper lobe TB. *A.* Posterior-anterior chest radiograph with volume loss of the right upper lobe is indicated by the elevated minor fissure. Small cavities are not clearly seen but there is endobronchial spread to the superior segment of the right lower lobe, suggesting cavitary formation. *B.* A CAT scan of the same patient that clearly demonstrates extensive bilateral cavitary disease.

The combination of patchy pneumonitis, fibrosis, and calcification is always suggestive of chronic granulomatous disease, usually TB.

Table 13-3. Criteria for Activity in Pulmonary TB

Symptoms
Change in roentgenogram
Evidence of cavitation
Positive sputum by smear or culture
Response to therapeutic trial

The cavities that develop in TB are characterized by a moderately thick wall, a smooth inner surface, and the lack of an air-fluid level (Fig. 13-4). Cavitation is frequently associated with endobronchial spread of disease. Radiographically, it appears as multiple small acinar shadows.

Chest Computed Tomography (CT) Findings in Pulmonary Tuberculosis

CT scans allow practitioners to examine both the pulmonary parenchyma and the lymph nodes in greater details than can be done with plain chest x-ray alone. The Chest CT in patients with primary TB typically

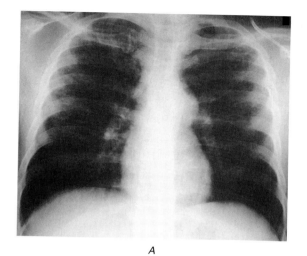

A

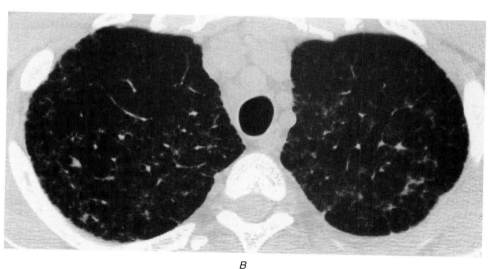

B

Fig. 13-4. Miliary TB. *A*. Characteristic diffuse small nodules are seen in the posterior-anterior radiograph. *B*. CT scan of the lung in the same subject demonstrates the diffuse small nodular disease.

demonstrate lobar consolidation in association with mediastinal or hilar adenopathy. The consolidation is usually well defined, dense, homogeneous, and confined to a segment or lobe. Small cavities may be appreciated on the CT that were not seen on plain chest x-ray (Fig. 13-4). In reactivation TB one can see centrilobular nodules or branching linear structures ("tree in bud") with or without bronchial wall thickening, lobular consolidation, cavity formation, bronchiectasis, and/or fibrotic changes.[20,21] Controversy exists over whether CT

scans can reliably distinguish active TB from latent infection with several authors arguing that findings such as the "tree in bud" and/or areas of centrilobular nodules predict active disease.[20,21]

DIAGNOSIS

The diagnosis of TB often can be very difficult. Some of the problems that occur are listed in Table 13-4. A firm diagnosis of TB requires bacteriologic confirmation. It is

Table 13-4. Diagnostic Difficulties

Lack of organisms for culture
Slow growth of TB culture
Chest x-ray findings absent or misinterpreted
Biopsy material may not be specific
Decreased tuberculin sensitivity
Symptoms and signs of TB easily attributed to
    a preexisting disease

important to remember that a positive acid-fast smear is not specific for *Mycobacterium tuberculosis*. Other mycobacteria, both saprophytes and potential pathogens, can be acid-fast. Thus, culture of *M. tuberculosis* is the only absolute way of confirming the diagnosis.

Freshly expectorated sputum is the best sample to stain and culture for *M. tuberculosis*. Sputum samples 24 hours old are frequently overgrown with mouth flora and are much less useful. If the patient is not spontaneously producing sputum, induced sputum is the next best specimen for study. It can be obtained by having the patient breathe an aerosol of isotonic or hypertonic saline for 5–15 minutes. If the patient cannot cooperate to give a spontaneous sputum sample, a gastric aspirate to obtain swallowed sputum may be useful. This sample must be obtained in the morning before the patient arises or eats.

In the majority of patients, the above procedures will be successful in obtaining positive material for culture. Smears of gastric contents for acid-fast bacilli are of limited value because of the presence of nontuberculous ingested acid-fast bacilli. In a few cases, one may have to resort to bronchoscopy. In 41 patients proven to have TB, cultures of specimens, taken during fiberoptic bronchoscopy, were positive in 39 cases.[22] Stainable mycobacteria were seen in 14 of the cases, and in eight cases granulomas were seen on biopsy. Similar results have been obtained in another study of 22 patients with proven mycobacterial disease and negative smears prior to bronchoscopy.[23] The local anesthetics used during fiberoptic bronchoscopy may be lethal to *M. tuberculosis*, so specimens for culture should be obtained using a minimal amount of anesthesia; however, irritation of the bronchial tree during the fiberoptic bronchoscopy procedure will frequently leave the patient with a productive cough. Thus, collection of the postbronchoscopy sputum can be another valuable source of diagnostic material. In nine (13%) of the above cases, the postbronchoscopy sputum was the only source of positive material.

In 2003, as reported to the Centers for Disease Control,[24] 45% of pulmonary cases of TB were smear positive, 41% were negative and 14% were not done or unknown. Sputum culture was positive in 69%, negative in 16% and unknown in 16% of cases. Thus, in a significant number of cases, the diagnosis of TB had been made in the absence of bacteriologic confirmation. In these cases, the diagnosis was made by a combination of a positive skin test, a compatible chest radiograph, and a therapeutic trial.

Differential Diagnosis

Since TB today is a disease frequently present in older individuals, one major differential diagnosis is usually between TB and carcinoma of the lung. An important concept to remember is that carcinoma may cause a focus of TB to spread; thus, carcinoma of the lung and TB may be present simultaneously. In cases with the simultaneous presentation of carcinoma and TB, the diagnosis of TB frequently is made first, and the diagnosis of carcinoma is delayed for several months. Thus, if radiograph and clinical findings suggest carcinoma but the sputum has acid-fast bacilli, further procedures to diagnose carcinoma may still be indicated. Isolated involvement of the anterior segment of the upper lobe, isolated lowerlobe involvement, or the presence of irregular cavities would suggest carcinoma, and further diagnostic workup may be indicated despite acid-fast bacilli in the sputum smear.

Any type of infectious or granulomatous disease may be radiologically identical to TB. Three broad categories must be distinguished: fungi (histoplasmosis, coccidioidomycosis, and blastomycosis), bacteria (*Pseudomonas pseudomallei*), and atypical mycobacteria (mainly *Mycobacterium kansasii* and *Mycobacterium intracellulare*). Culture of the organism from the patient's sputum is the best way to differentiate these diseases, although serum antibody titers to fungi are also valuable.

Common bacterial pneumonias are usually easily differentiated from TB. The localized alveolar infiltrate on the chest radiograph and the prompt response to antibiotic therapy usually differentiate bacterial pneumonia from TB. When in doubt, treatment for a bacterial pneumonia should be given first and TB therapy withheld until adequate sputum has been obtained and the response to antibiotics determined. Lung abscesses can usually be differentiated from tuberculous cavities by (a) prominent air-fluid level, (b) more common lower-lobe distribution, and (c) clinical findings (i.e., associated with seizures, alcoholism, dental caries, etc.).

Tuberculosis and Acquired Immune Deficiency Syndrome (AIDS)

A consensus has emerged that human immunodeficiency virus (HIV) infection is the explanation for the resurgence of TB in the United States since 1984.[25] Prior to 1984, there had been a consistent decline in the numbers of newly reported active cases of TB. Since 1984, there has been a slight increase in the number of newly reported active cases and this has resulted in an excess of 27,000 cases over what would have been expected.

Several lines of evidence link the current HIV epidemic and the resurgence of TB.[26] First, since AIDS is associated with depressed cell-mediated immunity, it would not be surprising for it to be associated with active TB. Second, epidemiological evidence suggests that the two diseases are related. The counties with the greatest increase in active TB also have the greatest number of cases of AIDS. In addition, the ethnic groups with the largest number of cases of AIDS also have the largest number of cases of TB. Third, several studies have now documented that the incidence of TB among patients with AIDS is increased.[27–30] Finally, the clinical presentation of patients with HIV infection and TB suggests a strong correlation.

Several important differences have emerged about the clinical presentation of subjects with TB with and without HIV infection. As previously mentioned, patients with HIV infection are more likely to present with disseminated disease. Additionally, they tend to have increased number and severity of symptoms, and a more rapid progression to death unless treatment is begun.[4]

Radiographic findings of TB in HIV have been found to correlate with the degree of immunosuppression due to the HIV virus itself.[5] Lower CD4 counts (ie. <200/mm^3) are associated more often with hilar and mediastinal lymphadenopathy while higher CD4 counts are more frequently associated with cavitation. Additionally, some studies have suggested that HIV subjects are more likely to have non-apical infiltrates, pleural effusions, and miliary infiltrates.[6]

In patients with HIV infection but without the manifestations of AIDS, the tuberculin skin test will be positive in 50–80% of patients with TB. Once an individual has developed AIDS, the tuberculin skin test will be less likely to be positive, but reactivity may be seen in as many as 30 to 50% of patients. Active TB should be considered in any HIV-infected patient with a tuberculin skin test that has greater than 5 mm of induration.

The diagnosis of TB in patients with HIV infection is made by collecting respiratory secretions or other clinically relevant specimens. The proportion of positive sputum smears and cultures is similar for both HIV-infected and noninfected patients. If spontaneous or induced sputum are negative, then bronchoscopy with lavage and biopsy may be necessary to obtain material for histologic study and culture. Whenever an acid-fast organism is identified, the assumption must be that the organism is *M. tuberculosis* and treatment should be initiated until definitive identification of the organism occurs.

Tuberculosis in the Elderly

As the population ages, increasing attention has been paid to how disease behaves differently in the elderly. Some studies have begun to suggest that not only is increasing age a risk factor for the development of active TB,[31] but that the disease itself may present differently in the elderly making it harder to recognize and therefore diagnose. One study prospectively examined 93 consecutive patients over the age of 60 admitted with pulmonary TB to a hospital in South Africa.[32] Among these patients "atypical" radiographic findings were the norm rather than the exception. For instance, only 7% had purely apical infiltrates, while 48% had mid- and lower-lung zones only, and 46% had mixed infiltrates between upper and lower lung fields. A pleural reaction was common (46%) and cavities were not (33%), with half of those seen in the lower- and mid-lung fields. In addition, the investigators found that systemic abnormalities of routine blood work were common, including anemia (66%), elevated erythrocyte sedimentation rates (90%), hyponatremia (60%), and hypoalbuminemia (83%); however, not all studies have confirmed these differences.[33] One recent meta-analysis of 12 studies of TB found that the elderly were less likely to have symptoms such as fever, sweating, hemoptyis, and cavitary lung disease. They were more likely to have dyspnea and significant co-morbidities.[34] In this study, the only differences seen in radiographic patterns between young adults and the elderly was an increased incidence of miliary disease in the older population.

Pleural Effusions Due to Tuberculosis

Pleural effusion is a relatively uncommon manifestation, particularly of primary TB, occurring in only 3% of clinical cases. Tuberculous pleural effusions are almost always due to rupture of subpleural foci of TB, which may not be evident radiologically. The effusions in TB are unilateral and mild to moderate in extent. The presence of bilateral effusions in TB usually means a miliary spread.

The natural course of a tuberculous pleural effusion is to gradually resorb and frequently disappear completely or with minimal changes on the chest radiograph.

Tuberculous pleural effusions must be differentiated from effusions due to congestive heart failure, carcinoma, and other types of infections. Pleural fluid protein is most useful for differentiating tuberculous effusions from transudates.[35] Almost without fail, the pleural fluid protein in TB will be greater than 4 g/dL (exudate), whereas it is most unusual for congestive heart failure fluid to have protein levels this high (transudate). The differentiation of carcinomatous from tuberculous effusions is more difficult. Both may appear exudative with high levels of lactic dehydrogenase (LDH) and protein in the pleural fluid. In tuberculous effusions, the differential count of the cells in the pleural fluid usually does not contain any mesothelial cells. A low pleural fluid glucose (less than 30 mg/dL) is common in TB and rare in carcinoma. Similarly, elevated adenosine deaminase (ADA) is frequently found in tuberculous effusions but is rare in carcinoma.[36,37] Additionally, pleural biopsies should be done in all cases to establish the diagnosis. It is usually easy to differentiate tuberculous effusion from bacterial effusions, since bacterial effusions usually contain a predominance of neutrophils. Tuberculous effusions are predominantly lymphocytic.[38] However, early in the course of tuberculous effusions, neutrophils may be seen. A Gram's stain of the pleural fluid and a culture of the fluid, sputum, and blood will usually establish the etiologic agent of bacterial effusions. More difficult is the differentiation of a viral pleural effusion from an effusion due to TB. When patients have a positive 5-TU tuberculin test (greater than 10-mm induration), their effusions should be presumed to be tuberculous until proven otherwise. If a patient has an undiagnosed exudative effusion and a negative tuberculin test, the tuberculin test should be repeated within two weeks, since it is not uncommon for patients with tuberculous effusions to have an initially negative tuberculin test.[16,39] Pleural biopsies and mycobacterial cultures of the pleural fluid and biopsy should be performed in all cases.

The diagnosis of pleural effusions due to TB can be accomplished by appropriate studies of the pleura and fluid in approximately 80% of cases.[40] These studies involve evaluation of the character of the fluid, which is an exudate with a prominent lymphocytosis. Smears of the fluid usually are negative for tubercle bacilli, but positive cultures are found in more than half of the cases. Repeated thoracenteses with culture of large quantities of fluid combined with centrifugation may also increase

bacteriological yield. Combining the histological examination and culture of the pleural biopsy specimen with study of the fluid yields the highest rate of diagnosis (80%). For each undiagnosed pleural effusion, in addition to the studies for TB, studies for malignant cells, fungi, and bacteria should be performed on the aspirated fluid and any biopsy material. At times, a video-assisted or standard thoracotomy with pathologic examination of the pleura for TB, fungi, malignant cells and bacteria may be necessary to establish the cause of a pleural effusion.

In the absence of a diagnosis and the presence of a compatible pleural effusion, consideration should be given to a trial of chemotherapy on the basis of a presumptive diagnosis of TB. Many patients with an undiagnosed pleural effusion will later develop progressive parenchymal TB if they are not treated. However, a therapeutic trial in pleural TB is not as helpful diagnostically as one in pulmonary TB, since the natural course of pleural TB is toward resolution.

Nevertheless, in contrast to tuberculous pleurisy, which does not require surgery, tuberculous empyema is usually accompanied by a thick pleural peal and requires surgical drainage or decortication (Fig. 13-5) in addition to anti-tuberculosis therapy.

ACTIVITY

Table 13-3 lists criteria for activity in TB. Since TB is a chronic disease with multiple exacerbations and remissions, it is important to determine if the disease is "healed," quiescent, or progressive. Decisions concerning infectiousness and the need for chemotherapy depend on this evaluation. The bases for these decisions are (a) clinical signs of infection (fever, weight loss, cough, sputum, etc.), (b) progressive x-ray changes, and (c) a positive sputum smear or culture. An improving x-ray study is also presumed to represent prior active TB. In the appropriate setting, the presence of any one of these findings is an indication for full therapy.

Therapy for pulmonary or pleural TB is discussed in Chapter 6. Corticosteroids are used as an adjunct to specific chemotherapy only in the most severe cases of active pulmonary TB. In the patient who is in danger of dying from TB, corticosteroids can be lifesaving by causing a rapid defervescence, symptomatic improvement, and weight gain. However, the routine use of corticosteroids has been shown to have no effect on the late effects of pulmonary or pleural TB.

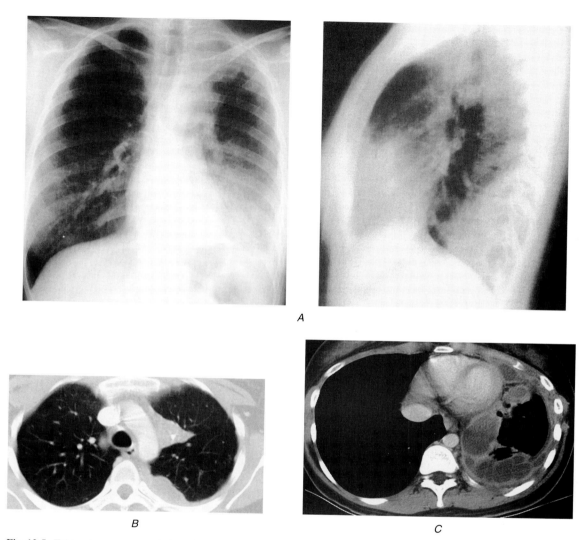

Fig. 13-5. Tuberculous empyema. *A.* Posterior-anterior and lateral chest radiographs demonstrating a left lower lobe effusion. *B.* CT scan of upper lobe showing calcific density in a consolidated and scarred-down left upper lobe. *C.* CT scan of lower lobe demonstrating thickened peal of a chronic empyema.

Predicting Who Has Active Tuberculosis

Several recent studies have focused on predicting which subjects admitted to the hospital with suspicion of TB should be placed immediately in respiratory isolation versus those who may not need it, given its high cost. Initial efforts to stratify subjects on the basis of risk factors had inadequate sensitivity from a public health perspective.[41] However, two recent groups have published prediction rules that may be more clinically useful (see Table 13-5). The first assigned points are based on immigration status, history of BCG immunization, HIV status, homelessness, compatible clinical symptoms, and

Table 13-5. Predicting Active Pulmonary TB

Study	Risk Factor	Points
Tattevin et al.[42]	Immigrant from Eastern or Southern Europe, South America, or French Guyana	1
	BCG immunization >10 yr earlier	1
	No HIV infection	5
	Homelessness	1
	Compatible symptoms	6
	Compatible chest x-ray	7
	Immigrant from sub-Saharan Africa, North Africa, Haiti, Southeast Asia	2
	No BCG	2
	No HIV infection	5
	Homelessness	1
	Typical clinical symptoms	12
	Typical chest x-ray	14
	Total 100% sensitivity	≥18
Wisnivesky, et al.[43]	TB risk factors* or chronic symptoms[†]	4
	Positive PPD	5
	Shortness of Breath	−3
	Temperature °C	
	<38.5	0
	38.5–39.0	3
	>39.0	6
	Crackles noted during examination	−3
	Upper lobe consolidation	6
	Total 98% sensitivity	1

* TB risk factors = recent immigration, recent institutionalization, known TB exposure
† TB chronic symptoms = weight loss, malaise, weakness, and/or night sweats for 3 or more months

compatible chest x-rays to define a risk score.[42] In their derivation cohort, this scoring system had a sensitivity of 100% and a negative predictive value of 100%. When this scoring system was tested in two other groups that sensitivity was not as good (91%) but within an acceptable range.

A second scoring system was developed at NYU.[43] This system factored in TB risk factors (recent immigration, institutionalization, and history of TB exposure) and chronic symptoms (weight loss, malaise, weakness and night sweats for 3 or more months), positive PPD, shortness of breath (protective), low or high grade temperatures, crackles on examination (protective), and upper lobe consolidation into a single score that could be used to determine who should be isolated. In their derivation cohort, a cut-off value of one or higher could be used to determine who to isolate (98% sensitivity, 46% specificity). This scoring system needs to be confirmed in another cohort to determine how well it functions in a different population.

COMPLICATIONS

Although a relatively uncommon complication of tuberculous infection, the development of a pneumothorax requires rapid attention. One of the postulated theories of etiology is the rupture of a cavity that then connects the tracheobronchial tree with the pleural space, creating a bronchopleural fistula. In this occurrence, contamination of the pleural space with caseous material results in spread of the infection to the pleura and should be corrected immediately because of the tendency to produce pleural fibrosis with expansion failure.

A second possible mechanism is the development of a submucosal bronchiolar lesion with air trapping in an acinus or subsegment that causes the development of a bleb. Rupture of this bleb allows air to enter the pleural space, but often without tuberculous infection of the pleura. However, both occurrences should be treated with rapid expansion of the lungs by tube suction to avoid the possibility of further infection and fibrosis of the pleura with trapping of the lung. A bronchopleural fistula may persist after these episodes of pneumothorax, and especially if untreated, often results in major problems owing to the tuberculous infection complicated by secondary invaders ("mixed" empyema).

Minor endobronchial disease is a common occurrence in TB but usually involves the distal bronchi. Resected lung specimens frequently show either ulceration or stenosis of the draining bronchioles or bronchi. Bronchial stenosis of significance may occur in the major bronchi but is rare. At times, it results from involvement of the central lymph nodes draining into the lobar bronchi, with caseation, ulceration, and fibrosis. Since fibrosis due to TB tends to contract and aggravate the stenosis, resection of the involved lung segment may be required after chemotherapy has produced inactivity of the acute inflammatory reaction.

The same endobronchial processes may result in bronchiectasis due to destruction of the bronchial wall. This usually is distal and frequently is in the upper lobes. The so-called "dry" bronchiectasis (without sputum) often is the result of prior pulmonary TB and may manifest itself chiefly as low-grade hemoptysis.

Empyema due to TB may result uncommonly from a primary infection with an associated tuberculous pleural effusion; however, the latter usually clears; Empyema is more common later in the disease, associated with debility and loss of resistance to infection (Fig. 13-5). It is usually a part of a progressive, extensive parenchymal infection with caseation and cavitation, the presumed sources for pleural contamination.

After treatment of extensive TB, the patient is often left with open, healed cavities as well as with areas of bronchiectasis. Colonization of these areas may occur with a variety of infectious agents. Usual oro-respiratory flora may produce the syndrome of "wet" bronchiectasis, i.e., with sputum production. Other mycobacteria may be recovered during the development of inactivity, and were, at one time, considered to be a sign of healing. The presence of other pathogenic mycobacteria brings up the possibility of a dual infection, especially when found early in the disease.

Aspergillus species are common in badly damaged lung areas, especially those that are cavitary. In England, a prospective study[44] revealed that 25% of clinically healed TB patients who had residual cavities developed positive precipitins to *Aspergillus* species; 11% had demonstrable cavitary "balls" presumed to be aspergillomas or "fungus balls." Three years later, these numbers had risen to 34%

and 17%, respectively. This high incidence may be due in part to the increased incidence of *Aspergillus* noted in the United Kingdom, both in the environment and as an infective agent, probably as a result of the more humid environment.

Massive hemorrhage, a dramatic event occurring in advanced cases of TB, is frequently terminal. Mild hemoptysis itself is very common in acute infection and not infrequently calls the attention of an otherwise unconcerned patient to the presence of serious disease. Rupture of a mycotic aneurysm of a branch of the pulmonary artery (Rasmussen's aneurysm) has been well publicized as a cause of death; an aspergilloma may be associated with severe and fatal hemorrhage; however, less well-defined major hemorrhages may also occur.

Resection of the involved area has been the most widely used method of control; unhappily, many patients die before this can be accomplished, and often (as in the case of aspergillomas) the areas are multiple, thus not lending themselves to excisional therapy. The extensive disease found in these patients often contraindicates surgery, since functional lung tissue necessary for survival must often be removed along with the diseased area at the time of surgery.

During the acute infectious phase of the disease, two interesting complications have been reported, the syndrome of inappropriate antidiuretic hormone excretion (SIADH) and a reset osmostat.[45] Both manifest themselves by abnormally low sodium; however, the former is associated with all of the clinical and renal abnormalities associated with SIADH. A reset osmostat is characterized by decreased serum osmolality without clinical symptoms, and the obligatory renal salt-wasting found in SIADH. Both conditions disappear with control of the infection; however, they should be differentiated from each other since SIADH requires metabolic control.

REFERENCES

1. Farer L, Lowell A, Meador M. Extrapulmonary tuberculosis in the United States. *Am J Epidemiol.* 1979;109(2): 205–217.

2. Arango L, Brewin AW, Murray JF. The spectrum of tuberculosis as currently seen in a metropolitan hospital. *American Review of Respiratory Disease.* 1973;108:805–812.

3. Small P, Schechter GF, Goodman PC. Treatment of tuberculosis in patients with advanced human deficiency virus infection. *N Engl J Med.* 324:289–294.

4. Shafe RW, Kim DS, Weiss JP, et al. Extrapulmonary tuberculosis in patients with human immunodeficiency virus infection. *Medicine.* 1991;70(6):384–397.

5. Perlman DC, El-Sadr WM, Nelson ET, et al. Variation in chest radiographic patterns in pulmonary tuberculosis patients by degree of human immunodeficiency virus-related immunosuppression. *Clinical Infectious Disease.* 1997;25: 242–246.

6. Shafer RW, Edlin BR. Tuberculosis in patients infected with human immunodeficiency virus: perspective on the past decade. *Clinical Infectious Disease.* 1996;22: 683–704.

7. Glassroth J, Robbins AG, Snider DE. Tuberculosis in the 1980's. *N Engl J Med.* 1980;302:1441–1450.

8. Mayock RL, MacGregor RR. Diagnosis, prevention and early therapy of tuberculosis. *Disease A Month.* 1976;22: 1–60.

9. Comstock G W, Livesay VT, Woolpert SF. The prognosis of a positive tuberculin reaction in childhood and adolescence. *Am J Epidemiol.* 1974;99:131.

10. Choyke PL, Sostman HD, Curtis AM, et al. Adult-onset pulmonary tuberculosis. *Radiology.* 1983;148:357–362.

11. Kiblawi SSO, Jay SJ, Stonehill RB, et al. Fever responses of patients on therapy for pulmonary tuberculosis. *Am Rev Respir Dis.* 1981;123:20–24.

12. Leung AN, Muller NL, Pineda PR, et al. Primary tuberculosis in childhood: radiographic manifestations. *Radiology.* 1992;182:87–91.

13. Chung DK. Hyponatremia in untreated active pulmonary tuberculosis. *Am Rev Respir Dis.* 1969;99:595–597.

14. MacGregor RR. A year's experience with tuberculosis in a private urban teaching hospital in the post-sanatorium era. *Am J Med.* 1975;58:221.

15. Garibaldi RA, Drusin RE, Ferebee SH et al. Isoniazid-associated hepatitis. Report of an outbreak. *Am Rev Respir Dis.* 1972;106:357.

16. Holden M, Dubin MR, Diamond PH. Frequency of negative intermediate-strength tuberculin sensitivity in patients with active tuberculosis. *N Engl J Med.* 1971;285:1560.

17. Fraser RG, Pare JAP. Diagnosis of diseases of the chest. Philadelphia, PA: WB Saunders; 1977:731–764.

18. Weber AL, Bird KT, Janower WL. Primary tuberculosis in childhood with particular emphasis on changes affecting the tracheobronchial tree. *Am J Roentgenol.* 1968; 103:123.

19. Poppius H, Thomander K. Segmentary distribution of cavities. A radiologic study of 500 consecutive cases of cavernous pulmonary tuberculosis. *Ann Med Intern Fenn.* 1957;46:113.

20. Lee KS, Hwang JW, Chung MP, et al. Utility of CT in the evaluation of pulmonary tuberculosis in patients without AIDS. *Chest.* 1996;110:977–984.

21. Hatipoglu ON, Manisali MM, Ucan ES, et al. High resolution compute tomographic findings in pulmonary tuberculosis. *Thorax.* 1996;51:397–402.

22. Wallace JM, Deutsch AL, Harrell JH et al. Bronchoscopy and transbronchial biopsy in evaluation of patients with suspected active tuberculosis. *Am J Med.* 1981;70:1189.

23. Danek SJ, Bower JS. Diagnosis of pulmonary tuberculosis by flexible fiberoptic bronchoscopy. *Am Rev Respir Dis.* 1979;119:677.

24. Centers for Disease Control. Reported Tuberculosis in the United States, 2003. Atlanta, GA: U. S. Department of Heatlh and Human Services; 2004.

25. Barnes PF, Bloch AB, Davidson PT, et al. Tuberculosis in patients with human immunodeficiency virus infection. *N Engl J Med.* 1991;324:1644–1650.

26. Bloch AB, Rieder HL, Kelly GD, et al. The epidemiology of tuberculosis in the United States. *Sem Respir Infect.* 1989;4: 289–296.

27. Chaisson RE, Schecter GF, Theuer, et al. Tuberculosis in patients with the acquired immunodeficiency syndrome. *Am Rev Respir Dis.* 1987;136:570–574.

28. Handwerger S, Mildvan D, Senie R, et al. Tuberculosis and the acquired immunodeficiency syndrome at New York City Hospital:1978–1985. *Chest.* 1987;91:176–180.

29. Louie E, Rice LB, Holzman RS. Tuberculosis in non-Haitian patients with acquired immunodeficiency syndrome. *Chest.* 1986;90:542–545.

30. Selwyn PA, Hartel D, Lewis VA, et al. A prospective study of the risk of tuberculosis among intravenous drug abusers with human immunodeficiency virus infection. *N Engl J Med.* 1989;320:545–550.

31. Stead WW, Lofgren JP. Does the risk of tuberculosis infection increase in old age? *J Infect Dis.* 1983;147:951–955.

32. Morris CDW. The radiography, haematology and biochemistry of pulmonary tuberculosis in the aged. *Quaterly Journal of Medicine.* 1989;266:529–535.

33. Korzeniewska-Kosela M, Krysl J, Muller NL, et al. Tuberculosis in young adults and the elderly: a prospective comparison study. *Chest.* 1994;106:28–32.

34. Perez-Guzman C, Vargas M, Torres-Cruz A, et al. Does aging modify pulmonary tuberculosis? A meta-analytical review. *Chest.* 1999;116:961–967.

35. Light RW, MacGregor MI, Luchsinger PC et al. Pleural effusions. The diagnostic separation of transudates and exudates. *Ann Intern Med.* 1972;77:507–555.

36. van Keimpema A R, Slaats EH, Wagenaar JP. Adenosine deaminase activity, not diagnostic for tuberculous pleurisy. *Eur J Respir Dis.* 71:15–18.

37. Valdes L, San Jose E, Alvarez D, et al. Adenosine deaminase (ADA) isoenzyme analysis in pleural effusions: diagnostic role, and relevance to the origin of increased ADA in tuberculous pleurisy. *Eur Respir J.* 1996;9:747–751.

38. Yam LT . Diagnostic significance of lymphocytes in pleural effusions. *Am Rev Respir Dis.* 1972;105:458–460.

39. Berger H W, Mejei E. Tuberculous pleurisy. *Chest.* 1973;63:88–92.

40. Scerbo J, Keltz H, Stone DJ. A prospective study of closed pleural biopsies. *JAMA.* 1971;218:377.

41. Bock N, McGowan Jr J, Ahn J, et al. Clinical predictors of tuberculosis as a guide for respiratory isolation procedures. *Am J Respir Crit Care Med.* 1996;154:1468–1472.

42. Tattevin P, Casalino E, Fleury L, et al. The validity of medical history, classic symptoms and chest radiographs in predicting pulmonary tuberculosis. *Chest.* 1999;115:1248–1253.

43. Wisnivesky J, Kaplan J, Henschke C, et al. Evaluation of clinical parameters to predict mycobacterium tuberculosis in inpatients. *Archives of Internal Medicine.* 2000;160: 2471–2476.

44. British Thoracic and Tuberculosis Association, R. C. Aspergilloma and residual tuberculous cavities—the results of a survey. *Tubercle.* 1970;51:227–245.

45. Mayock RL, Goldberg M. Metabolic considerations in disease of the respiratory system, *Diseases of metabolism.* Philadelphia, PA: WB Saunders;1964.

14

Upper Respiratory Tract Tuberculosis

Surinder K. Jindal
Ritesh Agarwal

Tuberculosis (TB) is traditionally regarded as a pulmonary disorder, although in the recent years, the incidence of extra pulmonary tuberculosis (EPTB) has increased worldwide. Over the last four decades, EPTB has gradually risen as a percentage of the total TB cases.[1] Upper respiratory tract TB is one of the rare forms of EPTB. In the prechemotherapeutic era, patients with active pulmonary TB often developed laryngeal, otologic, nasal, paranasal and pharyngeal involvement, and deteriorated progressively; however, with the advent of effective antituberculous drugs, the incidence came down significantly.

Upper respiratory tract is the portal of entry of all inhaled matter in the lungs. It also constitutes the first line of defense against inhalational insults; since inhalation is the most common and important route of mycobacterial infection, it should not be surprising to find tubercular involvement of the upper respiratory tract. On the other hand, it is the relative rarity of upper respiratory tract TB, which is somewhat puzzling. Nevertheless, it is the continuous airflow and smooth mucosal lining that do not allow mycobacteria to settle down in the respiratory tract and cause infection. Infection will occur more frequently in the entrapment areas, such as the larynx, or as part and parcel of pulmonary or disseminated TB.

Almost all parts of upper respiratory tract from the nose to the vocal cords and larynx can get involved although the frequency of involvement may vary to a great degree. Patients with tuberculosis of different components of upper respiratory tract may first report to a general physician, an otorhinolaryngologist, or a pulmonologist. It is an area that concerns all these specialists alike. Chest physicians, who also handle TB in developing countries, are frequently confronted with and consulted for upper respiratory tract TB. Factually speaking, TB of upper respiratory tract should be considered and handled at par with that of the lungs.

Symptoms and signs of upper respiratory tract TB depend upon the site of organ involvement (Table 14-1). Concurrent pulmonary involvement is frequent. Systemic manifestations such as fever and weight loss are uncommon but may occasionally be seen, especially, in the presence of involvement of lungs and/or other organs. Nodules or ulcerative lesions are seen on morphological examination. Endoscopic examination is required for mucosal lesions. Most of these lesions are initially missed as either nontubercular infections or malignant in nature. Diagnosis of TB is suspected on epidemiological basis in high prevalence countries or on failure to respond to routine treatment. Smear and/or histopathologic examinations help in establishing the final etiologic diagnosis.

Tuberculous involvement of upper respiratory tract was seen in less than two percent of TB admissions in the past.[2] More recently however, there is an increased occurrence of EPTB especially in patients with human immunodeficiency virus (HIV) infection. For example, of the 538 EPTB cases (28.6%) in a total of 1878 enrollees, the risk for EPTB in HIV seropositive patients, in a multivariate model was high; African American ethnicity was an independent risk factor for EPTB.[3] The most common sites of EPTB in this study were lymph nodes (43%) and pleura (23%).[3] There are several other reports which suggest the increase in incidence and change in spectrum of upper respiratory tract TB with an increase in diseases (such as HIV infection) and drugs causing general immunosuppression.[4,5] The association of HIV infection with TB is going to have impact on the practice of otolaryngologists as well.[6]

Tuberculosis of the upper respiratory tract is also a common cause of cervical lymph node enlargement.[7-10] Any presence of lymph nodes in the neck calls for careful search for a lesion in the upper respiratory tract and vice versa. In a recent series of 17 cases of TB of nasopharynx from Hong Kong, cervical lymphadenopathy was present in 59% of patients.[11] Similarly, in Thailand, the most common site of TB in the head and neck involved the cervical lymph nodes and the nasopharynx.[12] In addition, pulmonary lesions are present in about 20% of adults and about 50–60% of children.[13-16]

NASAL TUBERCULOSIS

Tuberculosis of the nose and paranasal sinuses is uncommonly reported, but a well described entity in otorhinolaryngology practice.[17,18] In 1997, only 35 cases were identified in a search of the English language medical literature of the last 95 years.[19] Several other reports of isolated cases have appeared since after 1997, mostly from the developing countries.[20-23] Recently, a series of ten cases were described from Pakistan, none of whom had any evidence of pulmonary TB.[24] Similarly, a large series of 17 cases was reported from Hong Kong.[11] Its reemergence as a major health problem in the United States

Table 14-1. Common Symptoms and Signs of Upper Respiratory Tract Tuberculosis

1. Nose:	Nasal discharge/obstruction
	Epistaxis, pain
	External nodule, ulcer (Lupus vulgaris) or deformity
	Mucosal ulcer/s
	Septal perforation
2. Oral cavity:	Ulcers—painless/painful on tongue, buccal or pharyngeal mucosa
	Localized swelling
	Tonsillar infiltration/ulcer
	Sore throat, dysphagia, white patches
	Secondary otitis media—otorrhea
3. Larynx:	Hoarseness
	Odynophagia, dysphagia
	Mucosal ulcers, localized swelling, abscess
	Upper airway obstruction—rare

was attributed to HIV infection, homelessness and deterioration of the social infrastructure.[19] Maxillary sinuses are commonly involved in nasal TB. Very rarely, involvement of other sinuses has been described. Tuberculosis of sphenoid sinuses established on magnetic resonance imaging and endoscopic biopsy was recently reported in two children.[25]

Clinical Features

Patients with nasal TB commonly present with nasal obstruction and purulent rhinorrhea. Epistaxis is another important manifestation.[26,27] Lupus vulgaris, a slow-growing, indolent ulcerative lesion caused by *M. tuberculosis* may affect nasal vestibule, the septum and the alae. Occasionally, lupus vulgaris with papulo-necrotic TB is reported.[28] External deformity may result in about one third of patients. Physical examination may reveal pallor of nasal mucosa with multiple, minute apple jelly nodules on diascopy. Perforation of septal cartilage can occur. Tuberculosis can also manifest as a polypoid lesion in the nasal cavity.[29,30] Sinonasal TB can invade the surrounding bones and result in osteomyelitis and abscess formation.[31] Intracranial extension can cause neurological manifestations such as epilepsy and optic neuritis.[26,32] In a large series of 18 cases of intrasellar tuberculomas, 6 had involvement of sphenoid sinus.[33] Cervical lymph node enlargement is present in about 30% of patients.

Most of the clinical manifestations can be seen in other diseases involving the nose such as the fungal infections, leprosy, syphilis and malignancies. Septal perforations have

been reported in patients on inhalational corticosteroids, allergic bronchopulmonary aspergillosis, and following chronic exposures to metal fumes in welders.[34,35] Granulomatous involvement of nose and sinuses can occur in several other conditions.[36] Wegener's granulomatosis, fungal infections, mid-line granulomatous disease, and leprosy are some such examples. Radiotherapy administered for undifferentiated carcinoma can also cause granulomatous inflammation which in many instances is attributable to TB.[37] Differential diagnosis is achieved on histologic and microbiologic parameter. Confirmation of diagnosis is made on mycobacterial culture since the acid-fast bacilli on smear examination may occasionally represent *Mycobacterium leprae*—an important cause of nasal involvement in endemic zones. Mycobacteria were detected on polymerase chain reaction (PCR) of nasal swabs in 6 out of 16 smear positive from TB patients and one out of 10 household contacts.[38] But the efficacy of PCR on nasal swabs in clinical diagnosis of nasal TB is not known. Although *Mycobacterium tuberculosis* is the most common organism, other mycobacteria have been rarely implicated. *Mycobacterium africanum* had been isolated in a case of cutaneous TB with nasal sinus invasion, nasal perforation and bilateral nodular scleritis.[39]

Treatment of nasal TB is given on standard lines. Surgical interventions may occasionally be required.

ORAL CAVITY AND PHARYNX

The oral cavity, a rare site of involvement, is generally resistant to TB. Infection of the oral cavity requires mucosal injury and is associated with poor dental hygiene and other causes which result in mucosal injury. Most patients have concomitant pulmonary TB and the lesions are believed to result from infected sputum being coughed out. Infection could also be acquired by the hematogenous route. Oral TB, diagnosed on histologic criteria in 15 patients in China occurred most commonly in association with pulmonary tuberculosis.[40] Tongue is the most common site of involvement. Several isolated cases of lingual TB have been reported in the recent past.[41–47] Very rarely, TB of the lips has been described.[48] Similar to TB of the nose, many of these cases are seen in patients with HIV infection.[44,48,49] Almost any part of the tongue such as the tip, the borders, dorsum and base of the tongue may be involved. Other sites in the oral cavity include the floor of the mouth, soft palate, tonsils, anterior pillars of fauces, and uvula.[50]

Clinical Features

The lesions can manifest as ulcers or nodules, which can be located anywhere in the mouth. These can be either single or multiple. Similarly, there can be painful or painless lesions. The lesions are usually well circumscribed but can also be irregular simulating malignant ulcers. The draining lymph nodes in the neck may also be palpable.

Tuberculosis of the pharynx can be ulcerative of the *lupus vulgaris* type or secondary to pulmonary involvement (so-called miliary TB of pharynx). Nasopharynx is the most common site of pharyngeal involvement.[22,23,51,52] Symptoms of nasopharyngeal TB include nasal obstruction, rhinorrhea, and nasal twang of voice, while physical findings may be limited to adenoid hypertrophy without any distinguishing features. Several atypical presentations have been described. Snoring which disappeared after antitubercular therapy, was the only complaint reported in a 58 year old patient.[53] Two different patterns of nasopharyngeal TB were identified on magnetic resonance imaging: the pattern of a discrete polypoid mass in the adenoids and the second pattern of a more diffuse soft tissue thickening of one or two walls of nasopharynx.[54] Extension outside the confines of nasopharynx was not seen.[54] Most infections are primary and fewer than 20% demonstrate pulmonary involvement.[52] Postradiation granulomatous inflammation in patients with nasopharyngeal carcinoma should be suspected as occult tubercular infection and diligently investigated.[37]

Oropharyngeal TB is likely to present with symptoms of sore throat.[55,56] Commonly, there is simultaneous involvement of larynx causing severe dysphagia and odynophagia.[56] Local hyperemia and irregularity of mucosa, erythematous papules, and swelling of cheek have been described in different case reports.[57–59] Cercial

lymphadenopathy is frequently present. Similarly, cutaneous *lupus vulgaris* and scrofuloderma may also be seen.

Tonsils constitute another important site of involvement with TB. Again, the involvement may occur in isolation or along with TB of the larynx and the lungs. Tonsillar TB was common in the era of unpasteurized milk and was acquired by drinking milk infected with *M. bovis*. Tonsillar involvement may present with features of sore throat, lymphadenopathy, dysphagia, ulceration, masses, and white patches.[60–62] Pharyngeal TB can also spread to the middle ear through the eustachian tube.[63] Tympanic membrane perforations (especially multiple), painless otorrhea, and hearing loss may result. Preauricular lymph node enlargement and postauricular fistula are considered pathognomic of tubercular otitis media. Occasionally, TB might complicate a malignant lesion in this region.[64] Physical examination includes unilateral tonsillar enlargement, ulcerations, and fibrosis of the tonsils. Incisional biopsy confirms the diagnosis, which is based on histopathologic findings and the identification of acid-fast bacilli. Patient tends to respond quickly to antitubercular chemotherapy; if no response is seen in two weeks, the diagnosis should be questioned.[10]

Tuberculosis of the salivary glands occurs as a result of infection of oral cavity or secondary to pulmonary TB. Primary sialitis may occur but rarely. Although parotid involvement is the most common, submandibular glands may also be involved.[65] The clinical presentation can be either acute or chronic. Most patients would present with only parotidomegaly and no other systemic manifestations. In a few case reports, the diagnosis was not suspected until histopathologic evidence manifested.[66,67] When suspected however, diagnosis can be made by fine needle aspiration cytology (FNAC).

Diagnosis of most forms of extralaryngeal upper respiratory tract TB is difficult and requires biopsy procedures. In a series of 16 cases of TB with involvement of oral cavity and/or pharynx (8), ear (4), salivary glands (2), nose (1), and frontal sinuses (1), the average duration of symptoms was 11.5 months, and biopsy was required in all; purified protein derivative skin test was also positive in 15 out of 16 patients.[68]

Treatment for all these patients consists of antituberculous chemotherapy and is generally favorable.[68] Surgical intervention should be avoided.[9]

TUBERCULOSIS OF THE LARYNX

Larynx is the most important and vital part of the upper respiratory tract. It can be involved in different infective, neoplastic, granulomatous, and other conditions. Tuberculosis is

Table 14-2. Changes in Clinical Spectrum of Laryngeal Tuberculosis—Pre- and Post-Chemotherapeutic Era

	Prechemotherapeutic Era	Postchemotherapeutic Era
Occurrence:	Common	Uncommon
	15–37% of patients with pulmonary TB	Less than 1% of cases
Age:	<40 years	5th–6th decade
Constitutional symptoms:	Prominent	Less common
Pulmonary involvement:	Severe	Advanced disease less common
Lesions:	Multiple	Solitary (usually)
	Ulcerative	Hypertrophic
Predilection for post-laryngeal involvement:	Yes	No predilection for any laryngeal site
Pseudotumor form:	Uncommon	Common

perhaps the most common cause of granulomatous disease of the larynx.[69] The clinical presentation of tubercular laryngitis has changed significantly from what it was before the advent of chemotherapy (Table 14-2). Involvement of larynx by TB is now a relatively uncommon phenomenon. In the prechemotherapy era, it was a common complication of active cavitary pulmonary disease occurring in about one third of cases.[70,71] Presently, it is reported in 1–2% of cases.[2,10] The primary infection can involve any part of the larynx while the previously described direct mode of spread from the lungs along with airways, predominantly involved the posterior larynx. In some series, almost all patients of laryngeal TB were reported to have some evidence of pulmonary TB and many would demonstrate sputum smear positivity for AFBs.[72,73] In the postchemotherapy era, laryngeal TB especially in the low prevalence countries generally occurs as an isolated manifestation.[74–78]

Laryngeal involvement is especially common in patients with immunodeficiency such as the HIV infection. In a large series of 45 patients with upper aerodigestive tract TB, 16 had laryngeal and 23 nasopharyngeal TB; 4 out of 26 patients had positive serological tests for HIV infection.[12] Similarly, laryngeal TB has been described in other diseases. In a review of 283 patients of systemic lupus erythematosus in Korea, TB was documented in 15 patients, one of whom had laryngeal involvement.[79] Two cases of laryngeal TB were reported in renal transplant patients—both responded promptly to antitubercular therapy.[80] Epiglottic TB was recently reported in a patient with Addison's disease treated with glucocorticoids for four years.[81]

Clinical Features and Diagnosis

There is a shift in the age and sex distribution of laryngeal TB in the last 3–4 decades.[77,82] It is more common in old age and more common in males than females.[71,83] Above 50 years of age, the male predominance is even more marked. It is also more frequent in individuals of poor constitution and health, especially those who are alcoholics and undernourished.[84] Consumption of tobacco is also identified as a risk factor.[84]

Presence of laryngeal symptoms is generally quite bothersome and brings the patient to the physician early in the course of disease. The most common symptom is hoarseness of voice present in over 90% of patients.[69,77] Cough, dysphagia, odynophagia, pain in the throat, or referred pain in the ear are also common. Laryngeal involvement can present as an emergency situation with severe upper airway obstruction resulting from edema and granulomatous involvement of laryngeal mucosa. Stridor may be present because of the presence of granulation tissue at the level of glottis, subglottic stenosis and vocal cord paralysis secondary to mediastinal lymphadenopathy.[78] Involvement of posterior larynx was thought to result from pooling of infected saliva in the recumbent position; recent reports have shown no predilection for posterior laryngeal involvement. Most patients show anterior vocal-cord involvement with hypertrophic lesions being more common than the ulcerative lesions (Figs. 14-1a and 14-1b). Occasionally, there is isolated involvement of the epiglottic, supraglottic, or subglottic regions.[85,86] Solitary lesions are present four times more often than multiple lesions.

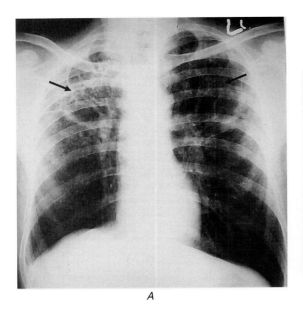
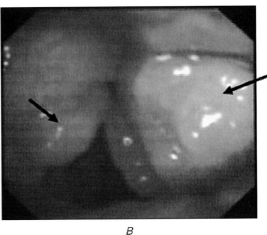

Fig. 14-1. (*A*) Chest roentgenogram (PA view) showing bilateral fibro-cavitary lesions and (*B*) fiberoptic laryngoscopic image showing bilateral nodular masses above the level of vocal cords. Biopsy from these masses confirmed TB.

Clinical picture in patients with underlying HIV infection and acquired immunodeficiency syndrome is somewhat different posing greater difficulties in diagnosis.[87] Systemic features such as fever, night sweats, and weight loss are common. Multiple agent infections are also more frequent. Laryngeal TB, especially the nodular presentation, sometimes with an abscess formation, may be difficult to differentiate from cancer on physical examination. A good lateral x-ray of the neck and computed tomography (CT) can help in diagnosis (Figs. 14-2a and 14-2b).[88,89] Although appearances of laryngeal TB are not specific, the possibility should be raised when there is bilateral involvement, thickening of the free margin of the epiglottis, and preservation of the preepiglottic and paralaryngeal spaces even in the presence of extensive mucosal involvement.[89] Any non-specific chronic laryngitis of poor evolution should lead to a suspicion of laryngeal TB.[84] Cartilage destruction is more common in malignancies but TB can occasionally masquerade.[90] Bacterial and fungal infections, Wegener's granulomatosis, sarcoidosis, and malignancies need to be considered in differential diagnosis.

Histopathologic examination is required for a definite diagnosis. Sputum microscopy may be positive in 20% of patients with laryngeal TB. A laryngeal swab smear positive for mycobacteria alone should not be considered to indicate laryngeal TB. It is frequently so in patients of pulmonary TB, especially in case of children. In a report on 116 children with suspected pulmonary TB, mycobacteria were seen on either smear examination or culture in one-third of 51 patients in whom laryngeal swabs were examined.[91] Direct laryngoscopic examination with biopsy provides the most conclusive evidence for diagnosis. The sample should be sent for both histopathologic examination and culture. It is the presence of mycobacteria on culture of biopsy specimen which provides the conclusive etiological evidence of TB. However in clinical practice, histologic demonstration of epithelioid cell caseating granulomas is considered enough to initiate antitubercular therapy.

Treatment and Outcome

The laryngeal lesions of TB respond quickly to standard antituberculous regimens within weeks. Vocal-cord immobility due to fibrosis and adhesion may produce permanent hoarseness in a minority of patients.[71,92] Occasionally, the disease may remain undiagnosed and untreated for long periods which would result in causing significant damage. Coexistence of laryngeal TB and carcinoma is reported in 1–2% cases.[93,94] In such patients, antituberculous drugs should be given for at least three to six weeks before treatment for laryngeal carcinoma

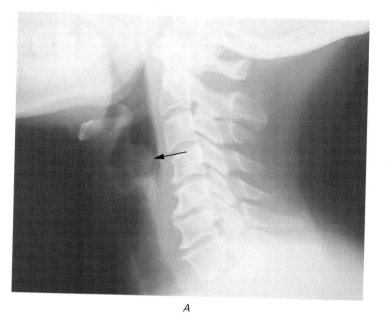

A

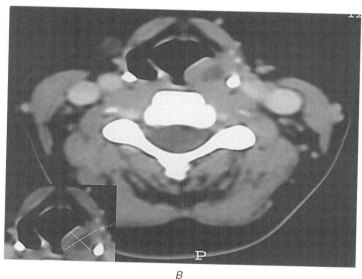

Fig. 14-2. (*A*) Roentgenogram of soft tissue neck and (*B*) CT scan of the neck showing well defined tubercular abscess in the left aryepiglottic fold obliterating the left piriform fossa.

B

is initiated.[93] Treatment includes antitubercular chemotherapy for at least six months, modified on the basis of culture and sensitivity reports in cases of suspected drug resistance. Laryngeal TB generally responds well to multiple drug antituberculous chemotherapy.[95] Surgical intervention such as tracheostomy, partial or complete laryngectomy or laryngo-tracheoplasty may be required in some patients with abscess formation and progressive disease

unresponsive to medical therapy. Airway obstruction, although rare, even in fulminant cases may require tracheostomy for relief.[96]

In conclusion, TB should be kept in the differential diagnosis of upper airway diseases and/or cervical lymphadenopathy whenever a patient presents with insidious onset of symptoms, ulcerative or granulomatous lesions and failure of response to therapy of more common lesions.

Classic clinical features may not always be present. Early diagnosis and treatment are essential to prevent long-term complications.

REFERENCES

1. Iseman MD. Extrapulmonary tuberculosis in adults. In: Iseman MD, ed. *A Clinician's Guide to Tuberculosis.* Philadelphia, PA: Lippincott William & Wilkins; 2000: 145–198.
2. Rohwedder JJ. Tuberculosis of the upper respiratory tract. Sixteen cases in a general hospital. *Ann Intern Med.* 1974; 80:708.
3. Gonzalez OY, Adams G, Teter LD, et al. Extra-pulmonary manifestations in a large metropolitan area with a low incidence of tuberculosis. *Int J Tuberc Lung Dis.* 2003;7:1178–1185.
4. Kandiloros DC, Nikolopoulos TP, Ferekidis EA, et al. Laryngeal tuberculosis at the end of the 20th century. *J Laryngol Otol.* 1997;111:619–621.
5. Burns JL. Laryngeal tuberculosis. *J Otolaryngol.* 1993; 22:398.
6. Cleary KR, Batsakis JG. Mycobacterial disease of the head and neck: current perspective. *Ann Otol Rhinol Laryngol.* 1995;104:830–833.
7. Kumar A. Lymph node tuberculosis. In: Sharma SK, Mohan A, eds. *Tuberculosis.* New Delhi, India: Jaypee Publishers; 2001:273–284.
8. Al-Serhani AM. Mycobacterial infections of the head and neck: presentation and diagnosis. *Laryngoscope.* 2001;111: 2012–2016.
9. Munck K, Mandpe AH. Mycobacterial infections of the head and neck. *Otolaryol Clin North Am.* 2003;36:569–576.
10. Williams GR, Phil M, Douglas-Jones T. Mycobacterium marches back. *J Laryngol Otol.* 1995;109:5–13.
11. Tse GM, Ma TK, Chan AB, et al. Tuberculosis of the nasopharynx: a rare entity revisited. *Laryngoscope.* 2003;113: 737–740.
12. Srirompotong S, Yimtae K. Tuberculosis in the upper aerodiagestive tract and human immuno-deficiency virus coinfections. *J Otolaryngol.* 2003;32:230–233.
13. Thompson MM, Underwood MJ, Sayers RD, et al. Peripheral tuberculous lymphadenopathy: a review of 67 cases. *Br J Surg.* 1992;79:763–764.
14. Jha BC, Dass A, Nagarkar NM, et al. Cervical tuberculous lymphadenopathy: changing clinical pattern and concepts in management. *Postgrad Med J.* 2001;77:185–187.
15. Seth V, Kabra SK, Jain Y, et al. Tubercular lymphadenitis: clinical manifestation. *Indian J Pediatr.* 1995;62:565–570.
16. Reviglion MC, Snider DE Jr, Kochi A. Global epidemiology of tuberculosis morbidity and mortality: a worldwide epidemic. *JAMA.* 1995;273:220–226.
17. Kukreja HK, Sacha BS, Joshi KC. Tuberculosis of maxillary sinus. *Indian J Otolaryngol.* 1977;29:27–28.
18. Krishnan E, Rudraksha MR. Paranasal sinus tuberculosis. *Indian J Otolaryngol.* 1978;30:124–126.
19. Butt AA. Nasal tuberculosis in the 20th century. *Am J Med Sci.* 1997;313:332–335.
20. Purohit SD, Gupta RC. Primary tuberculosis of nose. *Indian J Chest Dis Allied Sci.* 1997;39:63–64.
21. Hup AK, Haitjema T, de Kuijper G. Primary nasal tuberculosis. *Rhinology.* 2001;39:47–48.
22. Koktener A, Koktenera A. Nasopharyngeal tuberculosis. *Eur J Radiol.* 2001;39:186–187.
23. Percodani J, Braun F, Arrue P, et al. Nasopharyngeal tuberculosis. *J Laryngol Otol.* 1999;113:928–931.
24. Nawaz G, Khan MR. Primary sinonasal tuberculosis in north-west Pakistan. *J Coll Physicians Surg Pak.* 2004;14: 221–224.
25. Sharma SC, Baruah P. Sphenoid sinus tuberculosis in children—a rare entity. *Int J Pediatr Otorhinolaryngol.* 2003;67:399–401.
26. Batra K, Chaudhary N, Motwani G, et al. An unusual case of primary nasal tuberculosis with epistaxis and epilepsy. *Ear Nose Throat J.* 2002;81:842–844.
27. Choi YC, Park YS, Jeon EJ, et al. The disappeared disease: tuberculosis of the nasal septum. *Rhinology.* 2000;38:90–92.
28. Senol M, Ozcan A, Aydin A, et al. Disseminated lupus vulgaris and papulonecrotic tuberculid: case report. *Pediatr Dermatol.* 2000;17:133–135.
29. Blanco Aparicio M, Verea-Hernando H, Pombo F. Tuberculosis of the nasal fossa manifested by a polypoid mass. *J Otolaryngol.* 1995;24:317–318.
30. Nayar RC, Al Kaabi J, Ghorpade K. Primary nasal tuberculosis: a case report. *Ear Nose Throat J.* 2004;83:188–191.
31. Jha D, Deka RC, Sharma MC. Tuberculosis of the maxillary sinus manifesting as a facial abscess. *Ear Nose Throat J.* 2002;81:102–104.
32. Das JC, Singh K, Sharma P, et al. Tuberculous osteomyelitis and optic neuritis. *Ophthalmic Surg Lasers Imaging.* 2003;34:409–412.
33. Sharma MC, Arora R, Mahapatra AK, et al. Intrasellar tuberculoma—an enigmatic pituitary infection: a series of 18 cases. *Clin Neurol Neurosurg.* 2000;102:72–77.
34. Deepak D, Panjabi C, Gudwani S, et al. Nasal septal perforation in a patient with allergic bronchopulmonary aspergillosis and rhinitis on long term corticosteroids. *Asian Pac J Allergy Immunol.* 2001;19:287–290.
35. Lee CR, Yoo CI, Lee J, et al. Nasal septum perforation of welders. *Ind Health.* 2002;40:286–289.
36. Hughes RG, Drake-Lee A. Nasal manifestations of granulomatous disease. *Hosp Med.* 2001;62:417–421.
37. Chan AB, Ma TK, Yu BK, et al. Nasopharyngeal granulomatous inflammation and tuberculosis complicating undifferentiated carcinoma. *Otolaryngol Head Neck Surg.* 2004;130:125–130.
38. Warndorff DK, Glynn JR, Fine PE, et al. Polymerase chain reaction of nasal swabs from tuberculosis patients and their contacts. *Int J Lepr Other Mycobact Dis.* 1996;64: 404–408.
39. Baril L, Caumes E, Truffot-Pernot C, et al. Tuberculosis caused by *Mycobacterium africanum* associated with involvement of

the upper and lower respiratory tract, skin and mucosa. *Clin Infect Dis.* 1995;21:653–655.

40. Eng HL, Lu SY, Yang CH, et al. Oral tuberculosis. *Oral Surg Oral Med Oral pathol Oral Radiol Endod.* 1996;81:415–420.

41. Memon GA, Khushk IA. Primary tuberculosis of tongue. *J Coll Physicians Surg Pak.* 2003;13:604–605.

42. Carnelio S, Rodrigues G. Primary lingual tuberculosis: a case report with review of literature. *J Oral Sci.* 2002;44:55–57.

43. Iype EM, Ramdas K, Pandey M, et al. Primary tuberculosis of the tongue: report of three cases. *Br J Oral Maxillofac Surg.* 2001;39:402–403.

44. Anil S, Ellepola AN, Samaranayake LP, et al. Tuberculous ulcer of the tongue as presenting feature of pulmonary tuberculosis and HIV infection. *Gen Dent.* 2000;48:458–461.

45. Aktogu S, Eris FN, Dinc ZA, et al. Tuberculosis of the tongue secondary to pulmonary tuberculosis. *Monaldi Arch Chest Dis.* 2000;55:287–288.

46. Gupta A, Shinde KJ, Bhardwaj I. Primary lingual tuberculosis: a case report. *J Laryngol Otol.* 1998;112:86–87.

47. Jawad J, El-Zuebi F. Primary lingual tuberculosis: a case report. *J Laryngol Otol.* 1996;110:177–178.

48. Ilyas SE, Chen FF, Hodgson TA, et al. Labial tuberculosis: a unique cause of lip swelling complicating HIV infection. *HIV Med.* 2002;3:283–286.

49. Ceballos-Salobrena A, Aguirre-Urizar JM, Bagan-Sebastian JV. Oral manifestations associated with human immunodeficiency virus infection in a Spanish population. *J Oral Pathol Med.* 1996;25:523–526.

50. Brennan TF, Vrabec DP. Tuberculosis of the oral mucosa. *Ann Otol Rhinol Laryngol.* 1970;79:601–605.

51. Mair IWS, Johannessen TA. Nasopharyngeal tuberculosis. *Arch Otolaryngol.* 1970;92:392–393.

52. Sharma HS, Kurl DN, Kamal MZ. Tuberculoid granulomatous lesion of the pharynx—review of the literature. *Auris Nasus Larynx.* 1998;25:187–191.

53. Aktan B, Selimoglu E, Ucuncu H, et al. Primary nasopharyngeal tuberculosis in a patient with the complaint of snoring. *J Laryngol Otol.* 2002;116:301–303.

54. King AD, Ahuja AT, Tse GM, et al. MR imaging features of nasopharyngeal tuberculosis: report of three cases and literature review. *AJNR Am J Neuroradiol.* 2003;24:279–282.

55. Al-Serhani AM, Al-Mazrou K. Pharyngeal tuberculosis. *Am J Otolaryngol.* 2001;22:236–240.

56. Caylan R, Aydin K. Oropharyngeal tuberculosis causing severe odynophagia and dysphagia. *Eur Arch Otorhinolaryngol.* 2002;259:229–230.

57. Magina S, Lisboa C, Resende C, et al. Tuberculosis in a child presenting as asymptomatic oropharyngeal and laryngeal lesions. *Pediatr Dermatol.* 2003;20:429–431.

58. Cakan A, Mutlu Z, Ozsoz A, et al. Tuberculosis of oral mucosa. *Monaldi Arch Chest Dis.* 2001;56:315–317.

59. Hajioff D, Snow MH, Thaker H, et al. Primary tuberculosis of the posterior oropharyngeal wall. *J Laryngol Otol.* 1999;113:1029–1030.

60. Srirompotong S, Yimtae K, Srirompotong S. Clinical aspects of tonsillar tuberculosis. *Southeast Asian J Trop Med Public Health.* 2002;33:147–150.

61. Yamamoto K, Iwata F, Nakamura A, et al. Tonsillar tuberculosis associated with pulmonary and laryngeal foci. *Intern Med.* 2002;41:664–666.

62. Sutbeyaz Y, Ucuncu H, Murat Karasen R, et al. The association of secondary tonsillar and laryngeal tuberculosis: a case report and literature review. *Auris Nasus Larynx.* 2000;27:371–374.

63. Greenfield BJ, Selesnide AH, Harrison WG. Aural tuberculosis. *Am J Otol.* 1995;16:175–182.

64. Raman R, Bakthavizian A. Tuberculosis associated with malignancy of the nasopharynx. *Indian J Otolaryngol.* 1981;33:149–150.

65. Kumar S, Dev A. Primary tuberculosis of bilateral submandibular salivary glands. *Indian J Otolaryngol.* 1990;42:69–70.

66. El Hakim IE, Langdon JD. Unusual presentation of tuberculosis of the head and neck region. Report of three cases. *Int J Oral Maxillofacial Surg.* 1989;18:194–196.

67. Kant R, Sahi RP, Mahendra NN, et al. Primary tuberculosis of the parotid gland. *J Indian Med Assoc.* 1977;68:212.

68. Sierra C, Fortun J, Barros C, et al. Extra-laryngeal head and neck tuberculosis. *Clin Microbiol Infect.* 2000;6:644–648.

69. Ramadan HH, Tarazi AE, Baroudy FM. Laryngeal tuberculosis: presentation of 16 cases and review of the literature. *J Otolaryngol.* 1993;22:39–41.

70. Nishike S, Irifune M, Doi K, et al. Laryngeal tuberculosis: a report of 15 cases. *Ann Otol Rhinol Laryngol.* 2002;111:916–918.

71. Lindell MM, Jing GS, Wallace S. Laryngeal tuberculosis. *Am J Roentgenol.* 1977;129:677–680.

72. Lee K, Schecter G. Tuberculous infection of the head and neck. *Otolaryngol Head Neck Surg.* 1995;74:395–399.

73. Rupa V, Bhanu TS. Laryngeal tuberculosis in the eighties—an Indian experience. *J Laryngol Otol.* 1989;103:864–868.

74. Kilgore TL, Jenkins DW. Laryngeal tuberculosis. *Chest.* 1983;83:139–141.

75. Sode A, Rubio J, Salazar M, et al. Tuberculosis of the larynx: clinical aspects in 19 patients. *Laryngoscope.* 1989;99:1147–1150.

76. Thaller SR, Gross JR, Pitch BZ, et al. Laryngeal tuberculosis as manifested in the decades 1963–1983. *Laryngoscope.* 1987;97:848–850.

77. Shin J, Nam SY, Yoo SJ, et al. Changing trends in clinical manifestations of laryngeal tuberculosis. *Laryngoscope.* 2000;110:1950–1953.

78. Smallman LA, Clark DR, Raine CH, et al. The presentation of laryngeal tuberculosis. *Clin Otolaryngol.* 1987;12:221–225.

79. Yun JE, Lee SW, Kim TH, et al. The incidence and clinical characteristics of *Mycobacterium tuberculosis* infection among systemic lupus erythematosus and rheumatoid arthritis patients in Korea. *Clin Exp Rheumatol.* 2002;20:127–132.

80. Tato AM, Pascual J, Orofino L, et al. Laryngeal tuberculosis in renal allograft patients. *Am J Kidney Dis.* 1998;31: 701–705.

81. Egeli E, Oghan F, Alper M, et al. Epiglottic tuberculosis in a patient treated with steroid for Addison's disease. *Tohoku J Exp Med.* 2003;201;119–125.

82. Agarwal P, Bais AS. A clinical and videostroboscopic evaluation of laryngeal tuberculosis. *J Laryngol Otol.* 1998;112:45–48.

83. Levenson MJ, Ingerman M, Grimes C, et al. Laryngeal tuberculosis: review of twenty cases. *Laryngoscope.* 1984;94: 1094–1097.

84. Porras Alonso E, Martin Mateos A, Perez-Requena J, et al. Laryngeal tuberculosis. *Rev Laryngol Otol Rhinol.* 2002;123: 47–48.

85. Galli J, Nardi C, Contucci AM, et al. Atypical isolated epiglottic tuberculosis: a case report and a review of the literature. *Am J Otolaryngol.* 2002;23:237–240.

86. Richter B, Fradis M, Kohler G, et al. Epiglottic tuberculosis: differential diagnosis and treatment. Case report and review of the literature. *Ann Otol Rhinol Laryngol.* 2001;110: 197–201.

87. Singh B, Balwally AN, Nash M, et al. Laryngeal tuberculosis in HIV infected patients: a difficult diagnosis. *Laryngoscope.* 1996;106:1238–1240.

88. Bailey CM, Windle-Taylor PC. Tuberculous laryngitis: a series of 37 patients. *Laryngoscope.* 1981;91:93–100.

89. Kim MD, Kim DI, Yune HY, et al. CT findings of laryngeal tuberculosis: comparison to laryngeal carcinoma. *J Comput Assist Tomogr.* 1997;21:29–34.

90. Kenmochi M, Ohashi T, Nishino H, et al. A case report of difficult diagnosis in the patient with advanced laryngeal tuberculosis. *Auris Nasus Larynx.* 2003;30:S131–S134.

91. Thakur A, Coulter JB, Zutshi K, et al. Laryngeal swabs for diagnosing tuberculosis. *Ann Trop Paediatr.* 1999;19: 333–336.

92. Getson WR, Park YW. Laryngeal tuberculosis. *Arch Otolaryngol Head Neck Surg.* 1992;118:878–881.

93. Feld R, Bodey GP, Groschell D. Mycobacteriosis in patients with malignant disease. *Arch Intern Med.* 1976;136:67–70.

94. Kaplan MH, Armstrong D, Rosen P. Tuberculosis complicating neoplastic disease. A review of 201 cases. *Cancer.* 1974;33:850–858.

95. Riley EC, Amundson DE. Laryngeal tuberculosis revisited. *Am Fam Physician.* 1992;46:759–762.

96. Tong MCF, Hasselt AV. Tuberculous laryngitis. *Otolaryngol Head Neck Surg.* 1993;11:965–966.

15

Otologic Tuberculosis

George A. Pankey

OTOLOGIC TUBERCULOSIS

One year after the isolation of the tubercle bacillus by Koch in 1882, the organism was cultured from a middle-ear lesion. *Otologic tuberculosis* has been relegated to the status of "other" in the list of localizations of TB by the American Thoracic Society in their *Diagnostic Standards and Classification of Tuberculosis and Other Mycobac-terial Diseases, 1981.* Presumably it was given this status because TB of the ear is extremely uncommon in the United States; however, there are still occasional patients who have chronically draining ears due to *Mycobacterium tuberculosis.*[1] In addition, the incidence of TB is high in the refugee population, especially those from Indochina (1138 cases/100,000 refugees on arrival and 407/100,000 refugees per year thereafter).[2] These sources of patients with TB as well as those associated with human immunodeficiency virus (HIV) infection will undoubtedly spawn some other cases of otologic TB; therefore, a brief summary of the problem is justified.

INCIDENCE

Tuberculous otitis media and tuberculous mastoiditis occur together as a single disease process and will be referred to as tuberculous otitis media. Most of the medical literature on tuberculous otitis media is from Europe where the disease is more prevalent.

Between 1967 and 1979, 4000 biological specimens of the middle ear were examined in Pubinge, West Germany. Tuberculosis was found in 14 (0.1%), the youngest patient being 10 months and the oldest 69 years.[3] In a review of patients of the Massachusetts General Hospital and the Massachusetts Eye and Ear Infirmary from 1962 through 1984, there were four cases of TB otitis media/mastoiditis out of 6310 cases of chronic otitis media and out of 1850 cases of TB.[4] Vaamonde, et al. diagnosed 10 cases from 1996–2002 in Spain.[5] Laryngitis and otitis media remain the most frequent ear, nose, and throat (ENT) diseases of tuberculous origin.[6]

PATHOGENESIS AND PATHOLOGY

Pathogenesis of TB of the middle ear may be a primary focus in the area of the shorter and large-bored eustachian tube in neonates who have aspirated infected amniotic fluid or in older patients who have ingested and regurgitated tuberculous materials such as contaminated milk. Most cases occur secondarily, however, when organisms are coughed into the nasopharynx from pulmonary lesions or as the result of hematogenous spread. Preauricular or anterior cervical lymphadenopathy and facial nerve paralysis occur infrequently but are more likely with tuberculous than other types of bacterial otitis media.

Pathologically, the disease always involves the mucosa first, with extensive edema, infiltration by round and giant cells, granuloma formation, and finally cessation. Thickening of the tympanic membrane is followed by perforation with associated destruction of the ossicles and purulent discharge. Secondarily, the periostium becomes involved, followed months later by bone necrosis with resultant complications that are similar to those occurring with other infections of the middle ear and mastoid. The labyrinth appears to be at greatest risk in adults, and the facial nerve and meninges are the greatest risk areas in children.[7] Hearing loss with a large neurosensory component is frequent in all patients.

DIAGNOSIS

The history and physical findings in both primary and secondary tuberculous otitis media are frequently non-specific. Smoler and colleagues[8] believe that in secondary tuberculous otitis the classic findings of chronic ear infection (otorrhea, absence of pain, and profound hearing loss) are never well defined because of supra-infection with other bacteria. An exception is damage to the facial nerve, paralysis of which is usually associated with TB. Tympanic membranes are often extensively damaged, with one or more perforations. Older patients may complain of tinnitus and "funny noises."[9]

Tuberculous otitis media has to be considered in the differential diagnosis of chronic otitis media in tuberculous patients as well as in those who have no evidence of TB elsewhere and whose otorrhea does not improve with the usual medical treatment. A history of TB in a family member should arouse suspicion and lead to confirmatory studies. Tuberculous otitis media may be masked by suprainfection with other bacteria as well as by systemic antituberculous therapy. Skin testing for TB in children and adults with chronic otorrhea should be mandatory, although results may be falsely negative.[10] The diagnosis of tuberculous otitis media is confirmed by culture of *M. tuberculosis* from the local discharge or biopsy. However, the diagnosis can be assumed if pulmonary TB is confirmed to be associated with chronic otitis media in the absence of other pathogens. Positive acid-fast staining (auramine and Ziehl-Neelsen) of otorrhea is strongly suggestive. Nucleic acid amplification techniques (polymerase chain reaction, etc.) may be useful in patients in whom acid-fast stains are negative.[11] Histopathologic study of tissue as well as improvement following specific antituberculous therapy may support the diagnosis.

Primary TB of the middle ear is most difficult to diagnose. The tympanic membrane before perforation is swollen, yellowish, and hyperemic. Perforation follows in the untreated patient, and multiple perforations follow in 20–30%. In tuberculous otitis media of both primary and secondary types, abnormalities on x-ray films of the mastoid are less common than with other types of chronic otitis media, but computerized tomography shows a full tympanic cavity without bony erosion. Propagation to the inner ear may occur in older children and adults when the disease is subacute and is manifested by slowly progressive hearing loss (initially of the high tones) as a result of cochlear destruction. Extension and hematogenous dissemination from tuberculous otitis media are rare, as evidenced by the frequent chronicity of the disease for many years without such spread.[5] The dura mater usually resists direct extension to the brain; however, tuberculous meningitis is definitely associated with chronic tuberculous otitis media.[12,13]

The frequency of signs and symptoms in patients with tuberculous otitis media before and after 1953 is shown in Table 15-1.

Differential diagnosis is broad, including histoplasmosis, North American blastomycosis, South American blastomycosis, syphilis, midline granulomas (lethal), Wegener's granulomatosis, sarcoidosis, histiocytosis X, eosinophilic granuloma, nocardiosis, necrotizing external otitis, lymphoma, nontuberculous mycobacterial otitis media, and cholesteatoma.

TREATMENT

Once the diagnosis of tuberculous otitis media is confirmed, the combined talents of the primary care physician, an ENT surgeon, and an infectious disease specialist are required for optimum therapy. Isoniazid plus

Table 15-1. Frequency of Signs and Symptoms in Patients with Tuberculous Otitis Media (TOM)

Symptom or Sign	Number of Patients with TOM with Indicated Feature (%)		
	Pre-1953	**Post-1953–1986**	**2004[†]**
Otorrhea	103 (82)	93 (92)	10 (100)
Loss of hearing	18 (62)*	78 (90)[†]	10 (100)
Ear pain	10 (0.08)	24 (6.2)	3 (30)
Perforations	27 (21)	71 (70)	9 (90)
Granulations	22 (30)[‡]	64 (63)	5 (50)
Facial palsy	37 (30)	16 (16)	1 (10)
Aural polyp	4 (3.2)	13 (13)	1 (10)
Preauricular lymph node	68 (54)	2 (0.02)	1 (10)
Tinnitus	—	—	4 (40)

Note: Fever, cough, weight loss, night sweats, and periauricular fistulae occurred in <1% of cases both before and after 1953. The percentages are based on the study population as described in Skolink PR, et al.

*Ninety-six additional cases were excluded because of lack of adequate documentation.
[†]Fourteen additional cases were excluded because of lack of adequate documentation.
[‡]Fifteen additional cases were excluded because of lack of adequate documentation.

Source: Data from Skolink PR, et al. Tuberculosis of the middle ear: Review of the literature with an instructive case report. *Rev Infect Dis.* 1996;8:403–410, and from Vaamonde P, et al. Tuberculous otitis media: a significant diagnostic challenge. *Otolaryngol Head Neck Surg.* 2004;130:759–766.

rifampin is the preferred antituberculous therapy with pyrazinamide added for the first 2 months. Ethambutol is usually added until multidrug-resistant *M. tuberculosis* is ruled out. Final therapy is based on in vitro susceptibility studies. There have now been at least 12 cases of tuberculous otitis media treated with short-course therapy with favorable response. Ten were treated with isoniazid, rifampicin and pyrazinamide for 2 months followed by 4 months (8 patients) or 7 months (2 patients) of rifampicin. Two other patients[14] received isoniazid, rifampin, ethambutol and pyrazinamide for 9 months. There are not enough cases of tuberculous otitis media to conduct any treatment trials, but based on reported data most patients should be treated medically for 6–9 months.

In addition to obtaining tissue for diagnosis, the surgeon may have a role in therapy by removing a nidus of infected debris. Complications mandating surgical approach include facial nerve paralysis, subperiosteal abscess, labyrinthitis, persistent postauricular fistula, and extension of infection into the central nervous system.[15] After therapy is completed, reconstructive procedures may improve hearing in certain patients.

REFERENCES

1. Kirsch CM, Dhner JH, Jensen WA, et al. Tuberculous otitis rnedia. *South Med J.* 1995;88:363–366.
2. Tuberculosis among Indochinese refugees—an update. *MMWR Morb Mortal Wkly Rep.* 1981;30:603–606.
3. Plester D, Pulsakar A, Steinbeck E. Middle ear tuberculosis. *J Laryngol Otol.* 1980;94:1415–1421.
4. Skolnik PR, Nadol JR Jr, Baker AS. Tuberculosis of the middle ear: Review of the literature with an instructive case report. *Rev Infect Dis.* 1986:8:403–410.
5. Vaamonde P, Castro C, García-Soto N, et al. Tuberculous otitis media: a significant diagnostic challenge. *Otolaryngol Head Neck Surg.* 2004;130:759–766.
6. Sellars SL, Seid AB. Aural tuberculosis in childhood. *S Afr Med J.* 1973;47:216–218.
7. Rice DH. Pathologic quiz case 2. *Arch Otolaryngol.* 1977; 103:112–115.
8. Smoler J, Pinto SL, Vivar G, et al. Tuberculous otitis media. *Laryngoscope.* 1969;79:488–493.
9. Smith MHD, Starke JR, Marquis JR. Tuberculosis and other mycobacterial infections. In: Feigin RD, Cherry JD, eds: *Textbook of Pediatric Infectious Diseases*, 3rd ed, vol 1. Philadelphia, PA: WB Saunders; 1992:1339.
10. Saltzman SJ, Feigin RD. Tuberculous otitis media and mastoiditis. *J Pediatr.* 1971:79:1004–1006.
11. Garcovich A, Romano L, Zampetti A, et al. Tumour-like ear lesion due to Mycobacterium tuberculosis diagnosed by polymerase chain reaction-reverse hybridization (letter). *Br J Dermatol.* 2004;150:370–371.
12. Cawthon T, Cox RH, Pankey GA. Tuberculous otitis media with complications. *South Med J.* 1978:71:602–604.
13. Mongkolrattanothai K, Oram R, Redleaf M, et al. Tuberculous otitis media with mastoiditis and central nervous system involvement. *Pediatr Infect Dis J.* 2003;22:453–456.
14. Awan MS, Salahuddin I. Tuberculous otitis media: two case reports and literature review. *Ear Nose Throat J.* 2002;81: 792–794.
15. Lucente FE, Tobias GW, Parisier SC, et al. Tuberculous otitis media. *Laryngoscope.* 1978;88:1107–1116.

16

Ocular Tuberculosis

Daniel M. Albert
Matthew J. Thompson

HISTORICAL CONSIDERATIONS

Maitre-Jan[1] is often credited with the earliest description of ocular tuberculosis (TB) (1711). Major contributions to the understanding of the disease mechanism were not made until the latter part of the 19th century. In 1855, Eduard von Jaeger first described the ophthalmoscopic appearance of choroidal tubercles.[2] Cohnheim, in 1867,[3] showed that choroidal tubercles were similar microscopically to tubercles found elsewhere in the body and postulated that ocular involvement was a metastatic manifestation of systemic disease. In addition, Cohnheim produced similar lesions in guinea pigs by injecting them with tuberculous material. In 1882, Koch identified the tubercle bacillus as the causative agent,[4] and one year later Julius van Michel identified the organism in the eye.[5]

INCIDENCE

The reported incidence of ocular involvement varies considerably, depending on the criteria used for diagnosis and the population sampled. Early medical writers considered the infection rare. However, the diagnosis was usually reserved for patients with obvious clinical tubercles. In 1890, Terson[6] reported two cases of tuberculous iritis in a population of 30,000 patients with ocular disease. In patients with known systemic TB, the incidence of ocular involvement is obviously much higher.[7–9] A study reported in 1967 found an incidence of ocular TB of 1.4% in 10,524 patients at a TB sanitarium.[8] In this group, 74 patients had uveal involvement; 54 had scleral or corneal involvement, including 3 cases of corneal ulcers; and 12 patients showed disseminated retinitis. Rarer manifestations were retinal periphlebitis (7 cases); phlyctenular conjunctivitis (6 cases); and TB of the optic nerve (1 case). This study illustrates the variety of ocular tissues that can be affected by TB.

More recent reports include that of Rosen et al which, in 1990, reported 12 patients with intraocular TB, 9 of whom presented with retinal vasculitis, 2 with choroidal tubercles, and 1 with chronic anterior uveitis.[10] A prospective study from Spain by Bouza et al examined 100 randomly chosen patients from a population of 300 patients with proven systemic TB.[11] Ocular involvement was diagnosed in 18 patients (18%). Choroidal involvement was present in all but one of these, and retinal involvement was found in 6 patients. The anterior segment, sclera, and orbit were only affected in single cases. There was an association between miliary TB and ocular involvement but no association between human immunodeficiency virus (HIV)-positivity and ocular TB.[11] Ocular involvement was associated with decreased visual acuity and other ocular symptoms.

A prospective study from Malawi, Africa, reported a 2.8% incidence of choroidal granulomas in 109 patients presenting with fever and TB.[12] In patients presenting with uveitis in India, 0.6% of cases were felt to be caused by TB.[13] In a prospective case series in Japan, 20.6% of 126 patients with uveitis had a positive TB skin test, and 7.9% were believed to have intraocular TB.[14] In Saudi Arabia, TB was the cause in 10.5% of cases of uveitis seen in a major ophthalmic referral center.[15] In patients presenting with uveitis in Boston from 1982 to 1992, TB caused this disease in 0.6% of cases.[16] These studies reflect the wide variation in the reported incidence of ocular TB in differing populations and at varying times.

BASIC MECHANISMS OF INFECTION

The eye can become infected with TB through several different mechanisms.

1. The most common form of ocular involvement is from hematogenous spread. The uveal tract (composed of the iris, ciliary body, and choroid) is the coat of the eye most frequently involved, presumably because of its high vascular content.

2. Primary exogenous infection of the eye, while unusual, can occur in the lids or in the conjunctiva. Other external tissues more rarely infected include the cornea, sclera, and lacrimal sac.

3. Secondary infection of the eye may occur by direct extension from surrounding tissues or by contamination with the patient's own sputum.

4. Additionally, some forms of ocular TB, such as phlyctenular disease and Eales disease, are thought to be the result of a hypersensitivity reaction. Attempts to establish an animal model for phlyctenular disease have led to varying conclusions.[17–19]

Rich's law states that the extent of a tuberculous lesion is directly proportional to the number and virulence of the bacilli as well as the degree of hypersensitivity of the infected tissue.[20] It is inversely proportional to the host's native and acquired resistance to the organism. Dr. Alan Woods was the first to utilize Rich's law to divide ocular TB into 4 distinct categories.[21] Woods' 4 categories can be summarized as follows:

1. Foreign body-like reaction (e.g., miliary tubercles of the iris and choroid)

2. Acute circumscribed inflammation that may recur if the patient's resistance decreases (e.g., sclerokeratitis, Eales disease)

3. Chronic inflammation with multiple recurrence (e.g., ciliary body tuberculoma)

4. Acute, rapidly spreading inflammation with necrosis, caseation, and occasionally a ruptured globe (tuberculous panophthalmitis)

EXTERNAL DISEASE

Tuberculosis can involve the lid, conjunctiva, cornea, and sclera. Tuberculous lid disease is rarely an isolated ocular finding, but it can present as an abscess known as a "cold abscess" or as a soft fluctuant mass without acute inflammation that usually occurs in children.[22] The skin of the lids may also display lupus vulgaris, the most common form of cutaneous TB, which is characterized by reddish-brown nodules that blanch to an "apple-jelly" color when pressure is applied.[10,23] Primary infection of the conjunctiva, although reported,[24,25] is unusual. Typically, primary tuberculous conjunctivitis is a chronic disease that may lead to scarring of the involved tissue. The young are more susceptible to this form of TB than are the elderly. Patients with tuberculous conjunctivitis usually present with nonspecific complaints such as ocular redness and discomfort. Examination may reveal mucopurulent discharge and lid edema. There is often an accompanying marked lymphadenitis (more common in the secondary form), which is absent in most other bacterial and allergic conjunctivitis and less prominent in viral conjunctivitis. In cases of primary conjunctival TB, the organism can be detected via traditional acid-fast stains or polymerase chain reaction (PCR) on either a conjunctival smear or a biopsy[26] (Figs. 16-1–16-3).

Corneal involvement can have the appearance of either phlyctenular keratoconjunctivitis or an interstitial keratitis.

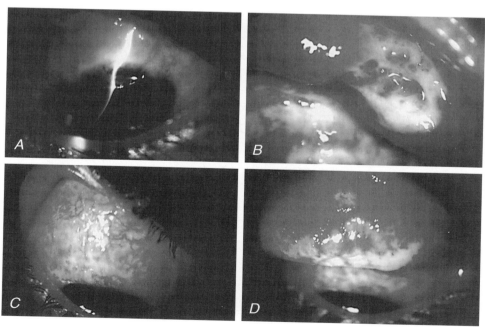

Fig. 16-1. (*A*) Bulbar conjunctival mass contiguous with a peripheral corneal ulcer with 80% stromal thinning. (*B*) Everted upper eyelid shows diffuse papillary reaction with tarsal necrosis laterally. (*C*) Down-gaze shows ulcerated bulbar conjunctiva. (*D*) Everted upper eyelid shows diffuse velvety appearance, with cheesy white areas of necrosis involving the upper tarsal border. (From: American Medical Association. All Rights reserved. Fernandes et al.[27])

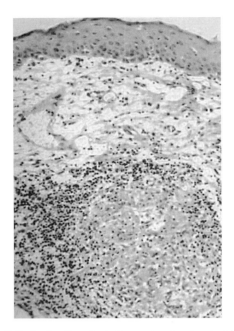

Fig. 16-2. Section from the bulbar conjunctiva shows an intact epithelium with discrete epithelioid cell granuloma in the deeper stroma, rimmed by lymphocytes (hematoxylin-eosin; original magnification × 250). (From: American Medical Association. All Rights reserved. Fernandes et al.[27])

In phlyctenular keratoconjunctivitis, a small nodule is first noted at the limbus. The nodule generally migrates centrally, "dragging" superficial vessels along. Initially the overlying epithelium is intact, but it often erodes,

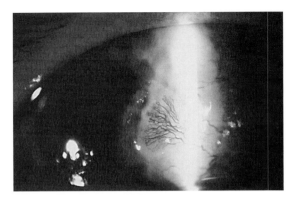

Fig. 16-4. Slit lamp picture of the left cornea showing a peripheral corneal ulcer and a heavily vascularized nodule. (From: American Medical Association. All Rights reserved. Frueh et al.[28])

leading to an epithelial defect. The presentation includes photophobia, foreign body sensation, redness, and tearing. The severity of symptoms usually corresponds to the degree of corneal involvement (Fig. 16-4). As previously noted, phlyctenular disease is believed to be a hypersensitivity reaction to a mycobacterial protein. Phlyctenulosis appears to be associated with a positive tuberculin skin test.[29] It is, however, rare among patients with proven systemic TB.[8] Attempts have been made to reproduce phlyctenular disease in animal models with mixed success.[17–19] In confirmed TB cases, treatment consists of a systemic antituberculous chemotherapy in conjunction with topical steroids. Cycloplegia substantially relieves discomfort, and topical antibiotics may be used as

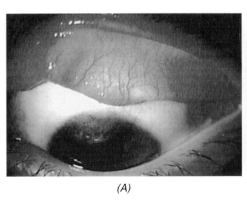

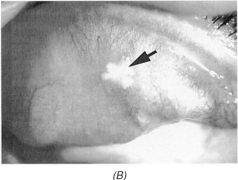

(A)   *(B)*

Fig. 16-3. (*A*) At 1-year follow-up, the left eye shows a superior vascularized corneal scar with normal-appearing bulbar and tarsal conjunctiva. (*B*) At 3-months follow-up, the everted right upper eyelid shows a residual area of necrosis (arrow) with mild persistent papillary reaction. (From: American Medical Association. All Rights reserved. Fernandes et al.[27])

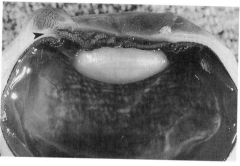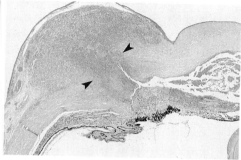

Fig. 16-5. Left, Gross appearance of the enucleated right eye. Note the scleral necrosis and the perilimbal scleral rupture (arrowhead) located interiorly. The limbal conjunctiva covers a dome-shaped, brown mass. Right, Histopathologic appearance of the enucleated right eye with a subconjunctival necrotic and inflammatory mass. There is necrosis of the iris and the anterior chamber contains necrotic debris (arrowheads) (hematoxylin-eosin, original magnification × 5). (From: American Medical Association. All Rights reserved. Rosenbaum et al.[33])

prophylaxis against secondary bacterial superinfection if epithelial defects are present.

Interstitial keratitis is a term used to describe inflammation and vascularization of the corneal stroma without endothelial or epithelial involvement. It is characteristically unilateral and is seen clinically as a sectorial, peripheral stromal infiltrate with vascularization. Treatment of tuberculous interstitial keratitis consists of systemic as well as topic antituberculosis chemotherapy and cycloplegia. As in the case with phlyctenular kerato-conjunctivitis, mycobacterial proteins are postulated as antigens that induce a corneal hypersensitivity reaction.[30]

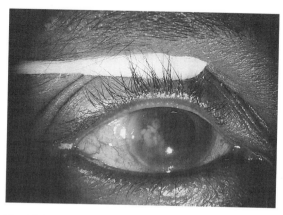

Fig. 16-6. Clinical appearance of a right eye shows mild conjunctival vasodilation and numerous confluent, temporal, tan iris nodules. (From: American Medical Association. All Rights reserved. Rosenbaum et al.[33])

Tuberculous scleritis is rare, but it should be considered in cases of scleritis that are unresponsive to the usual traditional therapy for scleritis. Bloomfield and associates[31] reported a case of tuberculous scleritis in an 82-year-old female with extensive pulmonary TB. This type of scleritis usually presents as a localized area of dark red discoloration of the sclera with chronic granulomatous inflammation and caseous necrosis. Nanda and coworkers[32] discussed a case of an 81-year-old male with culture-proven scleral TB. The patient initially presented with a scleral ulcer that worsened after initiation of oral prednisone (a medication often used for necrotizing scleritis). Examination of scrapings of the ulcer subsequently revealed numerous acid-fast bacilli. The patient quickly responded to topical amikacin and the combination of oral rifampin and isoniazid (Figs. 16-5 and 16-6).

UVEITIS

In the past, much emphasis was put on TB as a cause of uveitis; however, with the appreciation that brucellosis, sarcoidosis, toxoplasmosis, and other agents can also cause uveitis, together with the realization that uveitis in a TB patient may not be tuberculous uveitis, the apparent incidence of TB as the etiology of uveitis at the Wilmer Institute fell from 79% in 1944 to 22% in 1953.[21] The incidence of uveitis caused by TB at the Massachusetts Eye and Ear Infirmary from 1982 through 1992 was only 0.6%.[16] In parts of the world where the prevalence of TB infection is higher in the general population, uveitis is still more likely to be attributed to TB. In patients presenting with uveitis in India, 0.6% of cases were felt to be caused by TB.[13] In a prospective case series in Japan, 20.6% of 126 patients with uveitis had a positive TB skin test, and 7.9% were felt to have intraocular TB.[14] In Saudi Arabia, TB was stated to be the cause in 10.5% of uveitis cases seen in referral centers.[15]

Tuberculous uveitis is classically a chronic granulomatous disease and is often accompanied by other ocular manifestations of chronic granulomatous inflammation, such as mutton fat keratic precipitates (collections of inflammatory cells and macrophages) on the posterior aspect of the cornea as well as iris nodules. A nongranulomatous uveitis also occurs in TB, usually presenting with small white keratic precipitates and an absence of iris nodules.[34] In both granulomatous and nongranulomatous inflammation, there is inflammation of the anterior segment, and inflammatory cells and flare (the slit-lamp manifestation of protein in the aqueous humor) can be seen in the anterior chamber. Uveitis can also present as simple iritis, which is limited to cells and flare in the anterior chamber, or as iridocyclitis with involvement of the ciliary body. Iridocyclitis occurs clinically with inflammatory cells in the ciliary body and anterior vitreous and is associated with ciliary body pain and ciliary vasodilation. Alternatively, the inflammation may involve primarily the posterior part of the uvea (choroid), leading to choroiditis which is the most common manifestation of ocular TB.

CHOROIDITIS

Choroidal tubercles are seldom solitary. In 1 out of 2 recently reported cases of tuberculous choroiditis associated with acquired immunodeficiency syndrome (AIDS), the posterior pole was riddled with innumerable tubercles[35] whereas in the second case only two tubercles were seen.[36] The tubercles may appear as white, gray, or yellow lesions and may be accompanied by hemorrhages or exudates. Choroidal tubercles have indistinct borders with surrounding edema, and their size varies from about 0.5–3.0 mm in diameter. A useful way for clinicians to estimate size is by comparing the extent of the lesions to the optic disc, which is about 1.5 mm in diameter. Choroidal tubercles are usually found in the posterior pole and, when present, they should be revealed on a careful examination with the direct ophthalmoscope (Fig. 16-7).

Paton[38] described the sudden appearance of choroidal tubercles in a patient 4 days after admission. The lesions were not observed on careful examinations on previous days. Thus, multiple and frequent examinations may be required to demonstrate choroidal tubercles. In one series, only a single case of choroidal tubercles had been observed clinically in a series of 63 autopsy cases with acute miliary TB.[39] The authors suggested that this low incidence was the result of inadequate ophthalmoscopic examinations. Another study found a 60% incidence of choroidal tubercles.[40] To permit an adequate examination, all pupils were dilated, small children were sedated, and the average time for each fundus examination in a child was 30 minutes.

Choroidal tubercles should always be looked for on funduscopic examination when a patient is suspected to have TB or has a fever of unknown origin. The finding of choroidal tubercles is specific and allows the early institution of antituberculosis therapy even before the diagnosis is confirmed by positive sputum specimens. Although it has been claimed that choroidal tubercles occur only in terminally ill patients with miliary TB or tuberculous meningitis,[38] they can occur in a variety of clinical circumstances. Illingsworth and Wright[40] reported choroidal tubercles in very young children with acute miliary TB. A case was described in which miliary tubercles were associated with optic neuropathy but without other systemic lesions.[41] Massaro and colleagues[42] emphasized that tubercles occasionally occur in patients with pulmonary TB without evidence of miliary TB. Choroidal tubercles may be one of the earliest signs of disseminated disease. There have been reports of other manifestations of tuberculous infection of the choroid, including multifocal choroiditis[43] and serpiginous-like choroiditis.[44]

Recently, several cases of tuberculous choroiditis in patients with AIDS and systemic TB have been reported.[45,46] The choroidal tubercles in 3 patients were discovered after the initiation of systemic antituberculous chemotherapy when they were considered to be in a healing stage.[45] One patient with central nervous system TB and TB choroiditis improved dramatically after initiation of a triple antituberculous therapy. The cerebrospinal fluid findings returned to normal, and visual acuity improved from 20/200 to 20/20.[46]

It has been suggested that ocular TB may occur more often in immunocompromised patients. In a study of eyes from the autopsies of AIDS patients, however, intraocular TB was found in 2 eyes of 235 patients.[47] Additionally, ocular involvement appears not to be associated with the HIV status of TB patients. HIV is, of course, a risk factor for having systemic TB.[11]

Before the advent of chemotherapy, the prognosis for patients with choroidal tubercles was uniformly poor. However, the prognosis is much improved with the rapid use of systemic antituberculous agents. No specific local therapy is needed. Many of these lesions regress completely with minimal residual damage.[42,48,49] Other lesions heal with focal chorioretinal scars. An exception to this rule may

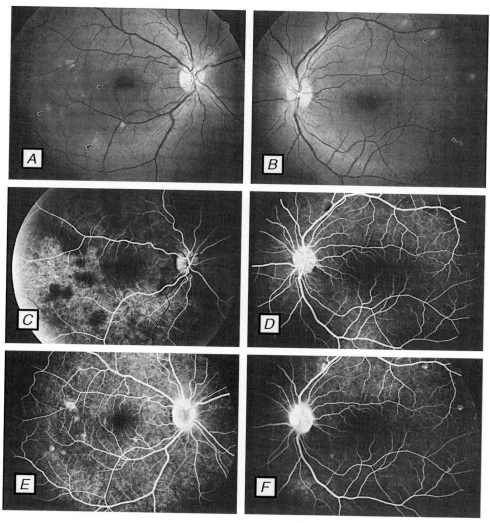

Fig. 16-7. Fundus photographs of the right (*A*) and left (*B*) eyes show bilateral, multifocal choroiditis (arrowheads). Serial fluorescein angiographic photographs (*C–F*) show early blocking hypofluorescence and late-staining hyperfluorescence corresponding to areas of choroidal infiltrate, as well as mild, late leakage from the optic nerve heads in each eye. (From: American Medical Association. All Rights reserved. Grewel et al.[37])

be the tuberculous choroiditis in the setting of AIDS. In these patients the ocular changes can progress in spite of vigorous antituberculous chemotherapy.[36] Reports of acquired resistance of mycobacteria are increasing,[50] and such resistance may be caused by several mechanisms. In the case reported by Snider and coworkers,[50] "resistance" was thought to be the result of incomplete antibiotic treatment and occurred after 8 months of isoniazid and rifampin therapy.

CHOROIDAL TUBERCULOMAS

Whereas choroidal tubercles are generally small and multiple, tuberculomas are usually solitary and better defined. They may measure up to 7 mm in diameter and have less surrounding edema than tubercles (Figs. 16-8 to 16-12). Tuberculomas have a predilection for the foveal and perifoveal area. Large tubercles have been confused with metastatic tumors, leading to unnecessary enucleation.[52]

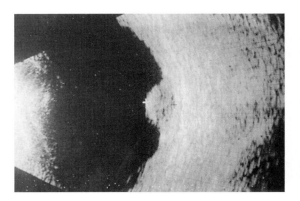

Fig. 16-8. B-scan ultrasonogram of the left eye showing an acoustically dense choroidal lesion with no choroidal excavation. (From: American Medical Association. All Rights reserved. Mason.[51])

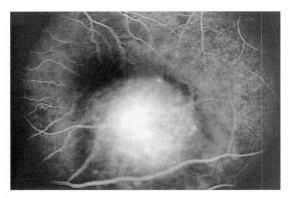

Fig. 16-10. Fluorescein angiogram in the late phase revealing late staining of the choroidal lesion. (From: American Medical Association. All Rights reserved. Mason.[51])

Tuberculomas of the uveal tract have a chronic course and tend to occur in young adults.[53] The duration of symptoms can be months to years. Affected patients often have a history of old, healed pulmonary TB. Sometimes, however, the presumed diagnosis of choroidal TB may lead to the diagnosis and treatment of pulmonary TB.[54]

Fluorescein angiography in patients with choroidal TB shows early hyperfluorescence with choroidal leakage, normal or slightly dilated overlying retinal vessels, late leakage, and in some cases associated serous neurosensory retinal detachment.[54–56] Fluorescein angiography is useful in differentiating among choroidal hemangiomas, foreign body, metastatic disease, and melanoma; however, fluorescein angiography cannot distinguish between TB and other granulomatous inflammations such as sarcoid. Serial fluorescein angiography may also be useful to assess the patient's responses to therapy.[56] Ultrasound has also been found to be useful in the diagnosis of choroidal tuberculomas.[11] The prognosis for resolution of the lesion is usually good with systemic treatment, but if the macular region is involved, visual loss may be permanent.[57]

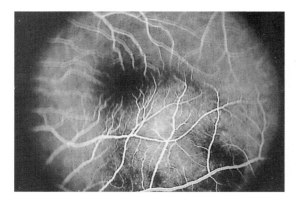

Fig. 16-9. Fluorescein angiogram in the early venous phase showing early blockage at the edges of the lesion and early hyperfluorescence within the central aspect of the choroidal lesion; the overlying retinal vessels are normal and in focus. The other retinal vessels are not in focus secondary to the thickness of the lesion. (From: American Medical Association. All Rights reserved. Mason.[51])

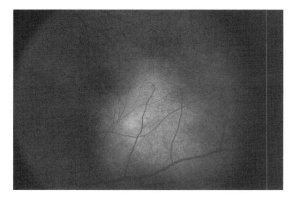

Fig. 16-11. Fundus photograph showing a white choroidal lesion causing the fovea to be ectopic. (From: American Medical Association. All Rights reserved. Mason.[51])

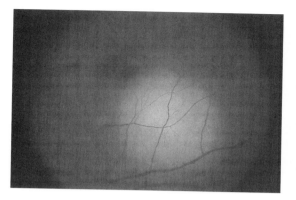

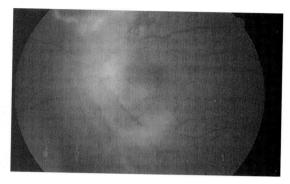

Fig. 16-12. Fundus photograph of the left eye showing resolution of the choroidal tubercle with retinal pigment epithelium stippling within the resolving choroidal tubercle. (From: American Medical Association. All Rights reserved. Mason.[51])

Fig. 16-13. Retinitis and retinal neovascularization obscuring clear view of optic disc in fundus photograph. (From: American Medical Association. All Rights reserved. Sarvananathan et al.[59])

CILIARY BODY TUBERCULOMA

Ciliary body tuberculoma is a rare but aggressive form of uveal TB. It occurs most frequently before the fourth decade of life and tends to follow a chronic, smoldering course with intermittent recurrences. Ni and associates[53] reported 3 cases that were enucleated at the Shanghai First Hospital. Results of the purified protein derivative (PPD) test were positive in all 3 patients. Two patients presented with painless loss of vision and a 1-month to 5-year history of intraocular inflammation. All patients were in generally good health, and only one patient had signs of systemic TB on examination. There was evidence of granulomatous anterior uveitis in all 3 patients. On histopathologic examination, the eyes showed inflammatory infiltrates of the iris consisting of plasma cells, monocytes, lymphocytes, and typical caseous granulomas in the ciliary body. The authors reported that the fellow eyes of 2 patients did well after the initiation chemotherapy; the third patient was lost to follow-up.

TUBERCULOUS RETINITIS

Tuberculosis of the retina most commonly results from the direct extension from the underlying uvea but may also be caused by hematogenous spread. Retinal lesions may take the form of either focal tubercles or diffuse retinitis. The clinical features of tuberculous retinitis include vitreous opacification and gray-white retinal lesions.[30] In rare instances, retinal TB can present as isolated vasculitis.[58]

Neovascularization and peripheral capillary occlusion have been described in cases of choroiditis, chorioretinitis, and retinal vasculitis (Figs. 16-13 to 16-15).[10,60,61] A combination of systemic treatment and retinal photocoagulation has been advocated for treatment of retinal neovascularization related to TB.[10,60]

Fountain and Werner[62] described a case of central retinal vein occlusion associated with active pulmonary TB. Fundus examination revealed engorged and tortuous retinal veins, sheathing of retinal vessels, and dot and blot hemorrhages in the posterior pole, as well as the typical gray-white retinal lesions.

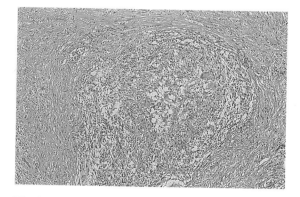

Fig. 16-14. Noncaseating granuloma from transvitreal biopsy specimen. (From: Copyrighted (c) 1998, American Medical Association. All Rights reserved. Sarvananathan et al.[59])

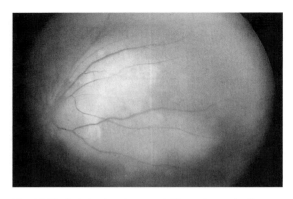

Fig. 16-15. Left fundus photograph illustrating optic disc new vessels with choroidal mass nasally. (From: American Medical Association. All Rights reserved. Sarvananathan et al.[59])

Eales disease, a poorly understood form of retinal perivasculitis, has sometimes been linked to TB.[21,63] The disease predominately affects the peripheral retina and is most common in young and otherwise healthy adults.[64] The initial presenting event in Eales' disease is often a sudden painless decrease in vision secondary to a vitreous hemorrhage. After the vitreous hemorrhage clears, perivascular exudates and hemorrhages are visible along the retinal vessels. The vasculitis can progress to venous thrombosis, neovascularization, glial tissue proliferation, and eventual tractional retinal detachment. There have been reports recently of patients with Eales' disease who have had PCR examination of vitreous and epiretinal membrane tissue that was positive for TB DNA, which lends weight to TB being causative for the disease.[64,65]

TUBERCULOUS PANOPHTHALMITIS

Acute tuberculous panophthalmitis usually occurs in children or severely ill adults with evidence of systemic TB. The ocular involvement and duration of symptoms is relatively short (1–2 months). Presentation includes painless, progressive visual loss, decreased motility of the eye, cloudy cornea, signs of granulomatous ocular inflammation, and low intraocular pressure. Perforation of the globe can occur, usually at a site near the equator. Predisposing factors for systemic spread to the eye include poor nutrition, chronic illness, and intravenous drug abuse.[53,54]

There have been reports of tuberculous panophthalmitis and endophthalmitis masquerading as ocular tumors.[66,67] A case of tuberculous panophthalmitis has been described in a woman with systemic lupus erythematosus. She initially presented with a serous retinal detachment that progressed to panophthalmitis with no light perception and glaucoma. Tuberculosis was diagnosed after enucleation, and recurring postoperative orbital abscesses improved after administration of systemic antituberculous therapy.[68]

ORBITAL TUBERCULOSIS

Tuberculosis of the orbit is extremely rare in the United States and Europe. A review of the literature revealed only 5 cases reported in the Western literature over the past 50 years.[69] Three cases were associated with pulmonary TB,[70–72] one with tuberculous sinusitis, and one with tuberculous pericarditis.[69] Four of the five cases presented with ocular symptoms: pain and proptosis,[69] lid swelling,[70] and intermittent periorbital swelling associated with headache and epistaxis.[71] In 1 case, proptosis was an incidental finding in a patient who presented with fatigue, dry cough, and fever.[69] Other clinical findings in the 5 cases included decreased vision and visual field abnormalities, chemosis, Marcus Gunn pupil, epiphora, increased orbital resistance to retropulsion, and an orbital mass visualized on computerized tomography. Diagnosis was confirmed in 4 cases by orbital tissue biopsy and culture. In 4 cases the orbital masses were followed by computed tomography and observed to resolve over the 3–6 months following the initiation of systemic antituberculous chemotherapy; 1 case was treated with additional surgery.

A case of orbital TB in a 37-year-old American man[72] presented with a recurring orbital abscess that was not responding to repeated drainage and broad-spectrum antibiotic therapy and steroids. Tuberculosis was diagnosed by histopathologic examination of an orbital biopsy obtained 1 month after initial presentation.

In India, where TB is endemic, cases of orbital TB are more common. In one report, three cases of isolated presumed orbital tuberculoma in children were described. The patients presented with painful proptosis, low-grade fever, lid swelling, mechanical ptosis, and decreased vision. In all three cases, TB mycobacteria were found in orbital fine-needle aspiration specimens. Symptoms improved with systemic antituberculous therapy.[73,74] There have also been reports from Europe of a Somalian child with an orbital TB abscess and a woman presenting with dacryoadenitis secondary to TB.[75,76]

DIAGNOSIS

Before the introduction of PCR technology, a definitive diagnosis of ocular TB was often elusive because it required the demonstration of the Mycobacterium TB bacilli in ocular tissues or secretions by microscopy or culture. Opportunities for culture and biopsies may arise in the case of lid involvement, keratitis, or orbital TB. The majority of ocular cases, however, present with intraocular involvement wherein a biopsy is not practical. Aqueous and vitreous paracentesis have generally failed to yield positive bacterial cultures.[21] In addition to the difficulty of isolating the organism, the extreme variability of ocular manifestations makes routine clinical diagnosis difficult. Finally, the similarity to the presentation of other granulomatous inflammations adds to the diagnostic challenge. As a result, the vast majority of ocular TB cases should more correctly be labeled "presumed ocular TB."

Woods[21] outlines a thorough diagnostic approach to suspected ocular TB. Because the majority of ocular cases are associated with systemic findings, a complete history (including exposures and systemic symptoms); physical examination; sputum smear and culture; PPD test; and chest radiography should be performed. Other possible causes of granulomatous inflammation, such as syphilis, brucellosis, toxoplasmosis, Toxocara infection, and sarcoid, must be ruled out by history, examination, and appropriate serologic testing.

An initial workup that yields negative results should not eliminate TB from the differential diagnosis. Abrams and Schlaegel point out that the chest radiograph showed no active or inactive evidence of TB in 17 of 18 cases of tuberculous uveitis. They caution against requiring a strongly positive PPD response to make the diagnosis of ocular TB.[77] The PPD is less likely to be reactive in immunosuppressed patients. These authors report that of 18 patients with presumed tuberculous uveitis (based on history, physical examination, tests to rule out other etiologies, tuberculin skin test, and the isoniazid therapeutic test) who were tested with intermediate-strength (5TU) PPD, only 9 experienced at least 5 mm of induration, 5 experienced no reactivity at all, and 4 had erythema only. The 5 with no reaction to the intermediate PPD were retested with the second-strength PPD (250 TU). Only two patients experienced more than 5 mm of reaction. All of the reported cases improved clinically with an isoniazid therapeutic test (3 weeks of 300 mg of isoniazid per day) and remained inflammation-free, without relapse, during 1 year of antituberculous treatment. An isoniazid therapeutic trial was recommended for patients with uveitis in whom TB was the suspected etiology on the basis of either history or a positive reaction to an intermediate-strength PPD test. An isoniazid test result is considered positive if there is "dramatic improvement" in 1–3 weeks of therapy. This trial, however, may be falsely negative in patients with AIDS or in cases of drug-resistant disease (Fig. 16-16).

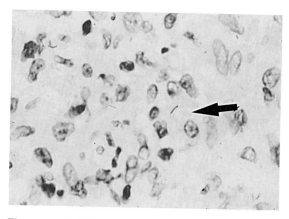

Fig. 16-16. Acid-fast stain of conjunctival biopsy specimen shows acid-fast positive rods within epithelioid histiocytes.

With the development of diagnostic molecular biology techniques, diagnosis based on detection of mycobacterial deoxyribonucleic acid (DNA) is becoming the method of choice (PCR). There have also been reports of testing for TB antigens via ELISA, such as the cord factor antigen.[78] PCR yields results much faster than mycobacterial cultures, which can require several weeks for a positive result. Detection of mycobacterial DNA has been successful in a variety of nonocular tissues.[79] In the past decade, there have been several reports of PCR being used to detect TB in a host of ocular tissues, including eyelid skin, conjunctiva, aqueous and vitreous humor, fixed choroidal tissue, subretinal fluid, and epiretinal membranes.[64,65,80–84] While further investigations are needed to determine the sensitivity and specificity of PCR and ELISA testing for TB in ocular tissues, these techniques have added a valuable alternative for the diagnosis of intraocular TB infection.

TREATMENT

Once the diagnosis of ocular TB is made, systemic antituberculosis therapy should be initiated at once. Systemic treatment is successful in the vast majority of cases, with subsequent resolution of symptoms, inflammation, and often an improvement in visual acuity to near premorbid levels; however, cases are reported in which traditional therapies fail to check the ocular infection. In one case, a choroidal tuberculoma did not respond to chemotherapy, and the eye eventually became blind and painful, necessitating enucleation.[55] Blodi and colleagues[35] reported that choroidal TB rapidly progressed despite treatment in an HIV-positive patient. The increasing prevalence of acquired drug resistance of mycobacteria in response to incomplete chemotherapy should also be kept in mind in patients not responding to conventional antituberculous therapy.

Any patient with disease highly suspicious for ocular TB should be treated with a multidrug regimen of proven efficacy. Because pulmonary infection and other foci of infection may coexist, primary treatment should always be systemic. Ocular penetration of these drugs varies, and additional topical treatment may be useful in patients with external disease.

Topical ointment and subconjunctival injection of isoniazid can lead to adequate intraocular drug levels, especially in the anterior segment. Parenteral administration, however, causes higher vitreous drug levels that make this route of administration the method of choice in posterior intraocular TB.[85]

Topically administered streptomycin is absorbed by the corneal stroma and penetrates the aqueous at high levels, but only in the presence of an epithelial defect. Parenteral administration of high doses can lead to detectable levels in all ocular tissues.[86] Intravitreal injection is more successful in generating therapeutic intraocular levels but may lead to retinal damage with high doses.[87]

Rifampin administered orally attained an aqueous concentration of 2–9% of its serum level, which may be a therapeutic level against some organisms.[88] Studies regarding the ocular penetration of pyrazinamide have not yet been published.

It should be noted that ethambutol, one of the staples of antituberculous pharmacotherapy, has significant ocular toxicity.[89] Toxicity is dose-related and is rare with a daily dose not exceeding 15 mg/kg. One to two percent of patients on a daily dose of 25 mg/kg or more experience significant ocular effects. The most common ocular side effect is optic neuritis. This toxicity can occur in axial and periaxial forms. Axial optical neuritis is associated with macular degeneration that manifests with decreased central visual acuity and is associated with decreased green color perception. Periaxial optic neuritis leads to paracentral scotomas (visual field defects) with normal visual acuity and color perception. Other side effects include photophobia, extraocular muscle paresis, and toxic amblyopia. Symptoms of optic neuritis are most often abrupt in onset and begin 3–6 months after the onset of ethambutol therapy.

All patients to be started on ethambutol should undergo a baseline ophthalmic examination including visual acuity, color vision, and visual fields. Patients should be examined every 2–4 weeks when doses greater than 15 mg/kg/day are used and every 3–6 months for lower doses. The patient should be given a vision card and instructed to stop the ethambutol and seek an ophthalmic examination immediately if there is a decrease in visual acuity. Most symptoms resolve over a period of 3–12 months, but cases with permanent vision loss have been reported. If the vision does not improve after 10–15 weeks of drug discontinuation, treatment with parenteral hydroxocobalamin, 40 mg daily over a 10- to 28-week period, should be considered.

The role of laser therapy in the treatment of ocular TB has yet to be defined. Balashevich[90] has used argon laser photocoagulation on tuberculous chorioretinitis lesions near the fovea and concluded that such treatment results in better visual acuity than conventional treatment does. Jabbour and associates[54] reported; however, that a subretinal granulomas-like lesion had grown outside previously placed photocoagulation scars. Gur and colleagues[60] and Rosen and coworkers[10] reported on the successful use of sector photocoagulation for the treatment of subretinal neovascularization in a case of chorioretinitis. Laser therapy should never be used as primary treatment without systemic antituberculosis chemotherapy. Laser treatment should be delayed until the diagnosis is established and the response to chemotherapy is confirmed in order to avoid further confusion of the clinical picture and course.

REFERENCES

1. Maitre-Jan A. Traite des maladies des yeux. Troyes: Jacques le Febvre; 1707.
2. von Jaeger E. Ueber choroidealtuberkel. *Desterr Ztschr f Pract heilke.* 1855;1:9–10.
3. Cohnheim J. Ueber tuberkulose der choroiden. *Virchows Arch (Pathol Anat).* 1867;39:49–69.
4. Koch R. Die Aetiologe der Tuberculose. *Berliner Klin Wochenschr.* 1882;15:221–230.
5. von Michael J. Ueber iris and iritis. *Graefes Arch Clin Exp Ophthalmol.* 1881;27(2):171–282.
6. Terson A. Tuberculose oculaire: Excision d'un tubercule de l'iris suive de success. *Arch Ophthalmol.* 1890;10:7–14.
7. Goldenberg M, Fabricant ND. The eye in the tuberculous patient. *Trans Sect Ophthalmol Am Med Assoc.* 1909;135.
8. Donahue HC. Ophthalmic experience in a tuberculosis sanatorium. *Am J Ophthalmol.* 1967;64:742–748.
9. Glover LP. Some eye observations in tuberculosis patients at the State Sanatorium, Cresson, Pennsylvania. *Am J Ophthalmol.* 1930;13:411–412.
10. Rosen PH, Spalton DJ, Graham EM. Intraocular tuberculosis. *Eye.* 1990;4:486–492.
11. Bouza E, Merino P, Munoz P, et al. Ocular tuberculosis: A prospective study in a general hospital. *Medicine.* 1997;76(1):63–61.

12. Beare NA, Kublin JG, Lewis DK, et al. Ocular disease in patients with tuberculosis and HIV presenting with fever in Africa. *Br J Ophthalmol.* 2002 Oct;86(10):1076–1079.

13. Biswas J, Narain S, Das D, et al. Pattern of uveitis in a referral uveitis clinic in India. *Int Ophthalmol.* 1996–1997; 20(4):223–228.

14. Morimura Y, Okada AA, Kawahara S, et al. Tuberculin skin testing in uveitis patients and treatment of presumed intraocular tuberculosis in Japan. *Ophthalmology.* 2002 May; 109(5):1–857.

15. Islam SM, Tabbara KF. Causes of uveitis at The Eye Center in Saudi Arabia: a retrospective review. *Ophthalmic Epidemiol.* 2002 Oct;9(4):239–249.

16. Rodriguez A, Calonge M, Pedroza-Seres M, et al. Referral patterns of uveitis in a tertiary eye care center. *Arch Ophthalmol.* 1996 May;114(5):593–599.

17. Gibson WS. The etiology of phlyctenular conjunctivitis. *Am J Dis Child.* 1918;15:81–115.

18. Rosenhauch E. Ueber das Verhaeltnis phlyctaenularer Augenentzuendungen zu Tuberkulose, Albert v Graefes. *Arch Ophthalmol.* 1910;76:370–396.

19. Thygeson P. Phlyctenulosis: Attempts to produce an experimental model with BCG. *Invest Ophthalmol Vis Sci.* 1962; 1:262–266.

20. Rich A, McCordock H. An enquiry concerning the role of allergy, immunity and other factors of importance in the pathogenesis of human tuberculosis. *Bull Johns Hopkins Hosp.* 1929;44:273.

21. Woods AC. *Endogenous Uveitis.* Baltimore: Williams & Wilkins; 1961.

22. Mehta DK. Bilateral tubercular lid abscess—a case report. *Indian J Ophthalmol.* 1989;37:98.

23. Domonkos AN, Arnold HL, Odom RB. *Andrews' Diseases of the Skin, Clinical Dermatology* (7th ed). Philadelphia, PA: WB Saunders; 1982.

24. Chandler AC, Locatcher-Khorazo D. Primary tuberculosis of the conjunctiva. *Arch Ophthalmol.* 1964;71:202–205.

25. Fernandes M, Vemuganti GK, Pasricha G, et al. Unilateral tuberculous conjunctivitis with tarsal necrosis. *Arch Ophthalmol.* 2003 Oct;121(10):1475–1478.

26. Cook CD, Hainsworth M. Tuberculosis of the conjunctiva occurring in the association with a neighboring lupus vulgaris lesion. *Br J Ophthalmol.* 1990;74:315–316.

27. Fernandes M, Vemuganti GK, Pasricha G, et al. Unilateral tuberculous conjunctivitis with tarsal necrosis. *Arch Ophthalmol.* 2003;121:1475–1478.

28. Frueh BE, Dubuis O, Imesch P, et al. Mycobacterium szulgai keratitis. *Arch Ophthalmol.* 2000; 118:1123–1124.

29. Philip RN, Comstock GW, Shelton JH. Phlyctenular keratoconjunctivitis among Eskimos in Southwestern Alaska. *Am Rev Respir Dis.* 1965;91:171–187.

30. Spencer WH. *Ophthalmic Pathology: An Atlas and Textbook.* Vol 1. Philadelphia, PA: WB Saunders; 1996.

31. Bloomfield SE, Mondino B, Gray GF. Scleral tuberculosis. *Arch Ophthalmol.* 1976;94:954–956.

32. Nanda M, Pflugfelder SC, Holland S. Mycobacterium tuberculosis scleritis. *Am J Ophthalmol.* 1989;108:736–737.

33. Rosenbaum PS, Mbekeani JN, Kress Y. Atypical mycobacterial panophthalmitis seen with iris nodules. *Arch Ophthalmol.* 1998;116:1524–1527.

34. Abrams, AB, Schlaegel TF. The role of the isoniazid therapeutic test in tuberculosis uveitis. *Am J Ophthalmol.* 1982; 94:511–515.

35. Blodi BA, Johnson NW, McLeish WM. Presumed choroidal tuberculosis in a human immunodeficiency virus infected host. *Am J Ophthalmol.* 1989;103:605–607.

36. Croxatto JO, Mestre C, Puente S, et al. Nonreactive tuberculosis in a patient with acquired immune deficiency syndrome. *Am J Ophthalmol.* 1986;102:659–660.

37. Grewal A, Kim RY, Cunningham ET Jr. Miliary Tuberculosis *Arch Ophthalmol.* 1998;116:953–954.

38. Paton RT. The clinical significance of choroidal tubercles. *Ann Intern Med.* 1932;5:997–999.

39. Chapman CB, Whorton CM. Acute generalized miliary tuberculosis in adults. *N Engl J Med.* 1946;235:239–248.

40. Illingsworth RS, Wright T. Tubercles of the choroids. *Br Med J.* 1948;2:365–368.

41. Mansour AM, Haymond R. Choroidal tuberculomas without evidence of extraocular tuberculosis. *Graefes Arch Clin Exp Ophthalmol.* 1990;228:382–385.

42. Massaro D, Katz S, Sachs M. Choroidal tubercles. *Ann Intern Med.* 1964;60:231–241.

43. Grewal A, Kim RY, Cunningham ET Jr. Related Articles, Links. Miliary tuberculosis. *Arch Ophthalmol.* 1998 Jul; 116(7):953–954.

44. Gupta V, Gupta A, Arora S, et al. Presumed tubercular serpiginousline choroiditis: clinical presentations and management. *Ophthalmology.* 2003 Sep; 110(9):1744–1749.

45. Perez Blazquez E, Montero Rodriguez M, Mendez Ramos J: Tuberculous choroiditis and acquired immunodeficiency syndrome. *Ann Ophthalmol.* 1994;26:50–54.

46. Muccioli C, Belfort R. Presumed ocular and central nervous system tuberculosis in a patient with acquired immunodeficiency syndrome. *Am J Ophthalmol.* 1995;121(2): 217–219.

47. Morinelli EN, Dugel RU, Riffenburg R, et al. Infectious multifocal choroiditis in patients with acquired immunodeficiency syndrome. *Ophthalmology.* 1993;100:1014–1021.

48. Olazabal F. Choroidal tubercles. *JAMA.* 1967;200:374–377.

49. Dollfus MA. Fundus lesions in tuberculosis meningitis and miliary pulmonary tuberculosis treated with streptomycin. *Am J Ophthalmol.* 1949;32:821–824.

50. Snider DE Jr, Cauthen GM, Farer LS, et al. Drug-resistant tuberculosis [letter]. *Am Rev Respir Dis.* 1991;144:732.

51. Mason JO. Treatment of large macular choroidal tubercle improves vision, *Arch Ophthalmol.* 2000;118: 1136.

52. Seward DNL. Tuberculoma of the ciliary body. *Med J Aust.* 1973;1:297–298.

53. Ni C, Papale JJ, Robinson NL. Uveal tuberculosis. *Int Ophthalmol Clin.* 1982;22(3):103–124.

54. Jabbour NM, Farris B, Trempe CL. A case of pulmonary tuberculosis presenting with a choroidal tuberculoma. *Ophthalmology.* 1985;92:834–837.

55. Lyon CE, Crimson BS, Peiffer RL. Clinico-pathological correlation of a solitary choroidal tuberculoma. *Ophthalmology.* 1985;92:845–850.

56. Cangemi FE, Friedman AH, Josephberg R. Tuberculoma of the choroids. *Ophthalmology.* 1980;84:252–258.

57. Goldberg MF. Presumed tuberculous maculopathy. *Retina.* 1982;2:47–50.

58. Shah SM, Howard RS, Sarkjes NJC, et al. Tuberculosis presenting as retinal vasculitis. *J R Soc Med.* 1988;81:232–233.

59. Sarvananthan N, Wiselka M, Bibby K. Intraocular Tuberculosis without detectable systemic infection, *Arch Ophthalmol.* 1998;116:1386–1388.

60. Gur S, Silverstone BZ, Zylberman R, et al. Chorioretinitis and extrapulmonary tuberculosis. *Ann Ophthalmol.* 1987;19:112–115.

61. Chung Y, Yeh T, Sheu S, et al. Macular subretinal neovascularization in choroidal tuberculosis. *Ann Ophthalmol.* 1989;21:225–229.

62. Fountain JA, Werner RB. Tuberculous retinal vasculitis. *Retina.* 1984;4:48–50.

63. Eliot A. Recurrent intraocular hemorrhage in young adults. *Trans Am Ophthalmic Soc.* 1954;52:811–875.

64. Biswas J, Therese L, Madhavan HN. Use of polymerase chain reaction in detection of Mycobacterium tuberculosis complex DNA from vitreous sample of Eales' disease. *Br J Ophthalmol.* 1999 Aug;83(8):994.

65. Madhavan HN, Therese KL, Gunisha P, et al. Polymerase chain reaction for detection of Mycobacterium tuberculosis in epiretinal membrane in Eales' disease. *Invest Ophthalmol Vis Sci.* 2000 Mar;41(3):822–825.

66. Darrell RM. Acute tuberculosis panophthalmitis. *Arch Ophthalmol.* 1967;78:51–54.

67. Demirci H, Shields CL, Shields JA, et al. Ocular tuberculosis masquerading as ocular tumors. *Surv Ophthalmol.* 2004 Jan–Feb;49(1):78–89.

68. Anders N, Wollensack G. Ocular tuberculosis in systemic lupus erythematosus and immunosuppressive therapy. *Klin Monatsbl Augenheilkd.* 1995;204:368–371.

69. Khalil M, Lindley S, Matouk E. Tuberculosis of the orbit. *Ophthalmology.* 1985;92:1624–1627.

70. Sheridan PH, Edman JB, Starr SE. Tuberculosis presenting as an orbital mass. *Pediatrics.* 1981;67:847–875.

71. Spoor TC, Harding SA. Orbital tuberculosis. *Am J Ophthalmol.* 1981;91:644–647.

72. Pilai S, Malone TJ, Abad JC. Orbital tuberculosis. *Ophthal Plast Reconstr Surg.* 1995;11(1):27–31.

73. D'Souza P, Garg R, Dhaliwal RS, et al. Orbital-tuberculosis. *Int Ophthalmol.* 1994;18:149–152.

74. Maurya OPS, Patel R, Thakur V, et al. Tuberculoma of the orbit—a case report. *Ind J Ophthalmol.* 1990;38:191–192.

75. Roberts BN, Lane CM. Orbital tuberculosis. *Eye.* 1997;11 (Pt 1):138–139.

76. van Assen S, Lutterman JA. Tuberculous dacryoadenitis: a rare manifestation of tuberculosis. *Neth J Med.* 2002 Sep;60(8):327–329.

77. Abrams AB, Schlaegel TF. The tuberculin test in the diagnosis of tuberculosis uveitis. *Am J Ophthalmol.* 1983;96:295–298.

78. Sakai J, Matsuzawa S, Usui M, et al. New diagnostic approach for ocular tuberculosis by ELISA using the cord factor as antigen. *Br J Ophthalmol.* 2001 Feb;85(2):130–133.

79. Peneau A, Moinard D, Berard I, et al. Detection of mycobacteria using the polymerase chain reaction. *Eur J Clin Microbiol Infect Dis.* 1992;11:270–271.

80. Salman A, Parmar P, Rajamohan M, et al. Subretinal fluid analysis in the diagnosis of choroidal tuberculosis. *Retina.* 2003 Dec;23(6):796–799.

81. Biswas J, Kumar SK, Rupauliha P, et al. Detection of mycobacterium tuberculosis by nested polymerase chain reaction in a case of subconjunctival tuberculosis. *Cornea.* 2002 Jan;21(1):123–125.

82. El-Ghatit AM, El-Deriny SM, Mahmoud AA, et al. Presumed periorbital lupus vulgaris with ocular extension. *Ophthalmology.* 1999 Oct;106(10):1990–1993.

83. Arora SK, Gupta V, Gupta A, et al. Diagnostic efficacy of polymerase chain reaction in granulomatous uveitis. *Tuber Lung Dis.* 1999;79(4):229–233.

84. Bowyer JD, Gormley PD, Seth R, et al. Choroidal tuberculosis diagnosed by polymerase chain reaction. A clinicopathologic case report. *Ophthalmology.* 1999 Feb;106(2):290–294.

85. Kratka WH. Isoniazid and ocular tuberculosis: An evaluation of experimental and clinical studies. *AMA Arch Ophthalmol.* 1955;54:330–344.

86. Leopold IH, Nichold A. Intraocular penetration of streptomycin following systemic and local administration. *Arch Ophthalmol.* 1946;35:33–38.

87. Gardiner PA, Michaelson IC, Rees EJW, et al. Intravitreous streptomycin: Its toxicity and diffusion. *Br J Ophthalmol.* 1948;32:449–456.

88. Outman WR, Levitz RE, Hill DA, et al. Related Articles, Links. Intraocular penetration of rifampin in humans. *Antimicrob Agents Chemother.* 1992 Jul;36(7):1575–1576.

89. Fraundelder FT. *Drug-Induced Ocular Side Effects and Drug Interactions,* 3rd Ed. Philadelphia, PA: Lea & Febiger; 1989.

90. Balashevich LI. Argon laser-coagulation in focal chorioretinitis. *Oftalmologia.* 1984;7:414–416.

17

Central Nervous System Tuberculosis

John E. Kasik

PATHOGENESIS

Many of the symptoms, signs, and sequelae of tuberculosis (TB) meningitis (TBM) are the result of an immunologically directed inflammatory reaction to the infection.[1] It is the immune reaction to the infection that produces damage to blood vessels, scarring, edema, and exudates in the central nervous system that produces the clinical manifestations of this disease.

The clinical events in TBM, as with all forms of TB, usually begin with inhalation of an infected droplet of aerosolized sputum generated by the cough of a person with active pulmonary TB. In the nonimmune host, the inhaled organisms multiply in the lung and are then dispersed throughout the body, carried by the lymphatics of the lung to the thoracic duct into the general circulation. As a result, multiple emboli of mycobacteria escape from their original pulmonary focus and are spread to various organs in the body, including the meninges.[2–4]

These metastatic mycobacteria form tuberculids, small foci of infection. But in most instances, immunity develops and they become dormant, usually for the life of the patient. In some instances, however, a tuberculid may persist, enlarge, and caseate. Caseation occurs as a part of the immune response, and only after the development of immunity in TB does the disease produce its classic picture of a caseating granuloma containing epithelioid cells, macrophages, giant cells, and acid-fast bacilli (AFB), as are found in a typical tuberculous lesion in an immunocompetent person.[5,6]

When the caseous content of a tuberculid on the meninges leaks into the cerebral spinal fluid (CSF), the released material contains a significant amount of mycobacterial antigen. In the immunologically competent individual, this produces an intense immune reaction. As a result, severe inflammatory changes occur with accumulation of cells and the onset of hyperemia, edema, capillary damage, exudates, and fibrosis. This inflammatory reaction damages nerves, blocks the circulation of CSF and thrombose small blood vessels, and produces multiple cerebral infarcts. Because of the predilection of these changes to occur in the basilar portion of the brain, the inflammatory reaction tends to interfere with the function of cranial nerves, to produce hydrocephalus and injure blood vessels in that area.[5–7] Because of the potential variety of these pathologic changes and the differences in intensity of the reaction, there can be a wide variation in the clinical presentation of TBM. In addition, there can be a further variation in clinical presentation imposed by the immunologic status of the patient.

It has been known for over a quarter of a century that immunosuppression can modify, and prevent, some of the sequelae of TBM.[8] If TBM were to occur in an immunosuppressed patient, a further modification of the clinical picture occurs and causes additional difficulties in establishing the diagnosis. In addition, a tuberculoma, located in a crucial area, may produce localized symptoms and signs, like any intracranial space-occupying lesion.[9–11]

The changes in the incidence and epidemiology of TB in the United States further underscore these observations.[12,13] As documented elsewhere in this book, TB has emerged as another, important complication of the acquired immunodeficiency syndrome (AIDS). Either typical or atypical mycobacteria can be present and involve the central nervous system (CNS).

The combination of AIDS and latent TB is an explosive clinical problem. AIDS is often encountered in those populations which commonly have a positive skin reaction to purified protein derivative (PPD).[13,14] In this population, the appearance of active TB may be the first indication of AIDS. While the atypical mycobacterial infections such as *Mycobacterium avium complex* (MAC) usually appear late in the course of AIDS, TB caused by M. TB often develops before the signs or symptoms of AIDS are discernible.[14]

Another facet of this problem is the reported increased incidence of multidrug resistance in this population, usually involving the widely used mainstays of drug therapy such as isoniazid and rifampin.[15,16]

These events were very frightening and stimulated a vigorous response in the Public Health community. Programs to control TB, that had been discontinued or had been given a very low priority, were given fresh effusions of talent, money and interest. The advent of DOTS (directly observed therapy short course) and increasingly effective anti-AIDS therapy has controlled this resurgenal of TB at least in the developed countries.[17–19]

OCCURRENCE

In general, it could be said that in developed countries there has been a steady decline in the incidence of active TB for almost a century and that all form of TB, including TBM, have reached the status of a rare disorder.

As mentioned above, there was a small but very discon-
certing increase in reported cases of TB in the United
States,[12,14] which appeared to be, in part, connected to the
prevalence of AIDS and social problems such as drug
addiction, homelessness, and immigration. These changes
have produced considerable publicity and much concern.[16]

In other countries, the impact of widespread AIDS
infection will have a very serious effect on TB control
and will have long-term implications. Any increase in the
prevalence of TB will increase the incidence of skin-test
conversion and attendant TBM.[17]

Another serious problem involving tuberculous
infection in patients with AIDS is the progressive disease
produced by MAC.[18] In the past, atypical mycobacteria
have been the cause of lung disease in patients with
apparently normal immunity, but extrapulmonary
infection in these individuals was rare. In immunosuppressed persons, MAC produces a disseminated disease
that is often unresponsive to therapy. Despite the spread
of this organism throughout the body of patients with
AIDS, meningeal involvement has been reported to be
only a minor feature of this devastating situation.[18]

When CNS TB has occurred in patients with AIDS, it
has been reported as a part of disseminated disease and
appears as cerebral abscesses or tuberculomas[19,20] and
the usual manifestation of classical TBM are muted,
obscured, or absent. MAC infections have been shown to
respond to anti-AIDS therapy. With improved CD4
counts MAC infection is attenuated, with clearing of the
infection from the lung and else where.[18]

Bishburg and others[21,22] have reported that in 4,200
patients with AIDS and the AIDS-related complex, 52 had
TB in some form, ten of whom had CNS involvement. In
most of the patients, there was cutaneous anergy to PPD
and the presentation of their illnesses was modified by their
immunosuppressed state. Most of these patients were
intravenous-drug abusers, a group of individuals known to
have a high risk of exposure to TB as well as the AIDS
virus. Other studies have yielded similar results.[14,16,23]

Clinical Presentation

Tuberculomas usually present with the symptoms and
signs of a space-occupying lesion. As a result, the clinical
picture depends on the size and location of the tumor and
the pressure it produces on adjacent structures. Headache,
seizures, paralysis, personality changes, all symptoms
compatible with a space-occupying lesion, may be
seen.[10,11] Laboratory findings, including abnormalities in
the CSF, may be minor or absent, especially if the lesion is
parenchymal. Elevation of CSF protein is common, but

pleocytosis and low CSF sugars are rare unless the subarachnoid space is also involved. The PPD skin test is often
positive unless immunosuppression is present.

Radiographic studies, including computerized axial
tomography (CT scan), and magnetic-resonance imaging
(MRI) are useful in establishing the presence of this space-
occupying lesion, but identification of the lesion as a
tuberculoma rather than a tumor can be difficult and usually
requires a high index of clinical suspicion (Figs. 17-1 and 17-2).
Attempts at biopsy or removal create the risks of contaminating the meninges but frequently must be done because of
the inherent difficulties in establishing a definitive diagnosis.
Coverage with antituberculous drugs and steroids may limit
the risks incurred with a biopsy and these drugs probably
should be used routinely in this situation. Removal of the
mass, as opposed to biopsy, depends on the surgical risks
involved.

TBM generally has an insidious onset.[7,17,22] Apathy,
lethargy, fever, headache, malaise, mental changes such as
an ability to comprehend, personality changes, confusion,
and increasing obtundation are common presenting complaints. Seizures may occur, and symptoms of increased

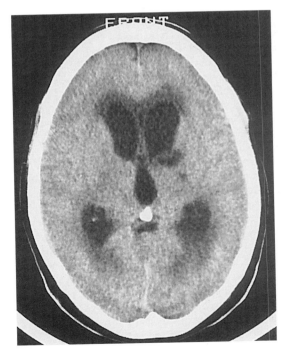

Fig. 17-1. Computerized axial tomograms of a patient with
TBM. Note enlarged ventricles and thickening of the meninges.

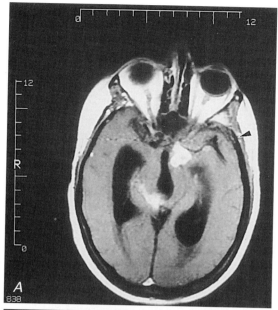

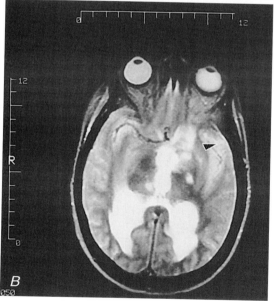

Fig. 17-2. Magnetic resonance imaging of the same patient depicted in Figure 17-2 before (*A*) and after (*B*) contrast enhancement with gadolinium. The enlarged ventricles and inflammatory changes in the basal area of the brain (*arrowheads*) are compatible with tuberculous meningitis and demonstrate the predilection of this disorder for producing damage to the cranial nerves and obstruction of cerebrospinal fluid.

intracranial pressure, such as vomiting, may be present. Occasionally diplopia, photophobia, anorexia, neck stiffness, or speech problems predominate. The course of TBM is usually downhill, but occasionally there may be temporary remissions and exacerbations of symptoms during this period.[22–24] These symptoms usually exist for days or even weeks, but on occasion can develop rapidly. There is evidence that an abrupt onset and rapid course of the disease are more common in children than in adults.[23,25]

Findings on physical examination can range from no objective findings to an obtuned patient with multiple neurologic defects, depending on the stage of the disorder. Common findings are a blunted sensorium, a stiff neck, and cranial-nerve defects, particularly of the fourth (trochlear) cranial nerve. The second (optic), third (oculomotor), sixth (abducens), and eight (acoustic) cranial nerves may also be involved. Cerebellar and pyramidal tract signs may be present.[17,22]

Examination of the retina in patients with suspected TBM can be difficult because of poor co-operation, but the findings can be sufficiently important to warrant perseverance by the clinician. Papilledema, for example, especially in the adult, may be the only indication of increased intracranial pressure. In addition, patients with TBM occasionally have a retinal tuberculid, a small, grayish-white, choroidal nodule. This is an important finding[22] since it is highly suggestive of TB. These lesions are said to be more common in miliary disease than in other types of TB (up to 80% in one report) and as a result are not necessarily diagnostic of TBM.[26–28] Very occasionally, they can also be seen in pulmonary TB, usually during the hematogenous phase of a primary infection.

The remainder of the examination is usually limited to various neurologic defects related to the diffuse and patchy nature of the damage to the brain that occur in TBM. Nystagmus or other features of cerebellar involvement may be noted[17,23] Because the disorder is progressive, in the later stages of TBM, patients may develop decorticate or decerebrate posturing or the signs of cerebral herniation as a result of their increased intracranial pressure. Thus, the important considerations on physical examinations are reasonably straightforward but variable. The salient features to look for in suspected TBM are the signs of meningitis, cranial-nerve damage, patchy neurologic defects, and signs of increased intracranial pressure.[27]

Laboratory Diagnosis

The usual methods used for the laboratory diagnosis of TBM are simple, but the definitive diagnosis can be difficult to establish. Because of the variety in the clinical presentations and its potential for misdiagnosis, it is one of those disorders that requires a high index of suspicion and clinical vigilance in order to obtain useful data to confirm the diagnosis.[29]

Although the patient's chest x-ray is often negative in TBM, it should be carefully evaluated. Klein and colleagues[7] found abnormalities suggestive of TB in 11 of 21 patients with TBM, at least retrospectively. In primary TB, the findings on chest x-ray often appear as a simple pneumonia, usually as a small infiltrate in a lower lobe. Hilar adenopathy may be present, especially in children. Occasionally, TBM may be present in patients with reactivation TB with the classical findings of a fibronodular infiltrate and cavities most commonly in the apical posterior portion of the upper lobe or in the superior segment of the lower lobe. A pleural effusion or a pleural scar suggestive of old pulmonary disease can be another useful clue to the diagnosis. If an effusion is present, a plural tap with the biopsy of the pleura should be done.

Miliary TB is difficult to identify on chest film unless it is specifically looked for by an experienced observer. It presents as a generalized fine nodular pattern.[28,30] Remote inactive pulmonary disease usually appears as fibrotic scarring, pleural disease, calcification of regional lymph nodes, or as a primary complex.

The tuberculin skin test is of limited diagnostic value. It is very useful if it is positive,[29] but if it is negative, it does not rule out TBM. It must always be done if TB of any kind is suspected; and in TBM, it must be applied with the recognition that it is often negative despite the presence of active disease. Two studies have reported that approximately 40% of patients with TBM had a negative tuberculin test when using 5TU of PPD.[31,32] If the 5TU test is negative, it is useful to repeat the test with 250 TU (second-strength PPD), but frequently this test is also nonreactive in TBM.[33,34]

It is common practice to apply a tuberculin test with another skin test using an antigen that is usually reactive in the normal general population. These control tests are used in an attempt to assess the state of delayed-type, cell-mediated immunity in these patients, and the results may have some value.[35] Mumps and monilia antigens appear to be most commonly used for this purpose. Despite its widespread use, the data to support the value of this practice are sparse. Even if a patient were found to have a positive mumps or monilia skin test and a negative reaction to second-strength PPD, the clinician should not eliminate TBM from the differential diagnosis.

Evidence has been presented to indicate that an initially negative reaction to tuberculin may become positive after therapy.[33] This sequence of events is logical if one considers the course of the disorder. In the instances where the disease occurs as a part of a primary infection with mycobacteria, later testing may allow time for cell-mediated immunity to tuberculin to develop. In other instances, individuals whose skin test has been suppressed because of the severity of their illness or other medical problems should have sufficient improvement in their general condition to allow their suppressed cell-mediated immunity to be restored. In cases where therapy has been instituted without the confirmation of the diagnosis by biopsy or bacteriologic examination, a positive PPD skin test obtained after a few weeks of treatment would be of considerable diagnostic importance and a significant inducement to continue therapy in a patient who is also improving on appropriate antituberculous therapy.[34,36]

The PPD skin test can be suppressed as a part of overwhelming TB, in malnutrition, as a side effect of immunosuppressive drugs, irradiation, as the result of certain tumors, particularly the lymphomas, AIDS, or of some of the viral exanthems such as measles.[33–37] Suppression may not be complete, but it may be sufficient to diminish the size of the reaction to a point where the clinician considers it negative. While a weakly positive test or a reaction to second-strength PPD can be the result of previous exposure to atypical mycobacteria and of little diagnostic value, one should also remember that the weak reaction may represent the most vigorous response the patient's immune system can develop under the stress of TBM, immunosuppressive drugs, lymphoma, or AIDS.

Assessment of the sequelae of patients who have recovered from TBM has indicated that postinfection cranial-nerve palsies, blindness, seizures, impairment of cognitive function, and hydrocephalus are common. These reports[33,35,37–39] indicate that overall about half of the patients with TBM who survive will have some residual damage.

Taken together, the incidence of serious sequelae of this infection and the correlation between prognosis and the amount of CNS damage evident at the time appropriate chemotherapy is started, emphasizes the need for prompt initiation of adequate chemotherapy whenever the diagnosis of TBM is seriously considered. In view of the penalties that result if there is a delay in treatment of TBM, if an error is to be committed in treatment, it should be the error of instituting early chemotherapy while continuing efforts to establish a definitive diagnosis.[7,17,40]

Therapy of TBM

The chemotherapy of TBM is, in most circumstances, simple and straightforward, as outlined in the chapter

"Chemotherapy of Tuberculosis": an initial 2-month (8 weeks) phase of treatment with isoniazid (INH), rifampin (RIF), and pyrazinamide (PZA) followed by a continuation phase with INH and RIF. Ethambutol (EMB) or streptomycin (SM) should be included in the initial phase until the results of drug susceptibility studies confirm susceptibility to INH and RIF. Since the number of tuberculous organisms involved in TBM are small, two-drug therapy with isoniazid (INH), 300 mg a day (in adults), and 600 mg rifampin (RIF) is often sufficient, although organism susceptibility should be assured. Some recommend prolonging the total course of therapy to 9–12 months for TBM.

In comatose individuals, injectable INH and parenteral rifampin can be used. In the absence of injectable drugs, oral drugs by nasogastric tube can be used. Ethambutol, in parenteral form is available. Streptomycin, an older injectable drug, is also available. The common companion drugs are pyrazinamide (PZA), ethambutol (ETB), Streptomycin(SM) and a fluoroquinolone. In suspected MDR PZA, a fluoroquinolone and SM are useful. It should be pointed that these drugs are more toxic than INH or RIF, and must be more carefully monitored than INH or RIF. Hepatic function is especially important. In the case of ETB the effective dose (20mg/kg) has considerable ophthalmic toxity, causing RFT. As a result the high dose of ETB must be limited to 60 days and then reduced to 15m per kg. SM is ototoxic and this is especially common when renal function is reduced.

The use of intrathecal tuberculin in TBM is of some historical interest. It was found to limit destructive inflammatory response in TBM that is the cause of much of the damage to the CNS. This relatively old idea[8,41] has been fairly well documented as being effective.[42] In the light of more recent understanding of immunology, the effect of intrathecal tuberculin would appear to be related to producing an antigen overload in the CSF and suppressing the immune reaction. Limitation of the immune reaction and its inflammatory response and prevention of internal hydrocephalus would be very useful.[43,44]

Anti-inflammatory, immunosuppressive drugs should have the same effect as tuberculin if used appropriately. Steroids have been widely employed in this therapeutic context, particularly to treat cerebral edema, as, for example, dexamethasone administered in patients with head injuries.

Although the use of steroids in TBM has been widely advocated, no definitive, well-controlled study has demonstrated their beneficial effect. Anecdotal evidence suggests that as predicted, they reduce edema, inhibit the inflammatory response, and prevent CFS block.

Certainly, steroids are known to suppress both immunity and inflammation, an action that would be desirable in patients with TBM. Against their use are the known complications of steroids in large doses, especially in complex clinical situations such as meningitis, where the diagnosis may not have been established. In general, it seems best to use steroids and accept the risk, especially if the situation appears reasonable clear and the patient's condition is critical. Prednisone, 60mg/day, given in two divided doses, is usually employed in adults[45] and then tapered over a period of weeks as the patient improves. Thalidomide has significant immunosuppressive activity and may be useful in TBM, replacing or enhancing the activity if steroids.[46,47]

The usefulness of a skin test reaction <5 mm but >10 mm in diameter has been acknowledged.[48] At present, a person with a test reaction of this diameter, >10 mm but <5 mm, who has AIDS or suspected AIDS, has been in close contact with a known case of TB or a person with a chest x-ray suspicious for TB, should be treated with anti-tuberculosis drugs while being evaluated further or given prophylaxis depending on the clinical situation.[48] Patients with suspected TB in any form should be tested for AIDS.

Cerebrospinal Fluid

An examination of the spinal fluid is usually the most valuable diagnostic procedure in TBM. Although the results may not be definitive, the basic studies are simple, use commonly available equipment, and can be repeated as often as needed to either establish diagnosis or follow the progress of therapy.[23,48–50]

As in any instance where an increased intracranial pressure may exist, a spinal puncture carries some risk of herniation of the medulla, but if meningitis is suspected, the procedure must be done regardless of the risk. The physician should be aware of the complications of a spinal puncture, use suitable precautions, and obtain informed consent.

Spinal fluid in TBM is usually a clear or slightly opalescent fluid, under increased pressure, with an elevated CSF protein, as may be found in a number of other intracranial diseases. In individuals with a tuberculoma of the CNS, as opposed to meningitis, this may be all that is found.[9,10]

When tubercle bacilli and their cellular products are first leaked into the CSF, polymorpholeukocytes appear initially, usually in low moderate numbers. These are replaced by mononuclear cells within a few days, and this cell type is the one classically found in TBM. The cell count is usually in the low hundreds and seldom greater than 1,000 cells/mm^3.

The initial appearance of polymorphonuclear leukocytes in the CSF of some patients with TBM may be a significant trap for the unwary and illustrates the degree of caution and perseverance needed to evaluate patients suspected of having TBM, as well as the importance of not relying on a single spinal puncture in suspected cases when the initial evaluation is inconclusive.

CSF glucose is low in TBM, often less than half of normal, in the range of 45–50 mg/dl.[7,17,22–24] CSF glucose should be determined after the CSF and blood glucose levels have had an opportunity to equilibrate, and a blood glucose should always be obtained to allow comparison with the CSF value. A useful rule of thumb is to consider the normal CSF glucose value as greater than half the serum concentration. A ratio of CSF to blood glucose below 1:2 is a significant abnormality, particularly if the CSF value is marginally low. Nevertheless, a small percent of individuals with TBM may have CSF glucose levels that are normal, particularly during the early stages of the disease. In one series, over 10% had levels above 50 mg/dL, and in another study 4 of 21 patients had CSF sugar above 60 mg/dl.[7,20,23,48] The presence of hyperglycemia, glucose infusion, or the administration of insulin can obscure the diagnosis of TBM by producing rapid changes in serum glucose levels. These factors must be considered in the evaluation of the CFS findings.[38–40] It takes about two hours for CFS and blood glucose levels to equilibrate.

The presence of acid-fast bacilli in the CSF should be diagnostic for the disease. Unfortunately, AFB can be found in the CSF on smear only in a minority of the patients who have subsequently been shown to have TBM.[49] Klein and coworkers[7] have reported that in a major teaching hospital, only 4 positive smears for AFB were found in 36 examinations of spinal fluid submitted from 21 patients with TBM. This fact is not surprising, The number of bacilli, usually present in the CSF in tuberculous meningitis is never large,[1] the volume of the sample obtained at tap for examination is small, and the fraction of the sample viewed through an oil-immersion lens is miniscule. Centrifugation of the CSF to concentrate the bacilli in a sediment is helpful, and a diligent examination of the stained slides by a skilled microbiologist is essential.[14] The technique of placing a drop of unconcentrated CSF on a slide that is then stained and briefly examined by an inexperienced observer is not satisfactory.

Newer tests, designed to provide rapid and sensitive diagnostic tools are available, at least in developed countries. In general tests, such as rapid DOT immunoassay (DOT) appear to be useful additions to the diagnostic tools used to identify TBM. There are nucleic acid amplification (NAA) techniques that appear to be more sensitive and more rapid than traditional tests.[51–55]

A major problem with the newer methods used to identify TBM is their limited availability in the countries where TB and TBM are most common. The lack of equipment and trained personal are serious deficits. Budgets are very limited in some areas of the world and the costs of treating AIDS impose additional burdens.

Cultures of the CSF for mycobacteria in suspected TBM are of limited value since they are retrospective. Unfortunately, 3–8 weeks are needed for cultures to become positive because of the slow in vitro growth of *Mycobacterium tuberculosis*. Reports indicate that 50–80% of cases of TBM have positive CSF cultures.[6,7,17,22]

The widespread availability of computerized axial tomography (CT) has provided another valuable diagnostic instrument for the evaluation of patients with suspected TBM.[56–59] While it cannot establish the diagnosis of TBM, it is useful to rule out other serious CNS diseases in patients who have an obscure illness or evidence of increased intracranial pressure. The CT in TBM with contrast enhancement often shows dilated ventricles, an exudate with thickened meninges, particularly in the basilar areas of the brain. The vasculitis and thrombosis associated with TBM are seen on the CT scan as multiple areas of radiolucency secondary to ischemia. These changes are usually located in the basal ganglia and adjacent to the sylvian fissure.[42] Another technique useful in TBM that has become increasingly available in the United States and other developed countries is magnetic-resonance imaging (MRI). It has a significant advantage over CT because it allows better visualization of the bases of the brain, where TBM is most likely to occur (See Figs. 17-1 and 17-2).

It has been reported[42] that TBM produces focal infarcts with circumscribed edges, usually in gray matter, together with thickened meninges, often at the base of the brain, with dilated ventricles. White-matter infarcts and infarction of the midbrain and brain stem are also visible. Obstruction of CSF circulation can be identified and followed, and the response of the therapy can be followed.

While these findings, both CT and MRI, can be produced by a variety of other infectious meningeal diseases such as cryptococcal meningitis,[60] they are sufficiently distinct to provide useful information and may allow the clinician enough information to consider chemotherapy.

Meningeal biopsy is another approach to establishing the diagnosis of TBM by obtaining tissue submitting the specimen to laboratory for histologic and bacterial study.

Although this procedure may seem overly aggressive, one should remember that in some instances, particularly where immunosuppression is present, the diagnosis of TBM can be difficult and a delay in therapy can be followed by deterioration of the condition of the patient and permanent CNS damage.

Differential Diagnosis

The list of diseases that should be considered in the differential diagnosis of TBM is long, but in reality the number of those that create major diagnostic problems is limited.[31,35] Certain groups of clinical problems can be discarded using simple, well-defined criteria (see Tables 17-1 and 17-2).

For example, acute bacterial meningitis such as a meningococcal infection can be included in the differential diagnosis of TBM, but bacterial infections usually occur as acute illnesses with large number of polymorphic leukocytes and identifiable bacteria in the CSF. In general, this diagnosis can be almost eliminated from consideration by the patient's history and results of culture of CSF. Partially treated bacterial meningitis can be a diagnostic problem on some occasions, but again the type of cells in the CSF, the history, and an element of caution on the part of the clinician should suffice to identify this problem.

Another bacterial illness that can be a more serious problem is subacute bacterial endocarditis (SBE), which often results in multiple mycotic emboli that produce successive infected infarcts that mimic some of the findings in TBM. The disease can be associated with low-grade fever and meningeal signs. In this instance, the symptoms and signs of SBE, such as a heart murmur and evidence of mycotic emboli, should be evident. The CSF sugar should be normal unless there is a cerebral abscess that has contaminated the subarachnoid space. Echocardiography of heart valves and blood cultures would identify this problem in most instances.

The major clinical problems that must be seriously considered in the differential diagnosis of TBM are the viral and fungal infections of the CNS and infiltration of the meninges by metastatic carcinoma, particularly a lymphoma, or leukemic cells.

Viral infections of the CNS must always be considered in the differential diagnosis of TBM.[36] Viral meningoencephalitis can be caused by herpes simplex, mumps, West Nile fever or eastern equine encephalitis, and can be associated with a low CSF sugar. Herpes encephalitis produces focal neurologic deficits, CSF lymphocytosis, and seizures. The fact that antiviral therapy for this serious disease has been found to be effective and that both TB and this viral infection occur as opportunistic diseases adds weight to the recommendation that a biopsy of the brain and meninges might be useful.

While fungal infections of the CNS are rare, they are becoming more common since they are one of the many infectious complications of immunosuppression. They, like TBM, are associated with a low sugar and the appearance of lymphocytes in the CSF. The key points in eliminating this group of infections from consideration in this context would appear to be to consider the history, to search for a potential source of fungal infection, and to identify the organism in the CSF on smear, by culture, or by appropriate serologic tests. Cryptococcal meningitis is an excellent example. It mimics the clinical picture of TBM,[61] including the history of relatively slow progression with occasional spontaneous remissions, and the CSF findings are similar. It can be identified by obtaining appropriate cultures, an India-ink preparation of a centrifugal specimen of CSF and an immunoassay for cryptococcal antigen.

Amebic infections, rickettsial diseases, trypanosomiasis, echinococcus, or leptospirosis might be considered in the differential of TBM, but only in unusual circumstances. Again, a history of exposure to the organism and the

Table 17-1. Differential Diagnosis for TBM

Infectious	Fungal: Cryptococcus, histoplasmosis
	Viral: herpes, mumps, encephalitis, West Nile fever
	Bacterial infection (partially treated): brain abscess, leptospirosis
	Trypanosomal
Vascular	Multiple emboli, subacute bacterial endocarditis, thrombosis of sagital vain
Collagen vascular	Lupus erythematous, polyarteritis, collagen vascular disease
Other meningeal diseases	Sarcoid, metastatic carcinoma, acute hemorrhagic, leukoencephalopathy, lymphoma

Table 17-2. Points to Stress in Evaluating a Patient with Suspected TBM

Medical and Social History
History of significant TB contact or residence in an area with a high incidence of TB.
History of positive PPD skin test, especially a recent conversion.
A history of diseases or therapy associated with immunosuppression.
A history of BCG immunization.

Physical Examination
Search for BCG scar.
Fundal examination for tuberculids and papilledema.
Neurologic examination, with special reference to signs of meningeal irritation, state of
    consciousness, and demonstration of focal signs.

Laboratory
Hematocrit, hemoglobin/WBC and diff., urinanalysis, sedimentation rate, serology for syphilis,
    serum Na+, Cl+, creatinine, complement fixation test (or equivalent) for fungal infections,
    AIDS test.
Chest x-ray, CT scan of head, MRI.
Spinal puncture
    Manometrics.
    Gross inspection.
    Specimens for cell count, differential, and cytology.
    CSF glucose with simultaneous blood glucose.
    CSF protein.
    Specimen for AFB smear and culture. Gram stain of smear and appropriate bacterial culture.
    India-ink preparation and appropriate assay for cryptococcal and herpes antigen.
    Submit specimen for mycobacterial antigen.
    CFS for syphilis serology.
Tuberculin skin test 5 TU; if negative, apply 250 TU.

spinal-fluid findings should be helpful. Other disorders to remember in the differential diagnosis of TBM are the collagen vascular diseases; sarcoidosis with involvement of the meninges is associated with a low spinal-fluid sugar on occasion. Venous thrombosis of superior longitudinal sinus, and neurosyphilis are possibilities that can be dealt with by evaluating the history, doing appropriate laboratory testing, and, in the case of a suspected venous thrombosis, obtaining an angiogram and MRI.

In those instances where there is meningeal involvement by a malignant lymphoma or leukemic cells, a CSF cytology can be very helpful to establish the diagnosis. It should be recalled that malignant involvement of the meninges often produces a low CSF glucose and the cells of the tumor can be misidentified as lymphocytes. A history of a known malignancy or other findings compatible with a malignant tumor will alert the physician to this possibility.

Acute hemorrhagic necrotizing leukoencephalitis is rare. It may be associated with meningeal signs, a low CSF sugar, and pleocytosis. It presents as an acute,

rapidly progressive disorder without the more protracted features of TBM. It is also reported to produce a lower CSF protein value in association with internal hydrocephalus than does TBM. Because it has been reported as a complication of leukemia, lymphomas, sarcoidosis, and immunosuppressive therapy, it could be confused with TBM in certain instances.

The occurrence of AIDS imposes an additional burden on the physician involved in a suspected TBM. Tests may be altered, be absent or have a false negative result in a situation that occurs where accurate data is most needed.

Clinical Course and Prognosis

The result of untreated TBM is the death of the patient, usually in four to six weeks. While there were sporadic reports of survivors in the era before specific antituberculous therapy, these cases were reported because of their distinct rarity. Patients with CNS TB can have temporary partial remissions of their symptoms, but their course is downhill with worsening of their condition and increasing disability. The partial improvement in the patient's condition can be another trap for the unwary since it may mimic the expected clinical course of other infections producing meningitis where recovery is expected. This may lead to delays in the diagnosis of a disease whose prognosis is adversely affected by delays in therapy.[6,32]

In the recent past, treated meningeal TB has been reported to have an overall mortality of between 15–30%.[7,38,39,62] Unfortunately, residual damage is common in the survivors.

A poor prognosis for the patient with TBM, either death or severe and permanent brain damage, has been clearly linked to the patient's status at the time therapy is initiated. The critical factor is the level of consciousness on admission and the number of evident focal neurologic signs noted before effective therapy is begun.[7,23,38] Since it is usual for patients with TBM to have continued worsening of their symptoms, at least for some days after the initiation of adequate chemotherapy, those admitted with severe CNS damage will have much poorer prognosis. The multiple infarctions of the brain, the presence of an inflammatory exudate, and the resulting nerve damage are often permanent and illustrate the widely held opinion that a patient with serious neurologic deficits on admission will probably be left with serious residual central nervous damage.[7]

The other useful supportive measures in TBM are those normally used in severely ill patients, including careful fluid management, protection of the airway, and support of ventilation. Anticonvulsant therapy may be necessary. It should be recalled that inappropriate antidiuretic hormone (ADH) might be present.

It should be pointed out that TBM is not contagious unless simultaneous active pulmonary disease is present. The care of patients with TBM and a normal chest x-ray is greatly simplified if they are not unnecessarily isolated.

Other Mycobacteria

TBM produced by species of mycobacteria other than *M. tuberculosis* has been reported in people with presumed normal immunity, most commonly *Mycobacterium kansasii*.[63] Unfortunately, these rare mycobacterial infections may be identified on culture. Most species of the so-called atypical mycobacteria are resistant to conventional chemotherapy, but clinical treatment of pulmonary TB caused by *M. kansasii* with INH and rifampin has produced reasonable results despite this species' frequent in vitro resistance to these drugs.

As will be discussed elsewhere in this book MAC is commonly associated with AIDS. In the past this combination had a very poor prognosis. It is now apparent that highly active antiviral therapy (HAAT) restores the CD4 count and may help control the infection.

Drug Resistance

Mycobacterial resistance to antituberculous drugs is a growing problem.[15] There are reports of TBM with AFB resistant to one or more of the commonly used antituberculous drugs. This situation usually arises when a child or a non-immune adult is exposed to a patient with infectious TB who is excreting a strain of mycobacterium resistant to one or more antituberculous agents. As a result, the primary infection and subsequent meningeal disease would involve resistant organisms.

Identification of this serious condition is not easy. A careful history of the patient's tuberculous contacts must be obtained and evaluated. An example of such a contact would be an alcoholic relative who had been in and out of TB therapy for many years and who recently has been living in the same home with the patient.

If there is a suspicion of this problem, initial therapy for TBM should include at least two drugs to which there is reasonable evidence that the organism is sensitive. This sensitivity can be inferred by carefully evaluating the drug history of the contact and obtaining the most recent drug-sensitive profile of the source case, if available. The so-called second line drugs are less effective, often more toxic and have side effects such as nausea which hinders compliance. CDC recommends[48] using INH, rifampin, pyrazinamide (PZA), a fluoroquinolone, and two other drugs.

The problems, social and economic, commonly associated with AIDS, TB, and especially MDR-TB, have been and continue to be a particular problem in Southeast Asia and much of Africa. Even when anti-AIDS therapy is available, compliance may be poor because of the large number of medications involved, potential side effects and costs.

ACKNOWLEDGMENT

The author wishes to thank Dr. J. Cowdery for his support and consul during the preparation of the manuscript. He would also like to thank Heidi Vekemans for her help with the manuscript.

REFERENCES

1. Rich AR. *The Pathogenesis of Tuberculosis,* 2nd ed. Springfield, IL.; CC Thomas; 1951.
2. Myers JA. The natural history of tuberculosis in the human body. *JAMA.* 1965;194:1084–1092.

3. Stead WW. Pathogenesis of the sporadic cases of tuberculosis. *N Engl J Med.* 1967;227:1008–1012.

4. Stead WW, Kenby GR, Schleuter DP, et al. The clinical spectrum of primary tuberculosis. *Ann Int Med.* 1968;68: 731–745.

5. Rich AR, McCord HA. The pathogenesis of tuberculous meningitis. *Bull Johns Hopkins Hosp.* 1933;52:5–27.

6. Meyes BR. Tuberculous meningitis. *Med Clin North Am.* 1982;66:155–162.

7. Klein NC, Damskr B, Hirschman SZ. Mycobacterial meningitis: retrospective analysis 1970 to 1983. *Am J Med.* 1985;79:29–34.

8. Smith HV, Vollum RL. Effects of inthrathecal tuberculin and streptomycin in tuberculous meningitis. *Lancet.* 1950;2:275–286.

9. Decuns P, Garre H, Pheline C. Tuberculoma of the brain and cerebellum. *J Neurosurg.* 1954;11:243–250.

10. Demergis JA, Liftwitch EL, Curtin JA, Witorsch P. Tuberculoma of the brain. *JAMA.* 1978;239:413–415.

11. Hildebrant G, Agnoli AL. Differential diagnosis and therapy of intracerebral tuberculomas. *J Neurol.* 1982;118:201–208.

12. Reichman LB. The U-shaped curve of concern. *Am Rev Respir Dis.* 1991;144:741–742.

13. Brundy K, Dobkin J. Resurgent tuberculosis in New York City: Human immunodeficiency virus, homelessness and decline of tuberculosis control programs. *Am Rev Respir Dis.* 1991;144:745–749.

14. Modilevsky T, Sattler F, Barnes P. Mycobacterial disease in patients with human-deficiency virus infection. *Arch Intern Med.* 1989;149:2201–2205.

15. From Centers for Disease Control, Leads from the Mobility and Mortality Weekly Report. Nosocomial transmission of multidrug-resistant tuberculosis among HIV-infected persons—Florida and New York, 1988–1991. *JAMA.* 1991; 266:1483–1484.

16. Selwyn PA, Hartel D, Lewis VA, et al. A prospective study of the risk of tuberculosis among intravein drug abuses with immunodeficiency virus infection. *N Engl J Med.* 1989;320: 545–550.

17. Molovi A, LeFock JL. Tuberculous meningitis. *Med Clin North Am.* 1985;69:315–331.

18. Hawkin CC, Gold JWM, Whimbey E, et al. *Mycobacterium avium complex* infection in patients with acquired immunodeficiency syndrome. *Ann Int Med.* 1986;105:184–188.

19. Sunderarm G, McDonald RJ, Manatis T, et al. Tuberculosis as a manifestation of the acquired immunodeficiency syndrome (AIDS). *JAMA.* 1986;256:362–366.

20. Kim HS, Hong SJ, Kim SJ, et al. Treatment of multi resistant pulmonary tuberculosis in a chest clinic. *Int J Tuberc Lung Dis.* 2001;5:1129–1136.

21. Bishburg E, Sunderarm G, Reichman L, et al. Central nervous system tuberculosis with acquired immunodeficiency and its related complex. *Ann Int Med.* 1986;105:210–213.

22. Parsons M. Diagnosis not to be missed, tuberculosis meningitis. *Br J Hosp Med.* 1982;27:682–684.

23. Dostur KD, Lalitha VS. The many facets of neurotuberculosis: an epitome of neuropathology. *Prog Neuropathol.* 1973;2:351–408.

24. Crocco JA, Bleckel MJ, Rooney JJ, et al. Tuberculous meningitis in adults, *NY State J Med.* 1980;80:1231–1234.

25. Castleman B (ed.). Weekly clinicopathological exercise. *N Eng J Med.* 1974;290:1130–1136.

26. Illingsworth RS, Wright T. Tubercles of the choroid. *Br Med J.* 1948;2:356–370.

27. Kocen RS, Parsons M. The neurological complications of tuberculosis: some unusual manifestations. *Q J Med.* 1970;34:17–31.

28. Munt PW. Miliary tuberculosis in the chemotherapy area. *Medicine.* 1971;51:139–155.

29. Kasik JE, Schuldt S. Why tuberculosis is still a health problem in the aged. *Geriatrics.* 1977;3:63–72.

30. Gelb AF, Leffler C, Brewin A, et al. Miliary tuberculosis. *Am Rev Respir Dis.* 1973;108:1327–1333.

31. Haas EJ, Modhaven T, Quinn EL, et al. Tuberculous meningitis in an urban general hospital. *Arch Int Med.* 1977;137:1518–1521.

32. Fitzsimons JM. Tuberculous meningitis: a follow-up study on 198 cases. *Tubercle.* 1963;44:87–102.

33. Rooney JJ, Crocco JA, Kramer S, et al. Further observations on tuberculin reactions in active tuberculosis. *Am J Med.* 1976;60:517–522.

34. Schacter EH. Tuberculin negative tuberculosis. *Am Rev Respir Dis.* 1972;106:587–593.

35. Barret-Connor E. Tuberculous meningitis in adults. *South Med J.* 1967;60:1061–1067.

36. Grieco MH, Chmel H. Acute disseminated tuberculosis as a diagnostic problem. *Am Rev Respir Dis.* 1974;109: 554–560.

37. Collins FM. The immunology of tuberculosis. *Am Rev Respir Dis.* 1982;125:42–49.

38. Shah AK, Gandhi VK. Prognosis of tubercular meningitis. *Indian J Pediatr.* 1984;21:791–795.

39. Fallon RJ, Kennedy DH. Treatment and prognosis in tuberculous meningitis. *J Infect.* 1981;3:39–44.

40. Kasik JE. Tuberculosis and other mycobacterial diseases. In: Rakel RE, ed. *Conn's Current Therapy.* Philadelphia, PA: WB Saunders; 1984:125.

41. Smith HV, Vollum RL. The treatment of tuberculous meningitis. *Tubercle.* 1956;37:301–320.

42. Acheson RM. Smith RV. Radiological technique in the management of tuberculous meningitis. *Q J Med.* 1958;27: 83–101.

43. Lorber J. Treatment of tuberculous meningitis. *Br Med J.* 1960;1:1309–1312.

44. American Trudeau Society. A statement by the Committee on Therapy: tuberculous meningitis. *Am Rev Tubc.* 1970;70: 756–758.

45. Weg JG. Tuberculosis and other mycobacterial disease. In: Conn WE, ed. *Conn's Current Therapy.* Philadelphia, PA: WB Saunders; 1981:137.

46. Sokal K, Freedman VH, Kaplan D, et al. A combination of thalidomide and antibiotics protects rabbits from mycobac- terial associated death. *J Infect Dis.* 1998;177: 1563–1572.

47. Shoeman F. Thalidomide therapy of childhood meningitis. *J Child Neurol.* 2000;15:838.

48. Horsburg CR, Priorities for the treatment of latent tuberculosis and infection in the United States. *N Engl J Med.* 2004;350:2060–2067.

49. Kennedy DH, Fallon RJ. Tuberculous meningitis. *JAMA.* 1979;241:264.

50. Hooker AJ, Muhindi DW, Amyo DW, et al. Diagnostic utility of cerebral spinal fluid in clinically suspected tuberculous meningitis. *Int J Tuberc Lung Dis.* 2003;7:287–326.

51. Daniels TM. Antibody and antigen detection of immunodiagnosis of tuberculosis. Why not, What more is needed, Where do we stand. *J Infect Dis.* 1988;158:678–680.

52. Soda E, Ruiz-Palacios GM, Lopez-Vidal Y. Detection of mycobacterial antigens in cerebral spinal fluid of patients with tuberculous meningitis by enzyme-linked immunoabsorbent assay. *Lancet.* 1983;2:651–652.

53. Kashyap RS, Kainthla RP, Biswas SS, et al. Rapid diagnosis of tuberculous meningitis using simple DOT enzyme-linked immunoabsorbent assay (DOT-ELISA). *Med Sci Monit.* 2003;9:123–126.

54. Thwait ES, Cows M, Chau TT, et al. Comparison of conventional bacteriology with nucleic acid amplification for diagnosis of tuberculous meningitis. *J Clin Microbiol.* 2004;42:996–1002.

55. Seshadri S. Nucleic acid amplification tests for tuberculous meningitis: a systematic review of diagnostic accuracy (Review). *Natl Med J India.* 2003;16:260–261.

56. Teah R, Humphries MJ, Hoare RD, et al. Clinical correlation of CT changes in 64 Chinese patients with tuberculous meningitis. *J Neuro.* 1989;236:48–51.

57. Nai-Shin C. Tuberculous meningitis. Computerized tomographic manifestations. *Arch Neurol.* 1980;37:458–460.

58. Bullock MR. Diagnostic and prognostic features of tuberculous meningitis on CT scanning. *J Neurol Neurosurg Psychiatry.* 1982;45:1098–1101.

59. Price HI, Danziger A. Computerized tomograph in cranial tuberculosis. *AJR Am J Roentgenol.* 1978;130:769–771.

60. Stockstill MT, Kaufmann CA. Comparison of cryptococcal and tuberculous meningitis. *Arch Neurol.* 1983;40:81–85.

61. Schoeman J, Hewlett R, Donald P. MR of childhood tuberculous meningitis. *Neuroradiol.* 1988;30:473–477.

62. Kennedy DH. Tuberculosis meningitis (letter). *Lancet.* 1981;1:261.

63. Wolinsky E. Nontuberculous mycobacterial infections of man. *Med Clin North Am.* 1974;58:639–648.

18

Tuberculous Lymphadenitis and Parotitis

Dwight A. Powell

HISTORICAL PERSPECTIVES

"What great difficulty we meet with in the cure of the King's Evil, with the daily experience both of Physicians and Chirurgeons doth shew....When upon trial he shall find the contumaciousness of the disease which frequently diluded his best care and industry, he will find reason of acknowledging the goodness of God; who hath dealth so beautifully with this nation, in giving the Kings of it at least from Edward the Confessor downward (if not for a longer time) an extraordinary power in the miraculous Cure thereof"-Richard Wiseman, 17th century surgeon.[1]

Scrofula, defined as tuberculosis (TB) of the lymphatic glands, has afflicted humans for thousands of years. Hippocrates (460–377 B.C.) mentioned scrofulous tumors in his writing, and Herodotus (5th century B.C.) described the exclusion of those afflicted with leprous or scrofulous lesions from the general population. This illness was known as the King's Evil during the Middle Ages in Europe because of the apparent cure of many cases following the king's royal touch. Clovis I of France (466–511 A.D.) is the first recorded king to use the royal touch to cure scrofula after his baptism in 496 A.D. English sovereigns from Edward the Confessor to Queen Anne[2] practiced the royal touch and historians have recorded vivid accounts of the crushing mobs who gathered to see the royal touch. Charles II of England is reputed to have applied the royal touch 90,798 times. After being touched, patients received a gold piece, which was to protect them from subsequent scrofulous attacks. It was often the job of the parish rector to select needy patients and to assure that they were more desirous of a cure of their scrofula than of the golden coin about their neck.[2]

Not until the 19th century, when pathology emerged as a science, was the tuberculous etiology of scrofula recognized. As late as the first half of the 19th century, the German physician, Johan Lucas Schulman differentiated scrofula from TB as a different family of blood borne diseases.[3] A variety of internal and external causes of scrofula were proposed, including hereditary lymphatic temperament, contagion, degeneration of the syphilitic virus, food and drink, dirt, excretions, and atmospheric influence. In 1846, in England, scrofula most frequently afflicted children between ages 2 and 15 years. Of 133,000 children examined, 24% showed obvious scars of scrofula or had enlarged cervical glands.[3] Once a scrofulous node erupted through the skin, the illness became a repulsive, long-term disability because the resulting ulcers intermittently exuded a thick, sour-smelling pus. It is little wonder that this sinister, chronic disease was regarded by the public and by some physicians as the manifestation of an inherited disordered constitution or even of degeneracy.[3]

EPIDEMIOLOGY

Tuberculosis of the lymph nodes is the most common form of extrapulmonary TB. Surveys in the United States and Canada have shown lymph node involvement to represent 5–9% of all reported cases of TB.[4] Despite declining rates of TB in the United States, during the past decade,[5] the incidence of TB has increased world-wide resulting in an increased incidence of tuberculous lymphadenitis.[6–8] In contrast, TB of the parotid glands, first described in 1894[9] remains a rare occurrence, reported primarily in single or small case studies and identified mostly in parotidectomy specimens.[9–11]

Lymph node TB has historically been a disease most common in children. However, in numerous recent studies from developed countries, the peak age range is between 20 to 40 years of age.[6] This shift in age probably reflects the falling incidence of childhood TB in developed countries because children still compose a high percentage of cases of scrofula in areas of endemic TB,[12] or areas where immigration from developing countries has increased.[7]

It has long been recognized that primary (childhood) versus secondary (adult) TB is distinctly different relative to lymph node involvement. In untreated primary TB of children, almost all patients will have enlargement of hilar or paratracheal lymph nodes (or both) apparent on chest roentgenograms.[13,14] Extrapulmonary lymphadenitis develops in 5% of patients within 6 months of tuberculous infection.[15] Infected nodes commonly become greatly enlarged and caseous. That node involvement occurs shortly after the onset of primary infection is supported by the fact that 50–80% of children with cervical lymph node involvement have radiographic evidence of active pulmonary TB.[7,13,14] In contrast, adult tuberculous cervical lymphadenitis is accompanied by an abnormal chest radiograph less than 30% of the time,[6] and these changes usually represent old, healed TB, suggesting that node disease results from reactivation of previous infection.

Ethnic origin and sex also seem to have a major bearing on the risk of developing tuberculous lymphadenitis. Within the United States, Canada, Australia, and the United Kingdom, a majority of cases occur in persons born on the Indian and Asian subcontinents. In a national British survey, tuberculous lymphadenitis accounted for about 40% of the cases of TB in immigrants of Asian origin.[16] The influx of Asian immigrants to Canada has been one of the major reasons for the sustained incidence of lymph node TB in that country despite a decline in pulmonary TB. In addition to a higher risk of TB, persons born in Africa or Southeast Asia appear to have a predilection for developing lymphadenitis.[17] Within a population of U.S. Naval personnel with active TB, Asians have a disproportionately high rate of lymph node versus pulmonary involvement[18] (Table 18-1). Although males predominate in cases of pulmonary TB, most studies of peripheral lymph node TB describe a greater than 2:1 female/male case rate.[17] In the developed world, then, those at highest risk for having lymph node TB are Indian, Asian, or African women between the ages of 20 and 40 years. Persons infected with the human immunodeficiency virus (HIV) have a high risk for developing TB. It has been estimated that among persons with active TB, HIV-1 infected patients represent 8% of the worldwide total and 30–60% of cases in Africa.[19,20] Extrapulmonary TB appears to be much more frequent in patients with HIV infection. Isolated extra pulmonary localizations, particularly lymphadenitis, are described in 53–63% of TB cases in HIV-1 infected patients, and more frequently in severely immunocompromised HIV patients.[20]

Table 18-1. Racial Distribution of Tuberculous Lymphadenitis and Pulmonary Tuberculosis in U.S. Navy Personnel

	Distribution of TB (%)	
Race	**Lymph node**	**Pulmonary**
White	7	55
Black	7	10
Asian	79	31
Other	7	4
	100	100

Source: Adapted from Cantrell RW, Hensen JH, Reid D. Diagnosis and management of tuberculous cervical adenitis. *Arch Otolaryngol.* 1975;101:53–57.

PATHOLOGY

A nearly uniform event following infection by *Mycobacterium tuberculosis* is spread from the primary focus to regional lymph nodes. This often results in a greater volume of diseased tissue in regional lymph nodes than at the original site of the infection. From the regional nodes, organisms may continue to spread via the lymphatic system to other nodes or may pass through the nodes and reach the bloodstream in small numbers, from whence they may spread to virtually any organ in the body. This form of lymphatic and hematogenous dissemination is usually self-limited, and more than 90% of primary infections in humans heal with a positive tuberculin reaction and perhaps a little pulmonary calcification as their only apparent vestige. Reactivation TB may develop as a late recrudescence from dormant organisms in lymph nodes that were invaded during the primary infection.

Tuberculous infection in the parotid gland usually develops following infection of intraparotid lymph nodes. The intraparotid lymphoid tissue becomes infected following spread up lymphatics from a focus of mycobacterial infection in a tonsil, gingival sulcus, or mucosal break. As the capsule of the infected lymph tissue breaks down, parotitis ensues. Direct infection of the parotid gland may also follow hematogenous seeding or by spread up the salivary ducts from autoinoculation with infected sputum.[10,11]

Historically, lymph node and parotid TB was caused mainly by *Mycobacterium bovis*, but nearly all tuberculous lymphadenitis is now due to *M. tuberculosis*. Because infection with this organism usually begins in the lungs, the regional nodes draining the pulmonary parenchyma are most commonly infected. These nodes include a para bronchial group, filling the hilar regions of both lungs; a subcarinal group, at the angle of the bifurcation of the trachea behind the right pulmonary artery; and a para-tracheal group, adjacent to the trachea within the posterior mediastinum. These nodes may all be involved in endobronchial TB, which occurs most commonly in children but is being described with increasing frequency in adults.[6,13,14]

Even though mediastinal nodes are the most common primary regional draining sites, they account for only 5% of reported lymph node TB. Instead, clinically apparent tuberculous lymphadenitis most frequently involves nodes of the head and neck, typically those in the anterior or posterior cervical chains and supraclavicular region.[6,7,13,14] Because localized primary infections of the head and neck are unusual, infection in these nodes probably results from the generalized lymphatic spread following a primary pulmonary infection. It has been suggested that paratracheal lymph nodes have communications with deep cervical nodes and abdominal nodes.[21] Among 54 patients with primary TB in the right upper lobe, a location that primarily causes drainage to the right paratracheal lymph node, 14 had involvement of the deep cervical nodes on the same side and 3 had involvement of the abdominal nodes.[21]

In the uncommon occurrence of axillary, inguinal, or other noncervical peripheral node TB, a focus of infection distal to the infected node will often be identified. Preauricular adenitis suggests a scalp, eye, or lacrimal duct infection.[22,23] Epitrochlear lymphadenitis may follow infections on the forearm or hand.[24] Axillary lymph nodes are involved with lesions on the arms, chest wall, or in mammary glands.[25,26] Inguinal lymph nodes may become infected following lesions on the feet or legs or following genital infection.[27]

The major pathological events of lymph node TB include compression of surrounding tissue, caseation and breakdown of nodes, and fibrosis from healing of the eroded nodes. Mortality is uncommon, but morbidity and chronic illness are the rule. Probably the best example of the severe pathologic events associated with lymph node TB is found in endobronchial disease of children.[13,28] In the child whose body is unable to contain the progressive multiplication and spread of tubercle bacilli, the onset of delayed hypersensitivity is accompanied by marked hyperemia and swelling of the regional nodes, with external compression of the trachea and bronchi. When the centers of the nodes develop necrosis and caseation, marked perinodal inflammation leads to node adherence to the outer surface of the airways (Fig. 18-1). As the

nodes begin to erode through the bronchial wall, submucosal tubercles, intraluminal polyps, and granulation tissue appear (Fig. 18-2). Ultimately, nodes may perforate the bronchial wall, causing caseous tissue to extrude into the bronchial lumen with possible bronchial obstruction or spread of caseous tissue to other areas of the lung. With healing of the involved nodes and bronchus, fibrosis usually leads to permanent bronchial stenosis or bronchiectasis. Lymph node enlargement within the mediastinum may also be accompanied by compression of major blood vessels, impingement on the phrenic or recurrent laryngeal nerves, occlusion of lymphatic drainage, or erosion into the chest wall and sternum.

Involvement of the superficial lymph nodes usually results in enlarging mass lesions. If untreated, swelling progresses and nodes within a group become matted together and adherent to the overlying skin. Eventually, the overlying skin develops a purplish discoloration, the center of the mass become soft, and caseous material soon ruptures into surrounding tissue or through the skin. This is the classical appearance of scrofula.

CLINICAL ILLNESS

More than 90% of superficial tuberculous lymph nodes are found in the head and neck regions.[6] In order of decreasing frequency, these include anterior and posterior cervical, supraclavicular, submandibular, and occasionally preauricular or submental nodes.[29] Several nodes within a group are usually involved, and bilateral adenitis is common, particularly in young children. Generalized lymphadenopathy and hepatosplenomegaly occur in less than 5% of most

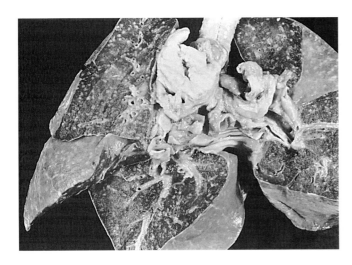

Fig. 18-1. Autopsy specimen of endobronchial TB. A large caseous lymph node is attached to and compresses the right mainstem and right upper-lobe bronchi.

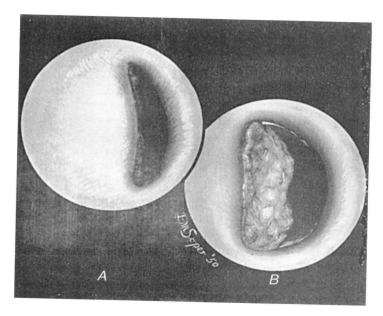

Fig. 18-2. A drawing of the bronchoscopic appearance of childhood endobronchial TB. *A*: Loss of lumen size owing to external compression by a tuberculous peribronchial lymph node. *B*: Erosion of the lymph node through the bronchial wall with intraluminal granulation tissue. (Reprinted with permission from Hardy JB. *Tuberculosis in White and Negro Children.* Cambridge, Mass: Harvard University Press; 1958.)

series. It should be noted, however, that in childhood miliary TB, generalized lymphadenopathy may be found in 10–15% of cases.[30]

The symptoms associated with tuberculous lymphadenitis depend largely on the location of involved nodes. In both adults and children, the primary presenting symptom of cervical lymphadenitis is a painless, slowly progressive swelling in the neck[31] (Fig. 18-3). Several weeks may pass before the nodes sufficiently enlarge to warrant medical attention. In less than 20% of patients, there are associated symptoms such as weight loss, temperature elevation, anorexia, fatigue, malaise, or pain. If the nodes are allowed to progress through the stages of caseation and erosion, the patient may seek medical attention because of the chronic damage from the resulting ulcer or sinus tract. In the more recent series, this occurs less than 10% of the time.[24]

With parabronchial or paratracheal lymph node enlargement, presenting symptoms are somewhat dependent on age. In the adult, enlarging nodes rarely impinge on the bronchial lumen to cause respiratory symptoms. Instead, illness is manifested as weight loss, fever, low grade night sweats, chronic chest pain, malaise, anorexia, or asymptomatic abnormal-looking pulmonary radiographs.[6] In children, symptomatic endobronchial TB is most common in children under 4 years of age and symptoms arise from airway compromise.[13,14] Coughing, often severe and paroxysmal, is the most frequent symptom. With progressive obstruction of the airway lumen the child may experience wheezing, stridor, dyspnea, and eventually respiratory distress with hypoxia and cyanosis due to pulmonary atelectasis.

Other uncommon presenting symptoms of tuberculous lymphadenitis include chyluria due to obstruction of the thoracic duct, chronic abdominal pain and low-grade fever due to retroperitoneal lymphadenitis, progressive jaundice due to biliary obstruction, chronic chest pain caused by intercostal lymph node involvement, a neck mass with dysphagia caused by a traction diverticulum of the

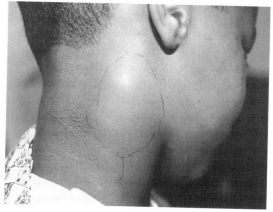

Fig. 18-3. A nine-year-old child with tuberculous lymphadenitis. (Copyright © by the President and Fellows of Harvard College.)

esophagus or retropharyngeal abscess, generalized lymph node enlargement suggesting reticulohistiocytic tumors, vocal card paralysis, or a nasopharyngeal mass.

On physical examination, peripheral tuberculous nodes are initially firm or rubbery, discrete, and nontender. The painless quality usually persists despite caseation and erosion through the skin. Occasionally, in young children, the nodes may be swollen and tender at the time of presentation owing to secondary bacterial infections.[15] The physical appearance of superficial tuberculous lymphadenitis has been classified into five stages by Jones and Campbell[32]: *stage 1*, enlarged, firm, mobile, discrete nodes showing nonspecific reactive hyperplasia; *stage 2*, larger, rubbery nodes fixed to surrounding tissue owing to periadenitis; *stage 3*, central softening due to abscess formation; *stage 4*, collar stud abscess formation; and *stage 5*, sinus tract formation. The majority of cases fall into stages 2 and 3 at the time of their initial presentation.[12]

Tuberculous parotitis rarely presents as acute glandular swelling. More often chronic parotitis develops as an asymptomatic localized lesion enlarging over months to years.[10,11,33–36] These masses are often difficult to distinguish from parotid tumors. In 25–50% of cases, chronically draining sinus tracts may develop which mimic a true branchial cleft fistula. Most patients show few signs of systemic or pulmonary TB. Mild tenderness or spontaneous pain may develop, and late in the course of the swelling, the size of the mass may increase rapidly.[34]

DIAGNOSIS

The differential diagnosis of tuberculous lymphadenitis or parotitis is extensive. Consideration must be given to infections (nontuberculous mycobacteria, viruses, chlamydia, bacteria, fungi, and toxoplasma), neoplasms (lymphoma, sarcoma, adenoma, Warthin tumor, Hodgkin's disease, and, metastatic carcinoma), drug reactions (hydantoin), sarcoidosis, nonspecific reactive hyperplasia, and nonlymphoid neck or parotid swelling (Sjögren's syndrome, sialosis, brachial arch cyst, cystic hygroma, carotid body tumor). In the differentiation of tuberculous disease from other forms of adenitis, medical or social history and chest radiographs may be helpful, particularly in the young child. More than 80% of children have a history of exposure to active TB and chest radiographs showing evidence of recent or active TB.[13–15,21] These findings are uncommon in adults, where less than 20% have a history of tuberculous contact, and less than 30% have chest radiograph abnormalities.[6] Tuberculin skin testing is the most definitive noninvasive diagnostic procedure, yielding positive results in more than 90% of persons with tuberculous lymphadenitis.

Occasionally, there may be difficulty distinguishing tuberculous lymphadenitis from that caused by nontuberculous mycobacteria (NTM), a more common problem in children.[37] Tuberculous lymphadenitis rarely presents as unilateral involvement of the superior anterior cervical nodes in the digastric triangle, a symptom typical of lymphadenitis caused by NTM. Other helpful clues in this distinction are shown in Table 18-2. Although differential skin testing with tuberculin and NTM antigens has proved useful, the NTM antigens are not currently available for routine use.

When diagnosis of tuberculous lymphadenitis remains in doubt, biopsy material must be submitted for histology and culture or polymerase chain reaction (PCR). Total excisional biopsy should be performed because an incomplete biopsy, nearly always results in ulcerations or sinus tract formation. Ideally the solid portion of the node should be cultured and processed for histologic sections, whereas the frankly caseous portion of the node should be stained with rhodamine-auramine and examined by fluorescent microscopy for mycobacteria. The histology

Table 18-2. Comparative Features of Tuberculous and Nontuberculous Mycobacterial Cervical Lymphadenitis

Feature	Tuberculous	Nontuberculous
Age	Any, but peak at 20–40 years	1–6 years
Sex	Females predominate	Equal between sexes
Race	Asians and blacks predominate	None
TB exposure	Common in children	Uncommon
Systemic symptoms	Uncommon	Uncommon
Node involvement	Anterior and posterior cervical, supraclavicular, bilateral	Jugulodigastric, unilateral
Chest roentgenogram	Abnormal in most children, one-third abnormal in adults	Normal
Tuberculin skin test	Usually positive	Commonly positive

of mycobacterial adenitis may include nonspecific lymphoid infiltrates, small noncaseating granulomas, or typical Langhans' giant cells in areas of extensive caseous necrosis. Tuberculous and NTM-infected nodes cannot be differentiated histologically, and distinction from other granulomatous diseases may be difficult. It is, therefore, essential that the biopsy specimen be handled expeditiously in a knowledgeable microbiology laboratory to maximize the possibility of positive culture results.

Fine-needle aspiration of lymph nodes or parotid glands for cytology and culture[38–40] in conjunction with tuberculin skin test results may be an effective method of diagnosis in geographical areas where tuberculous disease is prevalent. Cytologic findings identify granulomatous changes in 50–80% of patients with tuberculous lymphadenitis, but acid-fast bacilli are identified in only 30–60% and cultures are positive in only 20–80%.[39,40] Thus, other causes of granulomatous lymphadenitis must be excluded in a majority of patients unless the tuberculin skin test is strongly positive. The use of PCR dot-Elisa versus Ziehl-Neelson staining or culture of specimens from needle aspiration of tuberculous lymph nodes increased the identification of *M. tuberculosis* to 70–80%.[41,42]

When assessing hilar or mediastinal lymph node involvement, sputum and gastric aspirate cultures are usually negative, and diagnosis is best made by excisional biopsy of an involved lymph node with mediastinoscopy or open thoracotomy. If respiratory symptoms or chest radiographs indicate bronchial obstruction, bronchoscopy should be performed to remove any polyps or granulation tissue seen in the bronchial lumen[28] for histology and culture.

TREATMENT

Management of tuberculous lymphadenitis and parotitis involves appropriate use of antituberculous chemotherapy with the judicious use of surgical excision in a minority of patients. When superficial lymphadenitis is detected before extensive caseation, periadenitis, or erosion has occurred, chemotherapy is nearly always curative. During chemotherapy, up to 25% of patients may have the appearance of new nodes or enlargement, fluctuation or drainage of existing nodes. This complication usually occurs in the first few weeks or months of therapy, but occasionally it develops later, even after a year. Documented microbiologic treatment failure or relapse is rare, however, and these events do not usually require additional chemotherapy or surgery. The American Thoracic Society, Centers for Disease Control and Prevention, and Infectious Diseases Society of America,[43] as well as

the World Health Organization (WHO),[44] recommend a 6-month regimen of therapy for all patients with tuberculosis lymphadenitis caused by drug-susceptible organisms. For adult patients, four basic regimens are recommended including various combinations of isoniazid (H), rifampin (R), pyrazinamide (Z), and ethambutol (E). These recommendations are based on two prospective controlled studies that have demonstrated successful treatment with combinations of H, Z, R, and E or streptomycin (S), for 6 months versus 9 months. In 157 adults with cervical, axillary, or chest wall lymph node TB followed for 9–30 months after therapy, no differences in outcome were demonstrated between the group treated daily for 6 months (Z2H6R6) versus two groups treated daily for 9 months (Z2H9R9 or E2H9R9).[45] Similarly, in 91 adults with cervical lymph node TB followed for a median of 21 months, no differences in outcome were noted between groups treated thrice weekly for 6 months (S4Z4H6R6) versus 9 months (S4Z4H9R9).[46]

For pediatric patients, prospective, controlled trials are limited, but a recent critical review of evidence for short course therapy of tuberculous adenitis in children[47] has recommended following WHO guidelines.[44] These include 2 months HRZ and 4 months HR daily, or 3 times weekly.

It would thus appear that most patients infected with drug-sensitive *M. tuberculosis* can be effectively managed with a 6 month course of combination drug therapy. Data are too few to establish guidelines for treatment of drug-resistant organisms; such cases have generally been excluded from analysis in the published studies. For further details of therapy, please refer to Chapter 7. There are no published trials of therapy for parotitis, so guidelines for lymphadenitis should be followed.

If not done for diagnostic purposes, surgery should be limited to those individuals who fail to show improvement after an adequate course of chemotherapy or who have discomfort from enlarged or tense, fluctuant nodes.[48] Even nodes with sinus tracts and chronic drainage should undergo an attempted trial of chemotherapy prior to surgical removal because initial excision does not seem to affect outcome. The surgery of choice is always complete excision of the involved nodes and surrounding tissue. Incision and drainage carries the same risk of ulceration or chronic sinus drainage as partial surgical excision.

Tuberculous lymph nodes in the mediastinum should also be treated the same as pulmonary TB. Endobronchial TB in children, however, may represent a unique situation in which antituberculous chemotherapy alone may not result in prompt or satisfactory resolution of the illness.[28,49] It is speculated that extensive caseation in the peribronchial lymph nodes makes it difficult for drugs to reach all of the

Table 18-3. Prednisone Therapy for Children with Severe Endobronchial Tuberculosis.*

Dosage (mg/kg/d)	Duration (days)
3.0	3
2.0	3
1.0	24
0.5	4
0.25	3
	37

*To be used only in addition to antituberculous chemotherapy.
Source: Adapted from Nemir RL, Cardona J, Vaziri F, et al. Prednisone as an adjunct in the chemotherapy of lymph node bronchial tuberculosis in childhood: A double-blind study. *Am Rev Respir Dis.* 1967;95:402.

infected tissue. This condition may therefore merit the use of corticosteroids to help control the inflammatory response and resulting bronchial compression. In the only controlled study of its kind, Nemir and colleagues demonstrated that administering corticosteroids within the first 4 months of illness of children with endobronchial TB resulted in significantly more rapid resolution of disease.[49] Unfortunately, no data are available to determine whether there is a beneficial effect on the long-term outcome in terms of bronchiectasis and bronchial stenosis. The recommended corticosteroid regimen is outlined in Table 18-3.

Finally, surgery may also have a role in endobronchial TB in both adults and children. Bronchoscopy in skilled hands may be important for removing intraluminal polyps, granulation tissue and frank caseous necrotic tissue. In some children, repeated bronchoscopic procedures may be necessary to maintain bronchial potency.[28] Rarely, a child or adult with an eroded bronchial wall requires intrathoracic surgery to remove the caseous nodes and patch the bronchial wall erosion.[50]

CONCLUSIONS

Tuberculous lymphadenitis, a disease of great historical interest, may occur more frequently because of the high prevalence of TB and extrapulmonary TB in patients with HIV infection. It is most common in young adult Asian or black females. It usually presents as painless, slowly evolving lymph node enlargement in the head and neck region but may involve any nodes in the body, particularly those in the mediastinum. Tuberculous parotitis is a rare cause of parotid swelling usually detected following parotidectomy. Scrofula must be differentiated

from a variety of tumors, nontumor masses, and infectious diseases, particularly cervical lymphadenitis caused by NTM. Although history, epidemiology, clinical presentation, chest radiographs, and tuberculin skin testing may provide a satisfactory diagnosis, fine needle aspiration or excisional biopsy may be necessary for histology and culture. Partial biopsies or incision and drainage should be avoided to prevent ulceration or chronic sinus drainage. Treatment involves the use of antituberculous chemotherapy with occasional need for surgical excision.

REFERENCES

1. Major RH. *Classic Descriptions of Disease*, 3rd ed. Springfield, IL: Charles C. Thomas: 1945.
2. Maulitz RO, Maulitz SR. The King's Evil in Oxfordshire. *Med Hist.* 1973;17:87–89.
3. Lomax L. Hereditary or acquired disease? Early nineteenth century debates on the cause of infantile scrofula and tuberculosis. *J Hist Med.* 1977;32:356–374.
4. Farer LS, Lowell PM, Meador MP. Extrapulmonary tuberculosis in the United States. *Am J Epidemiol.* 1979;109: 205–217.
5. Trends in tuberculosis—United States, 1998-2003. *MMWR Morb Mortal Wkly Rep.* 2004;53:209–214.
6. Geldmacher H, Taube C, Kroeger C, et al. Assessment of lymph node tuberculosis in Northern Germany. *Chest.* 2002; 121:1177–1182.
7. Maltezou HC, Spyridis P, Kafetzis DA. Extra-pulmonary tuberculosis in children. *Arch Dis Child.* 2000;83: 342–346.
8. Global tuberculosis control. Surveillance, planning, financing, WHO Report 2004, (WHO/CDS/TB/2004). Geneva: WHO; 2004.
9. Chatterjee A, Meera V, Trent Q. Parotid abscess caused by *Mycobacterium tuberculosis. Pediatr Infect Dis J.* 2001;20: 912–914.
10. Hamdan AL, Hadi U, Shabb N. Tuberculous parotitis: A forgotten entity. *Otolaryngol Head Neck Surg.* 2002;126: 581–582.
11. Suoglu Y, Erdamar B, Colhan I, et al. Pathology in focus. Tuberculosis of the parotid gland. *J Laryngol Otol.* 1998; 112:588–591.
12. Kabra SK, Lodha R, Seth V. Tuberculosis in children—what has changed in last 20 years? *Indian J Pediatr.* 69 Suppl. 2002; 1:S5–S10.
13. Inselman LS and Kendig EL. Tuberculosis. In: Chernick V, Boat TF, eds. *Disorders of the Respiratory Tract in Children.* Philadelphia, PA: WB Saunders; 1998:883.
14. Starke TR. Tuberculosis. In: Gershon AA, Hotez PJ, Katz SL, eds. *Infectious Diseases in Children.* St. Louis: CV Mosby; 2004:731.
15. Lincoln EM, Sewell EM. *Tuberculosis in Children.* New York, NY: McGraw-Hill; 1963.

16. Medical Research Council Tuberculosis and Chest Diseases Unit. National survey of tuberculosis notifications in England and Wales. *Br Med J.* 1980;281:895–898.

17. Gonzalez OY, Teeter LD, Thanh BT, et al. Extrathoracic tuberculosis lymphadenitis in adult HIV seronegative patients: a population-based analysis in Houston, Texas, USA. *Int J Tuberc Lung Dis.* 2003;7:987–993.

18. Cantrell RW, Hensen JH, Reid D. Diagnosis and management of tuberculous cervical adenitis. *Arch Otolaryngol.* 1975;101:53–57.

19. Glynn JR, Crampin AC, Ngwira BM, et al. Trends in tuberculosis and the influence of HIV infection in northern Malawi, 1988–2001. *AIDS.* 2004;18:1459–1463.

20. Aaron L, Saadoun D, Calatroni I, et al. Tuberculosis in HIV-infected patients: a comprehensive review. *Clin Microbiol Infect.* 2004;10:388–398.

21. Starke JD, Smith KC. Tuberculous and other mycobacterial infections. In: Feigin RD, Cherry JD, Demmler GL, Kaplan SL, eds. *Textbook of Pediatric Infectious Diseases*, 5th ed. Philadelphia, PA: WB Saunders;2004:1337.

22. Whitford J, Hansman D. Primary tuberculosis of the conjunctiva. *Med J Aust.* 1977;1:486–487.

23. Abrol R., Nagarkar NM, Mohan H, et al. Primary bilateral tuberculous dacryocystitis with preauricular lymphadenopathy: A diagnostic difficulty of recent times. *Otolaryngol Head Neck Surg.* 2002;126:201–203.

24. Crum NF. Tuberculosis presenting as epitrochlear lymphadenitis. *Scand J Infect Dis.* 2003;35:888–890.

25. Khanna R, Prasanna GV, Gupta P, et al. Mammary tuberculosis: report on 52 cases. *Postgrad Med J.* 2002;78:422–424.

26. Prasoon D. Tuberculosis of the intercostal lymph nodes. *Acta Cytol.* 2003;47:51–55.

27. Thami GP, Kaur S, Kanwar AJ, et al. Isolated inguinal tuberculous lymphadenitis. *J Eur Acad Dermatol Venereol.* 2002;16:284–301.

28. Lincoln EM, Harris LC, Bovornkitti S, et al. Endobronchial tuberculosis in children. *Am Rev Tuberc.* 1958;77:271.

29. Jha BC, Dass A, Nagarkar NM, et al. Cervical tuberculous lymphadenopathy: changing clinical pattern and concepts in management. *Postgrad Med J.* 2001;77:185–187.

30. Schuit KE. Miliary tuberculosis in children: Clinical and laboratory manifestation in 19 patients. *Am J Dis Child.* 1979;133:583–585.

31. Al-Serhani AM. Mycobacterial infection of the head and neck: Presentation and diagnosis. *The Laryngoscope.* 2001;111:2012–2016.

32. Jones PG, Campbell PE. Tuberculous lymphadenitis in childhood: The significance of anonymous mycobacteria. *Br J Surg.* 1962;50:202.

33. Suleiman AM. Tuberculous parotitis: report of 3 cases. *Br J Oral Maxillofac Surg.* 2001;39:320–323.

34. Zheng JW, Zhang QH. Tuberculosis of the parotid gland: A report of 12 cases. *J Oral Maxillofac Surg.* 1995;53:849–851.

35. Hunter DC and Thomas JM. Tuberculosis in the parotid region. *Br J Surg.* 1993;80:1008.

36. Coen LD. Tuberculosis of the parotid gland in a child. *J Pediatr Surg.* 1987;22:367–368.

37. Powell DA. Nontuberculous mycobacteria. In: Behrman RE, Kliegman RM, Jenson HB, eds. *Nelson Textbook of Pediatrics.* Philadelphia, PA: WB Saunders; 2004:975.

38. Handa U, Kumar S, Punia RS, et al. Tuberculous parotitis: a series of five cases diagnosed on fine needle aspiration cytology. *J Laryngol Otol.* 2001;115:235–237.

39. Nataraj G, Kurup S, Pandit A, et al. Correlation of fine needle aspiration cytology, smear and culture in tuberculous lymphadenitis: a prospective study. *J Postgrad Med.* 2002;48:113–116.

40. Bezabih M, Mariam DW, Selassie SG. Fine needle aspiration cytology of suspected tuberculous lymphadenitis. *Cytopathol.* 2002;13:284–290.

41. Sung-sook K, Sung-min C, Jong-nam K, et al. Application of PCR from the fine needle aspirates for the diagnosis of cervical tuberculous lymphadenitis. *J Korean Med Sci.* 1996;11:129–132.

42. Jain A, Verma RK, Tiwari V, et al. Development of a new antigen detection dot-ELISA for diagnosis of tubercular lymphadenitis in fine needle aspirates. *J Microbiol Methods.* 2003;53:107–112.

43. Blumberg HM, Burman WJ, Chaisson RE, et al. American Thoracic Society/Centers for Disease Control and Prevention/ Infectious Diseases Society of America: treatment of tuberculosis. *Am J Respir Crit Care Med.* 2004;169:316–317.

44. World Health Organization. Treatment of tuberculosis. guidelines for national programmes, 3rd ed. WHO report 2003, (WHO/CDS/TB/2003). Geneva: WHO; 2003.

45. Campbell IA, Ormerod LP, Friend JAR, et al. Six months versus nine months chemotherapy for tuberculosis of lymph nodes: final results. *Respir Med.* 1993;87:621–623.

46. Yurn APW, Wong SHW, Tam CM, et al. Prospective randomized study of twice weekly six-month and nine-month chemotherapy for cervical tuberculous lymphadenopathy. *Otolaryngol Head Neck Surg.* 1997;116:189–192.

47. McMaster P and Isaacs D. Critical review of evidence for short course therapy for tuberculous adenitis in children. *Pediatr Infect Dis J.* 2000;19:401–404.

48. Ammari FF, Hani AHB, Ghariebeh KI. Tuberculosis of the lymph glands of the neck: A limited role for surgery. *Otolaryngol Head Neck Surg.* 2003;128:576–580.

49. Nemir RL, Cardona J, Vaziri F, et al. Prednisone as an adjunct in the chemotherapy of lymph node bronchial tuberculosis in childhood: A double-blind study. *Am Rev Respir Dis.* 1967;95:402.

50. Yurdakul Y, Aytac A. Surgical repair of the tracheobronchial compression by tuberculous lymph nodes. *Br J Dis Chest.* 1979;73:305–308.

19

Genitourinary Tuberculosis

Sarah J. McAleer
Christopher W. Johnson
Warren D. Johnson, Jr.

HISTORY

Consumption has been seen in humans for more than 6000 years. The remains of ancient skeletons show the characteristic changes of tuberculosis (TB), indicating that the disease has affected man since 4000 B.C.[1]

The first reference to renal involvement was in 1879, when Cohnheim proposed that tubercle bacilli in the blood were eliminated in the urine and became lodged within the urinary tract. Thirty years after Cohnheim's hypothesis, Ekehorn[2] proposed his direct hematogenous theory. He believed that the bacilli were transported, like emboli, to the renal capillaries, where they became trapped and formed tuberculous foci. This theory was accepted and formed on the basis of the belief that TB of the kidney could be treated by nephrectomy.

The pathogenesis of TB remained obscure until 1926 when Medlar[3] published his classic studies of 30 patients who had died from pulmonary TB, none of whom had any clinical evidence of genitourinary disease. He reviewed thousands of serial sections from the kidneys of these patients, which revealed microscopic lesions, almost all bilateral, and in the cortex.[3] Finally, in 1935 Coulaud[4] succeeded in producing primary TB in the renal cortex of rabbits. Two years later, Wildbolz[5] emphasized that renal and epididymal TB did not constitute separate diseases but were local manifestations of the same blood-borne infection.

Surgical intervention was introduced in 1870, when the first nephrectomy was performed for pyonephrosis. The prognosis for these patients was poor and 85% of them died prior to the introduction of antituberculous medications (streptomycin, 1943). Today, the outcomes are excellent with medical therapy alone and surgical intervention is only occasionally required.

INCIDENCE

In the United States, the number of reported cases of TB declined annually until 1985, at which time the trend was dramatically reversed due to the emergence of the HIV/AIDS epidemic.[6] Globally, TB is the most common opportunistic infection in AIDS patients. Other factors that contributed to this resurgence of TB included the increase in immigrant movement, drug abuse, and the development of multi-drug resistant strains of M. tuberculosis.[7] During the past decade, the implementation of stringent public health guidelines and surveillance has succeeded in reversing this trend. Nonetheless, TB remains a serious public health concern worldwide. For example, according to the World Health Organization, in 2002 there were 350 cases of TB per 100,000 people in Africa, as compared to 43 cases per 100,000 people in the Americas and 54 per 100,000 in Europe.[8]

The prevalence of genitourinary TB has decreased in the United States. The percentage of patients with extrapulmonary TB who had genitourinary involvement was 17.9% in 1977, 11.9% in 1986, and 5% in 2003.[9,10] Similarly, in Great Britain, there had been a reduction in the prevalence of genitourinary TB from 4.5% in 1983 to 2.6% in 1993. HIV-infected patients however may be at greater risk for the development of genitourinary TB.[11] The incidence of genitourinary TB is also much higher in developing countries where as many as 15–20% of TB patients have M. tuberculosis in their urine.

The male to female ratio for genitourinary TB is 2:1 and has remained relatively constant. Most patients are between ages 20 and 40 years, but recently more patients in the 45–55-year age group have been affected. Genitourinary TB is uncommon in children under the age of 5 because it typically has a latency period of 3–10 years after the primary infection.

PATHOGENESIS AND PATHOLOGY

Genitourinary TB is caused by metastatic spread of organisms through the blood stream during the initial infection. In urinary TB, the kidney is usually the primary organ affected with other parts of the urinary tract being infected by direct extension. The initial infection occurs in the renal cortex, where the bacilli can remain dormant within granulomas for decades. This dormant infection becomes activated due to failure of the local immune response caused by factors such as corticosteroid use, diabetes mellitus, or coexistent illness. The primary site for infection of the genital tract is often the epididymis in men and the fallopian tubes in women, both by hematogenous spread. Similar to urinary disease, the infection then spreads to adjacent organs by direct extension.

Urinary Tuberculosis

In renal TB progressive necrosis within the granulomas leads to ulceration and deformity of the calicies and can cause sloughing of the papillae. Healing of these lesions, results in fibrosis and infundibular stenosis. Calcification is another common finding in renal TB, seen in up to 60% of patients at the time of diagnosis, and is due to necrosis and healing of the granulomas. In one study, 28% of the excised areas of calcification had viable *M. tuberculosis* in the calcified matrix.[12] Extensive involvement of the kidney can lead to complete parenchymal destruction and loss of function (autonephrectomy).

Tuberculosis of the ureter is invariably an extension of disease from the kidney. Involvement leads to the development of fibrosis and strictures, which are most common at the ureterovesical junction (approximately 10% of patients) but can occur at the pelviureteral junction and rarely in the middle third of the ureter. Disease can spread from the kidney to the bladder causing inflammation and edema of the ureteral orifice. As the disease progresses, the ureteral orifice can become completely obstructed. Tuberculous ulcers are another pathologic feature in the bladder but are rare and always a late finding. Ulcers initially develop at the ureteral orifices and if the disease continues to progress, they disseminate throughout the bladder. Once the disease reaches this stage, even modern chemotherapy may not allow recovery of the bladder sufficiently to enable adequate capacity and reasonable function. In addition to ulceration, fibrosis of the detrusor occurs leading to contraction of the bladder and severe irritative symptoms. Vesicoureteral reflux can also develop due to detrusor fibrosis causing contraction around the ureteral orifices.

Genital Tuberculous

As with TB of the kidney, epididymal disease is caused by metastatic spread through the bloodstream. Retrovasal migration of organisms may occur in acute epididymitis after prostatectomy, but abnormalities in the posterior urethra and extensive destructive lesions in the prostate are rare. Renal and epididymal disease may occur in the same patient but it is by no means universal. Tuberculous orchitis is uncommon and due to infection from the epididymis. Involvement of the testicle without epididymal disease is exceedingly rare.

Another uncommon form of genital TB involves the prostate, which is usually diagnosed incidentally by the pathologist after a transurethral resection of the prostate. It can mimic neoplasia by causing nodularity of the prostate; however, this usually regresses after successful antituberculous therapy.[13] Infection is via hematogenous spread, rather than by contact with infected urine from the upper tracts. Other rare forms of genital TB are penile and urethral disease.

TB of the female pelvis is rare in developed countries, but in developing countries, it is commonly encountered. The true incidence is difficult to estimate because most patients are asymptomatic. Like epididymal and renal disease, it typically results from hematogenous spread of the organism at the time of primary infection. Less than 5% of cases result from direct spread from the bladder, rectum or peritoneum.[10] The fallopian tubes are the most commonly involved female genital organ and the disease is usually bilateral.[14] The infection can seed the endometrium and less frequently, the ovaries, cervix or vagina by direct extension. Pathologically, the fallopian tubes become thickened and scarred and synechiae can develop in the endometrium.[15] Caseating granulomas can be identified in any of these structures on microscopic examination, most commonly after endometrial biopsy or curettage. Occasionally patients can develop a tubo-ovarian abscess, which would also reveal granulomas and possibly bacilli.[16]

CLINICAL FEATURES

Genitourinary TB has a varied and insidious presentation. It is often difficult to diagnose because its symptoms are nonspecific. Therefore, TB should be considered in any patient with longstanding urinary tract symptoms of unknown etiology. Recurrent cystitis can indicate an underlying urinary tuberculous infection with urinary frequency and/or dysuria being common symptoms. In one study of 143 patients the most common presenting symptoms were flank pain (44%), dysuria (43%), hematuria (40%), and urinary frequency (34%).[17] Flank pain or suprapubic pain with urgency are usually indicative of advanced disease.

Urinary TB can also present with acute or chronic renal failure.[18,19] It is a rare presentation because in order to occur, the tuberculous lesions must be bilateral or involve a functionally solitary system. When renal failure does occur it usually is secondary to autonephrectomy or an obstructive uropathy caused by edema or stricture of the ureter.[18,20] Hypertension is a very rare complication of severe unilateral renal TB. It is due to significantly reduced renal blood flow, but can be cured by nephrectomy in select patients.[21,22]

Tuberculous epididymitis may be the presenting symptom of genitourinary TB. It usually presents as a painful, inflamed scrotal swelling but occasionally can present as a draining sinus on the posterior surface of the scrotum. The disease is most common in young, sexually active males with a previous history of active TB. Diagnosis can be difficult if organisms are not isolated from the urine, and the differential diagnosis of epididymo-orchitis must be considered. Tuberculous epididymitis can also present as infertility due to scarring of the epididymis or multiple vasal obstructions.[23,24]

Infertility is the most common presenting symptom of TB of the female genital tract. Other symptoms include abnormal uterine bleeding or pelvic pain. In one study of 72 females with genital TB, 47% presented with infertility, 32% with abdominal/pelvic pain, and 11% with metrorrhagia.[14]

Less common clinical presentations of genital TB include superficial ulcers on the glans of the penis in penile disease. They are indistinguishable from a malignant lesion or a sexually transmitted disease such as syphilis or chancroid. The diagnosis is confirmed by biopsy. These lesions respond rapidly to antituberculous chemotherapy. Vulvar disease also presents with ulcerous lesions on the genitalia. Urethral TB can present as a urethral stricture with a decreased urinary stream and a large postvoid residual. In very extensive disease, patients with genitourinary TB can present with fistulas to the rectum,[25] penis,[26] bladder,[27] or perineum.

DIAGNOSIS

Tuberculin Test

The tuberculin test is carried out by an intradermal injection of a purified protein derivative of tuberculin. An inflammatory reaction occurs at the site of injection, which is maximal between 48 and 72 hours. An area of induration larger than 10 mm is accepted as a positive reaction in the general population. False-positive reactions may occur due to the presence of mycobacteria other then *M. tuberculosis* or because of previous injections of Bacille Calmette-Guérin (BCG). A positive reaction indicates that a person has been infected but not whether the infection is currently active. (See Chap. 5 for details about skin testing).

Urine Examination and Culture

Urine is examined for red blood cells, white blood cells, pH, and concentration. Pyuria with negative routine urine cultures is a classic finding in genitourinary TB. Microscopic hematuria is present in up to 50% of patients, with gross hematuria in 10%. Hematospermia can be seen, although rarely. The urine should also be

routinely cultured for nontuberculous organisms since secondary bacterial infection is seen in about 20% of patients and is most commonly due to *Escherichia coli*.

At least three, and preferably five, consecutive first morning specimens of urine should be cultured for *M. tuberculosis.* Urine cultures are positive in 80–90% of patients with urinary TB. In contrast, cultures from the female genital tract[28] or male seminal fluid are usually negative and are therefore not reliable. It is important to collect all specimens in sterile containers, because unsterilized containers may be contaminated with environmental bacteria. Sensitivity tests should always be carried out on positive cultures.

Polymerase Chain Reaction (PCR)

PCR analysis can be used to rapidly identify *M. tuberculosis* in the urine. It takes approximately 1–2 days, as opposed to the 6–8 weeks required for culture results. In addition, PCR assays offer improved sensitivity and specificity when compared to AFB culture and smear.[29,30] Moussa et al. found that when analyzing pooled urine samples for a *M. tuberculosis* species-specific DNA insertion sequence, the sensitivity and specificity were 96% and 98%, respectively.[30] Pooled urine samples are recommended since urinary excretion of the organism is intermittent and may be missed with a single specimen. Hemal et al. reported that urinary PCR was positive in 94% of 35 patients with genitourinary TB documented by classic IVU findings and the presence of mycobacteria by smear, culture, or biopsy.[29] However, PCR technology has its disadvantages. It requires specialized equipment and trained personnel, which adds expense. Furthermore, the presence of enzyme inhibitors or sample contamination can lead to both false-negative and false-positive results.

RADIOGRAPHY

Plain Abdominal Radiography

The plain abdominal film is useful because it can show calcifications in the renal parenchyma and genitourinary tract (Fig. 19-1). Plain radiographs of the chest and spine are also important to exclude evidence of old or active pulmonary or spinal TB.

Intravenous Urography

High-dose intravenous urography (IVU) (Fig. 19-2) has traditionally been the gold standard for the radiographic diagnosis of genitourinary TB, but in many areas it is being supplanted by computed tomography (CT).

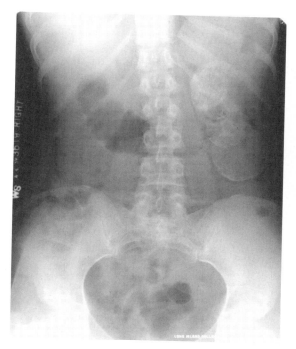

Fig. 19-1. A kidney-ureter-bladder (KUB) in a patient with left renal TB with a calcified nonfunctioning left kidney.

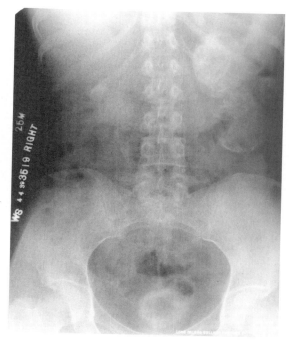

Fig. 19-2. An intravenous pyelogram (IVP) in a patient with left renal TB with no uptake of contrast in the calcified nonfunctioning left kidney.

Renal lesions vary in appearance on IVU. There may be distortion of a calyx secondary to erosion, revealing the typical trifoliate or "moth-eaten" appearance. The calyx may also fibrose, occluding the calyx itself (phantom calyx) or occluding a whole pole of the kidney. Other findings include multiple calyceal deformities or dilatation, cortical scarring and complete destruction of the kidney in advanced disease. Calcification may occur and is always associated with a calyceal lesion. Lastly, ureteral strictures may be visible and in advanced bladder disease, the cystographic phase may reveal a small and contracted bladder, classically referred to as a thimble bladder (Fig. 19-3).

Computed Tomography and Magnetic Resonance Imaging

CT of the abdomen and pelvis has become the imaging modality of choice for the radiological evaluation of genitourinary TB (Fig. 19-4). It is at least the equal of IVU in identifying caliceal abnormalities, hydronephrosis or hydroureter, autonephrectomy, amputated infundibulum, urinary tract calcifications, and renal parenchymal cavities.[31] In a retrospective study of 53 patients with the diagnosis of genitourinary TB, the most common findings on CT were parenchymal scarring (79%), hydrocalycosis, hydronephrosis or hydroureter (67%), and thickening of the walls of the renal pelvis, ureters or bladder (61%).[31] As with IVU, many of the radiographic findings of genitourinary TB are not specific and therefore one must look for multiple abnormalities and consider them in conjunction with the patient's history and presentation.

Unlike IVU, CT allows the identification of other extrapulmonary manifestations of TB. Furthermore, other genitourinary findings such as adrenal necrosis or calcification, a thickened or shrunken bladder, and calcification or caseation in the prostate or seminal vesicles can be identified.[32] Magnetic resonance imaging (MRI) has not provided any advantage over CT or IVU.

Ultrasonography

Ultrasound, while of limited value for the diagnosis of genitourinary TB, is useful to follow patients with

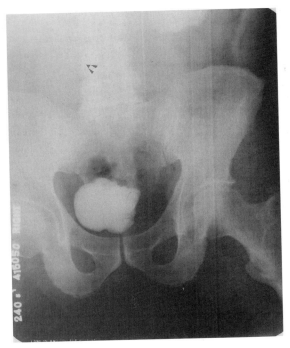

Fig. 19-3. The cystogram portion of an intravenous pyelogram (IVP) in a patient with left renal TB. Notice the contracted left side of the bladder that is secondary to fibrosis from TB.

known disease. Particular instances where ultrasound proves valuable include monitoring obstruction due to ureteral structures, demonstrating change in tuberculous cavities, and evaluating the volume of a contracted

bladder during treatment. Transrectal ultrasound (TRUS) can help in identifying tuberculous prostatitis, which appears as hypoechoic areas usually with an irregular pattern in the peripheral zone of the prostate.

Hysterosalpingography

For the diagnosis of pelvic TB in females, hysterosalpingography is the study of choice. There are no pathognomonic findings, but commonly seen abnormalities include fallopian tube constrictions or obstructions, hydrosalpinx, peritubal adhesions, adnexal or tubal calcifications and distortion of the uterine cavity.[15]

Pyelography, Endoscopy and Biopsy

Retrograde pyelography is rarely necessary because of the accuracy of the IVU and CT. There are however two indications for its use. The first is when there is a stricture of the lower end of the ureter and it is necessary to delineate its length and determine the amount of dilatation above the stricture. The second indication is for ureteric catheterization to obtain selected urine samples for culture from each kidney, when it is unclear which kidney is infected.

Percutaneous antegrade pyelography is an alternative to retrograde pyelography as a means to obtain urine samples from the renal pelvis for diagnostic examination. It also allows for decompression of the kidney when there is severe ureteral obstruction that cannot be bypassed in a retrograde manner.

Biopsy is not advised prior to the initiation of medical therapy due to the concern that it can lead to dissemination of the bacilli and tuberculous meningitis.[33] Biopsy is

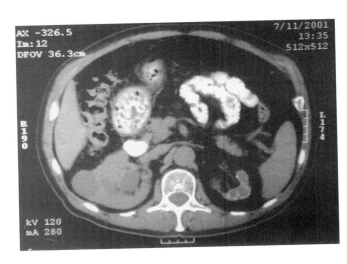

Fig. 19-4. A computerized tomography (CT) scan with oral contrast in a patient with bilateral TB. The right kidney is hydronephrotic secondary to infundibular stenosis, but has retained good function. The left kidney is an end-stage non-functioning atrophic kidney with calcification.

usually only necessary to rule out malignancy in lesions that are distant from the ureteral orifices.

BACILLE CALMETTE-GUÉRIN (BCG) INFECTION

Morales et al. introduced intravesical BCG to treat superficial bladder cancer in 1976.[34] The precise mechanism of action has not been delineated but the attenuated bacillus is thought to induce a cellular immune reaction, which is effective in reducing the recurrence rate of superficial transitional cell carcinoma of the bladder and carcinoma in situ.[35,36] There is no uniform agreement with regard to the treatment duration, however most data suggest that a 6 week course is optimal, followed by a second 3–6 week course as needed.[37]

Intravesical BCG treatment is generally well tolerated, with hematuria being the most common side effect. Persistent fever >38.5 for over 24 hours or fever greater that 39.5°C may warrant treatment with isoniazid for 3 months. Systemic BCG infection may result in hepatic or pulmonary dysfunction and requires treatment with isoniazid and rifampin (with or without ethambutol) for 6 months. Finally, BCG sepsis can rarely occur (<4%) and requires a full antituberculous treatment.[37]

MANAGEMENT

Medical Treatment

Chemotherapy is the cornerstone of treatment for genitourinary TB and is detailed in Chapter 6. The current recommendations for the medical treatment of genitourinary TB are comparable to those for pulmonary TB. Typically a regimen of isoniazid, rifampin, and ethambutinol or pyrazinamide is given for 2 months followed by isoniazid and rifampin for 4 months to patients with drug-sensitive disease. High concentrations of isoniazid, rifampin, and pyrazinamide are achieved in the urine and all the standard drugs penetrate the ureters, bladder and prostate in concentrations that are bactericidal for *M. tuberculosis*. In addition, the relatively small numbers of organisms in the GU tract, as compared to the lungs, contributes to the favorable response of medical treatment. Four-month regimens have been introduced, but have yet to be validated and are therefore not routinely advocated. Treatment for patients with multidrug resistant TB must be tailored to the organism's sensitivity and frequently requires treatment for 1–2 years.

After completion of the course of chemotherapy, the patient should be seen at 3-, 6-, and 12-month intervals, at which time the urine should be examined and cultured to exclude any recurrence. After 12 months without a recurrence, the usual patient can be discharged, unless there are significant calcifications present. Patients with calcifications should be imaged at yearly intervals to ensure that the calcifications are not increasing in size. In developing countries, a longer period of follow-up is indicated in patients with poor nutrition and under social conditions which may decrease compliance with medical treatment. For example, Gokce et al., in a retrospective review of 174 Turkish patients, reported a 19% relapse rate after 12 months of medical treatment.[17]

Corticosteroid therapy has been utilized as an adjunct to standard medical therapy to decrease inflammation and stricture formation;[38] however, this is largely based on anecdotal experience and is not universally advocated.[10,21]

Surgical Treatment

Since the advent of effective antimicrobials for the treatment of TB, the indications for surgical intervention have dramatically decreased. Chemotherapy is of the utmost importance in treatment, and surgery is typically delayed until after 4–6 weeks of antituberculous therapy.

When surgery is required, organ preservation and reconstruction are most common goals, with a shift away from organ resection.[39] Treatment failure despite an adequate course of chemotherapy remains an indication for surgery, however it is rarely required. The typical interventions include repair of ureteral strictures with ureteral reimplantation, dilation, or pyeloplasty to restore proper drainage of the kidney. Patients with severely contracted bladders secondary to longstanding disease may require augmentation cystoplasty, diversion, or neobladder reconstruction. Testicular TB occasionally requires removal of the epididymis after which the testicular lesion rapidly responds to medical therapy. Similarly, prostatic or renal abscesses not responding to medical management alone may require surgical, or more often, percutaneous drainage.

Unfortunately, male and female patients with genital disease who present with infertility do not typically improve with vasovasostomy or tubal reconstruction and therefore IVF is advised.[14,23,28] Additionally, many women with tuberculous endometritis will have difficulty with egg implantation due to the scarring of the endometrium.[28]

Nephrectomy was once commonly advocated for the treatment of nonfunctioning kidneys due to the concern that they harbored latent infection and without removal would allow for relapses. However, the development of effective chemotherapy has made that less of a concern and has called into question the need to perform a nephrectomy for nonfunctioning kidneys.[40,41] Current indications for nephrectomy include persistent fistula formation, hypertension, hemorrhage, or intractable pain. Some groups have also recommended nephrectomy to treat patients with persistent tuberculous cystitis and to prevent stone formation.[42] When nephrectomy is required, it has been shown that both open and laparoscopic removal of the kidney is appropriate and safe.[43,44]

ACKNOWLEDGMENTS

The authors acknowledge the contribution of James G. Gow, MD to the chapter on this subject in the previous edition of his book.

REFERENCES

1. Meyers JA. Chemotherapy in tuberculosis (Editorial). *Dis Chest*. 1952;22:598–600.
2. Ekehorn G. Die Ausbreitumgswerse der Nieren tuberkulose in der tuberkulosen Niere. *Folia Urol*. 1908;2:412.
3. Medlar EM. Cases of renal infection in pulmonary tuberculosis: Evidence of healed tuberculous lesions. *Am J Pathol*. 1926;2:401.
4. Coulaud MD. Etude experimentale de la tuberculose renale du lapin. *J Urol (Paris)*. 1935;39:572.
5. Wildboltz H. Ueber Urogenical tuberkulose. *Schweiz Med Wochenschr*. 1937;67:1125.
6. Small PM, Fujiwara PI. Management of tuberculosis in the United States. *N Engl J Med*. 2001;345:189–200.
7. Wise GJ, Marella VK. Genitourinary manifestations of tuberculosis. *Urol Clin North Am*. 2003;30:111–121.
8. World Health Organization. Estimated TB incidence and mortality, 2002. Available at:http://www.who.int/mediacentre/factsheets/fs104/en/.Accessed November 2004.
9. Centers for Disease Control. Extrapulmonary Tuberculosis Cases and Percentages by Site of Disease: States 2003. Available at:http://www.cdc.gov/nchstp/tb/surv/surv2003/PDF/Table27.pdf. Accessed November 2004.
10. Goldfarb DS, Salman L. Tuberculosis of the genitourinary tract. In: Rom WN, Garay SM, eds. *Tuberculosis*. 2nd ed. Philadelphia, PA: Lippincott Williams & Wilkins; 2004:549–563.
11. Shafer RW, Kim DS, Weiss JP, et al. Extrapulmonary tuberculosis in patients with human immunodeficiency virus infection. *Medicine*. 1991;70:384–397.
12. Wong SH, Lan WY. The surgical management of nonfunctioning tuberculous kidneys. *J Urol*. 1980;124:187–191.
13. Saw KC, Hartfall WG, Rowe RCG. Tuberculous prostatitis: Nodularity may simulate malignancy. *Br J Urol*. 1993;72:249.
14. Saracoglu OF, Mungan T, Tanzer F. Pelvic tuberculosis. *Int J Gynecol Obstet*. 1992;37:115–120.
15. Chavhan GB, Hira P, Rathod K, et al. Female genital tuberculosis: hysterosalpingographic appearances. *Br J Radiol*. 2004;77:164–169.
16. Jahromi BN, Parsanezhad ME, Ghane-Shirazi R. Female genital tuberculosis and infertility. *Int J Gynecol Obstet*. 2001;75:269–272.
17. Gokce G, Kilicarslan H, Ayan S, et al. Genitourinary tuberculosis: A review of. 174 cases. *Scand J Infect Dis*. 2002;34:338–340.
18. Conte G, Iavarone M, Santorelli V, et al. Acute renal failure of unknown origin. Don't forget renal tuberculosis. *Nephrol Dial Transplant*. 1997;12:1260–1261.
19. Nzerue C, Drayton J, Oster R, et al. Genitourinary tuberculosis in patients with HIV infection: Clinical features in an inner-city hospital population. *Am J Med Sci*. 2000;320:299–303.
20. Benn JJ, Scoble JE, Thomas AC, et al. Cryptogenic tuberculosis as a preventable cause of end-stage renal failure. *Am J Nephrol*. 1988;8:306–308.
21. Gow JG. Results of treatment in a large series of cases of genito-urinary tuberculosis and the changing pattern of disease. *Br J Urol*. 1970 ;42:647–655.
22. Flechner SM, Gow JG. Role of nephrectomy in the treatment of non-functioning or very poorly functioning unilateral tuberculous kidney. *J Urol*. 1980;123:822–825.
23. Paick J-S, Kim SH, Kim SW. Ejaculatory duct obstruction in infertile men. *BJU Int*. 2000;85:720–724.
24. Fraietta R, Mori MM, DeOliveira JM, et al. Tuberculosis of seminal vesicles as a cause of azospermia. *J Urol*. 2003;169:1472.
25. Patoir G, Spy E, Cordier R. Trois cas de fistules vesico ou rectales tuberculeuses. *J Urol Nephrol (Paris)*. 1969;75:210–217.
26. Karthikeyan K, Thappa DM, Shivaswamy KN. "Water can" penis caused by tuberculosis. *Sex Transm Infect*. 2004;80:75.
27. Goel A, Dalela D, Gupta S, et al. Pediatric tuberculous vesicovaginal fistula. *J Urol*. 2004;171:389–390.
28. Parikh FR, Nadkarni SG, Kamat SA, et al. Genital tuberculosis—a major pelvic factor causing infertility in Indian women. *Fertil Steril*. 1997;67:497–500.
29. Hemal AK, Gupta NP, Rajeev TP, et al. Polymerase chain reaction in clinically suspected genitourinary tuberculosis: Comparison with intravenous urography, bladder biopsy, and urine acid fast bacilli culture. *Urology*. 2000;56:570–574.
30. Moussa OM, Eraky I, El-Far MA, et al. Rapid diagnosis of genitourinary tuberculosis by polymerase chain reaction and non-radioactive DNA hybridization. *J Urol*. 2000;164:584–588.
31. Wang L-J, Wu C-F, Wong Y-C, et al. Imaging findings of urinary tuberculosis on excretory urography and computerized tomography. *J Urol*. 2003;169:524–528.
32. Harisinghani MG, McLoud TC, Shepard JO, et al. Tuberculosis from head to toe. *Radiographics*. 2000;20:449–470.
33. Naude JH. Reconstructive urology in the tropical and developing world: A personal perspective. *BJU Int*. 2002;89:31–36.

34. Morales A, Edinger D, Brice AW. Intercavity bacillus Calmette Guerin in the treatment of superficial bladder tumours. *J Urol.* 1976;116:180–183.

35. Alexandroff AB, Jackson AM, O'Donnell MA, et al. BCG immunotherapy of bladder cancer: 20 years on. *Lancet.* 1999;353:1689–1694.

36. Bevers RMF, Kurth K-H, Schamhart DHJ. Role of urothelial cells in BCG immunotherapy for superficial bladder cancer. *Br J Cancer.* 2004;91:607–612.

37. Malkowicz SB. Management of superficial bladder cancer. In: Walsh PC, Retik AB, Vaughan ED, Wein AJ, eds. *Cambell's Urology,* 8th ed. Philadelphia, PA: Saunders: 2002:2789–2792.

38. Horne NW, Tulloch WS. Conservative management of renal tuberculosis. *Br J Urol.* 1975;47:481–487.

39. Mochalova TP, Starikov IY. Reconstructive surgery for treatment of urogenital tuberculosis: 30 years of observation. *World J Surgery.* 1997;21:511–515.

40. Bloom S, Wechsler H, Lattimer JK. Results of a long-term study of non-functioning tuberculous kidneys. *J Urol.* 1970;104:654–657.

41. Wechsler M, Lattimer JK. An evaluation of the current therapeutic regimen for renal tuberculosis. *J Urol.* 1975;113:760–761.

42. Skutil V, Obsitnik M. Persistent tuberculous cystitis: The most common indication for nephrectomy in the management of urogenital tuberculosis. *Eur Urol.* 1987;13:57–61.

43. Hemal AK, Gupta NP, Kumar R. Comparison of retroperitoneoscopic nephrectomy with open surgery for tuberculous nonfunctioning kidneys. *J Urol.* 2000;164:32–35.

44. Lee K-S, Kim HH, Byun S-S, et al. Laparoscopic nephrectomy for tuberculous nonfunctioning kidney: Comparison with laparoscopic simple nephrectomy for other diseases. *Urology.* 2002;60:411–414.

20

Musculoskeletal Tuberculosis

Michael K. Leonard, Jr.
Henry M. Blumberg

INTRODUCTION

Musculoskeletal tuberculosis (TB) occurs in more than 10% of persons with extra-pulmonary disease. Vertebral involvement (tuberculous spondylitis or Pott's disease) is the most common type of skeletal TB, accounting for about half of all cases of musculoskeletal TB. The presentation of musculoskeletal TB may be insidious over a long period of time and the diagnosis may be elusive and delayed, as TB may not be the initial consideration in the differential diagnosis. Concomitant pulmonary involvement may not be present, thus confusing the diagnosis even further.

Ancient skeletal remains dating back several thousand years have preserved the history of skeletal TB. Egyptian mummies are some of the oldest specimens and demonstrate evidence of spinal TB, as well as psoas abscesses.[1] Polymerase chain reaction (PCR) has confirmed that these ancient lesions are due to *Mycobacterium tuberculosis* and not *Mycobacterium bovis* as others have suggested.[2] There is also evidence of skeletal TB in pre-Colombian, new world remains.[3] PCR studies have also confirmed these lesions as *M. tuberculosis*.[4,5] These findings also demonstrate that TB was present in the New World prior to arrival of Europeans, which had been a disputed for some time.

Hippocrates in ancient Greece described vertebral TB. Sir Percival Pott in 1779 was the first to describe the modern presentation of the clinical aspects of vertebral TB when he described a patient that had spinal deformity with paraplegia. He even proposed drainage of adjacent paraspinal abscesses, which frequently are seen in skeletal TB and reported improvement in symptoms after the procedure.[6] It was not until the late 19th century, after the description of the tubercle bacillus in 1882, that Pott's disease was linked to illness caused by *M. tuberculosis*.

EPIDEMIOLOGY

The incidence of TB in the United States declined significantly during the 20th century; however, in the mid-1980s there was a marked resurgence of this ancient disease.

Between 1985 and 1992 there were an additional 40,000 cases TB in the U.S. that were not expected. This resurgence of TB was due to several factors including the HIV epidemic, and a breakdown in the public health infrastructure in the U.S. for TB control due to decreases in funding. As cases of pulmonary TB increased, a rise in the number of extrapulmonary disease cases, including musculoskeletal TB, was seen. Enhanced efforts at TB control (including increased funding) were implemented in response to the resurgence and led to a subsequent decline in TB cases and incidence in the U.S. beginning in 1993. In 2003, there were 14,871 cases reported in the U.S. for a case rate which reached a record low of 5.1/100,000.[7] Despite a decline in TB cases nationwide, rates have increased in certain states, and elevated TB case rates continue to be reported in certain populations (e.g., foreign-born persons and racial/ethnic minorities).[7] The decrease in U.S. cases has been primarily due to decreases in U.S. born TB cases. The total number of foreign-borne TB cases has remained relatively stable and the proportion of TB cases occurring among the foreign born in the U.S. has increased and now represents more than half of all U.S. cases. In 2003, foreign-born persons with TB in the U.S. accounted for 53% of all reported cases.[7]

As the number of pulmonary cases has declined in the U.S., the extrapulmonary cases have remained relatively constant such that the percentage of extrapulmonary cases has actually risen. The proportion of U.S. TB cases that are extrapulmonary has gradually but steadily increased from 13.5% in 1975 to 20.4% in 2003.[7] Bone and joint TB have accounted for about 2% of all reported TB cases in the U.S. (Table 20-1); in some series reported from outside the U.S., >6% of TB cases have been due to bone and joint disease.[8] Data from the preantibiotic era demonstrated that half of those with musculoskeletal TB had evidence of coexisting pulmonary disease.[9] As the number of reported TB cases and incidence of TB disease has decreased in the U.S., an increasing racial disparity has been noted with the majority of cases occurring among minorities and the foreign born. For example, among 220 cases of musculoskeletal TB in Los Angeles County between 1990–1995, 72% were foreign borne.[10] This is important for clinicians to remember as multiple studies have shown that immigrants (e.g., foreign born persons) have accounted for an increasing percentage of extrapulmonary TB cases and the diagnosis is often delayed.[8,11] In a study from the United Kingdom of 1,120 TB cases from 1978 to 1987, 6.3% were musculoskeletal and musculoskeletal TB was two times more common in patients from India compared with Caucasian patients from the U.K.[8]

Table 20-1. Total Number of Bone/Joint and Skeletal Tuberculosis Cases in the United States, 1993–2003

Year	Bone/Joint or Skeletal TB cases	Percent of U.S. Cases Due to Bone/Joint or Skeletal TB	All Other Cases Reported	Total U.S. Cases of Tuberculosis
1993	644	2.56	24,464	25,108
1994	574	2.37	23,631	24,205
1995	547	2.41	22,181	22,728
1996	561	2.64	20,650	21,211
1997	514	2.60	19,237	19,751
1998	498	2.72	17,788	18,286
1999	482	2.75	17,019	17,501
2000	457	2.80	15,851	16,308
2001	439	2.75	15,506	15,945
2002	469	3.11	14,588	15,057
2003	436	2.93	14,435	14,871
Total	5621	2.66	205,350	210,971

Source: Centers for Disease Control and Prevention.

Diabetes mellitus, end-stage renal disease, chronic steroid use, and the presence of a hematologic malignancy have all been shown to increase the risk of developing disease after infection with *M. tuberculosis.*[12] HIV coinfection is the most powerful risk factor for progression from infection with *M. tuberculosis* to active disease. The risk of developing TB in a HIV-infected patient with latent TB infection (LTBI) is about 10% per year. Extrapulmonary TB is more common in patients with HIV, but musculoskeletal TB is not necessarily increased in HIV seropositive patients compared to those that are HIV seronegative.[13]

Historically, musculoskeletal TB was a disease of children often seen developing within a few years after primary infection. In developing countries this is still the case. In a series of 194 patients from India with musculoskeletal TB, 30% of cases occurred during the second decade of life, 22% occurred in the first decade, 185 in the third decade, and 14% in the fourth decade.[14] However, in developed countries with a lower prevalence of TB, musculoskeletal TB is seen more frequently in the adult age group, especially among foreign born persons.

Vertebral TB is the most common site for musculoskeletal TB accounting for about 50% cases in most series. In Los Angeles County, 220 cases of musculoskeletal TB were registered between 1990 and 1995; the distribution of sites was as follows: 118 (54%) had vertebral TB; 56 (26%) had joint involvement (29 cases or 13% with knee involvement and 18 or 8% with hip involvement, and 9 (4%) cases with wrist involvement); and 10 (4%) had

soft-tissue/muscle involvement (Table 20-2).[10] A report from India with 194 cases noted of musculoskeletal TB reported the distribution of cases as follows: 49% had vertebral disease (spondylitis), 34 (18%) had involvement of the knee, 32 (16%) had hip involvement, 15 (8%) ankle/foot, 8 (4%) elbow, 4 (2%) had hand involvement, and 3 (1%) had wrist involvement.[14] Other sites in this series with two or fewer cases included ileum, shoulder, rib, pubis, calcaneus, femur, and sacro-iliac joint. Tuberculosis affecting the peripheral joints, skull, and ribs is uncommon.[15]

PATHOGENESIS

In skeletal TB, the basic lesion generally consists of a combination of osteomyelitis and arthritis. Bone involvement usually occurs by hematogenous spread of *M. tuberculosis* (especially occurring following primary infection) but bone and joint involvement can also be due to lymphatic drainage or secondary to a contiguous focus of the disease. The growth plates (metaphyses) receive the richest blood supply and are most often the initial site of infection. Tubercle bacilli invade the end arteries causing an endarteritis and bone destruction through the epiphysis. After crossing the epiphysis, bacilli can drain into the joint space, resulting in tuberculous arthritis or form a sinus tract after being released from the destroyed bone. *M. tuberculosis* does not produce any cartilage destroying enzymes as is seen in pyogenic infections. If the infection progresses without treatment, abscesses surrounding the

Table 20-2. Anatomic Site of Musculoskeletal Tuberculosis Reported in Los Angeles County from 1990 to 1995

Group	Site	No.	% of Group	% of Total
I. Spine	Cervical	6	5.1	2.7
118 cases	Thoracic	45	38.1	20.5
	Lumbar	65	55.1	29.5
	Sacrum	2	1.7	0.9
II. Peripheral joints	Hip	18	23.1	8.2
78 cases	Knee	29	37.2	13.2
	Ankle	5	6.4	2.3
	Foot	7	9.0	3.2
	Shoulder	4	5.1	1.8
	Elbow	5	6.4	2.3
	Wrist	9	11.5	4.1
	Finger	1	1.3	0.5
III. Other	Other bone	14	58.0	6.4
24 cases	Soft tissue and muscle	10	42.0	4.4

joint or bone may develop. These are often described as being "cold" abscesses. The abscesses may rupture forming sinus tracts, which have long been associated with musculoskeletal TB. Healing of musculoskeletal TB, especially of the joints, involves the formation of fibrous scar tissue. Calcifications are also frequently seen in healed lesions, especially if an abscess, infected bursa, or paraspinous mass were involved. A calcified psoas muscle in someone with healed Pott's disease is a classic example of this. The same hematogenous spread of tubercle bacilli can also primarily infect the synovium, bursae, or tendon sheaths although this occurs much less frequently than bone involvement.

In children, the main route of infection in skeletal TB is through hematogenous spread from a primary source. Children may also experience musculoskeletal TB from reactivation of a quiescent focus after the development of latent TB infection as occurs not uncommonly among adults. Children historically have been most affected with musculoskeletal TB because of the increased vascularity of their bones during growth, thus making them more susceptible during the period of hematogenous dissemination (e.g., following primary infection). Large weight bearing bones and joints are the most commonly affected. Muscles are rarely primarily infected in adults or children, but tuberculous myositis may occur secondarily from contiguous bone infection or a draining sinus tract as is seen with psoas muscle involvement that occurs secondary to Pott's Disease.[16]

After the dissemination of bacilli to the bone, a granulomatous inflammatory response ensues. Biopsies of bone samples from those with skeletal TB reveal few organisms as compared with pulmonary TB. The infected area consists of abscess and granulation tissue and histologically, there are giant cells, epithelioid histiocytes, a mantle of lymphocytes and plasma cells, with an outer layer of proliferating fibroblasts and granulation tissue. As the area of infection enlarges, the center becomes necrotic resulting in an area of caseating necrosis. This caseation may progress to cause bone expansion and eventually destruction of the cortex. A pathologic feature of tuberculous osteomyelitis is that there is no bone regeneration (sclerosis) or periosteal reaction.[17]

PATHOPHYSIOLOGY

Tuberculous Spondylitis

Sir Percival Pott described the classic presentation of vertebral TB in 1779 as destruction of two or more contiguous vertebrae and apposed end plates, commonly associated with a paraspinal mass or abscess.[18] In 1936, Compere and Garrison from the University of Chicago provided classic descriptions of vertebral TB, comparing radiologic findings with pathology and autopsy findings.[19] They also compared findings at autopsy of patients with tuberculous spondylitis and pyogenic infections. Their descriptions of tuberculous spondylitis noted that the anterior portion of the vertebral body is much more commonly affected than the posterior components of the vertebrae. From this site, TB may spread to adjacent intervertebral disks. More than one vertebra is usually involved because of the contiguous spread along the anterior longitudinal ligaments. Skip lesions can also occur.

Tuberculous spondylitis begins with infection of the subchondral bone that spreads to the cortex. The cartilage resists destruction by *M. tuberculosis* and despite there being a rich blood supply to the vertebrae, there is no blood supply to the disk.[20] The anterior portion of the vertebral body is the most affected with sparing of the posterior components. Involvement of the posterior components (i.e., laminae, pedicles, transverse processes, and spinous processes) is rare.[21] In children, the intervertebral disk is vascularized—therefore tuberculous diskitis in children may be the result of primary infection. In adults, the disk is avascular and disk disease is due to the contiguous spread of infection from the vertebral body. The narrowing disk space visible in adults on plain radiography is more often due to collapse of the vertebral end plate rather than to destruction of the disk itself.[22] Collapse of the anterior spinal elements results in a kyphotic deformity giving the hunchback appearance and gibbus deformity associated with Pott's disease. Tuberculosis of the vertebral skeleton causes lytic destruction without new bone formation (sclerosis). The infection can extend to the soft tissue forming paraspinal abscesses. The degree of the kyphosis is proportional to the initial loss of vertebral body volume and continues until the vertebral bodies meet anteriorly or until the caseous material and granulation tissue mature into bone.[23]

The lower thoracic and upper lumbar vertebral bodies are the most affected in patients with skeletal TB.[17] Cervical and sacral involvement occurs less frequently. Historically, the thoracic vertebrae have been most commonly affected area of the spine but more recent reports have suggested that among adults, lumbar involvement is most common. Of 118 cases of vertebral TB reported from a series in Los Angeles, 65 patients had lumbar tuberculous spondylitis, 45 thoracic, 6 cervical, and 2 sacral. Cervical involvement though uncommon, is frequently associated with retropharyngeal abscess and severe neurologic defects.[24] In a series from South Africa where 25 children had spinal TB, 18 (72%) had involvement of thoracic vertebrae and 7 (28%) had involvement of lumbar vertebrae.[25]

Paraplegia is the most serious complication of tuberculous spondylitis. Rarely does it result directly from the kyphotic defect unless it is severe enough to cause subluxation of the spine. Paraplegia can be due to compression of the spinal canal by an adjacent abscess, sequestra of the vertebral body or disc or direct dural invasion. Cervical vertebral TB is highly associated with early and severe neurologic compromise.[26]

Paraspinal abscesses are quite common in vertebral TB occurring in more than 90% of cases. The abscess may extend anteriorly to adjacent ligaments and soft-tissues or it may also extend posteriorly into the epidural space. Because the abscesses can spread beneath the ligament, distant sites may be involved. There are also reports of tuberculous paraspinal abscesses eroding into internal organs or to the body surface.[27] Lumbar disease may spread into or beneath the psoas-iliac muscle causing abscesses in the thigh. Sacral lesions have been reported to extend into the perineum.

Pyogenic abscesses differ from vertebral TB in several ways. Pyogenic abscesses destroy the disc rapidly resulting in early disc space narrowing. Calcification of a large paraspinous abscess, which may be seen with TB, is not a prominent feature of a pyogenic abscess. In a study comparing pyogenic, tuberculous, and brucellar vertebral osteomyelitis in Spain, patients with vertebral TB were more likely to have a prolonged clinical course, thoracic segment involvement, absence of fever, presence of spinal deformity, neurologic deficit, and paraspinal or epidural masses.[28]

Tuberculous Osteomyelitis and Arthritis

Tuberculous osteomyelitis may extend to a joint or tendosynovium. In adults the lesion may be single and affect any bone, including long bones, the pelvis, ribs, and skull. In children, multiple lesions in long bones dominate but the bones of the hands and feet may be affected. Tuberculous dactylitis (involvement of the short bones of the hands or feet) is more common among children than adults. Tuberculous osteomyelitis has a predilection for the metaphysis of long bones such as the femur, tibia, and ulna. In children, TB may violate the growth plate and lesions of the epiphysis may extend into the joint space. Destruction of the epiphyseal growth plates in children can also result in shortening of the limb. Although uncommon, TB can also involve the ribs and skull. The skull contains little cancellous bone, which is usually affected by *M. tuberculosis*. Disease involving the skull occurs more often in children, and anecdotally may be associated with head trauma.[29] In a review of 223 cases of TB involving the skull, Strauss found that only 15 had associated central nervous system disease (10 with meningitis and 5 with cerebral TB). This is thought to be due to the dura being resistant to infection with *M. tuberculosis*.[30] Tuberculosis of the ribs can occur either by hematogenous seeding of the ribs or in some cases due to

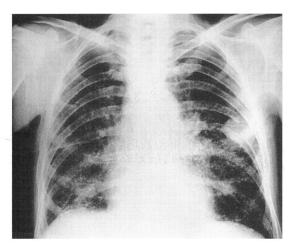

Fig. 20-1. Tuberculosis of the rib: A posteroanterior radiographic view of the chest of a man after 3 months of successful antituberculosis chemotherapy. Note the mass in the left chest with destruction of a portion of the adjacent rib. A biopsy and culture confirmed TB. The mass resolved with continued therapy.

contiguous spread in a patient with pulmonary disease. Tuberculosis of the ribs (Fig. 20-1) is an uncommon manifestation of the disease but is the second most common cause of nontraumatic rib lesions after malignancy.[31] A closed cystic form of skeletal TB can occur, especially in the long bones, and may not have associated sclerosis, osteopenia, or abscess/sinus tract formation as in other forms of skeletal TB. This form of TB is more likely to occur in children and may be misdiagnosed as a malignancy.[32,33]

Tuberculous osteomyelitis is frequently complicated by tuberculous arthritis (discussed below) as well as by the development of "cold" abscesses that may form around the adjacent bone process and can rupture creating draining sinus tracts (Fig. 20-2). Cold abscesses are composed of white blood cells, products of caseating necrosis from the tubercle, bone debris, and tubercle bacilli. Cold abscesses appear to occur commonly among HIV-infected patients.

Several reports have noted an association between mechanical factors such as trauma and the development of skeletal TB. In a Canadian study of 99 patients with skeletal TB, 30 had a history of trauma preceding their presentation and 7 had a recent history of intraarticular steroid injection.[34] This may also explain why weight-bearing joints are most frequently involved. Trauma may be associated with skeletal TB because of resulting increased vascularity, decreased resistance, or unmasking of latent infection.[29,35]

Tuberculous Arthritis

Tuberculous arthritis most typically involves large weight bearing joints such as the hip and the knee, although any other joint may be affected. Invasion of the joint space may be either hematogenous seeding or indirectly from lesions in epiphyseal bone (in adults) or metaphyseal bone (in children) eroding into the joint space. Contiguous spread of TB from other organs to bones may also occur. In long bones, hematogenous spread commonly affects the synovium, causing an erosive deforming arthritis that is

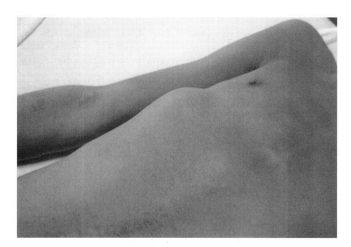

Fig. 20-2. A "cold abscess" of the chest wall in an HIV-negative patient.

monoarticular in about 90% of cases. Initially the synovium develops an inflammatory reaction followed by formation of granulation tissue, which leads to the development of a pannus. The pannus can erode the margins and surface of the joint. As the effusion develops, fibrin may precipitate forming "rice bodies" seen in the synovial fluid, bursae and tendon sheaths. Rice bodies are not unique to TB as they can also be seen in rheumatoid arthritis. The infection then spreads to the epiphysis and upper metaphysis on either side of the joint through the periarticular vasculature. The granulation tissue erodes and eventually destroys the cartilage, eventually leading to demineralization of the bone and caseating necrosis. In advanced and late disease, para-osseous cold abscesses develop surrounding the joints. Spontaneous drainage of cold abscesses results in sinus tract formation.

Poncet Disease (Poncet's Arthritis)

Poncet Disease is a reactive polyarthritis associated with visceral or disseminated TB in the absence of any evidence of mycobacterial infection of the joints. Poncet Disease was originally described by Charcot in 1864 and Lancereaeaux in 1871 but Anton Poncet first gave a detailed description of this syndrome when he described polyarthritis occurring in a 15 year-old with suppurative TB of the hip in 1897.[36] Poncet's arthritis is a reactive form of arthritis and is a separate entity from TB directly affecting joint spaces. Usually it occurs during acute TB infection and is a polyarticular process associated with fever. The pathogenesis is unclear. As noted, joint fluid analysis does not reveal the presence of *M. tuberculosis* in the joint space and clinical symptoms resolve with antituberculosis therapy.

Tuberculous Myositis

Tuberculous myositis is an uncommon manifestation of the disease and usually the result of contiguous infection, especially seen in Pott's disease.[37,38] Tuberculous myositis can also be "primary" (i.e., a cause of pyomyositis), resulting from hematogenous spread but this is a less common manifestation of disease and much less likely to occur than myositis due to secondary or contiguous spread.[16,39] The tuberculous lesion of primary myositis may present as a solitary nodule with epithelioid granuloma and caseating necrosis or a cystic formation containing a gelatinoid material enclosed by a thick wall.[40] The most common presentation of tuberculous myositis is a psoas abscess due to a complication of and contiguous spread from tuberculous spondylitis, and may extend below the inguinal ligament.[37] Tuberculous myositis has been reported more frequently among HIV-infected patients.[41]

CLINICAL FEATURES

The onset of musculoskeletal TB is usually an insidious process that takes months to years from the first symptoms to the time of diagnosis. Local pain and tenderness are generally the presenting symptoms followed by impairment of function and swelling of the affected part. Regional muscle wasting and joint deformity are common findings. A painless cold abscess (Fig. 20-2), may be the only presenting clinical feature for an extended period of time. Systemic symptoms such as fever, night sweats, and weight loss may be seen with early disease but are more likely to occur with advanced cases. About half of the cases of musculoskeletal TB have evidence of active or healed pulmonary TB.[14] A single site of involvement is generally seen, but multiple locations are not uncommon. Multiple lesions occur more often in those who are immunocompromised, including persons with HIV infection. Several studies have reported that >90% of patients with musculoskeletal TB were tuberculin skin test positive[34,42]; however, these studies were largely carried out in the pre-HIV era.

Tuberculous Spondylitis

Tuberculous spondylitis remains the most common manifestation of musculoskeletal TB. The progression of disease is usually slow and insidious and the main symptom, back pain, is not specific. This frequently results in delayed diagnosis resulting in diagnosis from weeks to years after the onset of symptoms. Pertuiset reported a median of 4 months duration of symptoms prior to diagnosis with a range of 1 week to 3 years among 103 patients with spinal TB and noted weight loss in 48%, fever (>38°C) in 31%, and night sweats in 18%.[43] As the disease advances cold abscesses, neurologic deficits, sinus tract formation, and kyphotic deformities can develop. Cold abscesses of the paraspinal tissues or psoas muscle abscesses may be large and protrude under the inguinal ligament when a patient is examined for the first time. Some degree of kyphosis is frequently present. Weakness and paralysis of the lower extremities may occur early during the course of the disease. HIV infection has not been shown to alter the clinical presentation or course of tuberculous spondylitis.[13]

On physician examination, there may be focal tenderness over the spinal processes as well as back spasm. Fluctuance, erythema, or focal warmth on examination are unusual findings as the spinal infection typically involves the anterior column of the spine.[44] Range of motion testing may produce severe pain and especially with advanced disease, focal kyphosis can be seen on physician examination. Neurologic symptoms may be subtle at first and progress over time. Initially these include numbness and tingling in the lower extremities or a subjective sense of weakness with activity. With more advanced disease there is evidence of spinal cord compression, which can result in paraplegia. Between 10 to 25% of patients in reported case series have had paraplegia.[43] Cervical lesions are prone to developing neurologic compromise very quickly and are almost always associated with retropharyngeal abscesses.[24,45,46] Cervical TB can also present with torticollis, dysphagia, hoarseness, and cranial nerve 12 palsy, depending upon which level of the cervical spine is affected.[47] The degree of neurologic damage correlates with prognosis with those presenting with complete motor loss are unlikely to recover neurologically. Extrinsic cord compression can occur due to vertebral subluxation, collapse of a vertebral body or an extradural abscess.

Tuberculous Arthritis

Tuberculous arthritis usually occurs as a monoarthritis usually of weight-bearing bearing joints. It is slowly progressive and characterized by painful, boggy swelling caused by synovial hypertrophy and effusion (Fig. 20-3). Eventually ankylosis of the joint may occur. Periarticular abscesses and draining sinus tracts are late findings. Pain is such a prominent symptom that it may lead to immobility of the affected joint. Prolonged immobility may eventually lead to deformity, especially of the knee and hip. Tuberculous arthritis clinically can mimic other processes such as gout or juvenile rheumatoid arthritis making the diagnosis confusing and delayed.[48] Polyarticular tuberculous arthritis has been reported but is rare.[49]

Tuberculous Osteomyelitis

Tuberculous osteomyelitis often occurs in conjunction with tuberculous arthritis, but can occur as a distinct entity without joint involvement. In adults, tuberculous osteomyelitis without joint involvement usually presents as a single lesion, usually in the metaphysis of long bones (e.g., femur and humerus) although ribs, pelvis, skull, mastoid and mandible can be affected. In children, older adults and immunocompromised persons including those with HIV infection, the lesions may be multiple.[50] In children the lesions may affect the short bones of the hand and feet; tuberculous dactylitis has been reported in adults but is unusual. Patients with widespread lesions may be misdiagnosed as having a malignant process. Bacterial superinfection can also mask the diagnosis and presentation as there are a number of reports of infection due to coexisting *Staphylococcus aureus* and TB.[51,52]

Tuberculous osteomyelitis usually presents with pain and swelling adjacent to the bone with eventual limitation of movement of the affected limb. Symptoms may be present for 6–24 months before a diagnosis is made. Fever, weight loss, and night sweats are often present. Abscesses and sinus tracts may occur, often later in the course. Tuberculous involvement of the skull may be associated with headaches and soft tissue masses. Tuberculosis involving the ribs presents with chest pain and sometimes with a "cold" chest wall mass (Fig. 20-2). Infection of bones of the head and neck, especially mastoids and mandible has been reported as a result of tuberculous otitis and disease involving the oral cavity. Facial paralysis can occur secondarily to tuberculous mastoiditis.[53] Tuberculosis of the temporomandibular joint (TMJ) has also been reported as a cause of chronic

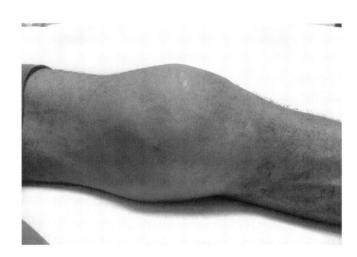

Fig. 20-3. An HIV-infected patient presented with a painful, swollen knee after being hit with a piece of wood. On examination the knee was warm and an effusion was present. At the time of presentation the patient had recently been started on INH for LTBI for about 2 months. Culture of the knee aspirate grew *Mycobacterium tuberculosis* that was susceptible.

TMJ pain.[54] Tuberculosis of the sternum can present with anterior chest pain.[55]

Tuberculous Tenosynovitis

Tuberculous tenosynovitis is rare and usually occurs in conjunction with another form of skeletal TB, i.e., TB of the carpal bones in the hand or rarely hematogenous spread to the synovium.[56] The most common presentation is carpal tunnel syndrome.[57] Carpal tunnel syndrome occurs when the median nerve, going through the flexor compartment of the wrist, is compressed secondarily to thickening and edema of the tendon sheath. Diagnosis is often made late in the course due to its slow progression, indolent symptoms, and the fact that the diagnosis may be delayed because infectious causes are not considered initially.[58] Presenting symptoms include swelling followed by wrist pain, numbness and tingling of the fingers, and decreased range of motion.[56] Other causes of carpal tunnel syndrome in the differential diagnosis include trauma, diabetes, amyloidosis, and sarcoidosis. Another presentation of tuberculous tenosynovitis is a ganglion formation along the volar carpal ligament that presents with soft-tissue swelling above the flexor retinaculum.[59]

DIAGNOSIS

In countries with a high burden of TB disease, musculoskeletal complaints may be attributed to TB correctly based on clinical and radiological examination. In the developed world with a lower prevalence of TB, the diagnosis may not be initially considered and the diagnosis is frequently delayed. Any bone or joint may be involved but the spine and weight-bearing joints are the most common sites of infection. Pain is the most common complaint that leads a patient to seek medical care and TB should be considered in the differential diagnosis of the cause of skeletal pain. Interestingly, local pain, swelling, and limitation of movement may even on occasion precede radiographic findings by up to 8 weeks.[60] Cold abscesses can occur and sometimes with draining sinus tracts, but this is usually seen in advanced, untreated disease or among patients with HIV infection. The differential diagnosis of musculoskeletal TB includes other infectious causes of musculoskeletal disease (bacterial, fungal, other mycobacterial pathogens), as well as malignancy, rheumatologic conditions, and sarcoidosis.

The tuberculin skin test (TST) is currently the most widely used diagnostic test for latent TB infection (LTBI) and until recently was the only diagnostic test for detection of LTBI. There are limitations of TST in sensitivity (e.g., anergy which is common in immunocompromised persons) and specificity; false positive tests can be seen due to cross reactivity with environmental nontuberculous mycobacteria. In addition, the tuberculin skin test is unable to distinguish between infection with *M. tuberculosis* and *Mycobacterium bovis* BCG among those who have received BCG vaccination.[12] The interpretation may also be reader dependent. A positive skin test result may be helpful but a negative result does not rule-out the presence of LTBI or active disease. A positive tuberculin skin test in the presence of bone or joint complaints should make one strongly consider musculoskeletal TB. However, a negative tuberculin skin test does not rule out active TB disease and definitive diagnosis of skeletal TB depends on recovery of *M. tuberculosis* from mycobacterial culture of appropriate specimens. The role of newer diagnostic tests for LTBI (such as the γ-interferon release assay or ELISPOT tests)[61,62] in diagnosing active TB remains to be determined.

Imaging techniques which include conventional radiography, computed tomography (CT), and magnetic resonance imaging (MRI) are useful in evaluation of the patient with suspected musculoskeletal TB and other skeletal diseases. Use of newer techniques such as CT, MRI, and CT-guided fine-needle aspiration biopsy have revolutionized the diagnostic approach and have resulted in more accurate results and much less invasive procedures than when only plain radiography and open biopsy were available.

Conventional radiography had been the mainstay in the diagnosis of tuberculous arthritis and osteomyelitis; however MRI may detect associated bone marrow and soft tissue abnormalities.[17] MRI is generally accepted as the imaging modality of choice for diagnosis of tuberculous spondylitis and can demonstrate the extent of the disease of tuberculous spondylitis and soft tissue TB.[17] Moreover, MRI may be very helpful in providing diagnostic clues in the evaluation of spondylodiscitis, as it may easily demonstrate anterior corner destruction, the relative preservation of the intervertebral disk, multilevel involvement with or without skip lesions, and a large soft tissue abscess, as these are all arguments in favor of a tuberculous spondylitis (vs. a pyogenic infection). On the other hand, CT is still superior in the demonstration of calcifications, which are found in chronic tuberculous abscesses. Fine needle aspiration biopsy of involved bone to obtain specimens for culture is useful diagnostically as well as for the draining of abscesses in certain situations. In addition to modern culture techniques performed on specimens obtained by biopsy of involved tissues, the use of molecular diagnostics has also added to the ability to detect the presence of *M. tuberculosis* and should continue to improve the ability to diagnosis skeletal TB as methods are further refined.[63] Establishing a definitive diagnosis by recovering *M. tuberculosis* is essential in order for susceptibility testing to be performed to help guide therapy.

Tuberculous Spondylitis

Plain radiography is often the first imaging technique employed when considering tuberculous spondylitis. At least 50% of the vertebra needs to be destroyed before it can be detected on plain radiography making it an insensitive diagnostic tool (Fig. 20-4).[17] Plain radiography may reveal several features indicative of tuberculous spondylitis such as osteoporotic end-plates, multiple levels involved, and

Table 20-3. Radiographic Characteristics of Tuberculous Spondylitis

Multiple levels involved
Lytic destruction of anterior portion of vertebral body
Disc space narrowing
Vertebral end-plate osteoporosis
Increased anterior wedging
Collapse of vertebral bodies
Paravertebral shadow of an abscess sometimes
    with calcification
Enlarged psoas muscle shadow often with calcifications

anterior destruction leading to collapse (Table 20-3). Sometimes a paravertebral abscess or enlarged psoas muscle may be observed on plain radiography. Plain radiography will show calcifications in abscesses if they are present. Atypical features that may be seen on radiography include involvement of posterior elements, single vertebral involvement, and an "ivory" vertebra, that is the result of diffuse sclerosis.[64]

Nuclear medicine imaging is not very useful in diagnosing tuberculous spondylitis because of low sensitivity and is not recommended as a diagnostic imaging modality in the evaluation of patients with spondylitis. CT scanning is superior to both plain radiography and nuclear medicine imaging. CT has also proved useful in determining the extent of soft-tissue infection such as abscesses and draining sinus tracts, as well as soft-tissue calcifications (Fig. 20-5). Irregular lytic lesions, sclerosis, and disc collapse all can be demonstrated on CT. CT is also very helpful in providing guidance for percutaneous drainage and biopsy of vertebral associated lesions and abscesses.[65]

However, as noted above, MRI is now generally accepted as the imaging modality of choice for the evaluation of patients with suspected tuberculous spondylitis and may be very useful in the evaluation of soft tissue TB.[17] MRI allows the entire spine to be viewed and provides high contrast resolution. By comparing T1-weighted and T2-weighted images, one can accurately differentiate various diseased tissues and delineate clearly vertebral bodies, detect marrow infiltration, intervertebral discs, intraspinal contents, posterior vertebral components, meningeal involvement, and paraspinal tissues[66] (Fig. 20-6). The early inflammatory, bone marrow changes that are able to be viewed with MRI also allow for an earlier radiologic diagnosis of tuberculous spondylitis.[17] MRI best demonstrates the origin of the pathologic tissue causing spinal cord compression (Fig. 20-6A) by differentiating pus and granulation tissue from the bony, discal, or fibrotic causes

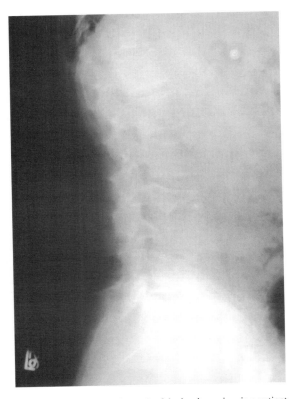

Fig. 20-4. Plain film radiograph of the lumbar spine, in a patient with culture positive TB, demonstrating anterior end-plate destruction, sclerosis, loss of disc space, and evidence of bony debris, which are all suggestive signs of TB spondylitis.

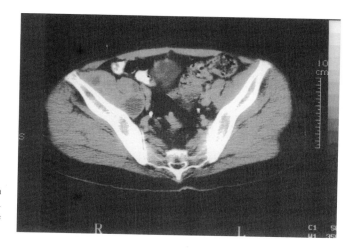

Fig. 20-5. A large right Psoas abscess is present in an HIV-infected patient with lumbar TB spondylitis. A percutaneous drain was placed and the fluid culture also grew *Mycobacterium tuberculosis.*

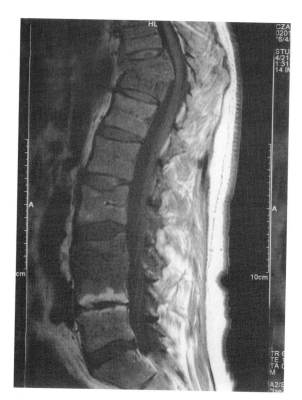

Fig. 20-6. MRI of a patient with known TB spondylitis. There is evidence of both thoracic and lumbar disease. The thoracic lesion reveals anterior collapse of adjacent vertebrae and a gibbus formation leading to kyphosis. There is also evidence of lumbar disease in this patient who has multi-focal TB spondylitis or "skip lesions".

of compression, thus helping to avoid unnecessary and aggressive surgical decompression.[58]

Newer imaging techniques are helpful distinguishing tuberculous spondylitis from other infectious etiologies and from neoplastic processes (Table 20-4). The combination of clinical findings, characteristic lesions on plain radiography, CT, and MRI, and sometimes either with a positive TST or evidence of pulmonary TB, strongly suggests the diagnosis of tuberculous spondylitis.

Table 20-4. Imaging Features Suggestive of Tuberculous Spondylitis versus other Infectious Etiologies

More than one vertebra involved
Multicentric involvement
Relative sparing of the disc
Large paravertebral abscess
Paravertebral osseous debris
Subligamentous spread
Heterogenous signal intensity on MRI
Rim enhancement pattern on MRI
Imaging features suggestive of tuberculous
  spondylitis versus neoplastic disease
Paravertebral abscess
Paravertebral osseous debris
Subligamentous spread
Predominant distribution adjacent to end plates
  or vertebral corners

Source: Table adapted from Griffith, Clin Orth Rel Res, 2002.

Diagnostic imaging modalities as described can also be helpful by providing means for a directed biopsy to definitively make the diagnosis by obtaining material for pathological examination and culture and susceptibility testing. It is essential to obtain appropriate specimens for mycobacterial cultures in order to establish a definitive diagnosis.

Tuberculous Arthritis

The classic triad of juxta-articular osteoporosis, peripheral osseous erosion, and gradual narrowing of the joint space are radiologic characteristics of tuberculous arthritis which were described by Phemister in 1933.[67] The joint space is preserved early in the course of tuberculous arthritis as opposed to most pyogenic infections in which there is early destruction of cartilage due to the production of proteolytic enzymes by bacterial pathogens. The radiologic characteristics of pyogenic, tuberculous, and rheumatoid arthritis are shown in Table 20-5. The differential diagnosis of tuberculous arthritis includes bacterial and fungal infections of the joint as well as noninfectious processes (e.g., rheumatologic). Pyogenic (bacterial) arthritis is usually a monoarticular process as is seen with tuberculous arthritis, but the time course is usually more acute in those with a pyogenic bacterial infection compared to the more chronic and initially indolent course seen among patients with tuberculous arthritis. Trauma or bacteremia is frequently associated with pyogenic arthritis. *Nocardia* spp., *Brucella* spp., and *Sporothrix schenckii* can also cause a chronic monoarthritis resembling TB. In addition to pyogenic and other inflammatory processes, pigmented villonodular synovitis, which can cause synovial thickening, and joint erosions, need to be included in the radiographic differential diagnosis.[64]

Radiologic studies may provide some clues to the diagnosis as discussed (Table 20-5) but cannot definitively differentiate bacterial from tuberculous arthritis. Because the process begins with synovial thickening and an effusion, joint space swelling is the first radiographic sign. Bone sequestration and dense triangular collections may be found at the edge of the joint. Marginal erosions are especially prominent in the weight-bearing joints (Fig. 20-7). Sclerosis is usually not seen in tuberculous arthritis except in children where a layered periosteal reaction can be seen.[17,68] Eventually severe joint destruction and fibrous ankylosis occurs when the process is untreated (Figs. 20-8, and 20-9).

Martini[41] summarized the radiologic changes of tuberculous arthritis in the following classification that also reflects the pathogenesis of the infectious process:

1. Stage I: No bony lesions, localized osteoporosis
2. Stage II: One or more erosions or lytic lesions in the bone; discrete diminution of the joint space
3. Stage III: Involvement and destruction of the whole joint without gross anatomic disorganization
4. Stage IV: Gross anatomic disorganization.

CT imaging of the joint may be useful for evaluating bony destruction and soft tissue swelling or abscess, and any evidence of bony sequestration (Fig. 20-10). MRI can detect earlier changes especially synovial thickening and periarticular soft tissue changes and has even been shown to demonstrate rice bodies in the joint space.[69] An absence of marrow enhancement on MRI along with bony erosions is suggestive of tuberculous arthritis rather than a pyogenic process.[68] MRI may reveal hemosiderin deposits in the synovium and demonstrate the erosions that occur with advanced disease and are often centrally located. As discussed below, a definitive diagnosis should be made. Pursuing arthrocentesis in order to obtain appropriate specimens (e.g., synovial fluid) or performing a synovial biopsy in order to obtain specimens for bacterial, fungal and mycobacterial culture is crucial in establishing a definitive diagnosis and in order to recover the organism so susceptibility testing can be performed.

Table 20-5. Radiologic Characteristics in the Differential Diagnosis of Tuberculous Arthritis

	Osteoporosis	**Marginal Erosions**	**Joint Space Narrowing**
Tuberculosis	+	+	Late, mild
Pyogenic	+/−	+	Early, significant
Rheumatoid arthritis	+	+	Early, significant
Gout	Mild, absent	+	0

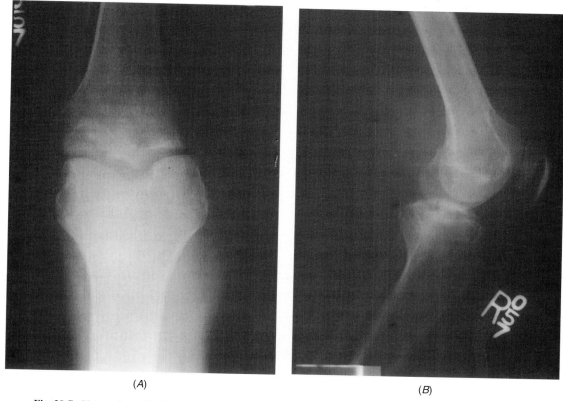

(A) (B)

Fig. 20-7. Plain radiograph of patient in Figure 20-3. Marginal erosions are well seen along with soft tissue swelling.

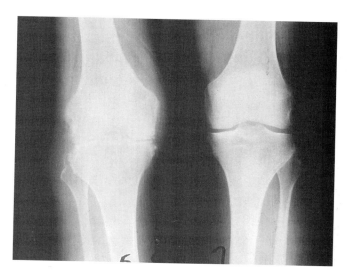

Fig. 20-8. Tuberculosis of the knee. The radiograph shows the normal knee on the reader's right. Note the narrowed joint space, lytic bone destruction in the distal femur and proximal tibia, and soft tissue swelling in the abnormal knee, which has shown clinical evidence of TB for more than 10 years but the patient had not undergone treatment.

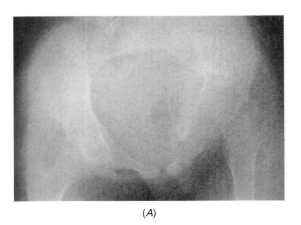

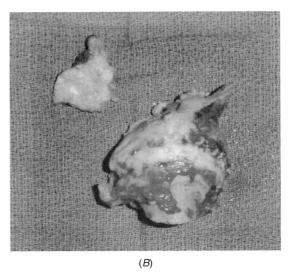

(A)

(B)

Fig. 20-9. (*A*) Plain radiograph of a 12-year-old female with who presented with an abnormal gait for several months. The left femoral head is completely destroyed. (*B*) Operative specimen of the destroyed femoral head.

Tuberculous Osteomyelitis

Radiographically, tuberculous osteomyelitis is often confused with malignancy, especially if the lesions are diffuse and lytic. Plain radiographs may show osteoporosis, lytic lesions, sclerosis, and periostitis. Sequestrae may appear as spicules of increased radiodensity within the area of destruction. Cystic lesions may be seen, especially in children and young adults. The differential diagnosis of cystic bone lesions is in Table 20-6. The lesions in children are less well defined as in adults where well defined margins of sclerosis are usually present.[32] Multifocal disease is an uncommon presentation and occurs primarily in children and the immunocompromised.[70] MRI is useful in detecting osteomyelitis early because of changes in the bone marrow. The normal marrow fat signal on T1-weighted images is replaced by low signal intensity, with corresponding high signal

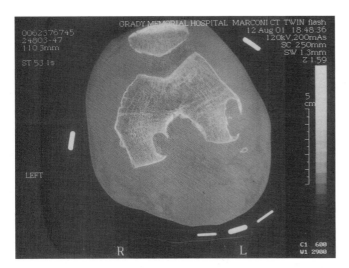

Fig. 20-10. CT of patient with culture positive TB of the knee showing extensive marginal destruction.

Table 20-6. Differential Diagnosis of Cystic Bone Lesions

Cystic TB
Syphilis
Eosinophilic granuloma
Sarcoidosis
Cystic angiomatosis
Multiple myeloma
Neoplasm
    Metastatic, lymphoma, neuroblastoma
Fungal infection
    Blastomycosis and coccidioidomycosis

Table 20-7. Differential Diagnosis of Primary Myositis.

Tuberculosis
Actinomycosis
Sarcoidosis
Malignancy (sarcoma)
Bursa or tendon cyst
Hematoma
Pyogenic myositis
Melioidosis

intensities on T2-weighted images and enhancement of T1-weighted images after gadolinium.[17] Tuberculous lesions are rarely seen in the hands and feet but tuberculous dactylitis occurring in children is a well recognized entity. The typical radiologic appearance is a ballooned-out configuration of "spina ventosa" in which the dissolution of bone causes absorption of trabeculae and expansion of the affected digit.[70]

Tuberculous Myositis

Tuberculous myositis is usually discovered secondary to a known skeletal focus. Primary myositis can occur, especially in the immunocompromised patient whereas secondary tuberculous myositis which is much more common is usually seen in conjunction with vertebral TB. The differential diagnosis of primary myositis or pyomyositis is shown in Table 20-7. Plain radiography may show calcifications or in the case of a psoas abscess, an enlarged psoas shadow. CT imaging shows a well-marginated tumor-like lesion, either hypodense or isodense, compared with normal muscle (Figs. 20-5 and 20-11). MRI shows a distinct mass that can be either lower or higher density than the muscle depending on the T1-weighted or T2-weighted image. CT and MRI cannot really differentiate tuberculous myositis from other causes of muscle lesions but the diagnosis may be highly suspected in the proper clinical setting (e.g., TB at a contiguous or distant site.[40] Ultimately, a definitive diagnosis needs to based on histologic and microbiologic studies. Psoas abscesses are often associated with vertebral TB, but other etiologies should be considered as well (Table 20-8). CT and MRI are both useful in detecting a

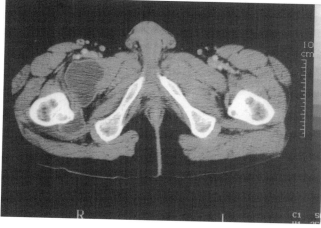

Fig. 20-11. CT of the lower extremities in a patient with TB lumbar spondylitis who had a Psoas abscess that extended in the right thigh. The patient actually presented with a "cold abscess" of the right thigh that required incisional drainage.

Table 20-8. Etiologies of a Psoas Muscle Abscess

Vertebral TB (Pott's Disease)
Diverticulitis
Appendicitis
Crohn's Disease
Postpartum infection
Neoplasm of spine or bowel
Renal calculi
Hematoma
Pyogenic infection (especially *Staphylococcus aureus*)
Actinomycosis

psoas abscess. A calcified psoas muscle on plain film is pathognomonic of a tuberculous abscess secondary to vertebral disease.[71]

Mycobacteriologic and Histologic Diagnosis

Radiologic methods may suggest a diagnosis of TB, but bacteriologic or histologic confirmation is required to prove the diagnosis. Every attempt should be made to establish a microbiologically confirmed diagnosis (i.e., recovery of *M. tuberculosis* from culture) so that an isolate is available for susceptibility testing. A presumptive diagnosis can be made by observing caseating granulomas with or without AFB on histologic examination of specimens; however, granulomas in musculoskeletal specimens do not always indicate infection with *M. tuberculosis*. Other diseases producing synovial granulomas include fungal diseases, nontuberculous mycobacteria, sarcoidosis, traumatic fat necrosis, brucellosis, and foreign body giant cell reactions. In developing countries where TB is highly endemic and resources including imaging and diagnostic capabilities are limited, the diagnosis of musculoskeletal TB is often based on the clinical and radiologic (e.g., plain film) findings.

Differentiating pyogenic, tuberculous, or inflammatory arthritis can be difficult radiographically and ultimately a microbiologic diagnosis needs to be made. For tuberculous arthritis, synovial fluid examination is the first procedure performed and if nondiagnostic, biopsies of the synovium are required to establish a diagnosis of tuberculous arthritis. Synovial fluid in early stages of disease appears xanthochromic and as the disease process advances the fluid becomes yellow-white and thick and gelatinous in nature because of the presence of degenerated cartilage and bony debris.[72] An elevated protein over 2.5gm/dL is a uniform finding. The joint fluid glucose level is thought to be low compared to serum levels. Enarson reported that in 61% of cases of tuberculous arthritis, the synovial fluid glucose was less than 50 mg/dL and 63% had a glucose 40 mg/dL less than the blood glucose.[34] The synovial fluid white blood cell count can vary widely with the average being in the 10,000–20,000/ml range but WBC counts up to 50,000–100,000/ml (in the range of what is often reported for bacterial or "septic arthritis") has been reported. All of these findings can also be consistent with rheumatoid arthritis as well. For these reasons, a bacteriologic and/or histologic diagnosis is imperative.

Acid-fast bacilli (AFB) staining of synovial fluid has a low-sensitivity but is thought to be higher than that seen in examination of fluid from other serosal membranes (e.g., pleura, pericardium, peritoneum). The sensitivity of the AFB smear of synovial fluid for tuberculous arthritis has been reported to be only 19% but was much higher for culture with up to 80% of cases being culture positive.[72] Synovial biopsy and culture had a higher yield with 94% specimens having a positive histology and yielding a positive culture for *M. tuberculosis*. Open biopsy and fine-needle aspiration biopsy also has a high likelihood of yielding a positive culture (>90%) but is generally not required. Mondal reported a series of 116 fine-needle aspiration biopsies in which TB was diagnosed in 38 patients; metastatic tumor was diagnosed in the remaining 78 patients. Thirty-four of the 38 patients with tuberculous arthritis had cultures positive for *M. tuberculosis* (89%) and 11 (39%) were smear-positive for AFB. The remaining four cases of tuberculous arthritis were confirmed histologically, and the patients demonstrated improvement with antituberculous treatment.[73] Masood performed fine-needle aspiration biopsy for diagnosis of bone and soft-tissue lesions in 11 patients and 64% were smear positive for AFB and 84% were culture positive; the author concluded that fine-needle biopsy is as good as open biopsy and less invasive[74] Molecular diagnostic techniques have promise for enhancing diagnostic capabilities.[63] For example, two recent case series each had a 100% sensitivity using PCR examination of synovial fluid and tissue specimens to diagnose tuberculous arthritis.[75,76]

Debeaumont showed that the total bacterial population of an infected spine may account for less than 1 million organisms, whereas an expectorated sputum specimen may produce up to 300,000 bacilli in 1 ml.[77] The lower burden of organisms may help explain why it is sometimes difficult to recover tubercle bacilli in paraspinal or psoas abscesses and draining sinus tracts. The yield from culturing material from a sinus tract can be increased if the specimen is collected with a syringe rather than a swab.[78] The low bacillary burden also implies that there is a lower chance of developing drug-resistant TB in skeletal disease than in pulmonary TB.

TREATMENT

Early diagnosis and initiation of appropriate antituberculosis therapy is important as early treatment can prevent loss of function and mobility. There is now abundant evidence to show that musculoskeletal TB detected early can be cured by chemotherapy without the previously expected, inevitable sequelae of deformity in the spine or ankylosis in the limb joints. Even if minor radiologic changes have occurred, full restoration of function without deformity can be confidently expected if the diagnosis is made early enough. Simple survival of the patient in a moderately disabled condition is no longer acceptable. Early diagnosis may indeed be the greatest contribution that surgery has to make to the modern management of musculoskeletal TB.

The basic principles that underlie the treatment of pulmonary TB also apply to extrapulmonary forms of the disease.[79] Regimens that are effective for the treatment of pulmonary TB are appropriate for the treatment of musculoskeletal TB. Several studies have examined the treatment of bone and joint TB and have shown that 6- to 9-month "short course" regimens containing rifampin are at least as effective as 18-month regimens that do not contain rifampin.[80–82] Because of the difficulties in assessing response, however, some experts tend to favor the 9-month duration.[79] Concomitant use of corticosteroids in the treatment of persons with bone and joint disease is not recommended.[79]

Tuberculosis Spondylitis

Historical Perspective

Before the availability of effective antituberculosis chemotherapy, Pott's disease was treated with immobilization using prolonged bed rest or a body cast. In Dobson's series of 914 patients, all received prolonged immobilization, either with a brace or a body plaster cast, and 54 underwent a spinal fusion.[83] The mortality rate was 20% and 22% were readmitted for relapses. Antituberculosis chemotherapy was gradually introduced into the treatment of osteoarticular TB after the studies of Canetti and Debeaumont demonstrated the effect of chemotherapy in osteoarticular disease.[77,84] Hodgson described the first series combining a surgical approach

using an anterior approach for decompression and autologous bone grafting for fusion with chemotherapy and reported a high success rate.[85] Konstam was the first to report an ambulatory, medical approach for tuberculous spondylitis.[86] He reported treatment of 207 patients with INH and PAS for at least 12 months (until there was radiographic improvement) and did not include bracing or immobilization as part of the therapy. Surgery was only performed in 27 patients who needed abscesses drained. Eighty-six percent of patients exhibited complete recovery. For the first time it was demonstrated that patients with vertebral TB could be cured with chemotherapy alone and without prolonged immobilization or a complicated surgical procedure.

It was this divergence of opinion and practice that led the British Medical Research Council to set up a series of randomized controlled clinical trials in different centers.[87–96] Patients included in these research studies had evidence of active TB of the thoracic or lumbar spine. These studies were carried out in Korea, Zimbabwe (then called Rhodesia), South Africa, and Hong Kong. All patients received chemotherapy (in most reports this consisted of 18 months of isoniazid and PAS supplemented with streptomycin during the first 3 months for some patients). The methods of treatment were determined by the therapy available at that time plus locally available resources and included outpatient antituberculosis therapy; chemotherapy with immobilization by bed rest or body casts; chemotherapy and conservative debridement of infected bone without fusion; and in Hong Kong and South Africa, chemotherapy with "radical surgery". The "radical" surgical therapy consisted of anterior resection, debridement of granulation tissue and nonviable bone, and autologous bone strut grafting.[94,95] Nonoperative treatment produced a favorable status in 67% of subjects at 18 months, 85% at 3 years, and 88% at 5 years. The continued improvement that became apparent with the passage of time, from 67% to 85–90% at 5–10 years is a valid warning against panic if all does not seem well at the end of the initial period of chemotherapy. No statistically significant difference could be shown at any stage between the results in patients who underwent 6 months of inpatient care, 9 months in plaster jackets, or neither. In addition, no statistically significant advantage could be shown from the addition of streptomycin to PAS and isoniazid. It was therefore concluded that in this series of cases, from the point of view of the preservation of life and health, ambulant outpatient chemotherapy gave excellent results, as judged over a period of 5 years, in patients whose drug-taking had been supervised as strictly as possible under the prevailing conditions. Debridement by open operation with or without anterior spinal fusion, in addition to chemotherapy, gave no better ultimate results than did ambulant outpatient treatment. Favorable outcome in these studies was defined as "full physical activity with clinically and radiographically quiescent disease, with no sinuses, abscesses or myelopathy with functional impairment, all without modification of the allocated regimen."[92]

Radical surgery, as performed in Hong Kong, gave similar results in the long term so far as preservation of life and health are concerned. The Hong Kong operation consisted of anterior resection, debridement of infected bone, and autologous bone grafting. At the end of the period of chemotherapy (18 months), 89% of patients had already reached a favorable status; at 3 years, 87% of patients and at 5 years, 89% were considered favorable. The Hong Kong operation in conjunction with nonrifampin based regimens (in the era before the availability of rifampin), however, produced certain distinct advantages: (1) abscesses, including mediastinal abscesses, resolved more rapidly than after conservative treatment and even after debridement, (2) bony fusion occurred much earlier, and (3) most importantly, kyphosis did not worsen.[94] The "Hong Kong" radical procedure was also performed in South Africa but unlike the reports from Hong Kong, did not show advantages over debridement alone. On the basis of the results of theses trials, in the era before the availability of rifampin, spinal TB was best treated by a combination of appropriate chemotherapy and the Hong Kong radical operation if, and only if, adequate surgical expertise, anesthesia, and nursing facilities were available. If not, surgery was to be avoided.

Modern Therapy for Tuberculous Spondylitis

Stimulated by the efficacy of short-course chemotherapy for pulmonary TB with isoniazid and rifampin, the British Medical Research Council Working Party started a second series of trials in Hong Kong, Korea, and south India.[95,97,98] In Hong Kong, all patients underwent the radical operation with either 6 months or 9 months of chemotherapy with isoniazid and rifampin supplemented by streptomycin for 6 months. In Korea, only ambulatory chemotherapy with a regimen of 6 months or 9 months of isoniazid plus rifampin was compared with a regimen of 9 months or 18 months of isoniazid plus PAS or ethambutol. In Madras (now Chennai), South India, ambulatory chemotherapy with a regimen of 6 months or 9 months of isoniazid and rifampin was compared with a regimen of 6 months or 9 months of isoniazid plus rifampin and the Hong Kong radical operation. After 3 years, all studies showed >95% had favorable results for regimens containing isoniazid and rifampin.[95,97,98] These results confirmed the efficacy of a short-course regimen of rifampin based regimens for 6 or 9 months for spinal TB. The resolution of sinuses and abscesses present on admission was more rapid in patients treated with isoniazid plus rifampin compared with patients treated with isoniazid plus PAS or ethambutol. There was no recurrence in patients prescribed rifampin-containing regimens. The resolution of myelopathy was very good in ambulatory regimens, with 83%–88% of patients making a full recovery. There was no clear evidence that 9 months of treatment with isoniazid plus rifampin had any advantages over 6 months of treatment. Primary drug resistance to isoniazid and streptomycin was a problem, particularly in the Hong Kong studies.

Thus, on the basis of the results of these more recent randomized trials carried out by the Medical Research Council (MRC) Working Party on tuberculosis of the spine; tuberculous spondylitis of the thoracolumbar spine due to drug susceptible organisms is best treated by a rifampin based regimens, including isoniazid and rifampin for a period of 6 to 9 months supplemented by pyrazinamide for two months (and ethambutol pending susceptibility results), similar to those regimens used in the treatment of pulmonary TB. Among patients taking rifampin-based short course regimens, there was no demonstrated additional benefit of surgical debridement or radical operation (resection of the spinal focus and bone grafting) in combination with chemotherapy compared with chemotherapy alone.[97] In addition, myelopathy with or without functional impairment most often responds to chemotherapy. In two studies conducted in Korea, 24 of 30 patients in one study[98] and 74 of 85 patients in an earlier study[99] had complete resolution of myelopathy or complete functional recovery when treated medically. In some circumstances, however, surgery appears to be beneficial and may be indicated. Such situations include failure to respond to chemotherapy with evidence of ongoing infection, the relief of cord compression in patients with persistence or recurrence of neurologic deficits, or instability of the spine.[79]

Despite the large number of patients enrolled in the MRC trials, patients with obvious myelopathy were excluded, so there are no controlled trials evaluating the role of surgery when paresis is present. Paresis is now generally considered a surgical indication.[79] Other accepted indications for surgery include failure to respond to chemotherapy with evidence of ongoing infection, the relief of cord compression in patients with neurologic deficits, paraspinal abscesses and psoas abscesses requiring drainage, or the instability of the spine. Late neurologic compromise resulting from kyphosis after the disease is no longer active is also an indication for surgical decompression.

Patients with tuberculous spondylitis of the cervical spine were not included in the MRC studies, in part because of the low incidence of cervical disease. In two case series which reported on a total of 46 patients with upper and lower cervical TB, all patients received antituberculosis chemotherapy and surgery.[100,101] Medical therapy consisted of isoniazid plus rifampin for 12–15 months or isoniazid plus PAS for 15–21 months. Of the six patients with upper cervical disease four of the six recovered without sequelae. There were 40 patients with lower cervical disease; all experienced a meaningful clinical and radiologic recovery. Twelve patients with cord compression experienced full neurologic recovery. Treatment recommendations for cervical TB are based on case series.[100–102] Surgical intervention of the cervical spine is often indicated because of the likely association of neurologic deficits, frequent abscesses that can cause respiratory compromise, and the relative instability of the cervical spine although in some cases such as those reported by Jain et al.,[102] there can be recovery without surgical intervention as was reported in about two-thirds of the patients in their series. An anterior approach is considered the treatment of choice. A laminectomy should be avoided because it is not as effective in relieving cord compression and can further lead to instability of the cervical spine.

Tuberculous Arthritis and Osteomyelitis

There are no controlled trials assessing treatment of musculoskeletal TB with the exception of tuberculous spondylitis, which is discussed above. Based on experience from treating tuberculous spondylitis and the experience with treating other forms of extrapulmonary disease, it is recommended that treatment of drug susceptible tuberculous arthritis and osteomyelitis be carried out using rifampin based short course regimens similar to those that are used for the treatment of pulmonary disease. Surgery is generally reserved for diagnosis and when necessary to drain an abscess that is not responding to medical therapy or to drain a large abscess to relieve pressure.[103] Late treatment or inadequate treatment results in ankylosis of the affected joint by fibrosis or bony fusion. The function of the affected joint is compensated by other joints, which in the long term are overused and may become painful because of degenerative arthritis. Recent technical developments have stimulated interest in indications for arthroplasty in joints with old, healed TB.[104–106] Su reported 16 cases of patients with a history of TB of the knee who underwent total knee replacement; eight patients had a preoperative

diagnosis of TB and had received at least 2 months of antituberculous medications and eight were diagnosed at the time of the operation. Five patients, four of whom did not receive antituberculosis chemotherapy at the time of the operation, suffered a recurrence of disease after arthroplasty.[106] There are no formal recommendations but some experts have suggested that patients requiring total arthroplasty for quiescent TB should receive perioperative chemotherapy for at 3 weeks before and at least 6–9 months after surgery to minimize the risk of reactivation.[107]

Tuberculous Myositis

There are no controlled trials of the treatment of tuberculous myositis. Regimens similar to that used for the treatment of pulmonary TB and other forms of musculoskeletal TB (i.e., rifampin-based "short course regimens") are recommended for the treatment of tuberculous myositis. Therapy should be initiated with isoniazid, rifampin, pyrazinamide and ethambutol as is recommended for other forms of TB. There are no controlled trials specifically addressing the role of incision and drainage as a complement to chemotherapy of tuberculous myositis. Aspiration or drainage of an abscess (e.g., by CT direction) is generally indicated to obtain specimens for culture and aids in making a definitive diagnosis.

CONCLUSION

The diagnosis of musculoskeletal TB is often delayed because of failure to consider the diagnosis. Early diagnosis of bone and joint disease is important in order to minimize the risk of deformity and enhance outcome. The introduction of new imaging modalities including CT and MRI have enhanced the diagnostic evaluation of patients with musculoskeletal TB and for directed biopsies of affected areas of the musculoskeletal system. Obtaining appropriate specimens for culture is essential in an effort to establish a definitive diagnosis and recover *M. tuberculosis* for susceptibility testing. A total of 6–9 months of a rifampin-based regimen, similar to those used for the treatment of pulmonary TB, is recommended for the treatment of musculoskeletal disease. Randomized trials of tuberculous spondylitis have demonstrated that such regimens are efficacious. These data and that from the treatment of pulmonary TB have been extrapolated to form the basis of treatment regimen recommendations for other forms of musculoskeletal TB. Finally, ensuring adherence to chemotherapy is essential for good outcomes; therefore, directly observed therapy is recommended for the treatment of the all persons with musculoskeletal TB.

REFERENCES

1. Zink A, Haas CJ, Reischl U, et al. Molecular analysis of skeletal tuberculosis in an ancient Egyptian population. *J Med Microbiol.* 2001;50:355–366.

2. Crubezy E, Ludes B, Poveda JD, et al. Identification of Mycobacterium DNA in an Egyptian Pott's disease of 5,400 years old. *C R Acad Sci III.* 1998;321:941–951.

3. Konomi N, Lebwohl E, Mowbray K, et al. Detection of mycobacterial DNA in Andean mummies. *J Clin Microbiol.* 2002;40:4738–4740.

4. Salo WL, Aufderheide AC, Buikstra J, et al. Identification of *Mycobacterium tuberculosis* DNA in a pre-Columbian Peruvian mummy. *Proc Natl Acad Sci USA.* 1994;91:2091–2094.

5. Donoghue HD, Spigelman M, Greenblatt CL, et al. Tuberculosis: from prehistory to Robert Koch, as revealed by ancient DNA. *Lancet Infect Dis.* 2004;4:584–592.

6. Hodgson AR Yau A, Kwon JS, Kim D. A clinical study of 100 consecutive cases of Pott's paraplegia. *Clin Orthop Relat Res.* 1964;36:128–150.

7. Centers for Disease Control and Prevention (CDC). Trends in Tuberculosis—United States, 1998–2003. *MMWR Morb Mortal Wkly Rep.* 2004;53;209–214.

8. Hodgson SP, Ormerod LP. Ten-year experience of bone and joint tuberculosis in Blackburn 1978–1987. *J R Coll Surg Edinb.* 1990 Aug;35(4):259–262.

9. Lafond EM. An analysis of adult skeletal tuberculosis. *J Bone Joint Surg Am.* 1958;40-A:346–364.

10. Schlossberg D, et al. *Tuberculosis,* 4th ed. New York, NY: McGraw-Hill, 1999: Davidson chapter.

11. Colmenero JD, Jimenez-Mejias ME, Reguera JM, et al. Tuberculous vertebral osteomyelitis in the new millennium: still a diagnostic and therapeutic challenge. *Eur J Clin Microbiol Infect Dis.* 2004;23:477–483.

12. American Thoracic Society and Centers for Disease Control and Prevention. Targeted tuberculin testing and treatment of latent tuberculosis infection. American Thoracic Society. *MMWR Recomm Rep.* 2000;49(RR-6):1–51.

13. Leibert E, Schluger NW, Bonk S, et al. Spinal tuberculosis in patients with human immunodeficiency virus infection: clinical presentation, therapy and outcome. *Tuber Lung Dis.* 1996;77:329–334.

14. Agarwal RP, Mohan N, Garg RK, et al. Clinicosocial aspect of osteo-articular tuberculosis. *J Indian Med Assoc.* 1990; 88:307–309.

15. Evanchick CC, Davis DE, Harrington TM. Tuberculosis of peripheral joints: an often missed diagnosis. *J Rheumatol.* 1986;13:187–189.

16. Belzunegui J, Plazaola I, Uriarte E, et al. Primary tuberculous muscle abscess in a patient with systemic lupus erythematosus. *Br J Rheumatol.* 1995;34:1177–1178.

17. De Vuyst D, Vanhoenacker F, Gielen J, et al. Imaging features of musculoskeletal tuberculosis. *Eur Radiol.* 2003; 13:1809–1819.

18. Moore SL, Rafii M. Imaging of musculoskeletal and spinal tuberculosis. *Radiol Clin North Am.* 2001;39:329–342.

19. Compere EL, Garrison M. Correlation of pathologic and roentgenologic findings in tuberculosis and pyogenic infection of vertebrae; fate of intervertebral disk. *Ann Surg.* 1936;104:1038–1067.

20. Palmer PES. *The Imaging of Tuberculosis: With Epidemiological, Pathological, and Clinical Correlation.* New York, NY: Springer-Verlag, 2001.

21. Naim-Ur-Rahman J. Atypical forms of spinal tuberculosis. *J Bone Joint Surg Br.* 1980;62-B(2):162–165.

22. Calderone RR, Larsen JM. Overview and classification of spinal infections. *Orthop Clin North Am.* 1996;27:1–8.

23. Boachie-Adjei O, Squillante RG. Tuberculosis of the spine. *Orthop Clin North Am.* 1996;27:95–103.

24. Al Soub H. Retropharyngeal abscess associated with tuberculosis of the cervical spine. *Tuber Lung Dis.* 1996;77: 563–565.

25. Hoffman EB, Crosier JH, Cremon BJ. Imaging in children with spinal tuberculosis. A comparison of radiography, computed tomography and magnetic resonance imaging. *J Bone Joint Surg Br.* 1993;75:233–239.

26. Wurtz R, Quader Z, Simon D, et al. Cervical tuberculous vertebral osteomyelitis: case report and discussion of the literature. *Clin Infect Dis.* 1993;16:806–808.

27. Burke HE. The pathogenesis of certain forms of extrapulmonary tuberculosis; spontaneous cold abscesses of the chest wall and Pott's disease. *Am Rev Tuberc.* 1950;62(1-B): 48–67.

28. Colmenero JD, Jimenez-Mejias ME, Sanchez-Lora FJ, et al. Pyogenic, tuberculous, and brucellar vertebral osteomyelitis: a descriptive and comparative study of 219 cases. *Ann Rheum Dis.* 1997;56:709–715.

29. LeRoux PD, Griffin GE, Marsh HT, et al. Tuberculosis of the skull—a rare condition: case report and review of the literature. *Neurosurgery.* 1990;26:851–855.

30. Strauss DC. Tuberculosis of the flat bones of the vault of the skull. *Surg Gynecol Obstet.* 1933;57:384–398.

31. Asnis DS, Niegowska A. Tuberculosis of the rib. *Clin Infect Dis.* 1997;24:1018–1019.

32. Gonzalez Herranz J, Farrington DM, Angulo Gutierrez J, et al. Peripheral osteoarticular tuberculosis in children: tumor-like bone lesions. *J Pediatr Orthop B.* 1997;6: 274–282.

33. Zahraa J, Johnson D, Lim-Dunham JE, et al. Unusual features of osteoarticular tuberculosis in children. *J Pediatr.* 1996;129:597–602.

34. Enarson DA, Fujii M, Nakielna EM, et al. Bone and joint tuberculosis: a continuing problem. *Can Med Assoc J.* 1979; 120:139–145.

35. Davidson PT, Horowitz I. Skeletal tuberculosis. A review with patient presentations and discussion. *Am J Med.* 1970;48:77–84.

36. Isaacs AJ, Sturrock RD. Poncet's disease—fact or fiction? A re-appraisal of tuberculous rheumatism. *Tubercle.* 1974;55: 135–142.

37. Huang DY. Tuberculous muscle abscess: an unusual presentation of tuberculosis. *Am J Med.* 1990;88:57N–59N.

38. Plummer WW, Sanes S, Smith WS. Hematogenous tuberculosis of skeletal muscle; report of the case with involvement of gastrocnemius muscle. *J Bone Joint Surg.* 1934;16: 631–639.

39. Ahmed J, Homans J. Tuberculosis pyomyosits of the soleus muscle in a fifteen-year-old boy. *Pediatr Infect Dis J.* 2002;21:1169–1171.

40. Kobayashi H, Kotoura Y, Hosono M, et al. Solitary muscular involvement by tuberculosis: CT, MRI, and scintigraphic features. *Comput Med Imaging Graph.* 1995;19:237–240.

41. Lupatkin H, Brau N, Flomenberg P, et al. Tuberculous abscesses in patients with AIDS. *Clin Infect Dis.* 1992;14: 1040–1044.

42. Martini M, Ouahes M. Bone and joint tuberculosis: a review of 652 cases. *Orthopedics.* 1988;11:861–866.

43. Pertuiset E, Beaudreuil J, Liote F, et al. Spinal tuberculosis in adults. A study of 103 cases in a developed country, 1980–1994. *Medicine (Baltimore).* 1999;78:309–320.

44. McLain RF, Isada C. Spinal tuberculosis deserves a place on the radar screen. *Cleve Clin J Med.* 2004;71:543–549.

45. Neumann JL, Schlueter DP. Retropharyngeal abscess as the presenting feature of tuberculosis of the cervical spine. *Am Rev Respir Dis.* 1974;110:508–511.

46. Garcia S, Combalia A, Serra A, et al. Unusual locations of osteoarticular tuberculosis. *Arch Orthop Trauma Surg.* 1997; 116:321–323.

47. Lukhele M. Tuberculosis of the cervical spine. *S Afr Med J.* 1996;86:553–556.

48. Al-Matar MJ, Cabral DA, Petty RE. Isolated tuberculous monoarthritis mimicking oligoarticular juvenile rheumatoid arthritis. *J Rheumatol.* 2001;28:204–206.

49. Valdazo JP, Perez-Ruiz F, Albarracin A, et al. Tuberculous arthritis. Report of a case with multiple joint involvement and periarticular tuberculous abscesses. *J Rheumatol.* 1990;17:399–401.

50. Gros T, Soriano V, Gabarre E, et al. Multifocal tubercular osteitis in a female patient infected with the human immunodeficiency virus. *Rev Clin Esp.* 1992;191:35–37.

51. Babhulkar SS, Pande SK. Unusual manifestations of osteoarticular tuberculosis. *Clin Orthop.* 2002;398:114–120.

52. Franco-Paredes C, Blumberg HM. Psoas muscle abscess caused by *Mycobacterium tuberculosis* and *Staphylococcus aureus*. Case Report and Review of the Literature. *Am J Med Sci.* 2001;321:415–417.

53. Chernoff WG, Parnes LS. Tuberculous mastoiditis. *J Otolaryngol.* 1992;21:290–292.

54. Wu H, Wang QZ, Jin Y. Tuberculosis of the temporomandibular joint. *Oral Surg Oral Med Oral Pathol Oral Radiol Endod.* 1988;85:243.

55. McLellan DG, Philips KB, Corbett CE, et al. Sternal osteomyelitis caused by mycobacterium tuberculosis: case report and review of the literature. *Am J Med Sci.* 2000; 319:250–254.

56. Jaovisidha S, Chen C, Ryu KN, et al. Tuberculous tenosynovitis and bursitis: imaging findings in 21 cases. *Radiology.* 1996;201:507–513.

57. Klofkorn RW, Steigerwald JC. Carpal tunnel syndrome as the initial manifestation of tuberculosis. *Am J Med.* 1976; 60:583–586.

58. Hoffman KL, Bergman AG, Hoffman DK, et al. Tuberculous tenosynovitis of the flexor tendons of the wrist: MR imaging with pathologic correlation. *Skeletal Radiol.* 1996;25: 186–188.

59. Cramer K, Seiler JG III, Milek MA. Tuberculous tenosynovitis of the wrist. Two case reports. *Clin Orthop Relat Res.* 1991;262:137–140.

60. Tuli SM. General principles of osteoarticular tuberculosis. *Clin Orthop Relat Res.* 2002;398:11–19.

61. Barnes PF. Diagnosing latent tuberculosis infection: turning glitter to gold. *Am J Respir Crit Care Med.* 2004;170:5–6.

62. Pai M, Riley LW, Colford JM Jr. Interferon-gamma assays in the immunodiagnosis of tuberculosis: a systematic review. *Lancet Infect Dis.* 2004;4:761–776.

63. Shamputa IC, Rigouts And L, Portaels F. Molecular genetic methods for diagnosis and antibiotic resistance detection of mycobacteria from clinical specimens. *APMIS.* 2004;112: 728–752.

64. Griffith JF, Kumta Shekhar SM, Leung PC, et al. imaging of musculoskeletal; tuberculosis: a new look at an old disease. *Clin Orthop Relat Res.* 2002;398:32–39.

65. Clementsen P, Hansen M, Conrad C, et al. Percutaneous drainage of tuberculous abscess of the psoas muscle. *Tubercle.* 1988;69:63–65.

66. Sharif HS, Morgan JL, Al Shahed MS, et al. Role of CT and MR imaging in the management of tuberculous spondylitis. *Radiol Clin North Am.* 1995;33:787–804.

67. Phemister DB, Hatcher CH: Correlation of the pathological findings in the diagnostic of tuberculous arthritis. *Am J Roentgenol Radium Ther Nucl Med.* 1933;29:736–740.

68. Hong SH, Kim SM, Ahn JM, et al. Tuberculous versus pyogenic arthritis: MR imaging evaluation. *Radiology.* 2001;218:848–853.

69. Moore SL, Rafii M. Advanced imaging of tuberculosis arthritis. *Semin Musculoskelet Radiol.* 2003;7:143–153.

70. Morris BS, Varma R, Garg A, et al.: Multifocal musculoskeletal tuberculosis in children: appearances on computed tomography. *Skeletal Radiol.* 2002;31:1–8.

71. Graves VB, Schreiber MH. Tuberculous psoas muscle abscess. *J Can Assoc Radiol.* 1973;24:268–271.

72. Wallace R, Cohen AS. Tuberculous arthritis: A report of two cases with review of biopsy and synovial fluid findings. *Am J Med.* 1976;61:277–282.

73. Mondal A. Cytological diagnosis of vertebral tuberculosis with fine-needle aspiration biopsy. *J Bone Joint Surg Am.* 1994;76:181–184.

74. Masood S. Diagnosis of tuberculosis of bone and soft tissue by fine-needle aspiration biopsy. *Diagn Cytopathol.* 1992;8: 451–455.

75. Titov AG, Vyshnevskaya EB, Mazurenko SI et al. Use of polymerase chain reaction to diagnose tuberculous arthritis from joint tissues and synovial fluid. *Arch Pathol Lab Med.* 2004;128:205–209.

76. Verettas D, Kazakos C, Tilkeridis C, et al.: Polymerase chain reaction for the detection of Mycobacterium tuberculosis in synovial fluid, tissue samples, bone marrow aspirate and peripheral blood. *Acta Orthop Belg*. 2003;69:396–399.

77. Debeaumont A. Bacteriology of osteoarticular tuberculosis under chemotherapy. *Bibl Tuberc*. 1966;22:125–188. (French)

78. Mousa HA. Tuberculosis of bones and joints: diagnostic approaches. *Int Orthop*. 1998;22:245–246.

79. Blumberg HM, Burman WJ, Chaisson RE et al. American Thoracic Society/Centers for Disease Control and Prevention/Infectious Diseases Society of America: treatment of tuberculosis. *Am J Respir Crit Care Med*. 2003; 167:603–662.

80. Medical Research Council Working Party on Tuberculosis of the Spine. Five-year assessment of controlled trials of short-course chemotherapy regimens of 6, 9 or 18 months' duration for spinal tuberculosis in patients ambulatory from the start or undergoing radical surgery. *Int Orthop*. 1999;23:73–81.

81. Medical Research Council Working Party on Tuberculosis of the Spine. Controlled trial of short-course regimens of chemotherapy in the ambulatory treatment of spinal tuberculosis: results at three years of a study in Korea. *J Bone Joint Surg Br*. 1993;75:240–248.

82. Medical Research Council Working Party on Tuberculosis of the Spine. A controlled trial of six-month and nine-month regimens of chemotherapy in patients undergoing radical surgery for tuberculosis of the spine in Hong Kong. *Tubercle*. 1986;67:243–259.

83. Dobson J. Tuberculosis of the spine; an analysis of the results of conservative treatment and of the factors influencing the prognosis. *J Bone Joint Surg Br*. 1951;33-B:517–531.

84. Canetti G, Debeyre J, Seze SD. Sterilization of lesions in osteo-articular tuberculosis by antibacillary chemotherapy, (French). *Rev Tuberc*. 1957;21:1337–1344.

85. Hodgson AR, Stock FE, Fang HS, Ong GB. Anterior spinal fusion. The operative approach and pathological findings in 412 patients with Pott's disease of the spine. *Br J Surg*. 1960;48:172–178.

86. Konstam PG, Blesovsky A. The ambulant treatment of spinal tuberculosis. *Br J Surg*. 1962;50:26–38.

87. Medical Research Council Working Party on Tuberculosis of the Spine. A 10-year assessment of controlled trials of inpatient and outpatient treatment and of plaster-of-Paris jackets for tuberculosis of the spine in children on standard chemotherapy. *J Bone Joint Surg Br*. 1985;67:103–110.

88. Medical Research Council Working Party on Tuberculosis of the Spine. A controlled trial of anterior spinal fusion and debridement in the surgical management of tuberculosis of the spine in patients on standard chemotherapy: a study in two centres in South Africa. Seventh Report of the Medical Research Council Working Party on tuberculosis of the spine. *Tubercle*. 1978;59:79–105.

89. Medical Research Council Working Party on Tuberculosis of the Spine. Five-year assessments of controlled trials of ambulatory treatment, debridement and anterior spinal fusion in the management of tuberculosis of the spine. Studies in Bulawayo (Rhodesia) and in Hong Kong. Sixth report of the Medical Research Council Working Party on Tuberculosis of the Spine. *J Bone Joint Surg Br*. 1978;60-B:163–177.

90. Medical Research Council Working Party on Tuberculosis of the Spine. A five-year assessment of controlled trials of in-patient and out-patient treatment and of plaster-of-Paris jackets for tuberculosis of the spine in children on standard chemotherapy. Studies in Masan and Pusan, Korea. Fifth report of the Medical Research Council Working Party on tuberculosis of the spine. *J Bone Joint Surg Br*. 1976;58-B:399–411.

91. Medical Research Council Working Party on Tuberculosis of the Spine. A controlled trial of anterior spinal fusion and debridement in the surgical management of tuberculosis of the spine in patients on standard chemotherapy: a study in Hong Kong. Fourth report of the Medical Research Council Working Party on Tuberculosis of the Spine. *Br J Surg*. 1974;61:853–866.

92. Medical Research Council Working Party on Tuberculosis of the Spine. A controlled trial of ambulant out-patient treatment and in-patient rest in bed in the management of tuberculosis of the spine in young Korean patients on standard chemotherapy a study in Masan, Korea. First report of the Medical Research Council Working Party on Tuberculosis of the Spine. *J Bone Joint Surg Br*. 1973;55: 678–697.

93. Medical Research Council Working Party on Tuberculosis of the Spine. A controlled trial of plaster-of-paris jackets in the management of ambulant outpatient treatment of tuberculosis of the spine in children on standard chemotherapy. A study in Pusan, Korea. Second report of the Medical Research Council Working Party on Tuberculosis of the Spine. *Tubercle*. 1973;54:261–282.

94. Medical Research Council Working Party on Tuberculosis of the Spine. A 10-year assessment of a controlled trial comparing debridement and anterior spinal fusion in the management of tuberculosis of the spine in patients on standard chemotherapy in Hong Kong. *J Bone Joint Surg Br*. 1982;64:393–398.

95. Medical Research Council Working Party on Tuberculosis of the Spine. A controlled trial of six-month and nine-month regimens of chemotherapy in patients undergoing radical surgery for tuberculosis of the spine in Hong Kong. *Tubercle*. 1986;67:243–259.

96. Medical Research Council Working Party on Tuberculosis of the Spine. A controlled trial of debridment and ambulatory treatment in the management of tuberculosis of the spine in patients on standard chemotherapy. *J Trop Med Hyg*. 1974; 61:853–866.

97. Medical Research Council Working Party on Tuberculosis of the Spine. Five-year assessment of controlled trials of short-course chemotherapy regimens of 6, 9 or 18 months' duration for spinal tuberculosis in patients ambulatory from the start or undergoing radical surgery. *Int Orthop*. 1999;23:73–81.

98. Medical Research Council Working Party on Tuberculosis of the Spine. Controlled trial of short-course regimens of chemotherapy in the ambulatory treatment of spinal tuberculosis: results at three years of a study in Korea. *J Bone Joint Surg Br.* 1993;75:240–248.

99. Pattison PRM. Pott's paraplegia: an account of the treatment of 89 consecutive patients. *Paraplegia.* 1986;24:77–91.

100. Fang D, Leong JC, Fang HS. Tuberculosis of the upper cervical spine. *J Bone Joint Surg Br.* 1983;65:47–50.

101. Hsu LC, Leong JC. Tuberculosis of the lower cervical spine (C2 to C7). A report on 40 cases. *J Bone Joint Surg Br.* 1984;66:1–5.

102. Jain AK, Kumar S, Tuli SM. Tuberculosis of spine (C1 to D4). *Spinal Cord.* 1999;37:362–369.

103. Aguirre M, Bago J, Martin N. Tuberculosis of the knee. Surgical or conservative treatment? *Acta Orthop Belg.* 1989; 55:22–25.

104. Eskola A, Santavirta S, Konttinen YT, et al. Arthroplasty for old tuberculosis of the knee. *J Bone Joint Surg Br.* 1988; 70:767–769.

105. Laforgia R, Murphy JC, Redfern TR. Low friction arthroplasty for old quiescent infection of the hip. *J Bone Joint Surg Br.* 1988;70:373–376.

106. Su J, Huang T, Lui S. Total knee arthroplasty in tuberculous arthritis. *Clin Orthop Relat Res.* 1996;323:181–187.

107. Kramer SB, Lee SHS, Abramson SB. Nonverbral infections of the musculoskeletal system caused by *Mycobacterium tuberculosis.* In: Tuberculosis, 2nd ed. Rom WN, Gray SM, eds. Philadelphia, PA: Lippincott, Williams & Wilkins: 2004.

21

Cardiovascular Tuberculosis

John A. Crocco

Cardiovascular tuberculosis (TB) is an uncommon extrapulmonary manifestation of mycobacterial disease. With the advent of acquired immunodeficiency syndrome (AIDS), which has increased the incidence of mycobacterial disease,[1–7] particularly of the extrapulmonary type,[8–21] one can expect an increase in cardiovascular TB. Nevertheless, cardiovascular TB is a rare complication of AIDS in the United States.[7,8,20] Pericardial TB is the disease present in the greatest percent of patients with cardiovascular TB.[22–26] Tuberculosis of the aorta[27,28] and myocardium[29] are reported but extremely unusual forms of cardiovascular tuberculosis.

PERICARDIAL TUBERCULOSIS

Pericardial tuberculosis is defined as pericardial tissue or fluid culture positive for Mycobacterium tuberculosis, pericardial biopsy specimens demonstrating acid-fast organisms, caseating granulomata, or both, extrapericardial bacteriologic or histologic evidence of active tuberculosis in conjunction with major pericardial effusion or pericardial thickening by echocardiography, or a combination thereof. Tuberculosis of the pericardium arises by contiguous, lymphogenous, or hematogenous spread from areas separate from the pericardium. The acute manifestations are associated with polymorphonuclear followed in about 3–5 days by a lymphocytic exudative pericardial effusion. In the subacute stage, there is caseation necrosis with the lying down of a fibrinous exudate. Later in the course of the disease, organization occurs and constrictive pericarditis with tamponade can occur.

Pericardial tuberculosis is rare, occurring in less than 1% of cases of TB,[22–25] and may be life threatening. Since the 1960s, great strides have been made in the diagnosis and treatment of TB so that death from TB in the United States now occurs in less than 3% of all patients with this disease.[23] Pericardial TB is associated with a 14–40% mortality rate with most treatment regimens.[22,23,30–32]

There are two major reasons for the high death rate in pericardial TB. First, there is difficulty in establishing the diagnosis of tuberculous pericarditis. Second, pericardial inflammation often has dire effects on the mechanical efficiency of the heart.

The individual clinical features of tuberculous pericarditis are nonspecific. When they are analyzed together, however, they often suggest the diagnosis. Most patients are middle-aged.[24] There appears to be a predilection for Black males, as evidence by a 12:1 preponderance of Blacks in one series at a large New York City hospital, even after correction for geographic and racial distribution.[22]

The most common symptoms are weight loss, cough, dyspnea, orthopnea, chest pain, and ankle swelling.[6,22,33–35] The last four symptoms serve as diagnostic clues[6,22,33–35] because they occur more frequently in tuberculous pericarditis than in pulmonary TB without pericarditis.

The most prevalent signs are fever, tachycardia, cardiomegaly, and signs of a pleural effusion.[6,22,33–35] In a study of 35 patients with pericardial TB, 25 patients had a pleural effusion and 9 (36%) had tuberculous pleuritis on pleural biopsy or autopsy.[22] Percutaneous needle and thoracoscopic biopsy of the pleural space appears to be an aid in the diagnosis of pericardial infection. Distant heart sounds, pericardial friction rub, and paradoxical pulse, which are more specific signs of pericarditis and possible tamponade, occurred in a minority of patients.[6,22] They were much more common in patients with tamponade.

In the recent past, the enzyme adenosine deaminase (ADA) has been found to be specifically elevated in pleural,[36–38] peritoneal,[39] pericardial,[40–42] and meningeal[43] fluids of tuberculous origin. Martinez-Vazquez and colleagues[40] looked at ADA levels of pericardial fluid of tuberculous origin versus those of idiopathic, neoplastic, or miscellaneous nontuberculous origin. The mean pericardial fluid ADA levels in patients with tuberculous pericarditis were 96.8 (SD 1.54) IU/L. and the ADA levels for pericardial fluid of nontuberculous origin were 2–20 IU/L. Komsuoglu and coworkers[44] performed a similar study and found that those patients with tuberculous pericarditis had mean pericardial effusion ADA values of 126 + 16.68 IU/L. versus values of 29.5 + 13.4 IU/L. for patients with other causes of pericarditis. The difference was statistically significant between the groups (p < 0.0001), indicating that the ADA value has a 100% sensitivity and 91% specificity. The studies of Koh and coworkers[45] yielded similar results, showing that an ADA value in pericardial fluid of 40 IU/L. or more had a sensitivity of 93% and a specificity of 97% in the diagnosis of tuberculous pericarditis. They also showed that ADA levels could be of great value in the early diagnosis of pericardial TB, particularly when the results of the clinical and laboratory tests are negative. They also noted significant elevation of pericardial fluid carcinoembryonic antigen (CEA) values in patients with malignant disease involving the pericardium. Inoue and associates[46] and Isaka and colleagues[47] experienced similar results in their studies. It appears that pericardial effusion ADA levels may be helpful in the diagnosis of tuberculous pericarditis.

Other forms of testing have been used in addition to ADA. These include pericardial fluid and tissue lysozyme (LYS), interferon-gamma (IFN-gamma) and polymerase chain reaction (PCR) in the diagnosis of pericardial TB. Aggeli and associates[48] in Greece have used a combination of ADA and LYS levels in pericardial fluid in order to compare their effectiveness in the diagnosis of idiopathic, neoplastic, and tuberculous pericarditis. Seven patients had tuberculous, 4 had neoplastic, and 30 had idiopathic pericarditis. A cutoff value of 72 IU/L for pericardial fluid ADA was associated with 100% sensitivity and 94% specificity in the diagnosis of pericardial TB. A cutoff value of 6.5 ugms/dL for pericardial fluid LYS had a sensitivity of 100% and a specificity of 92% in the diagnosis of this disease. These authors felt that both pericardial ADA and LYS need to be taken into account for an early diagnosis. Burgess et al.[49] in South Africa studied the pericardial fluid obtained via pericardiocentesis with echocardiographic direction in 110 patients with large pericardial effusions from various causes. Their diagnosis varied from 64 with tuberculous pericarditis, 12 with malignant disease, 5 with nontuberculous effusions, 10 with idiopathic effusions, and 19 with effusions from other causes. ADA and IFN-gamma levels were significantly higher in effusions from patients with tuberculous pericarditis than in patients with other forms of pericarditis (p < 0.05 for ADA and p > 0.005 for IFN-gamma). A cutoff value of 30 IU/L for pericardial fluid ADA was associated with a sensitivity of 94%, a specificity of 68%, and a positive predictive value of 80% in the diagnosis of pericardial TB. A cutoff of 200 pg/L for pericardial fluid IFN-gamma was associated with a sensitivity and specificity of 100% in the diagnosis of pericardial TB. These authors concluded that pericardial fluid levels of ADA and IFN-gamma were useful in the diagnosis of pericardial TB. Cegielski et al.[50] at Duke examined 36 specimens of pericardial fluid and 19 specimens of pericardial tissue in 20 patients, 16 of whom has tuberculous pericarditis and 4 had another diagnosis. Culture studies (Lowenstein-Jensen and Middlebrook solid media and BACTEC radiometric broth), histologic studies, and polymerase chain reaction (PCR) studies were performed on these tissues. Tuberculosis was correctly diagnosed in 15 of 16 (93%)

by culture, 13 of 16 (81%) by PCR and 13 of 15 (87%) by histology. PCR was performed on fluid and tissue specimens using the IS6110-based primers for Mycobacterium TB complex. There was one false positive PCR reading in a patient with Staphylococcus aureus pericarditis. If individual specimens were considered as the unit of analysis Mycobacterium TB was found by culture in 30 of 43 (70%) specimens tested and by PCR in 14 of 28 (50%) specimens tested (p > 0.05). PCR was significantly higher with tissue specimens (12 of 15 or 80%) than with fluid specimens (2 of 13 or 15%) (p = 0.02). The authors concluded that the PCR accuracy came close to that of culture and histology, but was considerably better in tissue specimens than in fluid specimens. They felt that studies of PCR should be pursued and note the poor sensitivity of PCR in analyzing pericardial fluid. Lee and colleagues[51] in South Korea looked at pericardial fluid PCR and ADA in the diagnosis of pericardial TB. They collected 67 patients with pericarditis, 12(18%) with TB, 20 (30%) with neoplastic disease and 35 (52%) with idiopathic disease. ADA was significantly higher in pericardial fluid from patients with tuberculous pericarditis than it was in patients without TB. An ADA cutoff value of 40 IU/L was associated with 83% (10 of 12) sensitivity and 78% (43 of 57) specificity for pericardial TB. Pericardial PCR was positive for TB in 9 of 12 patients with pericardial TB (a 75% sensitivity and negative for TB in 55 of 55 patients with nontuberculous pericarditis (a specificity of 100%). These authors point out that PCR is as sensitive but more specific than ADA in the diagnosis of pericardial TB. They also point out that ADA levels are higher in rheumatoid arthritis, sarcoidosis and is some empyemas as well as in tuberculous pericarditis and is some PCR testing of pericardial fluid is a rapid reliable method of identifying pericardial TB. Further evaluation of PCR techniques in the diagnosis of pericardial TB using IS6110, as well as other primers of Mycobacterium TB complexes or mycobacterial interspersed repeat units (MIRUs) genotyping,[52] to detect DNA specific for Mycobacterium TB is needed. It is known that IS6110-base typing requires sub culturing the isolates for several weeks to obtain sufficient DNA. MIRUs genotyping has a discriminatory power almost equal to that of 6110-based genotyping. It is technically simpler and can be applied directly to Mycobacterium TB cultures without DNA amplification. It is hoped that in the future PCR techniques will be rapid, more specific, and less expensive than at present.

The chest radiograph is frequently characterized by cardiomegaly, especially in the presence of a pericardial effusion. A "water-bottle" configuration to the cardiac silhouette may be visible. Various studies have found cardiomegaly in up to 95% of patients.[6,32,53,54]

Pericardial effusion is a common finding in TB of the pericardium.[6,22,33–36] A pericardial effusion is clinically manifested by distant heart sounds, a friction rub that may disappear or become clearly audible, and an apical pulse that ceases to be palpable. If the pericardial effusion is large, percussion may reveal an area of dullness and auscultation may reveal an area of tubular breathing at the angle of the left scapula (Ewart's Sign), which are likely caused by compression of the underlying lung.

The most feared complication of pericardial effusion is cardiac tamponade wherein the accumulated fluid seriously obstructs the inflow of blood into the ventricles. The result is a fall in cardiac output and systemic venous congestion that are clinically manifest in falling arterial pressure, a rising venous pressure, distended cervical neck veins on inspiration (Kussmaul's sign), and a paradoxical pulse (a fall in systolic arterial pressure on inspiration). Although a paradoxical pulse is a hallmark of cardiac tamponade, it is not pathognomonic because it can occur in various forms of restrictive cardiomyopathy, chronic obstructive airway disease, and severe bronchial asthma. Various investigators[22,30,32,41,54–58] have recorded pericardial tamponade in 10–40% of patients with tuberculous pericarditis.

The procedure of significant value in diagnosing and following pericardial effusion is the echocardiogram, which is safe, rapid, and most sensitive in detecting small amounts of fluid.[59] An echo-free space may occur, most often posteriorly and frequently anteriorly as well. Larrieu and colleagues[24] showed that echocardiography was 100% accurate in diagnosing pericardial effusion. Chia and associates[60] thought that two-dimensional echocardiography allows better recognition of fluid distribution in the pericardial cavity when compared with the M-mode echocardiogram. Agrawal and coworkers[61] used echocardiography to demonstrate a resolving intrapericardial mass in a tuberculous pericardial effusion. Martin and associates[62] suggested that two-dimensional echocardiograms demonstrate not only anterior and posterior effusions in patients with TB but also echodense structures lining the visceral and parietal pericardium and protruding into the pericardial space. Komsuoglu and colleagues[44] followed 20 patients with tuberculous pericarditis with effusion for 12–18 months via echocardiography. Pre- and post-therapy studies revealed that only two patients still had small effusions. Gallium-67 scans of chest and computer tomography of chest (CT) have also been used to diagnose pericarditis

and pericardial effusion.[63–69] Angiocardiography is also an effective means of localizing a pericardial effusion, but it is time-consuming, invasive, often uncomfortable, and at times associated with significant morbidity. Radionuclide angiography shows a gated blood pool and a fluid-filled pericardial space when a pericardial effusion is present. Magnetic resonance imaging (MRI) can directly image the pericardium and thereby demonstrate abnormal thickening of the pericardium.[69,70]

Hemodynamic findings during cardiac catheterization are often normal in pericardial TB.[56] When constrictive pericarditis is present, however, ventricular filling is not impeded until later in diastole. If cardiac tamponade occurs, ventricular filling is impeded throughout diastole. Central venous and right and left atrial pressure pulses show an M-shaped contour in constrictive pericarditis as well as prominent "x" and "y" descents followed by a rapid rise in pressure during early diastole. In addition to reduced stroke volume, ventricular end-diastolic pressures, and mean atrial, pulmonary vein and systemic vein pressures are elevated to an almost equal amount. The ventricular pressure pulse shows the characteristic "square-root sign" in diastole. With cardiac tamponade, the most prominent deflection is the "x" trough, whereas there is absence of the "y" descent in the jugular venous pulse and absence of the "square-root sign" in the ventricular pulse during diastole.

Other significant procedures in diagnosis are electrocardiogram findings, purified protein derivative (PPD) intermediate skin testing, pericardial aspirate culture, and pericardial biopsy.[22] Electrocardiographic T-wave inversion consistent with but not diagnostic for pericarditis is a common abnormality (84%).[22] Low-voltage QRS waves may also be visible. PPD of intermediate strength (PPD-intermediate) yields positive results in most patients (80 to 100%).[22,32,53,54] A negative PPD-intermediate test result is common in a patient with pericardial TB and AIDS because of the increased degree of anergy in patients with AIDS.[71]

Pericardial fluid is obtained via pericardiocentesis that is performed to establish an etiology, relieve tamponade, or both. In tuberculous pericarditis, the effusion is usually a lymphocytic exudate that may be bloody or blood-tinged.[22,32,54] It usually has high protein content and a low sugar level. Culture of pericardial fluid was positive in up to 50% of patients in three studies.[22,32,42] This percentage could not be duplicated in other studies.

Pericardial biopsy has also been advocated in the diagnosis of pericarditis.[6,23,32,42,55] Between 1950 and 1970, many investigators thought that examination of the entire pericardium at pericardiectomy or autopsy was required to definitively diagnose TB.[66,72,73] Fredriksen and associates[74] reviewed the cases of 20 patients with pericardial effusion who underwent pericardiocentesis and percutaneous open pericardial window with pericardial biopsy. Biopsy provided a specific etiological diagnosis in two (10%) and 13 (65%) had at least one serious complication postoperatively. Pericardiocentesis was uncomplicated and yielded a specific diagnosis in four patients (20%).

In view of the significant morbidity and poor diagnostic yield from pericardial windows Fredriksen and associates[74] proposed specific recommendations for pericardiocentesis and percutaneous open pericardial window with biopsy. These included relief of tamponade and establishment of the causative factor of pericardial effusion as the main indications for pericardiocentesis. Percutaneous pericardial window with biopsy was indicated for drainage of a purulent pericardial effusion, for recurrent tamponade after pericardiocentesis and for chronic effusion after unproductive pericardiocentesis. More recent studies have attempted to shed more light on the usefulness of pericardial biopsy. In 1988, Strang and colleagues[32] found that 33 (70%) of 47 pericardial biopsy samples in the patients with pericardial TB had histologic evidence of TB (e.g., caseating granulomata). Sagrista-Sauleda and coauthors,[42] also in 1988, found evidence of TB in all three pericardial biopsies performed on patients with tuberculous pericarditis and the six pericardiectomies performed in this series. All showed the presence of TB on histologic examination.

Endrys and associates[75] have presented a new technique for multiple pericardial biopsies. In the cardiac catheterization laboratory the pericardium is punctured, air is allowed to enter the pericardial space and a bioptome is inserted to obtain multiple biopsy specimens (an average of eight) of the parietal pericardium. This is all performed under fluoroscopy. The air is aspirated from the pericardial space at the end of the procedure and a sheath is left in place until daily fluid drainage is less than 30 ml. Eighteen biopsies were performed with six revealing TB, two cancer and one mesothelioma. The other nine biopsies were noncontributory, but excluded malignancy. None of the nine patients exhibited malignancy during follow-up.

THERAPY

In the Rooney and associates study[22] of 35 patients with tuberculous pericarditis, 11 died, for a 35% mortality rate. Twenty-eight received antituberculosis therapy for at least 24 months. Seven patients never received adequate therapy. Four of the twenty-eight patients who were adequately treated died, for a 14% mortality rate. The primary

modes of death were congestive heart failure, advance TB or a combination of both. Autopsies performed on 10 of 11 patients revealed that each one had pericardial as well as mediastinal lymph node involvement. This distribution of lesions suggests that lymphatic dissemination may be significant in the pathogenesis of pericardial TB.

The study of Strang and coworkers[32] included 240 patients from the Transkei in South Africa with possible tuberculous pericarditis. Of the 198 patients with a pericardial effusion, 144 (73%) had evidence of active TB in the pericardium or elsewhere. Of these 144, 12 (8%) died because of pericarditis in the 24 months after admission. Treatment included INH, rifampin (RIF), streptomycin, and pyrazinamide (PZA) for 6 months.

The American Thoracic Society, the Centers for Disease Control, and the Infectious Diseases Society[76] recommend that patients with pericardial TB receive a 6-month regimen (2 months of INH, RIF, PZA and Ethambutol (EMB) followed by 4 months of INH and RIF) as initial therapy unless the organisms are known or strongly suspected of being resistant to first-line drugs. They also recommended as adjunctive therapy for tuberculous pericarditis corticosteroid therapy for the first 11 weeks of antituberculosis treatment. The dosage of corticosteriods used was prednisone 60 mg/day (or equivalent dose of prednisolone) for 4 weeks, followed by 30 mg/day for 4 weeks, 15 mg/day for 2 weeks, and 5 mg/day for the final week.

Because current antituberculosis treatment is most effective in eradicating mycobacteria, prompt diagnosis and institution of therapy are imperative. Difficulty in the diagnosis of pericardial TB often results in the late institution of therapy and therefore is, in part, responsible for the high mortality in this disease. Another major cause of high mortality is that the pericardial inflammation interferes with the mechanical efficiency of the heart, particularly when pericardial tamponade occurs.

Mycobacteria grow slowly and therefore there is a lag time between institution of antituberculosis medication and elimination of the organisms. Abortion of the inflammatory response is not immediate. This interval or lag time is critical in terms of mortality. The pericardial inflammation that occurs is a potential risk because the rapid accumulation of fluid with tamponade and induction of arrhythmias may compromise cardiac performance.

In order to suppress a pericardial reaction and minimize its sequelae, corticosteroids have been introduced. These drugs have been found to be efficacious in the treatment and control of pericardial effusions in many different varieties of pericarditides.[22,32,77–82] In pulmonary and pleural TB, the addition or corticosteroids together with antituberculosis drugs results in a more rapid resolution of disease.[22,78,83–87] Experimental evidence has shown that cortisone reduced the host reaction to mycobacterial infections and minimized exudation, fibrin deposition and proliferation of granulation tissue.[22,32,83–92]

In tuberculous pericarditis, corticosteroids nonspecifically suppress the inflammation, thereby lessening the hemodynamic sequelae as the antituberculosis drugs eliminate the organisms. The exudation of fluid abates and reabsorption of fluid commences. A noticeable decrease in heart size often occurs within 2–3 days, and it may return to normal within 2 weeks. Defervescence is rapid and arrhythmias are controlled within 2–3 days. The corticosteroids may be withdrawn over the next 11 weeks without recrudescence of symptoms of tuberculous pericarditis. At the same time the mycobacteria, which evoke the inflammatory reaction in this disease, are being eradicated by the concomitant use of antituberculosis drugs. Upon withdrawal of corticosteroids, occasionally pulmonary TB may be aggravated transiently, which abates quickly with continuous antituberculosis therapy.

A number of authors have had success with corticosteroid therapy in addition to antituberculosis treatment in the management of tuberculous pericarditis.[22,32,77,80–82,93–94] In a study of 28 patients who received chemotherapy for tuberculous pericarditis, 10 patients were treated with a three-drug regimen alone and 18 were treated with 3 antituberculosis drugs and prednisone.[22] In the first group 4 patients died, 2 of whom were in a group of 4 requiring pericardiectomy. There were no deaths in the prednisone-treated group, 14 improved without surgery and 4 required pericardiectomy.

In a controlled study, Strang[95] reviewed the effect of open surgical drainage and prednisolone in a dose of 60 mg/day in the treatment of tuberculous pericarditis. Strang reported that comparison of the prednisolone and placebo groups showed that prednisolone significantly reduced the death risk during the 24 hours after admission and the need for repeat pericardiocentesis. There was also a reduction in need for open surgical drainage that is often needed because of rapid reaccumulation of pericardial fluid despite repeated pericardiocenteses (4% vs. 9% for placebo). The conclusion of this study was that corticosteroids increase the rate of clinical improvement during antituberculosis chemotherapy and reduce the risk of death in active constrictive pericarditis.

In 2000, Hakim et al.[96] in Zimbabwe studied 58 patients with effusive tuberculous pericarditis who were infected with human immunodeficiency virus (HIV). All received antituberculosis therapy, but one-half received prednisolone for 6 weeks and one-half received placebo in a double-blind randomized placebo controlled trial.

Prednisolone was given in a dose of 60 mg/day for the first week and tapered by 10 mg/day each week thereafter. In this study 5 patients in the prednisolone group and 10 patients in the placebo group died over an 18 month period (p = 0.07). The prednisolone group had a significantly more rapid resolution of hepatomegaly and elevated jugular venous pressure and more rapid improvement in physical activity. The authors concluded that treatment of effusive tuberculous pericarditis in HIV infected patients should include not only standard antituberculosis therapy, but also prednisolone.

In 1999, Chen and colleagues[97] in Taiwan studied 22 patients with tuberculous pericarditis. These patients were evaluated by echocardiography and 17 showed a pericardial effusion (either "shaggy" in 8 or "non-shaggy" in 9) whereas 5 showed constrictive pericarditis. Patients with a "shaggy" tuberculous pericardial effusion had a medium duration between onset of symptoms and diagnosis compared to those with a "non-shaggy" effusion. Antituberculosis treatment and 20 to 30 mg/day of prednisolone were used in 11 patients, 2 of whom developed constrictive pericarditis. Treatment with antituberculosis medicine, but without prednisolone resulted in constrictive pericarditis in 5 of 6 patients. The authors concluded that antituberculosis medication with prednisolone resulted in a significant decrease in constrictive pericarditis particularly in patients with a "shaggy" tuberculous pericardial effusion as compared with those who did not receive prednisolone. However, they also showed that patients with a "non-shaggy" tuberculous pericardial effusion did not exhibit the same benefit.

In 2003 Ntsekhe and associates[98] as well as their colleague Mayosi et al.[99] reviewed 4 randomized or quasi-randomized trials[32,93,96,100] using meta-analysis to compare the effectiveness of corticosteroids versus placebo therapy in the treatment of tuberculous pericarditis. In 469 patients studied, the corticosteroid patients had a statistically higher chance of being alive with no functional impairment at 2 years after treatment than those receiving placebo. However, in a sensitivity analysis including patients lost to follow-up, the effect of treatment was not sustained. Furthermore, the benefits of corticosteroid treatments on reaccumulation of pericardial effusion and its progression to constrictive pericarditis did not reach statistical significance. The authors felt that corticosteroids might have a beneficial effect on mortality and morbidity in tuberculous pericarditis, but that these trials were nor large enough to be conclusive. They felt that a large placebo controlled trial was needed to conclusively prove that corticosteroid therapy results in a statistically significant improvement in the treatment of pericardial TB.

Corticosteroids are successful in suppressing on-going inflammation, but they cannot reverse damage that has occurred prior to treatment. Repair by fibrosis can still take place, and blood, fibrin, and other exudative substances that are already present can result in continuous deleterious influences. In such circumstances, surgical intervention in the form of pericardiectomy is the best method for controlling mechanical compression. There are many excellent descriptions of the surgical technique, but it must be emphasized that the earlier the pericardiectomy is performed in patients that do not respond to medical therapy the better the overall results.[6,22–24,32,42,55,57,58,101–109]

Whether or not corticosteroids will diminish the likelihood of late constrictive pericarditis is not known because resolution of this problem requires a large number of untreated patients as well as a large number of antituberculosis drug-treated patients, equal numbers of whom do and do not receive corticosteroids. Death among untreated patients with tuberculous pericarditis is common. Therefore, little information is available to gauge what percentage of patients that heal spontaneously, later develop pericardial constriction. The report of Hageman and colleagues[30] suggests that antituberculosis drug-treated patients infrequently developed constriction. This conclusion is not secure without a minimum follow-up of 5 years and preferably 20 years to assess the true incidence of this complication. If residual fibrosis resulting from TB can be used as an index for predicting the likelihood of late constriction, the use of corticosteroids in pleural and pulmonary TB would suggest that these drugs do not significantly alter these residues and therefore probably will not prevent constriction to any greater degree than antituberculosis drugs alone,

Any patient who experiences signs and symptoms of pericarditis, whose tuberculin skin test result is positive, and whose chest radiograph is characterized by a pulmonary infiltrate, a pleural effusion or both should be empirically regarded as having tuberculous pericarditis until proven otherwise. Prompt treatment with antituberculosis drugs should be initiated. Prednisone, 60 mgs/day or its equivalent, is administered concomitantly. This dose is maintained for 4 weeks and is progressively reduced to discontinuation in 11 weeks. It has to be recognized that corticosteroid treatment is not a panacea in the management of tuberculous pericarditis and does not always eliminate the necessity for pericardiocentesis, ancillary agents to control heart failure or even pericardiectomy. The need for the later is dictated by close evaluation of the clinical response to treatment.

The need for pericardiectomy is not universal in tuberculous pericarditis. In the majority of studies that address the need for pericardiectomy in this disease, this surgical procedure was performed in 10–50%.[6,22,30,32,55,58,103,109] The indication for the procedure was constrictive pericarditis, cardiac tamponade, or both.

In the recent past investigators have looked at idiopathic chronic pericardial effusions,[110] acute cardiac tamponade,[111] and effusive-constrictive pericarditis.[112] In reviewing large idiopathic pericardial effusions Sagrista-Sauleda[110] looked at the natural history and treatment of this problem. They defined this malady as a collection of pericardial fluid that persists more than 3 months and does not have an apparent cause. They concluded that this condition can be well treated for long periods in many patients, but severe tamponade can occur at any time. They noted that large pericardial effusions can resolve with pericardiocentesis alone, but that recurrence is common and that when a large pericardial effusion occurs after pericardiocentesis, pericardiectomy should be considered. Spodick[111] in reviewing pericardial tamponade considered this medical problem as a slow or rapid compression of the heart, due to pericardial accumulation of fluid, pus, blood, clots, or gas as a result of effusion, trauma, or rupture of the heart. He felt the causes of this situation are diverse with traumatic tamponade likely to occur after cardiac surgery and tuberculous tamponade more common in Africa, but rare in the United States. His recommendation for treatment included drainage of the pericardial contents, preferably by needle pericardiocentesis under the guidance of echocardiographic, fluoroscopic or CT imaging. If the heart cannot be reached by needle or catheter, surgical drainage is required. Surgical drainage is also needed for intrapericardial bleeding, clotted hemopericardium, and recurrences of tamponade. Sagrista-Sauleda[112] discuss the problem of effusive-constrictive pericarditis, an uncommon syndrome characterized by a concomitant tamponade caused by a tense pericardial effusion and constriction caused by the visceral pericardium. The hallmark of this abnormality is persistent elevation of diastolic pressures after the removal of pericardial fluid has returned the intrapericardial pressures to normal. They felt that evolution to persistent constriction was frequent and that the idiopathic form may resolve spontaneously, but that extensive pericardiectomy with particular attention to the extent of involvement of the visceral pericardium was the best treatment in patients requiring surgery. In the surgical patient special attention should be paid to the extent of visceral pericardial involvement and the need for extensive epicardiectomy.

In order to determine the need for pericardiectomy in tuberculous pericarditis, the following course of action has been promulgated.[22] The patient's heart size is followed by radiography at least every 2 weeks, usually more frequently, and this reading is correlated with determination of right-sided heart pressures. If there is a persistently large heart and decreased cardiac performance supervenes, pericardiectomy is performed. If no change in heart size is observed by the 12th week of therapy, pericardiectomy is recommended. Similarly if the heart size regresses but the venous pressure rises, the operation is performed. In this situation, extensive epicardiectomy may be needed with particular attention to the visceral pericardium as described by Sagrista-Sauleda.[112] In patients whose heart size is decreased but in whom elevated venous pressure is stable, careful frequent observation is continued until the venous pressure returns to normal. If heart failure supervenes and/or venous pressure is not normal by the 12th week of therapy, pericardiectomy is performed. Patients whose heart size has decreased but has not reached normal are maintained on antituberculosis chemotherapy and followed carefully as long as their venous pressure remains normal and they are asymptomatic.

The problem of AIDS has arisen in recent years and has had a great effect on TB.[71,113,114] AIDS has been associated with a significant worldwide increase in TB, especially of the extrapulmonary type.[71,113] Tuberculous pericarditis has not escaped this problem.[15–21,115,116] Fortunately, treatment of M. tuberculosis in patients with AIDS appears to be just as effective as in TB patients without AIDS.[3,5,114,117–119] Unfortunately, atypical mycobacteria, particularly of the Mycobacterium avium-intracellulare type, are often poorly responsive to chemotherapy. In 11 patients reported by Anderson and Virmani,[118] two had M. avium-intracellulare as the causative organism.

TUBERCULOSIS OF AORTA AND MYOCARDIUM

More than 100 patients with TB of the aorta have been reported.[120–123] About half of these patients experience aneurysmal dilation of the thoracic or abdominal aorta. Most of these patients are diagnosed on post-mortem examination. Those with aneursym formation usually die from rupture and exsanguination.

The mechanism of development of aortic TB is believed to be via contiguous spread from tuberculous lymph nodes, pulmonary TB, vertebral TB, pericardial TB, pleural TB, or a combination thereof. Hematogenous spread to the aortic intima or vasa vasorum is thought to be uncommon. The rarity of aortic TB in patients with miliary TB seems

to support this contention. Tuberculosis usually spreads from a contiguous focus into the aorta, usually creating a false aneurysm. The most frequent complication of these aneurysms is rupture, especially into the gastrointestinal tract.

Whenever signs and symptoms of an aortic aneurysm are present in a patient with active TB elsewhere in the body, particularly in the thorax, tuberculous aortitis must be considered. Aortography must be performed immediately for an early definitive diagnosis because the arterial wall can necrose rapidly.

Treatment should include antituberculosis drugs. With the diagnosis of an aortic aneurysm, management also involves resection of the aneurysm to prevent rupture.

Another form of cardiovascular TB that has been reported recently is TB of the myocardium.[29,124–126] It has usually been diagnosed post-mortem, although with the advent of endomyocardial biopsy, ante-mortem diagnoses have been made.[126] Treatment of myocardial TB is via antituberculosis chemotherapy.

Unless there is vigilance in seeking out these patients who have TB and cardiovascular disease the mortality rate will remain high. Proper management and prevention of complications requires early diagnosis as well as early treatment.

REFERENCES

1. Davidson PT. Treating tuberculosis: What drugs, for how long? *Ann Int Med.* 1990;112:393–395.
2. Mann J, Snider DE, Francis, et al. Association between HTLV-III/LAV-infection and tuberculosis in Zaire. *JAMA.* 1986;256:346.
3. Chaisson RE, Schecter GF, Theuer, et al. Tuberculosis in patients with acquired immunodeficiency syndrome: Clinical features, response to therapy and survival. *Am Rev Resp Dis.* 1987;136:570–574.
4. Rieder HL, Cauthen GM, Block AB, et al. Tuberculosis and acquired immunodeficiency syndrome-Florida. *Arch Int Med.* 1989;149:1268–1273.
5. Pitchenik AE, Burr J, Suarez M, et al. Human lymphotrophic T-cell virus-III (HTLV-III) seropositivity and related disease among 71 consecutive patients in whom tuberculosis was diagnosed. A prospective study. *Am Rev Resp Dis.* 1987;135:875–879.
6. Quale JM, Lipschik GY, Heurich AE. Management of tuberculous pericarditis. *Ann Thor Surg.* 1987;43:653–655.
7. Kramer F, Modilevsky T, Waliany AR, et al. Delayed diagnosis of tuberculosis in patient with human immunodeficiency virus. *Am J Med.* 1990;89:451–456.
8. Alvarez S, McCabe WR. Extrapulmonary tuberculosis revisited. A review of experience of Boston and other hospitals. *Medicine (Baltimore).* 1984;63:25–55.

9. Shafer RW, Kim DS, Weiss JP et al. Extrapulmonary tuberculosis in patients with human immunodeficiency virus infection. *Medicine (Baltimore)*. 1991;70:384–397.

10. Supervia A, Campodarve I, Shaath M, et al. Tuberculous pericarditis as the first manifestation of AIDS: The indication for diagnostic pericardiocentesis. *Rev Clin Esp*. 1993;192:150–151.

11. Taelman H, Kagame A, Batungwanayo J, et al. Pericardial effusion in HIV infection. *Lancet*. 1990;335:924.

12. deMiguel J, Pedriera JD, Campos V, et al. Tuberculous pericarditis and AIDS. *Chest*. 1990;97:1273.

13. Dalli E, Quesada A, Juan G, et al. Tuberculous pericarditis as the first manifestation of the acquired immunodeficiency syndrome. *Am Heart J*. 1987;114:905–906.

14. Kwan T, Karve MMM, Emerole O. Cardiac tamponade in patients infected with HIV. *Chest*. 1993;104:1059–1062.

15. Antony SJ, Haas DW. Tuberculous pericarditis in an HIV infected patient. Scand *J infect Dis*. 1995;27:411–413.

16. Serrano-Heranz R, Camino A, Vilacosta I, et al. Tuberculous tamponade and AIDS. *Eur Heart J*. 1995;16: 430–432.

17. Cegielski JP, Lwakatara J, Dukes CS, et al. Tuberculous pericardial effusion associated with and without HIV infection. *Tuberc Lung Dis*. 1994;75:429–434.

18. Posniak AL, Weinberg J, Mahari M, et al. Tuberculous pericardial effusion associated with HIV infection: A sign of disseminated disease. *Tuberc Lung Dis*. 1994;75:297–300.

19. Pedro-Botet J, Auguet T, Coll J, et al. Tuberculous pericarditis as the first manifestation of AIDS. *Infection*. 1993;21:334–335.

20. Coulter JB, Walsh K, King SJ, et al. Tuberculous pericarditis in a child. *J Infect*. 1996;32:157–160.

21. Richter C, Nodosi B, Mwammy AS, et al. Extrapulmonary tuberculosis-a simple diagnosis? A retrospective study at Dar es Salaam, Tanzania. *Trop Geogr Med*. 1991;43: 375–378.

22. Rooney JJ, Crocco JA, Lyons HA. Tuberculous pericarditis. *Ann Int Med*. 1970;72:73–78.

23. Ortbals DW, Avioli LV. Tuberculous pericarditis. *Arch Int Med*. 1979;139:231–234.

24. Larrieu AJ, Tyers GF, Williams EH, et al. Recent experience with tuberculous pericarditis. *Ann Thor Surg*. 1980;29:464–468.

25. Blake S, Bonor S, O'Neill H, et al. Aetiology of chronic constrictive pericarditis. *Br Heart J*. 1983;50:273–276.

26. Fowler NO. Tuberculous pericarditis. *JAMA*. 1991;266: 99–103.

27. Felson B, Akers T, Hall G, et al. Mycotic tuberculous aneurysm of the thoracic aorta. *JAMA*. 1977;237:1104–1108.

28. Schlossberg D, Aaron T. Aortitis caused by Mycobacterium fortuitum. *Arch Int Med*. 1991;151:1010–1011.

29. Rose AG. Cardiac tuberculosis: A study of 19 patients. *Arch Pathol Lab Med*. 1987;111:422–426.

30. Hageman JH, D'Esopo NH, Glenn WW. Tuberculosis of the pericardium: A long-term analysis of forty-four proved cases. *N Engl J Med*. 1964;270:327–332.

31. Schepers GHW. Tuberculous pericarditis. *Am J Cardiol*. 1962;9:248–276.

32. Strang JIG, Kakaza MMS, Gibson DG, et al. Controlled clinical trial of complete open surgical drainage and of prednisone in treatment of tuberculous pericardial effusion in Transkei. *Lancet*. 1988;2:759–764.

33. Martin RP, Bowden R, Filly K, et al. Intrapericardial abnormalities in patients with pericardial effusion: Findings by two-dimensional echocardiography. *Circulation*. 1980;61: 568–572.

34. Harris LF. Tuberculous pericarditis, a unique experience. *Ala Med*. 1987;57:16–23.

35. Girling DJ, Darbyshire JH, Humphries, MJ, et al. Extrapulmonary tuberculosis. *Br Med Bull*. 1988;44:738–756.

36. Piras MA, Gakis C, Budroni A, et al. Adenosine deaminase activity in pleural effusions: An aid to differential diagnosis. *Br Med J*. 1978;2:1751–1752.

37. Ocana I, Martinez-Vazquez JM, Segura RM, et al. Adenosine deaminase in pleural fluids: Test for diagnosis of tuberculous pleural effusion. *Chest*. 1983;84:51–53.

38. Petersson T, Ojala K, Weber TH. Adenosine deaminase in the diagnosis of pleural effusion. *Acta Med Scand*. 1984;215:299–304.

39. Martinez-Vazquez JM, Ocana I, Ribera E, et al. Diagnostico temprano de la tuberculosis pleuroperitoneal mediante to determinacion de adenosina desaminasa. *Med Clin (Barcelona)*. 1984;83:578–580.

40. Martinez-Vazquez JM, Ribera E, Ocana I, et al. Adenosine deaminase activity in tuberculous pericarditis. *Thorax*. 1986;41:888–889.

41. Isaka N, Tanaka R, Nakamura M, et al. A case of tuberculous pericarditis-use of adenosine deaminase activity (ADA) in early diagnosis. *Heart Vessels*. 1990;5:247–248.

42. Sagrista-Sauleda J, Permanyer-Miralda G, Soler-Soler J. Tuberculous pericarditis: Ten year experience with a prospective protocol for diagnosis and treatment. *J Am Coll Cardiol*. 1988;11:724–728.

43. Piras MA, Gakis C. Cerebrospinal fluid adenosine deaminase activity in tuberculous meningitis. Enzyme. 1973;14:314–317.

44. Komsuoglu B, Goldeli O, Kulan KK, et al. The diagnostic and prognostic value of adenosine deaminase in tuberculous pericarditis. *Eur Heart J*. 1995;16:1126–1130.

45. Koh KK, Kim EJ, Cho CH, et al. Adenosine deaminase and carcinoembryonic antigen in pericardial effusion diagnosis, especially in tuberculous pericarditis. *Circulation*. 1994;89: 2728–2735.

46. Inoue T, Iga K, Hori K, et al. Tuberculous pericarditis: importance of adenosine deaminase activity in pericardial fluid. *Intern Med*. 1993;32:675–677.

47. Isaka N, Tanaka R, Nakamura M, et al. A case of tuberculous pericarditis-use of adenosine deaminase activity (ADA) in early diagnosis. *Heart Vessels*. 1990;5:247–248.

48. Aggeli C, Pisavos C, Brili S, et al. Relevance of adenosine deaminase and lysozyme measurements in the diagnosis of tuberculous pericarditis. *Cardiology*. 2000;94:81–85.

49. Burgess LJ, Reuter H, Carstens ME, et al. The use of adenosine deaminase and interferon-gamma as diagnostic tools for tuberculous pericarditis. *Chest*. 2000;122:900–905.

50. Cegielski JP, Devlin B, Morris AJ, et al. Comparison of PCR, culture and histology for diagnosis of tuberculous pericarditis. *J Clin Microbiol.* 1997;35:3254–3257.

51. Lee JH, Lee CW, Lee SG, et al. Comparison of polymerase chain reaction with adenosine deaminase activity in pericardial fluid for the diagnosis of tuberculous pericarditis. *Am J Med.* 2002;113:519–521.

52. Barnes PF, Cave MD. Molecular epidemiology of tuberculosis. *N Engl J Med.* 2003;349:1149–1156.

53. Fowler NO. The Pericardium in Health and Disease. Mount Kisco, NY: Futura; 1985.

54. Fowler NO, Manitsas GT. Infectious pericarditis. *Prog Cardiovasc Dis.* 1973;16:323–336.

55. Desai HN. Tuberculous pericarditis: a review of 100 cases. *S Afr Med J.* 1979;55:877–880.

56. Braunwald E. Pericardial disease. In: Wilson D, et al., eds. *Harrison's Principles of Internal Medicine,* 12th ed. New York, NY: McGraw-Hill; 1991:981–987.

57. Permanyer G, Sagrista-Sauleda j, Soler-Soler J. Primary acute pericardial disease: A prospective study of 231 consecutive patients. *Am J Cardiol.* 1985;56:623–630.

58. Long R, Younes M, Patton N, et al. Tuberculous pericarditis: Long-term outcome in patients who received medical therapy alone. *Am Heart J.* 1989;117:1133–1139.

59. Berger M, Bobak I, Jelveh M, et al. Pericardial effusion diagnosed by echocardiography. *Chest.* 1978;72:1744–1779.

60. Chia BI, Chod M, Tan H, et al. Echocardiographic abnormalities in tuberculous pericardial effusion. *Am Heart J.* 1984;107:1034–1035.

61. Agrawal S, Radhakrishnan, Sinha N. Echocardiographic demonstration of resolving intrapericardial mass in tuberculous pericarditis. *Int J Cardiol.* 1990;26:240–241.

62. Martin RP, Rakowski H, French J, et al. Localization of pericardial effusion with wide-angle phase array echocardiography. *Am J Cardiol.* 1978;42:904–905.

63. Haase D, Marrie TJ, Martin R, et al. Gallium scanning in tuberculous pericarditis. *Clin Nucl Med.* 1981;6:275.

64. Lin DS, Tipton RE. Ga-67 Cardiac uptake. *Clin Nucl Med.* 1983;8:603–604.

65. Solomon A, Weiss J, Stern D, et al. Computerized tomography in pericardial disease. *Heart Lung.* 1983;12:513–515.

66. Scwartz MJ, May HR, Fitzpatrick HF. Pericardial biopsy. *Arch Int Med.* 1963;112:155–157.

67. Bertolaccini T, Chimenti M, Bianchi S, et al. Gallium-67 scintigraphy in an AIDS patient presenting with tuberculous pericarditis. *J Nucl Biol.* 1993;37:245–248.

68. Suchel IB, Horowitz TA. CT in tuberculous constrictive pericarditis. *J Comput Assist Tomogr.* 1992;16:391–400.

69. Winkler M, Higgins CB. Suspected intracardiac masses: Evaluation by MR imaging. *Radiology.* 1987;165:117–121.

70. D'Silva SA, Nalladaru ZM, Dalvi DB, et al. MRI as a guide to surgical approach in tuberculous pericardial abscess. *Scand J Thoracic Cardiovasc Surg.* 1992;26:229–231.

71. Centers for Disease Control. Tuberculosis and human immunodeficiency virus infection: Recommendations of the Advisory Committee for the Elimination of Tuberculosis (ACET). *MMWR Morb Mortal Wkly Rep.* 1989;38:236–238.

72. Cheitlin MD, Serfos LJ, Sbar SS, et al. Tuberculous pericarditis: Is limited pericardial biopsy sufficient for diagnosis. *Am Rev Resp Dis.* 1968;98:287–290.

73. Deterling RA Jr, Humphreys GH. Factors in the etiology of constrictive pericarditis. *Circulation.* 1955;12:30–33.

74. Fredriksen RT, Cohen LS, Mullins CB. Pericardial windows or pericardiocentesis for pericardial effusions. *Am Heart J.* 1971;82:158–162.

75. Endrys J, Simo M, Shalie MZ, et al. New non-surgical technique for multiple pericardial biopsies. *Cath Cardiovasc Dig.* 1988;12:92–94.

76. American Thoracic Society/Centers for Disease Control/Infectious Diseases Society of America: Treatment of tuberculosis. *Am J Resp Crit Care Med.* 2003;167:603–662.

77. Dressler W. The post-myocardial infarction syndrome. *Arch Int Med.* 1959;103:28–42.

78. Freedberg CK. Diseases of the Heart. 3rd ed., Philadelphia and London: WB Saunders; 1966:956.

79. Legrand R, Linquette M, Desruelles J, et al. A propos de deux cas de pericardite tuberculeuse traits par la cortisone. *Fr Med.* 1954;17:37–38.

80. Voegtlin R, Simler M, Hauswald R. Pericardite tuberculeuse aigue: effet de la cortisone. *Strasb Med.* 1955;6:242–246.

81. Tourniaire A, Blum J, Gros G. Pericardite tuberculeuse en voie d'organisation symphysaire guerie par l'association medicamenteuse streptomycin-deltacortisone. *Lyon Med.* 1958;90:5–10.

82. Angel JH, Chu LS, Lyons HA. Corticotropin in the treatment of tuberculosis: A controlled study. *Arch Int Med.* 1961;180:353–369.

83. Aspin J, O'Hara H. Steroid-treated tuberculous effusion. *Br J Tuberc.* 1958;52:81–83.

84. British Tuberculosis Association, Research Committee. Trial of corticotropin and prednisone with chemotherapy in pulmonary tuberculosis: A two year radiographic follow-up. *Tuberc.* 1963;44:484–486.

85. Mathur KS, Prasad R, Mathur JS. Intrapleural cortisone in tuberculous pleural effusion. *Tuberc.* 1960;41:358–362.

86. Ballabio CH, Sala G. Le Indicazione al trattamento locale della pleurite e pericarditiessudatie con idracortisone acetato. *Minerva Med.* 1954;45:1839–1846.

87. Paley SS, Mihaly JP, Mais EL, et al. Prednisone in the treatment of tuberculous effusions. *Am Rev Tuberc.* 1959;79:307–314.

88. Cummings MM, Hudgkins PC, Whorton MC, et al. The influence of cortisone and streptomycin on experimental tuberculosis in the albino rat. *Am Rev Tuberc.* 1952;65:596–602.

89. Ebert RH. In vivo observation of the effect of cortisone in experimental tuberculosis, using the rabbit ear chamber technique. *Am Rev Tuberc.* 1952;65:64–74.

90. D'Arcy Hart P, Rees RJW. Enhancing effect of cortisone on tuberculosis in the mouse. *Lancet.* 1950;2:391–395.

91. Ragan C, Howes EL, Plotz CM, et al. Effect of cortisone on production of granulation tissue in the rabbit. *Proc Soc Exp Biol Med.* 1949;72:718–721.

92. Spain DM, Molomut N. Effects of cortisone on the development of tuberculous lesions in guinea pigs and on their modification by streptomycin therapy. Am Rev Tuberc. 1950;62:337–344.

93. Shrire V. Experimental pericarditis at Groote Schuur Hospital, Cape Town: An analysis of 160 cases over a 6 year period. *S Afr J Med.* 1959;33:810–817.

94. Dooley DP, carpenter JL, Rademacher S. Adjunctive corticosteroid therapy for tuberculosis: A critical appraisal of the literature. *Clin Inf Dis.* 1997;25:872–887.

95. Strang JI. Rapid resolution of tuberculous pericardial effusion with high dose prednisone and antituberculosis chemotherapy. *J Infect.* 1994;28:251–254.

96. Hakim JG, Ternouth J, Mushangi E, et al. Double blind randomized placebo-control trial of adjunctive prednisolone in treatment of effusive tuberculous pericarditis in HIV seropositive persons. *Heart.* 2000;84:183–188.

97. Chen LY, Liaw YS, Kao HL. Constrictive pericarditis in patients with tuberculous pericarditis. *J Formos Med Assn.* 1999;98:599–605.

98. Ntsekhe M, Wiysonge C, Volmink JA, et al. Adjuvant corticosteroids for tuberculous pericarditis. *QJM.* 2003;96: 593–599.

99. Mayosi BM, Ntsekhe M, Volmink JA, et al. Interventions for treating tuberculous pericarditis. *Cochrane Database Syst Rev.* 2002:4:CD000526.

100. Strang JI, Kakaza HH, Gibson DG, et al. Controlled trial of prednisolone as adjunct in treatment of tuberculous pericarditis in Transkei. *Lancet.* 1987;2:1418–1422.

101. Alzeer AM, Fitzgerald AM. Corticosteroids and tuberculosis: Risks and use as adjunct therapy. *Tuberc Lung Dis.* 1993;74:6–11.

102. Hatcher CR Jr, Logue RB, Logan WD, et al. Pericardiectomy for recurrent pericarditis. *J Thorac Cardiovasc Surg.* 1971;62:371–378.

103. Carson TJ, Murray GF, Wilcox BR, et al. The role of surgery in tuberculous pericarditis. *Ann Thorac Surg.* 1974;17:163–167.

104. Miller JI, Mansour KA, Hatcher CR Jr. Pericardiectomy: Current indications, concepts and results in a university setting. *Ann Thor Surg.* 1982;34:140–145.

105. Bauer H, Sachs R, Cummings MM. Tuberculous pericarditis among veterans: Veteran's Administration Transactions of the Fifteenth Conference on Chemotherapy of tuberculosis. U.S. Government Document, 1956;15:138.

106. Blakemore WS, Zinsser MF, Kirby CK, et al. Pericardiectomy for relapsing pericarditis and chronic constrictive pericarditis. *J Thorac Cardiovasc Surg.* 1978;39:26–34.

107. Scannell JG. Surgical treatment of tuberculous pericarditis. In: Luisada AA, ed. *Cardiology, an Encyclopedia of the Cardiovascular System,* New York, NY: McGraw-Hill; 1959;3:7–59.

108. Scannell JG, Meyers GS, Friedlich AL. Significance of pulmonary hypertension in constrictive pericarditis. *Surgery.* 1952;32:184–194.

109. Sonnenberg FA, Parker SG. Elective pericardiectomy for tuberculous pericarditis: Should the snappers be snipped? *Med Decis Making.* 1986;6:110–123.

110. Sagrista-Sauleda J, Angel J, Permanyer G, et al. Long-term follow-up of idiopathic pericardial effusion. *N Engl J Med.* 1999;341:2054–2059.

111. Spodick DH. Acute Cardiac Tamponade. *N Engl J Med.* 2003;349:684–690.

112. Sagrista-Sauleda J, Angel J, Sanchez A, et al. Effusive constrictive pericarditis. *N Engl J Med.* 2004;350:469–475.

113. Tuberculosis and acquired immunodeficiency syndrome-New York City. *MMWR Morb Mortal Wkly Rep.* 1987;36: 785–795.

114. Ellner JJ Tuberculosis in the time of AIDS. The facts and the message. *Chest.* 1990;98:1051–1052.

115. Flora GS, Modilevsky T, Antoniskis A, et al. Undiagnosed tuberculosis in patients with human immunodeficiency virus infection. *Chest.* 1990;98:1056–1059.

116. D'Cruz IA, Sengupta EE, Abrahams C, et al. Cardiac involvement including tuberculous pericardial effusion, complicating acquired immunodeficiency syndrome. *Am Hear J.* 1988;112:1100–1102.

117. Louie E, Rich LB, Holzman RS. Tuberculosis in non-Haitian patients with acquired immunodeficiency syndrome in a New York City Hospital. *Chest.* 1987;91:176–180.

118. Anderson DW, Virmani R. Progress in pathology: Emerging patterns of heart disease in patients with acquired immunodeficiency syndrome. *Hum Pathol.* 1990;21:253–259.

119. Snider DE Jr, Hopewell PC, Mills J, et al. Mycobacterioses and the acquired immunodeficiency syndrome: A joint position paper of the American Thoracic Society and the Centers for Disease Control. *Am Rev Resp Dis.* 1987;136: 492–496.

120. Efredmidis SC. Lakshmanan S, Hsu JT, et al. Tuberculous aortitis: A rare cause of mycotic aneurysm of the aorta. *Am J Reontgenol.* 1979;127:859–861.

121. Estrera AS, Platt MR, Mills LJ, et al. Tuberculous aneurysms of the descending aorta. *Chest.* 1979;75:386–388.

122. Silbergleit A, Arbulu A, Defever BA, et al. Tuberculous aortitis: Surgical resection of an abdominal false aneurysm. *JAMA.* 1975;193:331–333.

123. Choudhary SK, Bhan A, Talwar S, et al. Tubercular pseudo-aneurysm of the aorta. *Ann Thor Surg.* 2001;72:1239–1244.

124. Halim MA, Mercer EM, Guinn GA. Myocardial tuberculoma with rupture and pseudoaneurysm formation-successful surgical treatment. *Br Heart J.* 1985;54:603–604.

125. Bennett JM, Nande DF, DeVilliers. Recurrence of two myocardial aneurysms infected with tuberculosis after a previous aneurysmectomy. *Clin Cardiol.* 1989;12:605–606.

126. Bali HK, Wahi S, Sharma BK. Myocardial tuberculosis presenting as restrictive cardiomyopathy. *Am Heart J.* 1990;120:703–706.

22

Gastrointestinal Tuberculosis

Walter J. Coyle*
Todd A. Sheer*

INTRODUCTION

Tuberculous intestinal involvement remains ever present in the differential diagnoses of physicians and surgeons. Whether the patient has HIV disease, is immunosuppressed with steroids and chemotherapy, or lives in an endemic area, we need to be always vigilant for the signs, symptoms, and historical clues that suggest active tuberculosis (TB) of the gut. This disease remains the great mimic despite centuries of experience and awareness of its manifestations.

Abdominal TB can be divided into three types based on the region of involvement: peritoneal, hepatobiliary, and enteric. The enteric subset includes infection of the hollow viscera of the abdomen and comprises roughly one-half of all cases.[1–13] Coexisting intestinal and peritoneal TB is uncommon.[5,9] The following chapter will focus on the varied presentations of enteric TB. Peritoneal and hepatobiliary disease will be discussed in detail in chapters 24 and 25.

EPIDEMIOLOGY

In North America, tuberculous enteritis occurs in less than 5% of all cases of TB and it is one of the least prevalent extrapulmonary sites of infection.[14,15] However, enteric TB remains a problem in Asia,[16] the Middle East,[12,17] and Africa.[10] This is at least in part due to overall higher rates of TB in these regions.[18] Risk factors include low socioeconomic status and immunocompromised states.[19,20] In the latter group, solid organ transplant recipients constitute a growing number, and many cases of intestinal TB are being reported in this population.[21–23] In industrialized nations, an additional risk factor is immigration from a high-prevalence country, and this risk persists twenty years after arrival.[8,15] In the U.S., half of all TB cases in 2002 were in foreign-born individuals, with Mexico, the Philippines, and Vietnam being the most likely countries of origin.[15] Despite reports of increased cases of abdominal TB in the early 1990's,[24] current CDC data suggests a downward trend in all forms of the disease, both pulmonary and extrapulmonary,[15] most likely due to increased awareness and improved treatment of both HIV and TB.

PATHOGENESIS

Mycobacteria infect the gastrointestinal tract in one of four ways: (1) swallowing of infected sputum in a patient with active pulmonary disease, (2) hematogenous or lymphatic spread from a distant focus, (3) direct extension from a contiguous site, and (4) ingestion of milk products infected with *Mycobacterium bovis*. The latter mechanism is nonexistent in the U.S. and other developed nations due to pasteurization of milk and tuberculin testing of the herd population; however, it remains a viable means of infection in some countries, especially those where raw milk is consumed as part of local tradition.[12] Other authors have described two types of enteric TB: a primary form, usually from the ingestion of the bovine bacillus, and a secondary form due to spread of the human bacillus from active pulmonary disease.[25] As mentioned, the primary form is extremely rare in the U.S., and when it does appear to occur, it probably represents reinfection from a previous and no longer apparent focus or failure to uncover the pulmonary infection.[26] Only 20–30% of patients with intestinal TB have evidence for concurrent active pulmonary involvement,[4–6,27] but this is highly variable[7,28] and may reflect the rigidity of the criteria used to make the diagnosis. On the other hand, almost 50% of patients with smear-positive cavitating pulmonary TB had proven or suspected tuberculous enteritis with a statistically significant correlation (in the proven cases) between severity of the lung disease and likelihood of intestinal involvement.[29] Other authors have suggested that many cases of subclinical enteric TB go unnoticed and resolve with appropriate treatment of the pulmonary disease.[5,8]

The entire gastrointestinal tract from the esophagus to anus can be involved. The ileocecal region is the most common location, affected in 44–93% of cases.[7,25] The colon and small bowel alone are the next most frequent sites of infection and the esophagus and stomach are rarely involved.[3,6] The *Mycobacteria* have a fatty capsule, which resists digestion and interferes with release early in the gastrointestinal tract, explaining the rarity of proximal lesions.[28] The narrow lumen and relative stasis of the ileocecal region allow digestion of the capsule and efficient absorption of the organism. Abundant lymphatic tissue for which the organism has an affinity further enhances infection at this site.[30] Once in the submucosa, the bacillus

*The opinions expressed herein are solely those of the authors and do not reflect those of the U.S. Navy, the Department of Defense or the U.S. Government.

CLINICAL MANIFESTATIONS

The clinical presentation of enteric TB is often vague and nonspecific and there are no pathognomonic symptoms or signs (see Table 22-1). As a result, TB is often not entertained in the differential diagnosis. One U.S. study showed that physicians considered the diagnosis in only 39% of patients on initial presentation.[13] Perhaps as common is the tendency to diagnose the patient with more common diseases such as Crohn's disease,[32] appendicitis,[8] carcinoma,[33] irritable bowel syndrome,[7] and amebic colitis.[9] In one series of tuberculous enteritis, 53% of the cases were detected unexpectedly during surgery for an unrelated diagnosis.[5] The most commonly noted symptom is abdominal pain, seen in 70–100% of patients,[1,3,4,6,7,17,25] although some authors note this less frequently.[12] The pain is usually colicky and intermittent in nature and may represent subacute intestinal obstruction. It is frequently localized in the right lower quadrant or periumbilical regions,[1,4] although it may be epigastric in the rare cases of gastric or duodenal involvement.[11] Anorexia and weight loss are not infrequent, with patients demonstrating some degree of these symptoms in the majority of cases. Low-grade fever and/or night sweats are common but are not the universal symptoms that they are traditionally believed to be. A review of several large series demonstrates fever and/or night sweats in less than 50% of cases.[3,4,6,7,12,17,25,27] A change in bowel habits is encountered in 41–76% of affected patients,[17,25] with diarrhea predominating over constipation in most.[6,25,27] Less frequently reported symptoms include melena, hematochezia, oligomenorrhea, and amenorrhea.[1,3,9,12,27] Fourteen percent of patients may be asymptomatic.[5] A history of previous TB or exposure was elicited in almost half of the patients in one series.[27] On physical examination, a right lower quadrant abdominal

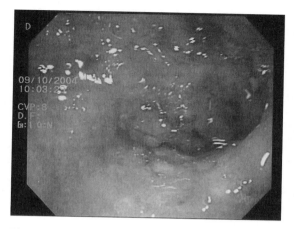

Fig. 22-1. Endoscopic image of tuberculous ulceration and nodularity of the duodenum.

colonizes the Peyer's patches and initiates an inflammatory response with granuloma formation. The tubercles undergo caseous necrosis and release organisms into the lymphatics with migration to regional nodes where further granulomata form. As the tubercles enlarge, the bowel wall becomes markedly thickened and small papillary elevations form in the mucosa. Combined with an associated endarteritis and lymphangitis, the superficial mucosa becomes edematous and circumferentially ulcerated (see Fig. 22-1). As the ulcers heal, deposition and contraction of collagen in the submucosa can lead to stricture formation.[26,28,30] Thus, tuberculous enteritis can be classified grossly as ulcerative, hypertrophic, mixed ulcerohypertrophic, and fibrotic.[6,31] The ulcerative form is more likely to be found in the small intestine and the hypertrophic form in the cecum.[3,28]

Table 22-1. Symptoms of Enteric Tuberculosis

	Fraki et al., 1975 (n = 33)[1]	Findlay et al., 1979 (n = 52)[4]	Al-Bahrani et al., 1982 (n = 50)[25]	Gilinsky et al., 1983 (n = 46)[6]	Al Karawi et al., 1995 (n = 84)[12]	Weighted Average
Pain	91%	81%	96%	80%	42%	72%
Nausea/vomiting	36%	19%	72%	50%	23%	37%
Weight loss	55%	40%	96%	83%	27%	56%
Fever	39%	16%	16%	50%	31%	37%
Diarrhea	42%	—	—	48%	15%	37%
Constipation	27%	—	—	20%	—	23%

mass or tenderness may be encountered, but these are variable. Frank abdominal distention is usually seen more often with the peritoneal form of the disease with associated ascites[10] but can been seen in enteric cases complicated by small bowel obstruction; these should be readily distinguishable by physical exam. Lymphadenopathy of the neck, axilla, and femoral regions is detectable 2–20% of the time.[3,4,6,12,25] The "classic" presentation of the doughy abdomen is rare and is an unreliable physical finding.[10,12,17] Routine laboratory testing is reflective of a chronic inflammatory process.[4] In 40%, a mild to moderate anemia with hemoglobin values of 10–11 mg/dl and microcytic indices is noted.[3,4,6,17,25,27,34] An elevation in the erythrocyte sedimentation rate (ESR) occurs in 19–92%.[7,25] Hypoalbuminemia is present in more than half of the cases[6,10,17] and is due to a combination of poor oral intake, liver dysfunction, malabsorption, and lymphatic disease. Leukocytosis is rare and usually signifies a complication.[1,27] Stool tested for occult blood is positive in 28–75% of those investigated.[6,27] Alkaline phosphatase has been reported to be elevated in some series,[34,35] but it is not clear if the source was liver, intestine, or bone, as fractionation was not performed. The results of skin testing with purified protein derivative (PPD) vary widely with the population studied. For example, only 23% were PPD positive in a series from Saudi Arabia[17] compared to 72% from the University of Michigan.[5] Besides its dubious sensitivity for enteric TB, the specificity of PPD testing is frequently compromised by a history of previous disease or prior vaccination with Bacille Calmette-Guérin (BCG).

The most common age at presentation is in the third or fourth decade[3,17,36] and most series do not support a tendency for higher rates at the extremes of age. The majority of patients present chronically, with symptoms for several weeks to several months duration.[3,17,27] The longest reported period of symptoms prior to presentation was 15 years.[27] Acute and acute-on-chronic presentations are also possible, and in a large case series by Bhansali,[3] these were seen 19% and 28% of the time, respectively. Despite a tendency for earlier reports to show a higher prevalence in females,[37–39] more recent collections show equal to slightly greater numbers of males affected.[2,3,5,6,10,25,27] One explanation for these differences is that depending on the social norms of a region and period of time, one sex may be more at risk for exposure to TB than the other.[4]

The most common complication of enteric TB is obstruction.[3] Malabsorption is also frequently present. Other complications include perforation, fistula formation, and hemorrhage. These will be discussed in more detail below.

ESOPHAGUS

Primary esophageal TB has been rarely reported.[40–43] The first primary case was described in 1950.[44] Most reports are cases in which there is extension of the infection from mediastinal lymph nodes or a pulmonary source.[45,46] The majority of these cases are reported from areas that are highly endemic for mycobacterial disease.

There are no specific symptoms that suggest esophageal TB. The most commonly reported symptoms are dysphagia, weight loss, cough, chest pain, and fever.[40,47–50] Interestingly, odynophagia is not a prominent complaint. The middle one third is the most common location for tuberculous involvement of the esophagus.[41,43,49] Severe complications occur in a small percentage of cases and include bleeding, perforation, and fistula formation.[51,52] Massive hematemesis from erosion into the thoracic aorta or aorto-esophageal fistula has been reported.[51,53–55] Bleeding may be spontaneous or develop after treatment is initiated. Fistulas between the esophagus and tracheobronchial tree and between the esophagus and mediastinum occur frequently.[56–58] In one series, 50% of subjects with tuberculous involvement of the esophagus had fistula formation.[57] Most patients had significant mediastinal lymphadenopathy and presented with dysphagia rather than cough.[57,59]

The endoscopic appearance of esophageal TB has been recently reviewed.[40] Mucosal ulceration is the most common lesion but mucosal infiltration with or without stricture formation is also seen. Occasionally, either the ulcerative or hypertrophied lesions are misdiagnosed as malignancy.[60–62] Extrinsic compression with overlying normal mucosa and intramural pseudo-diverticulosis has also been reported.[41,63] When performing endoscopy in any suspected case of TB, it is important to protect endoscopic personnel from possible aerosolized infection by using appropriate respiratory protection.

Radiographic tests can reveal displacement of the esophagus by mediastinal lymph nodes, sinus tracts and fistula into the mediastinum or bronchial tree. Mucosal architecture can be evaluated by barium studies. The most common finding on barium swallow is extrinsic compression of the esophagus, but traction diverticula, strictures, fistulas, and pseudotumoral mass lesions are reported.[59,64] CT provides details of mediastinal and pulmonary involvement. Esophageal wall thickening, fistulas, and nodal involvement are all well seen by chest CT.[46,59,65]

Endoscopic biopsies and diagnosis are discussed below. Antituberculous medical therapy can be found in a later section, also. Surgical therapy should be reserved for those individuals with large or nonhealing fistulas, recurrent or massive hemorrhage, or obstruction.[40] The first case of successful medical therapy alone as treatment for a tracheo-esophageal fistula was in 1976.[56] Drainage of a large mediastinal abscess and repair of an esophago-mediastinal fistula has been reported.[41] The usual approach to tuberculous fistulas that are large or unresponsive to medical therapy is a right thorocotomy with primary resection and closure.[58] A recent large series reports successful closure of esophageal fistulas in 90% of patients with antituberculous therapy alone.[57] There is limited literature on the use of esophageal or bronchial stents in the setting of TB; however, successful placement of an esophageal endoprosthesis was recently reported in a patient who refused surgery.[58]

STOMACH

The stomach is a rare site for mycobacterial infections. Earlier literature suggested an incidence of 0.1% in resected specimens and 0.5% in autopsy cases[66]; however, more recent literature reports greater incidence especially in patients with immunosuppression.[7,24,33] Gastric lesions usually are associated with concomitant pulmonary or disseminated disease.[8,67–69]

Primary gastric TB is extremely rare. As of 1987, only seven definite cases were reported,[67] and only a handful of cases have been published since.[70–73] The relative resistance of the stomach to tuberculous involvement has been attributed to multiple factors including the low pH, the absence of lymphatic tissue, and the rapid emptying process.[8,67,71]

The lesser curve portion of the antrum and the pylorus are the most frequent locations of tuberculous infection.[67,69–71,73] Gastric manifestations of TB include ulceration or infiltration and hypertrophy of the gastric wall. The ulcers can be single or multiple. Bleeding and rarely perforation have been noted by several authors.[67,70,71,73] Gastric outlet obstruction secondary to infiltration and fibrosis of the gastric outlet has been noted by several authors.[67,70,71]

In the reported cases, the diagnosis is either suspected or confirmed by endoscopic mucosal biopsies and cultures. Antimicrobial treatment is discussed in a later section but surgery remains an important adjunct to medical therapy. Surgery is usually required for gastric outlet obstruction and the most common procedures described are gastrojejunostomy or antrectomy with Billroth II reconstruction.[67,70,73] There is one reported case of successful treatment of outlet obstruction with medical and endoscopic therapy alone.[71]

SMALL INTESTINE

As mentioned previously, the small bowel is a frequent site of involvement with gastrointestinal TB. Duodeno-jejunal TB is rare, occurring in less than 5% of collected cases.[1,2,4,6,11] The likelihood of infection increases as one moves distally, and the ileum is involved three times as often as the jejunum.[3] Although the small bowel is usually involved in conjunction with the cecum, it may be the sole site of disease in up to one-third of cases.[1,6,9,11,25] Like tuberculous enteritis in general, isolated disease involving the small intestine often presents insidiously,[74,75] and symptoms are usually due to a specific complication.

Obstruction is the most frequent complication and was seen in almost one-third of cases in a surgical series.[9] It is often the result of circumferential stricturing,[75,76] but focal nodular mucosal inflammation[77] and extrinsic compression from adenopathy[3] are other potential causes. Strictures are usually multiple, with more than three present in 28% of cases.[3] The obstructive process is gradual and the bowel may be able to adapt to the progressive luminal narrowing.[1] The most common site of deformity and obstruction is the ileocecal valve. The classic appearance is described as a fish mouth deformity of the valve (see Fig. 22-2). Enterolith formation

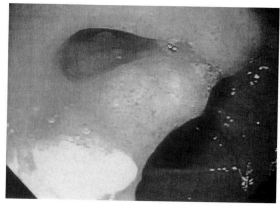

Fig. 22-2. Endoscopic appearance of the ileocecal valve with classic fish mouth deformity. (Courtesy of John Carethers, MD and Gregory Harmon, MD.)

proximal to a stricture may rarely occur.[78] Accordingly, symptoms may be acute or chronic and include nausea, vomiting, and abdominal pain.[76,79] Abdominal distention and hyperperistalsis are universally present but guarding is usually absent. The finding of abdominal tenderness on exam is highly variable.[3]

Due to the concomitant obliterative endarteritis seen in tuberculous intestinal ulcers, significant gastrointestinal hemorrhage is an uncommon complication, however, life-threatening upper and lower gastrointestinal bleeding from ulceration of the jejunum and ileum has been reported.[1,80,81] Fistulization from the small intestine to the aorta[82] and mesenteric arteries[83] can also cause massive hemorrhage. Bleeding from gastric varices secondary to jejunal TB with associated splenic vein thrombosis is another rare but documented presentation.[84]

Perforation in small intestinal TB is a rare event. Two case series, one of 52 patients and the other of 300 patients, both demonstrated an incidence of 7.6%.[3,85] Mortality after perforation is at least 30%.[26] The ileum is the most frequent site of perforation,[85] most likely a result of the higher rate of infection in this region. Perforation has been reported in the duodenum[86] and jejunum.[87] Multiple sites are not uncommon, occurring in 25–40% of the cases, and the mortality in these settings appears to be higher. This has been suggested to be the result of increased intraperitoneal soilage as well as a more aggressive infection or an immune deficiency pre-disposing to a higher rate of perforation.[87,88] Perforation is not limited to the small bowel and can also occur in the esophagus, stomach, colon, appendix, and rectum.[8,85,89] Multiple reports of perforation have been described during antituberculous therapy,[6,28,90] possibly due to a dramatic reduction in the intestinal wall inflammation before a sufficient fibrous response occurs.[28] Segal et al.[91] suggests that peritonitis in a patient with pulmonary TB should give reason to suspect a perforated tuberculous ulcer, but the absence of radiographic evidence of pulmonary disease does not rule out the diagnosis.[92] The clinical presentation may be surprisingly nonspecific but most reports suggest abdominal pain as the primary symptom in 85–100% of cases[3,92]; abdominal distention, guarding, and absent bowel sounds are less reliable.[3] Radiologic evidence of free air is not always noted, and this limitation in sensitivity may be due to adhesive disease limiting the spread of intraperitoneal air.[88] Accordingly, in a series of 28 patients with enteric TB and perforation (mainly small bowel), 23 were contained and only 5 showed free leakage into the peritoneum.[89] Fistulae are also rare, occurring in 1–33% of patients. Similar to perforation, they are most often seen originating

in the ileum but can also be found involving the esophagus, colon, and rectum. Enterocutaneous fistulae are the most common, followed by enteroenteric and enterocolonic.[89] Fistulae from the duodenum to the biliary tree[11,93,94] and from the duodenum to the renal pelvis[79] have been described. Since fistulae are also seen as a complication of Crohn's disease, their presence in tuberculous enteritis further adds to the difficulty in differentiating these two diseases.

Malabsorption is suspected to occur in approximately 20% of cases[13,19] but is more difficult to diagnose than the previous complications due to a lack of definitive radiologic or surgical findings. Intestinal TB is the second most common cause for malabsorption in South Africa and India.[6] The pathogenesis probably includes a combination of bacterial overgrowth from stricturing, decreased absorptive surface area secondary to diffuse mucosal ulceration and inflammation, lymphatic congestion, and bypassing of intestinal segments via fistulous tracts.[3] Tandon et al.[95] have shown greater rates of malabsorption, elevated quantitative small bowel bacterial cultures, and more bile salt deconjugation in patients with higher grades of obstruction compared to low-grade or no obstruction in enteric TB patients. These abnormalities reversed after surgical removal of the obstruction, suggesting that stagnant loops of intestine and bacterial overgrowth play a major role in malabsorption in intestinal TB. Besides causing diarrhea, malabsorption can cause a hypoproteinemic state, with subsequent higher post-surgical mortality, and may lead to subtherapeutic serum levels of antituberculous drugs. One author recommends using the lack of an expected urine color change with the use of rifampin as a screen for malabsorption.[13]

COLON

The colon is frequently involved with intestinal TB. As noted above, the ileocecal valve (Fig. 22-2) is the most common site of intestinal involvement followed by the ascending colon. The sigmoid colon and rectum are less commonly involved. Aoki first reported a case of colonic TB in 1971.[96] Multiple reports have been made since.

The classic endoscopic appearance of colonic TB is circumferential, white to yellow based ulcers with surrounding inflammation, nodules, and edema.[97–101] The ulcers of Crohn's disease are typically more linear but there is often confusion between the two diagnoses.[102–105] Tuberculous colitis has also presented as multiple small pink nodules with moderate erythema and friability of the surrounding mucosa (see Fig. 22-3). Pseudopolyposis and stenosis have also been described.[98–100,106]

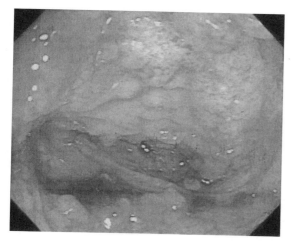

Fig. 22-3. Endoscopic view of colonic TB. (Courtesy of John Carethers MD, and Gregory Harmon MD.)

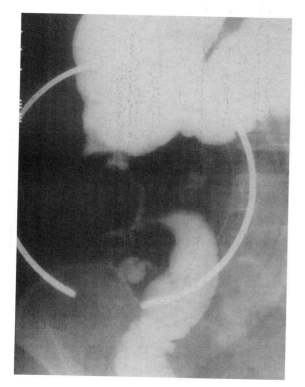

Fig. 22-4. Contrast barium enema demonstrating stricture and mass effect in the ileocecal region secondary to TB. (Courtesy of Sudha Praba MD.)

Segmental colitis involving every location of the colon has been reported in 19–26% with colonic TB.[106–109] In the largest published series of segmental colitis, 72% of subjects had only a single area of involvement measuring 4–8 cm. Marked hypertrophy of the mucosa along with stenosis due to TB has been misdiagnosed as malignancy.[91,98,110–112]

Both barium and CT imaging of the abdomen may suggest tuberculous involvement of the colon. The classic findings of ulceration, nodularity, tumor-like lesions, stricture, and fistula have been well described[12,103,113,114] (see Fig. 22-4).

Multiple complications of colonic TB have been reported including hemorrhage, obstruction, fistula formation, and perforation. Hemorrhage is unusual and massive bleeding is rare.[115–117] It is believed that obliterative endarteritis caused by the *Mycobacterial* infection lowers the risk for massive bleeding. Obstruction is the most common complication reported in 15–60% of series and tends to occur in short segmental areas with tight stenoses.[8,10,33,98,101,118] Colonic disease frequently requires surgical intervention for these complications. In a large surgical series, a variety of procedures were performed but 58% of subjects required either a hemi-colectomy or segmental resection. Fistulotomy was required in 10%, and in 12% of subjects the surgical procedure was only diagnostic.[100]

DIAGNOSIS

The diagnosis of intestinal TB should be considered in anyone with abdominal symptoms from an endemic area. Patients with prior exposure and infection should be evaluated if clinical clues suggest mucosal disease. With the increase in immunosuppression from medications and diseases, reactivation of latent infection is always a possibility. When there is clinical suspicion, the most useful diagnostic tests involve sampling of the intestinal mucosa or surrounding adenopathy. Endoscopic diagnosis is best facilitated by multiple biopsies, which should be sent for histology, AFB stain and culture, and polymerase chain reaction (PCR). The reported yield for endoscopic biopsies using multiple modalities is highly variable and ranges from 30–80%.[12,24,40,42,50,91,97,99,106,119] AFB staining has a very low sensitivity but remains a useful adjunct with high specificity.[12] The classic histology of noncaseating granulomas may not be seen if the endoscopic biopsies are superficial (see Fig. 22-5). The granulomas of TB are usually submucosal rather than mucosal.[29,120] Therefore, multiple deep biopsies are recommended in cases of suspected intestinal TB. AFB culture remains an important component of testing of

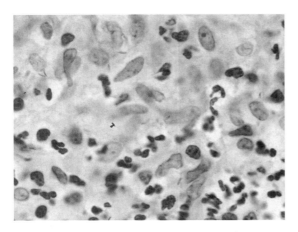

Fig. 22-5. Photomicrograph of ileal mucosal biopsy showing a poorly formed granuloma with multiple acid fast organisms. (Ziehl-Neelsen stain, × 1000) (Courtesy of Julie Steele.)

endoscopic biopsies. Most authors report a higher diagnostic yield from mycobacterial cultures compared to histology obtained from mucosal lesions and other sources.[121–123] PCR on biopsy specimens has recently become a very useful adjunct. Several studies have reported sensitivities as high as 75% with very high specificity.[39,124,125] One study reported the successful use of PCR on mucosal biopsies that were already embedded in paraffin.[126]

Cytology has also been a proven modality for the diagnosis of intestinal TB. Both endoscopic brush biopsies and percutaneous fine needle aspiration (FNA) of abdominal masses have been reported.[127–129] Cytology specimens can reveal both caseating and noncaseating granulomas and occasionally mycobacterial bacilli. Transesophageal endoscopic FNA has been reported to diagnose five cases of mediastinal TB.[130] Endoscopic ultrasound with FNA is a new modality, which allows directed sampling of lymph nodes surrounding the gut. Posterior mediastinal lymph nodes are readily accessible to this technique.[131,132] At our institution, two cases of tuberculous mediastinal lymphadenitis have been recently diagnosed by endoscopic ultrasound and FNA (unpublished data). Aspirated specimens can also be sent for PCR using this technique. EUS with FNA has also been used to diagnose tuberculous infection in splenic lesions.[133]

Immunoglobulin G antibodies to *Mycobacterium* TB antigen can be detected using an enzyme-linked immunosorbent assay.[134] This is a promising new method of rapid diagnosis of TB with reported sensitivity and specificity of 85% and 98%, respectively. More studies are required to determine the role of this test in clinical practice.

TREATMENT

Antituberculous therapy is extensively covered in chapters seven and eight. Most experts recommend similar type and duration of therapy used for active pulmonary TB. Surgery is used as an adjunct for significant bleeding, obstruction, abscess formation, and fistulas that are large or refractory to antimicrobial therapy. Surgery and endoscopic intervention need to be tailored to the specific site of involvement and the type of lesion.

SUMMARY

Tuberculous involvement of the gastrointestinal tract is uncommon but can be seen in both active pulmonary disease and as primary infection. An understanding of the pathogenesis and epidemiology of *M. tuberculosis* is crucial in order to avoid misdiagnosis and delay in treatment. Clinical suspicion remains a powerful tool and directs diagnostic testing and evaluation. Newer clinical tools for tissue acquisition and evaluation are now available to facilitate accurate diagnosis. Antimicrobial therapy is the mainstay of therapy but surgical and endoscopic intervention is frequently required for intestinal TB. Unfortunately, TB of the gastrointestinal tract will probably always remain the great mimic and will require astute clinical skills to diagnose and treat.

REFERENCES

1. Fraki O, Peltokallio P. Intestinal and peritoneal tuberculosis: report of two cases. *Dis Colon Rectum.* 1975;18: 685–693.
2. Mandal BK, Schofield PF. Abdominal tuberculosis in Britain. *Practitioner.* 1976;216:683–689.
3. Bhansali SK. Abdominal tuberculosis: experience with 300 cases. *Am J Gastroenterol.* 1977;67:324–337.
4. Findlay JM, Addison NV, Stevenson DK, et al. Tuberculosis of the gastrointestinal tract in Bradford, 1967–77. *J R Soc Med.* 1979;72:587–590.
5. Sherman S, Rohwedder JJ, Ravikrishnan KP, et al. Tuberculous enteritis and peritonitis: report of 36 general hospital cases. *Arch Intern Med.* 1980;140:506–508.
6. Gilinsky NH, Marks IN, Kottler RE, et al. Abdominal tuberculosis: a 10-year review. *S Afr Med J.* 64:849–857.
7. Palmer KR, Patil DH, Basran GS, et al. Abdominal tuberculosis in urban Britain—a common disease. *Gut.* 1985;26: 1296–1305.

8. Klimach OE, Ormerod LP. Gastrointestinal tuberculosis: a retrospective review of 109 cases in a district general hospital. *Q J Med.* 1985;56:569–578.

9. Glu AA, Bilgin I. Tuberculous enteritis and peritonitis. *Can J Surg.* 1988;31:55–58.

10. Lingenfelser T, Zak J, Marks IN, et al. Abdominal tuberculosis: still a potentially lethal disease. *Am J Gastroenterol.* 1993;88:744–750.

11. Walia HS, Khafagy AR, Al-Sayer HM, et al. Unusual presentations of abdominal tuberculosis. *Can J Surg.* 1994;37:300–306.

12. Al Karawi MA, Mohamed AE, Yasawy MI, et al. Protean manifestations of gastrointestinal tuberculosis: report on 130 cases. *J Clin Gastroenterol.* 1995;20:225–232.

13. Bernhard JS, Bhatia G, Knauer CM. Gastrointestinal tuberculosis: an eighteen-patient experience and review. *J Clin Gastroenterol.* 2000;30:397–402.

14. Enarson DA, Ashley MJ, Grzybowski S, et al. Non-respiratory tuberculosis in Canada: epidemiologic and bacterial features. *Am J Epidemiol.* 1980;112:341–351.

15. CDC Surveillance Reports. Reported Tuberculosis in the United States, 1999–2002. Available at (http://www.cdc.gov/nchstp/tb/surv/surv2002/default.htm). Accessed August 5, 2004.

16. Chen W, Leu S, Hsu H, et al. Trend of large bowel tuberculosis and the relation with pulmonary tuberculosis. *Dis Colon Rectum.* 1992;35:189–192.

17. Al Muneef M, Memish Z, Al Mahmoud S, et al. Tuberculosis in the belly: a review of forty-six cases involving the gastrointestinal tract and peritoneum. *Scand J Gastroenterol.* 2001;36:528–532.

18. World Health Organization. Global Tuberculosis Control: Surveillance, Planning, Financing. WHO Report 104:2004. Geneva, Switzerland.

19. Abdul-Ghaffer N, Ramadan IT, Marafie AA. Abdominal tuberculosis in Ahmadi, Kuwait: a clinico-pathologic review. *Trop Doc.* 1998;28:137–139.

20. Machado N, Grant CS, Scrimgeour E. Abdominal tuberculosis-experience of a university hospital in Oman. *Acta Trop.* 2001;80:187–190.

21. Zedtwitz-Liebenstein K, Podesser B, Peck-Radosavljevic M, et al. Intestinal tuberculosis presenting as fever of unknown origin in a heart transplant patient. *Infection.* 1999;27:289–290.

22. Kukura S, Viklicky O, Rudis J, et al. An unusual manifestation of tuberculosis in a female patient after kidney transplantation. *Vnitr Lek.* 2003;49:73–76.

23. Feriozzi S, Meschini L, Costantini S, et al. Fatal intestinal tuberculosis in a uremic patient with a renal transplant. *J Nephrol.* 2002;15:593–596.

24. Horvath KD, Whelan RL. Intestinal tuberculosis: return of an old disease. *A J Gastroentero.* 1998;93:692–696.

25. Al-Bahrani ZR, Al-Saleem T. Intestinal tuberculosis in Iraq: a study of 50 cases. *Int Surg.* 1982;67:483–485.

26. McGee GS, Williams LF, Potts J, et al. Gastrointestinal tuberculosis: resurgence of an old pathogen. *Am Surg.* 1989;55:16–20.

27. Schulze K, Warner HA, Murray D. Intestinal tuberculosis: experience at a Canadian teaching institution. *Am J Med.* 1977;63:735–745.

28. Tabrisky J, Lindstrom RR, Peters R, et al. Tuberculous enteritis: review of a protean disease. *Am J Gastroenterol.* 1975;63:49–57.

29. Pettengell KE, Larsen C, Garb M, et al. Gastrointestinal tuberculosis in patients with pulmonary tuberculosis. *Q J Med.* 1990;74:303–308.

30. Kasulke RJ, Anderson WJ, Gupta SK, et al. Primary tuberculous enterocolitis: report of three cases and review of the literature. *Arch Surg.* 1981;116:110–113.

31. Marshall JB. Tuberculosis of the gastrointestinal tract and peritoneum. *Am J Gastroenterol.* 1993;88:989–997.

32. Abel ME, Chiu YS, Russell TR, et al. Gastrointestinal tuberculosis: report of four cases. *Dis Colon Rectum.* 1990;33:886–889.

33. Panton O, Sharp R, English RA, et al. Gastrointestinal tuberculosis: the great mimic still at large. *Dis Colon Rectum.* 1985;28:446–450.

34. Croker J, Record CO, Wright JT. Ileo-caecal tuberculosis in immigrants. *Postgrad Med J.* 1978;54:410–412.

35. Monkemuller KE, Lewis JB. Massive rectal bleeding from colonic tuberculosis. *Am J Gastroenterol.* 1996;91: 1439–1441.

36. Sircar S, Taneja VA, Kansra U. Epidemiology and clinical presentation of abdominal tuberculosis—a retrospective study. *J Indian Med Assoc* 1996;94:342–344.

37. Wig, KL, Chitkara NL, Gupta SP, et al. Ileocecal tuberculosis with particular reference to isolation of mycobacterium tuberculosis. *Am Rev Respir Dis.* 1961;84:169–173.

38. Banerjea BN. Chronic hyperplastic ileocecal tuberculosis. *Ind J Surg.* 1950;12:33–41.

39. Anand SS, Pathak IC. Surgical treatment of abdominal tuberculosis with special reference to ileocecal tuberculosis: a record of one hundred cases treated surgically. *J Indian Med Assoc.* 1961;37:423–429.

40. Jain SK, Jain S, Jain M, et al. Esophageal tuberculosis: Is it so rare? report of 12 cases and review of the literature. *Am J Gastroenterol.* 2002;97:287–291.

41. Mokoena T, Shama DM, Ngakane H, et al. Oesophageal tuberculosis: a review of eleven cases. *Postgrad Med J.* 1992;68:110–115.

42. Gordon AH, Marshall JB. Esophageal tuberculosis: definitive diagnosis by endoscopy. *Am J Gastroenterol.* 1990; 85:174–177.

43. Seivewright N, Feehally J, Wicks AC. Primary tuberculosis of the esophagus. *Am J Gastroenterol.* 1984; 79:842–843.

44. Audouin J, Poulain J. Tuberculose stenosante de l' esophage d' appearance primitive, gueie par l' esophagetomie. *Arch Franc Malad Appareil Dig Nutr.* 1950;39:231–236.

45. Rosario MT, Raso CL, Comer GM. Esophageal tuberculosis. *Dig Dis Sci.* 1989;34:1281–1284.

46. Eng J, Sabanathan S. Tuberculosis of the esophagus. *Dig Dis Sci.* 1991;34(4):536–540.

47. Alatas F, Ozdemir N, Isiksoy S, et al. An Unusual Case of Esophageal Tuberculosis in an adult. *Respiration.* 1999;66: 88–90.

48. Abid S, Jafri W, Hamid S, et al. Endoscopic features of esophageal tuberculosis. *Gastrointest Endosc.* 2002;57(6): 759–762.

49. Annamalai A, Shreekumar S. Tuberculosis of the esophagus. *Am J Gastroenterol.* 1972;57(2):166–168.

50. Brullet E, Font B, Rey M, et al. Esophageal tuberculosis: early diagnosis by endoscopy. *Endoscopy.* 1993;25(7): 485.

51. Newman RM, Fleshner PR, Lajam FE, et al. Esophageal tuberculosis: a rare presentation with hematemesis. *Am J Gastroenterol.* 1991;86(6):751–755.

52. Fang HY, Lin TS, Cheng CY, et al. Esophageal tuberculosis: a rare presentation with massive hematemesis. *Ann Thorac Surg.* 1999;68:2344–2346.

53. Iwamto I, Tomita Y, Takasaki M, et al. Esophagoaortic fistula caused by esophageal tuberculosis: report of a case. *Surg Today.* 1995;25(4):381–384.

54. Catinella FP, Kittle CF. Tuberculous esophagitis with aortic aneurysm fistula. *Ann Thorac Surg.* 1988;45(1): 87–88.

55. Chase RA, Haber MH, Pottage JC, et al. Tuberculous esophagitis with erosion into aortic aneurysm. *Arch Pathol Lab Med.* 1986;110(10):965–966.

56. Wigley FM, Murray HW, Mann RB, et al. Unusual manifestation of tuberculous: TE fistula. *Am J Med.* 1976;60: 310–313.

57. Devarbhavi HC, Alvares JF, Radhikadevi M. Esophageal tuberculosis associated with esophagotracheal or esophagomediastinal fistula: report of 10 cases. *Gastrointest Endosc.* 2003;57(4):588–592.

58. Ramo OJ, Salo JA, Isolauri J, et al. Tuberculous fistula of the esophagus. *Ann Thorac Surg.* 1996;62(4): 1030–1032.

59. Ramakantan R, Shah P. Tuberculous fistulas of the pharynx and esophagus. *Gastrointest Radiol.* 1990;15(2): 145–147.

60. deMas R, Lombeck G, Riemann JF. Tuberculosis of the esophagus masquerading as ulcerated tumour. *Endoscopy.* 1986;18:153–155.

61. Laajam MA. Primary tuberculosis of the esophagus: pseudotumoral presentation. *Am J Gastroenterol.* 1984;79(11): 839–841.

62. Damtew B, Frengley D, Wolinsky E, et al. Esophageal tuberculosis: mimicry of gastrointestinal malignancy. *Rev Infect Dis.* 1987;9(1):140–146.

63. Upadhyay AP, Bhatia RS, Anbarasu A, et al. Esophageal tuberculosis with intramural pseudodiverticulosis. *J Clin Gastroenterol.* 1995;22(1):38–40.

64. Nagi B, Lal A, Kochhar R, et al. Imaging of esophageal tuberculosis. *Acta Radiol.* 2003;44:329–333.

65. Williford ME, Thompson WM, Hamilton JD, et al. Esophageal tuberculosis: Findings on barium swallow and computed tomography. *Gastrointest Radiol.* 1983;8: 119–122.

66. Palmer ED. Tuberculosis of the stomach and the stomach in tuberculosis. *Am Rev Tuberc.* 1950;61:116–130.

67. Subei I, Attar B, Schmitt G, et al. Primary gastric tuberculosis: a case report and literature review. *Am J Gastroenterol.* 1987;82(8):769–773.

68. Mathis G, Dirschmid K, Sutterlutti G. Tuberculous gastric ulcer. *Endoscopy,* (umlaut over 2nd U in Sutterlutti). 1987;19:133–135.

69. Weissman D, Gumaste VV, Dave PB, et al. Bleeding from a tuberculous gastric ulcer. *Am J Gastroenterol.* 1990;85(6): 742–744.

70. Tromba JL, Inglese R, Rieders B, et al. Primary gastric tuberculosis presenting as pyloric outlet obstruction. *Am J Gastroenterol.* 1991;86(12):1820–1822.

71. Gupta B, Mathew S, Bhalla S. Pyloric obstruction due to gastric tuberculosis-an endoscopic diagnosis. *Postgrad Med J.* 1990;66:63–65.

72. Wig JD, Vaiphei K, Tashi M, et al. Isolated gastric tuberculosis presenting as massive hematemesis: a case report. *Surg Today.* 2000;30(10):921–922.

73. Agrawal S, Shetty SV, Bakshi G. Primary hypertrophic tuberculosis of the pyloroduodenal area: report of two cases. *J Postgrad Med.* 1999;45(1):10–12.

74. Gleason T, Prinz RA, Kirsh EP, et al. Tuberculosis of the duodenum. *Am J Gastroenterol.* 1979;72:36–40.

75. Fukuya T, Yoshimitsu K, Kitagawa S, et al. Single tuberculous stricture in the jejunum: report of 2 cases. *Gastrointest Radiol.* 1989;14:300–304.

76. Brandt M, Bogner PN, Franklin GA. Intestinal tuberculosis presenting as a bowel obstruction. *Am J Surg.* 2002;183:290–291.

77. Schwartz DC, Pfau PR. Multifocal intestinal tuberculosis. *Gastrointest Endosc.* 2003;58:100.

78. Shiekh MY, Rizvi IH, Naeem SA, et al. Enterolithiasis secondary to intestinal tuberculosis. *J Pak Med Assoc.* 1991;41:286–287.

79. Nair KV, Pai CG, Rajagopal KP, et al. Unusual presentations of duodenal tuberculosis. *Am J Gastroenterol.* 1991;86:756–760.

80. Sherman HI, Johnson R, Brock T. Massive gastrointestinal bleeding from tuberculosis of the small intestine. *Am J Gastroenterol.* 1978;70:314–316.

81. Kuganeswaran E, Smith OJ, Quiason SG. Both massive upper and lower gastrointestinal hemorrhage secondary to tuberculosis. *Am J Gastroenterol.* 1999;94:270–272.

82. Kodaira Y, Shibuya T, Matsumoto K, et al. Primary aortoduodenal fistula caused by duodenal tuberculosis without an abdominal aortic aneurysm: report of a case. *Surg Today.* 1997;27:745–748.

83. Oran I, Parildar M, Memis A. Mesenteric artery aneurysms in intestinal tuberculosis as a cause of lower gastrointestinal bleeding. *Abdom Imaging.* 2001;26: 131–133.

84. Singh K, Zargar SA, Bhasin D, et al. Isolated splenic vein thrombosis with natural shunt caused by jejunal tuberculosis. *Trop Gastroenterol.* 1990;11:39–43.

85. Gilinsky NH, Voight MD, Bass DH, et al. Tuberculous perforation of the bowel: a report of 8 cases. *S Afr Med J.* 1986;70:44–46.

86. Berney T, Badaoui E, Totsch M, et al. Duodenal tuberculosis presenting as acute ulcer perforation. *Am J Gastroenterol.* 1998;93:1989–1991.

87. Friedenberg KA, Draguesku JO, Kiyabu M, et al. Intestinal perforation due to *Mycobacterium tuberculosis* in HIV-infected individuals: report of two cases. *Am J Gastroenterol.* 1993;88:604–607.

88. Porter KA, Henson J, Chong F. Perforated gastrointestinal tuberculosis [letter]. *Dig Dis Sci.* 1990;35:1046–1048.

89. Nagi B, Lal A, Kochhar R, et al. Perforations and fistulae in gastrointestinal tuberculosis. *Acta Radiol.* 2002;43:501–506.

90. Seabra J, Coelho H, Barros H, et al. Acute tuberculosis perforation of the small bowel during antituberculosis therapy. *J Clin Gastroenterol.* 1993;16:320–2.

91. Segal I, Ou Tim L, Mirwis J, et al. Pitfalls in the diagnosis of gastrointestinal tuberculosis. *Am J Gastroenterol.* 1981;75:30–35.

92. Eggleston FC, Deodhar MC, Kumar A. Tuberculous perforation of the bowel – results in 21 cases. *Trop Gastroenterol.* 1983;4:164–167.

93. Desta TT, Man KM, Bouvier D, et al. Choledocho-enteric fistula due to *Mycobacterium tuberculosis* in a patient with acquired immunodeficiency syndrome. *Gastrointest Endosc.* 1998;48:623–626.

94. Miyamoto S, Furuse J, Maru Y, et al. Duodenal tuberculosis with a choledocho-duodenal fistula. *J Gastroenterol Hepatol.* 2001;16:235–238.

95. Tandon RK, Bansal R, Kapur BM, et al. A study of malabsorption in intestinal tuberculosis: stagnant loop syndrome. *Am J Clin Nutr.* 1980;33:244–250.

96. Aoki G, Nagasaki K, Nakae Y. The fibercolonoscopic diagnosis of intestinal tuberculosis. *Endoscopy.* 1971;7:113–118.

97. Naga MI, Okasha HH, Ismail Z, et al. Endoscopic diagnosis of colonic tuberculosis. *Gastrointest Endosc.* 2001;53:789–793.

98. Singh V, Kumar J, Prakash V, et al. Clinicocolonoscopic profile of colonic tuberculosis. *Am J Gastroenterol.* 1996;91(3):565–567.

99. Shah S, Thomas V, Matham M, et al. Colonoscopic study of 50 patients with colonic tuberculosis. *Gut.* 1992;33:347–351.

100. Chen WS, Leu SY, Hsu H, et al. Trend of large bowel tuberculosis and the relation with pulmonary tuberculosis. *Dis Colon rectum.* 1992;35:189–192.

101. Sáenz EV, Magro PMH, Fernádez JFA, et al. Colonic Tuberculosis. *Dig Dis Sci.* 2002;47(9):2045–2028.

102. Healy JC, Gorman S, Kumar PJ. Case report: tuberculous colitis mimicking Crohn's disease. *Clin Radiol.* 1992;46:131–132.

103. Arnold C, Moradpour D, Blum HE. Tuberculous colitis mimicking Crohn's disease. *Am J Gastroenterol.* 1998;93(11):2294–2296.

104. Ehsannulah M, Isaacs A, Filipe MI, et al. Tuberculosis presenting as inflammatory bowel disease. *Dis Colon Rectum.* 1984;27:134–136.

105. Kaushik SP, Bassett ML, McDonald C, et al. Case report: gastrointestinal tuberculosis simulating Crohn's disease. *J Gastroenterol Hepatol.* 1996;11(6):532–534.

106. Bhargava DK, Kushwaha AHS, Dasarathy S, et al. Endoscopic diagnosis of segmental tuberculosis. *Gastrointest Endosc.* 1992;38:571–574.

107. Medina E, Orti E, Tome A, et al. Segmental tuberculosis of the colon diagnosed by colonoscopy. *Endoscopy.* 1990;22:188–190.

108. Horwath KD, Whelan RL, Weinstein S, et al. Isolated sigmoid tuberculosis. *Dis Colon Rectum.* 1195;38:1327–1330.

109. Breiter JR, Hajjar JJ. Segmental tuberculosis of the colon diagnosed by colonoscopy. *Am J Gastroenterol.* 1981;76(4):369–373.

110. Panton ONM, Sharp R, English RA, et al. Gastrointestinal tuberculosis The great mimic still at large. *Dis Colon Rectum.* 1985;28:446–450.

111. Murillo J, Wells GM, Barry DW, et al. Gastrointestinal tuberculosis mimicking cancer- a reminder. *Am J Gastroenterol.* 1978;70:76–78.

112. Devanesan JD, Sable RA, Pitchumoni CS, et al. Segmental tuberculosis of the colon mimicking carcinoma. *Arch Surg.* 1980;115(1):90–91.

113. Tishler JM. Tuberculosis of the transverse colon. *AJR.* 1979;133(2):229–232.

114. Balthazar EJ, Bryk D. Segmental tuberculosis of the distal colon: radiographic features in 7 cases. *Gastrointest Radiol.* 1980;5(1):75–80.

115. Veela P, Kapur BKLM. Massive rectal bleeding due to intestinal tuberculosis. *Am J Gastroenterol.* 1979;71:217–219.

116. Rabkin DG, Caiati JM, Allendorf JA, et al. Intractable hematochezia: an unusual presentation of intestinal tuberculosis. *Surgery.* 2002;133:592–593.

117. Monkemuller KE, Lewis JB. Massive rectal bleeding due to intestinal tuberculosis. *Am J Gastroenterol.* 1996;91:1439–1441.

118. Wong SS, Chow E. Endoscopic diagnosis of colonic tuberculosis: unusual presentation with two colonic strictures. *Endoscopy.* 1996;28:783.

119. Sheer TA, Coyle WJ. Gastrointestinal tuberculosis. *Curr Gastroenterol Rep.* 2003;5:273–278.

120. Pulimood AB, Ramakrishna BS, Kurian G, et al. Endoscopic mucosal biopsies are useful in distinguishing granulomatous colitis due to Crohn's disease from tuberculosis. *Gut.* 1999;45:537–541.

121. Shah I. Tuberculosis of the esophagus and the importance of bacterial tissue cultures. *Endoscopy.* 1986;18:254.

122. Gotuzzo E,Carillo C, Guerra J, et al. An evaluation of diagnostic methods for brucellosis—the value of boe marrow culture. *J Infect Dis.* 1986;153:122–125.

123. Kumar S, Seshadi MS, Koshi G, et al. Diagnosing tuberculous pleural effusion:comparative sensitivity of mycobacterial culture and histopathology. *Br Med J.* 1981;283:20.

124. Gan HT, Chen YQ, Ouyang Q, et al. Differentiation between intestinal tuberculosis and Crohn's disease in endoscopic biopsy specimens by polymerase chain reaction. *Am J Gastroenterol.* 2002;97:1446–1451.

125. Gan H, Ouyang Q, Bu H. The value of polymerase chain reaction in the diagnosis of intestinal tuberculosis and differentiation of Crohn's disease. *Chung-Hua Nei Ko Tsa Chih, Chin J Int Med.* 1995;34:30–33.

126. Moatter T, Mirza S, Siddiqui MS, et al. Detection of Mycobacterium tuberculosis in paraffin embedded intestinal tissue specimen by polymerase chain reaction: characterization of IS6110 element negative strains. *J Pak Med Assoc.* 1998;48:174–178.

127. Jain S, Kumar N, Das D, et al. Esophageal tuberculosis: endoscopic cytology as a diagnostic tool. *Acta Cytol.* 1999;43:1085–1090.

128. Misra SP, Misra V, Dwivedi M, et al. Diagnostic value of fine needle aspiration biopsy of palpable colonic masses. *Acta Cytol.* 1999;43:624–629.

129. Das DK, Pant CS. Fine needle aspiration cytologic diagnosis of gastrointestinal tract lesions. *Acta Cytol.* 1994;38:723–729.

130. Kochhar R, Sriram PVJ, Rajwanshi A, et al. Transesophageal endoscopic fine-needle aspiration cytology in mediastinal tuberculosis. *Gastrointest Endosc.* 1999;50(2): 271–274.

131. Wiersema MJ, Kochman ML, Chak A, et al. Real time endoscopic ultrasound guided fine needle aspiration of a mediastinal lymph node. *Gastrointest Endosc.* 1993;39: 429–431.

132. Wiersema MJ. The linear array echoendoscope, in Van Dam J, Sivak MV (eds.): *Gastrointestinal Endosonography*, 1st ed. Philadelphia, PA: WB Saunders; 1999:29.

133. Fritscher-Ravens A, Mylonaki M, Pantes A, et al. Endoscopic ultrasound-guided biopsy for diagnosis of focal lesions of the spleen. *Am J Gastroenterol.* 2003;98: 1022–1027.

134. Kashima K, Oka S, Tabata A, et al. Detection of anti-cord factor antibodies in intestinal tuberculosis for its differential diagnosis from Crohn's disease and ulcerative colitis. *Dig Dis Sci.* 1995;40:2630–2634.

23

Tuberculous Peritonitis

Ajay Shetty
Gregory C. Kane

INTRODUCTION

Gastrointestinal and peritoneal tuberculosis (TB) remain common problems in the developing world[1–6] but are uncommon in the United States and Europe. Still, the resurgence of TB in North America since the mid-1980's and early 1990's requires that clinicians continue to consider these relatively rare forms of extrapulmonary TB. Even with more recent declines in the incidence of active TB in the U.S., this presentation remains important because of its unique occurrence in special populations. Recent immigrants from endemic areas and patients with acquired immunodeficiency syndrome (AIDS) are two population groups at particular risk for abdominal TB in this country, as are the urban poor, the elderly, and Native Americans on reservations.[7,8] The symptoms and signs are nonspecific, and a high index of suspicion is necessary to avoid delay in establishing the diagnosis resulting in increased morbidity and mortality. Peritoneal TB is presently the sixth most common site of extrapulmonary TB in the United States, following lymphatic, genitourinary, bone and joint, miliary, and meningeal involvement. It accounts for 0.5–1.0% of all TB-related hospital admissions in the United States and has an overall mortality rate of 7%.[8] In this chapter we review the epidemiology, pathogenesis, and clinical features of this illness. Finally, diagnosis including recently available techniques and therapy are discussed.

DEFINITION

Tuberculous peritonitis represents intra-abdominal infection with *Mycobacterium tuberculosis* or *Mycobacterium bovis* that must include infection of ascites fluid or peritoneum with or without involvement of other intra-abdominal organs. Definitive cases require the demonstration of the causative agent from biopsy or paracentesis fluid, but clinical cases may be diagnosed by the clinical syndrome, pathology, and response to therapy even in the absence of a positive culture.

EPIDEMIOLOGY

Tuberculous peritonitis can occur at any age but appears most common in young adults, principally in their third and fourth decades of life. The growing number of extrapulmonary TB cases worldwide as a result of the human immunodeficiency virus (HIV) epidemic will likely amplify this pattern of age-incidence. In four large series of cases from the developing world, women were affected more frequently than men, accounting for 57–67% of reported cases.[1–3,9] Children under 10 years of age accounted for 10.5% of cases in one study, and a retrospective review between 1980 and 1993 from the University of California, San Diego, found 26 children with abdominal TB.[10] Interestingly, 80% of mycobacterial isolates from the latter study were identified as *M. bovis* and only 20% as *M. tuberculosis*.

Alcoholism appears to play an important role in the development of tuberculous peritonitis in North America. Nearly three quarters of Native Americans with tuberculous peritonitis were believed to be alcoholic in one series.[11] Additional studies have confirmed this.[12] In another series from Boston, 20 of 47 patients had coexistent alcoholic cirrhosis.[13] Still, the predominant group with tuberculous peritonitis in North America and Europe is the recently immigrated, especially those from Africa, South Asia, and Haiti.[14] Patients with end-stage renal disease on peritoneal dialysis also appear to be a group at risk, though this association is rare.[15–20] Although only 10–15% of non-HIV infected patients have extrapulmonary manifestations, the incidence is about 50% in patients with AIDS.[21] Tuberculous peritonitis as the initial manifestation of HIV infection was first reported in 1992, and further reports soon followed.[22–24]

PATHOGENESIS

Most cases of tuberculous peritonitis are thought to result from reactivation of latent foci in the peritoneum established previously via hematogenous spread from a primary focus in the lung (commonly to mesenteric lymph nodes). Up to a third of cases may be associated with active pulmonary TB, and old healed primary foci in the lung can be visible on chest radiograph in another third. Other, less common causes are hematogenous spread from *active* pulmonary disease or miliary TB and occasional contiguous spread from lesions in the gut (ileocecal) or fallopian tubes. *M. bovis* causing abdominal TB has been attributed to ingestion of nonpasteurized milk, though empiric data are lacking.[10,25]

CLINICAL FEATURES

The presentation of abdominal TB may occur jointly with active pulmonary TB, with evidence of old but inactive thoracic disease, or in the presence of a normal chest x-ray.[26] Thus, the clinician must be alert to the prospect of an abdominal presentation as the only site of disease activity.

The presentation of tuberculous peritonitis is often insidious; with patients reporting symptoms for weeks to months.[24] Abdominal distention and pain are the most common presentation (about 82% of cases). Fever (74%) and weight loss (62%) are also frequent. Diarrhea (16%) is not routinely noted.[9] Classically; affected patients experience intermittent fever, fatigue, and weight loss over several months, with increasing abdominal pain and distention.[25] Only a minority of patients have symptoms of coexistent active pulmonary disease with cough or hemoptysis. On examination, about 75% of patients have abdominal tenderness, and almost all have ascites.[26–28] Signs of chronic liver disease such as palmar erythema, spider angiomata, and evidence of elevated portal pressure (dilated abdominal wall veins, large hemorrhoidal veins) are not usually present unless there is coexistent liver disease. Two major clinical forms of the disease have been described—wet or ascitic, and dry or fibroadhesive peritonitis.

Anemia occurs in 48–68% of cases, and about 71% of patients experience a positive tuberculin skin test result. Approximately 48% of patients have an abnormal chest radiograph appearance (37–63% in a number of series), with 4–21% having evidence of active pulmonary TB and the others demonstrating old healed foci of infection. Ascitic fluid is characterized as "exudative" in greater than 95% of cases (protein >2.5 to 3 g/dl and serum-ascites albumin gradient <1.1),[29] with leukocytes at 150 to 4000/mm.[3] As might be expected, the differential cell count usually reveals 75–96% lymphocytes, except in peritoneal dialysis patients, in whom neutrophils may predominate.[1,16] Rarely, the fluid is grossly bloody, a feature that suggests malignancy.[2] Typical clinical and laboratory features are summarized in Table 23-1.

DIAGNOSIS

A number of diagnostic tests have been described but none have proved to be of sufficient sensitivity and specificity. The gold standard remains laparoscopy with directed biopsy.[9] Ultrasonography is a useful imaging modality in patients suspected of having abdominal TB for diagnosis and follow-up, but computed tomography (CT) is more sensitive in detecting bowel thickening and abdominal lymphadenopathy.[30–33] Barium studies may be useful in evaluating gastrointestinal tract disease. Various findings on ultrasound examination have been studied and include free or loculated ascites, intraabdominal abscesses, ileocecal masses, and retroperitoneal lymphadenopathy.[34,35] CT can distinguish tuberculous peritonitis from peritoneal carcinomatosis.[36] The diagnostic value of these imaging techniques can be enhanced by

Table 23-1. Clinical and Laboratory Features of Tuberculous Peritonitis

Symptoms		
General	Weight Loss	67–100%
	Anorexia	70%
Gastrointestinal	Abdominal pain	60–92%
	Nausea and vomiting	18–30%
	Diarrhea	12–30%
Signs	Fever	67–100%
	Abdominal tenderness	60%
	Ascites	67–100%
	Abdominal mass	6–40%
Laboratory		
Ascitic Fluid	Protein >3.0 g	84–100%
Other	Abnormal chest radiograph	52–65%
	Positive purified protein derivative (PPD) test result	56–100%

Source: Data References 1–5.

guided aspiration and biopsy. Fine-needle aspiration has been used (ultrasound-guided),[37] with one study reporting 45% positive results for acid-fast bacilli on Ziehl-Neelsen staining.[38] In most series, however, acid-fast staining of ascitic fluid identified the organism in only 3% of cases[1,27] with *M. tuberculosis* on culture in less than 20%[27,39] Singh and coworkers did report an 83% positivity rate by culturing 1 L of peritoneal fluid.[1] Another limitation is the prolonged duration (4–8 weeks) before a diagnosis is confirmed, even in those patients whose cultures ultimately turn positive.

Laparoscopic examination, supplemented by biopsy, confirms tuberculous peritonitis in 85–90% of cases.[39–43] Appearance on laparoscopy has been classified into three types: thickened peritoneum with *miliary* yellowish-white tubercles with or without adhesions, only thickened peritoneum with or without adhesions, and fibroadhesive pattern.[9,44,45] Some groups consider laparoscopy risky in the fibroadhesive type (recommending laparotomy instead); others characterize laparoscopy (with biopsy) as a safe, accurate, and uncomplicated method for diagnosis of fibroadhesive *and* ascitic tuberculous peritonitis.[45–47]

Other, noninvasive diagnostic tests are available. Adenosine deaminase has been reported to increase in ascitic fluid, with a sensitivity of 93% and a specificity of 96% in one study. Using a value of greater than 33 IU/L, others have reported sensitivity and specificity of 100% and 95%, respectively.[48–53] False positives may be seen in patients with hematologic malignancy and bacterial infections.[54] Ascitic fluid interferon-γ (sensitivity 93%, specificity 98%) is useful in differentiating tuberculous from sterile cirrhotic ascites.[48] Lactate and pH may be similarly helpful.[55]

A number of reports have also been published associating tuberculous peritonitis with increased *serum* CA-125.[56] Since ovarian dysgerminomas are an important differential diagnosis in women with ascites, abdominal pain, and constitutional symptoms; the recognition of this association is important.[57,58] In reported cases, CA-125 levels returned to normal after treatment confirming the association.[59]

The differential diagnosis of tuberculous peritonitis can be viewed from two perspectives. First, on initial presentation, malignant ascites is an important consideration. Both the time course and physical findings are similar. In addition, cirrhosis with spontaneous bacterial peritonitis (SBP) should also be considered, though constitutional complaints are much more acute in SBP. In general, these diagnoses can be differentiated from tuberculous peritonitis based on the characteristics of the ascitic fluid. Malignant ascites appears as a bloody exudate. SBP often shows increased neutrophils in the peritoneal fluid with a positive bacterial culture.

Other causes of granulomatous peritonitis are an important consideration for patients in whom biopsy material reveals granulomas but mycobacterial cultures are pending or negative. These include starch peritonitis from surgical gloves, peritoneal sarcoid, and nontuberculous mycobacterial peritonitis in patients undergoing peritoneal dialysis.[60–65] Thus, demonstration of *M. tuberculosis* on culture is necessary for specific or definitive diagnosis because the histopathology of these entities may be similar.

TREATMENT

The preferred treatment is medical,[66] using antituberculous therapy (with a regimen similar to that for pulmonary TB.) Surgery is reserved only for complications, aside from its use in diagnosis. Current rates of drug resistance necessitate initial four-drug therapy with a standard regimen of isoniazid, rifampin, pyrazinamide, and ethambutol (see Chap. 6). Surgery is required when complications occur. These include obstruction, perforation, abscess, fistula, and hemorrhage.

The role of corticosteroids is controversial, and empirical data on this issue are limited. Singh and coauthors reported intestinal obstruction in 3 of 24 patients treated with antituberculous therapy alone, whereas none of 23 patients receiving prednisone (30 mg daily for 3 months) experienced this complication.[1] A more recent report from Alrajhi and colleagues in Riyadh, Saudi Arabia, provided additional uncontrolled case series data involving nine steroid treated patients and 26 controls (who received antituberculosis treatment but no steroids).[67] Intestinal obstruction occurred in 5 of 26 patients receiving antituberculosis therapy alone, whereas zero of nine patients receiving steroids experienced such an event. Patients not treated with steroids were more likely to experience recurrent abdominal pain (17 of 26 patients), require emergency room attention for pain (7 of 26 patients), and to require laparotomy (4 of 26 patients). Three patients not treated with steroids died. By contrast only one patient receiving steroids (prednisone 0.5 mg/kg to 1mg/kg for 6 weeks on average) had recurrent abdominal pain.

While controlled trials are lacking and would be preferred, uncontrolled case series would support treatment with adjunctive corticosteroids in a dose of 0.5 mg/kg to 1 mg/kg for approximately 6–9 weeks in order to decrease the occurrence of adhesions, which could lead to abdominal pain and intestinal obstruction.

CONCLUSION

Tuberculous peritonitis is rare in the United Sates but continues to be reported in certain high-risk populations. The clinical presentation is often nonspecific, and a high index of suspicion is necessary to make the diagnosis. Tuberculosis should be suspected in any case of "exudative" ascites in patients with AIDS, immigrants from South Asia and Africa, Native Americans, and elderly nursing–home residents, and the inner-city poor. Laparoscopy with biopsy is the surest way to confirm the diagnosis. Antituberculous drugs are usually effective, except in cases of multi-drug resistance. Concomitant steroid therapy appears to diminish the occurrence of intestinal obstruction, perhaps by diminishing fibrous adhesions, though controlled trials are lacking. When obstruction does occur, surgical treatment is necessary. Other complications can include fistula, perforation, abscess formation, and hemorrhage.

REFERENCES

1. Singh MM, Bhargava AN, Jain KP. Tuberculous peritonitis. *N Engl J Med.* 1969;281:1091–1094.
2. Borhanmanesh F, Hekmat K, Vaezzadeh K, et al. Tuberculous peritonitis: prospective study of 32 cases in Iran. *Ann Intern Med.* 1972;76:567–572.
3. Ihekwaba FN. Abdominal tuberculosis: A study of 881 cases. *J R Coll Surg Edin.* 1993;38:293–295.
4. Lingenfelser T, Zak J, Marks IN, et al. Abdominal tuberculous: Still a potentially lethal disease. *Am J Gastroenterol.* 1993;88(5):744–750.
5. Al Karawi MA, Mohamed AE, Yasawy MI, et al. Protean manifestations of gastrointestinal tuberculosis: Report on 130 patients. *J Clin Gastroenterol.* 1995;20(3):225–232.
6. Chen YM, Lee PY, Perng RP. Abdominal tuberculosis in Taiwan: A report from Veterans' General Hospital, Taipei. *Tubercle Lung Dis.* 1995;76:35–38.
7. Rieder HL, Cauthen GM, Kelly GD, et al. Tuberculosis in the United States. *JAMA.* 1989;262(3):385–389.
8. Mehta JB, Dutt A, Harvill L, et al. Epidemiology of extra-pulmonary tuberculosis: A comparative analysis with pre-AIDS era. *Chest.* 1991;99:1134–1138.
9. Sandikci MU, Colakoglu S, Egun Y, et al. Presentation and role of peritoneoscopy in the diagnosis of tuberculous peritonitis. *J Gastroenterol Hepatol.* 1992;7:298–301.
10. Veeragandham RS, Lynch FP, Canty TG, et al. Abdominal tuberculosis in children: Review of 26 cases. *J Pediatr Surg.* 1996;31(1):170–176.
11. Marie TJ, Hershfield ES. Tuberculous peritonitis in Manitoba. *Can J Surg.* 1978;21:533–536.
12. Dineen P, Homan WP, Grafe WR. Tuberculous peritonitis: 43 years' experience in diagnosis and treatment. *Ann Surg.* 1976;184(6):717–722.
13. Burak WR, Hollister RM. Tuberculous peritonitis. *Am Med.* 1960;28:510–523.
14. Sheldon CD, Probert CSJ, Cock H, et al. Incidence of abdominal tuberculosis in Bangladesh migrants in East London. *Tubercle Lung Dis.* 1993;4:12–15.
15. Baumgartner DD, Arterbery EV, Hale AJ, et al. Peritoneal dialysis-associated tuberculous peritonitis in an intravenous drug user with acquired immunodeficiency syndrome. *Am J Kidney Dis.* 1989;14(2):154–157.
16. Cheng IKP, Chan PCK, Chan MK. Tuberculous peritonitis complicating long-term peritoneal dialysis. *Am J Nephrol.* 1989;9:155–161.
17. Mallat SG, Brensilver JM. Tuberculous peritonitis in a CAPD patient cured without catheter removal: Case report, review of the literature and guidelines for treatment and diagnosis. *Am J Kid Dis.* 1989;13(2):154–157.
18. Ong ACM, Scoble JE, Baillod RA, et al. Tuberculous peritonitis complicating peritoneal dialysis: A case for early diagnosis laparotomy? *Nephrol Dial Transplant.* 1992;7:443–446.
19. Ha SK, Lee CH, Park CH, et al. A case of tuberculous peritonitis associated with abdominal-wall peudocyst in a patient undergoing continuous ambulatory peritoneal dialysis (CAPD). *Nephrol Dial Transplant.* 1995;10:706–708.
20. Karayaylali I, Serek N, Akpolat T, et al. The prevalence and clinical features of tuberculous peritonitis in CAPD patients in Turkey, report of ten cases from multi-centers. *Renal Failure.* 2003;25(5):819–827.
21. Braun MM, Byers RH, Heyward WI, et al. Acquired immunodeficiency syndrome and extrapulmonary tuberculosis in the United States. *Arch Intern Med.* 1990;150:1913–1916.
22. Soubani AO, Glatt AE. Tuberculous peritonitis as an initial manifestation of HIV infection. *NY State J Med.* 1992;92(6):269–270.
23. Schanaider A, Madi K. Intra-abdominal tuberculosis in acquired immunodeficiency syndrome. *Int Surg.* 1995;80:147–151.
24. Chaisson RE, Schecter GF, Theuer CP, et al. Tuberculosis in patients with the acquired immunodeficiency syndrome. *Am Rev Respir Dis.* 1987;136:570–574.
25. Case records of the Massachusetts General Hospital. Case 35-1989. *N Engl J Med.* 1989;319:573.
26. Underwood MN, Thompson MM, Sayers RD, et al. Presentation of abdominal tuberculosis to general surgeons. *Br J Surg.* 1992;79:1077–1079.
27. Aguado JM, Pons F, Casafont F, et al. Tuberculous peritonitis: A study comparing cirrhotic and noncirrhotic patients. *J Clin Gastroenterol.* 1990;12(5):550–554.
28. Shakil AO, Korula J, Kane GC, et al. Diagnosstic features of tuberculous peritonitis in the absence and presence of chronic liver disease: A case control study. *Am J Med.* 1996;100:179–185.
29. Marshall JB, Vogele KA. Serum-ascites albumini difference in tuberculous peritonitis. *Am J Gastroenterol.* 1988;83:59–61.

30. Denton T, Hossain J. A radiological study of abdominal tuberculosis in a Saudi population, with special reference to ultrasound and computed tomography. *Clin Radiol.* 1993;47: 409–414.

31. Sheikh M, Abu-Zidan F, Al-Hilaly M, et al. Abdominal tuberculosis: comparison of sonography and computed tomography. *J Clin Ultrasound.* 1995;23(7):413–417.

32. Suri S, Gupta S, and Suri R. Computer tomography in abdominal tuberculosis. *Br J Radiol.* 1999;72(853):92–98.

33. Zissin R, Gayer G, Chowers M, et al. Computerized tomography findings of abdominal tuberculosis: report of 19 cases. *Isr Med Assoc J .* 2001;3(6):414–418.

34. Kedar RP, Shah PP, Shivde RS, et al. Sonographic findings in gastrointestinal and peritoneal tuberculosis. *Clin Radiol.* 1994;49:24–29.

35. Ramaiya LI, Walter DF. Sonographic features of tuberculosis peritonitis. *Abdom Imaging.* 1993;18:23–26.

36. Rodriguez E, Pombo F. Peritoneal tuberculosis versus peritoneal carcinomatosis: Distinction based on CT findings. *J Comput Assist Tomogr.* 1996;20(2):269–272.

37. Liu KW, Chan YL, Tseng R, et al. Childoood abdominal tuberculosis: the role of echo-guided fine-needle aspiration in its management. *Surg Endosc.* 1994;8:326–328.

38. Radhika S, Rajwanshi A, Kochar R, et al. Abdominal tuberculosis:diagnosis by fine needle aspiration cytology. *Acta Cytol.* 1993;37(5):673–678.

39. Wolfe JHN, Behn AR, Jackson BT. Tuberculous peritonitis and role of diagnostic laparoscopy. *Lancet.* 1979;1:852–853.

40. Manohar A, Simjee AE Hafffejee AA, et al. Symptoms and investigative findings in 145 patients with tuberculous peritonitis diagnosed by peritoneoscopy and biopsy over a five year period. *Gut.* 1990;31:1130–1132.

41. Bhargava DK, Shriniwas, Chopra P, et al. Peritoneal tuberculosis; laparoscopic patterns and its diagnostic accuracy. Am J Gastroenterol. 1992;87(1):109–112.

42. Reddy KR, DiPrima RE, Raskin JB, et al. Tuberculous peritonitis: Laparoscopic diagnosis of an uncommon disease in the United States. Gastrointest Endosc. 1988;34(5):422–426.

43. Hossain J, Al-Aska AK, Al-Mofleh I. Laparsocpy in tuberculous peritonitis. J R Soc Med. 1992;85(2):89–91.

44. Mimica M. Usefulness and limitations of laparoscopy in the diagnosis of tuberculous peritonitis. Endosc. 1992;24: 588–591.

45. Nafeh MA, Medhat A, Abdul-Hameed A, et al. Tuberculous peritonitis in Egypt: The value of laparoscopy in diagnosis. Am J Trop Med Hyg. 1992;47(4):470–477.

46. Levine H. Needle biopsy of tuberculous peritonitis. *Am Rev Respir Dis.* 1968;97:889–894.

47. Levine H. Needle biopsy in diagnosis of tuberculous peritonitis (Letter). *Am Rev Respir Dis.* 1968;98:519.

48. Sathar MA, Simjee AE, Coovadia YM, et al. Ascitic fluid gamma-interferon concentrations and adenosine deaminase activity in tuberculous peritonitis. *Gut.* 1995;36:419–421.

49. Ghargave K, Gupta M, Nijhawan S, et al. Adenosine deaminase (ADA) in peritoneal tuberculosis: Diagnostic value in ascitic fluid and serum. *Tubercle.* 1990;71:121–126.

50. Martinez-Vazquez JM, Ocana I, Ribera E, et al. Adenosine deaminase activity in the diagnosis of tuberculous peritonitis. *Gut.* 1986;27:1049–1053.

51. Banales JL, Pineda PR, Fitzgerald JM, Rubio H, Selman M, Salazar-Lezama M. "Adenosine deaminase in the diagnosis of tuberculous pleural effusions: a report of 218 patients and review of the literature." *Chest.* 1991;99:355–357.

52. Fernandez-Rodriguez CM, Perez-Arguelles BS, Ledo L, Garcia-Vila LM, Pereira S, Rodriguez-Martinez D. Ascites adenosine deaminase activity is decreased in tuberculous ascites with low protein content. *Am J Gastroenterol.* 1991;86:1500–1503.

53. Hillebrand DJ, Runyon BA, Yasmineh WG, Rynders GP. Ascitic fluid adenosine deaminase insensitivity in detecting tuberculous peritonitis in the United States *Hepatology.* 1996;24:1408–1412.

54. Burgess LJ, Maritz FJ, Le Roux I Taljaard JJ. Combined use of pleural adenosine deaminase with lymphocyte/neutrophil ratio. Increased specificity for the diagnosis of tuberculous pleuritis. *Chest.* 1996;109:414–419.

55. Sanchez-Lombrana JL, De La Vega J, Fernandez E et al. Tuberculous peritonitis: Diagnostic value of ascitic fluid pH and lactate. *Scand J Gastroenterol.* 1995;30:87–91.

56. O'Riordan DK, Deery A, Dorman A, et al. Increased CA-125 in a patient with tuberculous peritonitis: Case report and review of published works. *Gut.* 1995;36:303–305.

57. Adsuar N, Blanchette H, and Kilchevsky E. Tuberculosis peritonitis mimicking ovarian cancer in a 20-year-old woman. A case report. *J Reprod Med.* 2004;49(1):52–54.

58. Mahdavi A, Malviya VK, and Herschman BR. Peritoneal tuberculosis disguised as ovarian cancer: an emerging clinical challenge. *Gynecologic Oncology.* 2002;84(1):167–170.

59. Kiu MD, Hsuch S, Ng SH, Chen JS. Elevated serum CA-125 in tuberculous peritonitis: report of a case. *J. Formos Med Assoc.* 1994;93:816–818.

60. Bates B. granulomatous peritonitis secondary to corn starch. *Ann Intern Med.* 1965;62:335–347.

61. Hazards of surgical glove powders (Editorial). *Br Med J.* 1980;281:892–893.

62. Robinson EK, Ernst RW. Boeck's sarcoid of the peritoneal cavity. A case report. *Surgery.* 1954;36:986–991.

63. Wong M, Rosen SW. Ascites in sarcoidosis due to peritoneal involvement. *Ann Intern Med.* 1962;57:277–280.

64. Papowitz AJ, Lin KH. Abdominal sarcoidosis with ascites. *Chest.* 1971;59:692–695.

65. Pullien JP, Vernon DD, Alexander SR, et al. Non-tuberculous mycobacterial peritonitis continuous ambulatory peritoneal dialysis. *Am J Kidney Dis.* 1983;2:610–614.

66. American Thoracic Society. Treatment of tuberculosis and tuberculosis infection in adults and children. *Am Rev Respir Dis.* 1986;134:355–363.

67. Alrajhi AA, Halin MA, Al-Hokail A, et al. Corticosteroid treatment for peritoneal tuberculosis. *Clin Infect Dis.* 1998;27:52–56.

24

Tuberculosis of the Liver, Biliary Tract and Pancreas

Sushil K. Ahlawat
James H. Lewis

HISTORY OF HEPATOBILIARY TUBERCULOSIS

Involvement of the liver in patients with *Mycobacterium tuberculosis* has been described for more than a hundred years. Thomas Addison published one of the earliest descriptions in Guy's Hospital Reports in 1836.[1] Autopsy studies during the latter half of the 19th and early 20th century, an era of great interest in morbid anatomy, demonstrated granulomas and a variety of other lesions in the liver of patients dying with tuberculosis (TB).[1–4] The reports by Gillman & Gillman[5] and subsequently by many others[6,7] on the use of needle biopsy of the liver to demonstrate tuberculous lesions have made the procedure a valuable tool for diagnosis of the disease, especially in cases of cryptic miliary TB without recognized pulmonary involvement.[8] Although isolated hepatobiliary TB was described infrequently in years past,[9,10] a number of detailed reviews attest to its continued importance in the clinical spectrum of the disease.[11–15]

With the advent of the acquired immunodeficiency syndrome (AIDS) epidemic, the increase in homelessness, and increasing immigration of persons from developing countries, the rate of new cases of TB that had been declining began to increase between 1984 and 1994.[16] As many as two thirds of patients with AIDS and TB have extrapulmonary involvement.[17,18] The rate of new cases of TB, as described by Gordon Snider, is enormous with nearly 8 million new cases estimated to have occurred by the end of the 20th century, many of which were associated with human immunodeficiency virus (HIV) infection. Atypical mycobacteria, especially *Mycobacterium avium* complex, continue to play an important role in the course of AIDS, especially with respect to liver involvement.[19,20]

This chapter reviews the clinical, biochemical, and histopathologic spectrum of TB and atypical mycobacteria involving the liver and pancreaticobiliary tract, as well as the hepatotoxicity caused by antituberculosis therapy. Classic *M. tuberculosis* infection in persons not infected with HIV precedes the discussion of the disease in patients with HIV and AIDS and other immunocomprnised persons such as liver transplant recipients.

SPECTRUM OF HEPATOBILIARY AND PANCREATIC TUBERCULOSIS

The liver can be involved in all forms of TB (i.e., pulmonary, extrapulmonary, and miliary). In addition, infection confined predominantly to the liver or biliary tract has been recognized with some regularity, especially in areas where TB remains endemic. A variety of hepatic lesions have been recorded (Table 24-1). These include the lesions long known to be regularly associated with TB (i.e., granulomas, Kupffer cell hyperplasia, sinusoidal infiltration, caseous necrosis, and steatosis), as well as the less common ones, peliosis hepatitis and amyloidosis. Additional lesions associated with TB that have come into focus are those caused by adverse effects of drugs used for treatment. With the advent of effective therapy for TB after World War II, the pattern and prognosis of TB have undergone striking changes,[21,22] as will be discussed.

EVIDENCE OF HEPATIC INVOLVEMENT

Granulomas

Prevalence

The reported prevalence of hepatic granulomas (tubercles) in biopsy material from patients with TB has ranged from 0–100% of studied cases (Tables 24-2, and 24-3).

Pulmonary TB involves the liver less frequently than does miliary TB, with an average of approximately 20% for pulmonary TB and 68% for extrapulmonary or miliary disease. It has been suggested that hepatic invasion in patients with pulmonary TB occurs only terminally, a view based on the observations of Torrey[4] and Mather and colleagues[27] that no granulomas could be demonstrated in autopsy material from patients with active pulmonary TB dying of unrelated causes. Indeed, in most series employing liver biopsy, staining (see Fig. 24-4) or culture is positive far less frequently in patients with pulmonary TB than among those with the miliary form of the disease. Identification of the organism in patients with pulmonary TB has ranged from 0% in several large series to a high of almost 20% in others (Table 24-4). The figures for demonstrating the organism among patients

Table 24-1. Histopathologic Spectrum of Hepatobiliary Tuberculosis

Granulomas
Granulomatous hepatitis
Tuberculomas
Caseous necrosis
Tuberculous abscess
Cholangitis
Cholecystitis
Pancreatitis
Fulminant hepatic failure
Nonspecific changes
    Fatty change
    Focal necrosis
    Kupffer cell hyperplasia
    Sinusoidal inflammation
    Free acidophilic bodies
    Portal fibrosis
    Giant hepatocytes
    Amyloideosis
    Glycogenated nuclei
    Peliosis hepatis
Conincidental lesions
    Alcoholic liver disease and cirrhosis
    viral hepatitis
    Nodular regenerative hyperplasia
    Hemosiderosis
Hepatotoxicity secondary to antituberculous therapy
    Bacille Calmette-Guérin-induced granulomatous hepatitis
    Drug-induced hepatitis (isoniazid, para-aminosalicylic acid, rifampin, pyrazinamide)
    Drug-induced fibrosis (streptomycin)

with miliary TB range from 20–50% (Tables 24-4, and 24-5). The ability to demonstrate mycobacteria by staining is usually associated with the presence of caseous necrosis.[12,34] Caseation is thought to occur as a result of overwhelming acute dissemination of mycobacterial organisms; hence its presence more often in cases with miliary involvement.

The relative rarity of caseation in hepatic granulomas in nonmiliary TB is presumably the reason for the difficulty in demonstrating the acid-fast bacilli (AFB). Nevertheless, Alexander and Galambos[43] were able to identify acid-fast organisms in the liver of 2 of 11 patients with pulmonary TB (18%) with and without hepatic granulomas. They have also reported the greatest success

in demonstrating the organisms by stain and culture in miliary cases, doing so in 53 of 67 cases with hepatic granulomas. In their series, liver biopsy afforded the first morphologic evidence of TB in 82.5% of cases and provided the first bacteriologic proof of TB in 52.5% of miliary cases. In 45% of their patients, a positive liver biopsy provided the only laboratory evidence for systemic granulomatous disease. Granulomas have been demonstrated in an appreciable proportion of patients surviving their disease. The wide variation in reported prevalence has been attributed to the relative diligence with which granulomas had been sought. For example, the 93% prevalence reported by Haex and Van Beek[26] seems attributable to their having examined more than 100 sections from each biopsy specimen as well as having included "epithelioid cell subtubercles" as granulomas. An increased yield of hepatic granulomas also has been reported with a fluorescent staining technique as described by Yamaguchi and Braunstein.[46] The inclusion of patients, in some series, who had undergone previous antituberculous chemotherapy,[6] on the other hand, could lead to a falsely low estimate of the prevalence of granulomas because complete resolution of diffuse granulomatosis following successful therapy may occur within a few months.[12,47–49]

Character of Granulomas

Tuberculous granulomas are composed of mononuclear (epithelioid) cells, surrounded by lymphocytes with or without Langerhans' multinucleated giant cells (Figs. 24-1, and 24-2). They range in size from 0.05-mm microgranulomas[50] to 12-cm tuberculomas[49] but are generally 1–2 mm in diameter. Central necrosis of the tubercle sometimes develops. It is characteristically granular and cheesy; hence the term "caseous." Caseous necrosis (Figs. 24-3, and 24-4) occurs with more regularity in miliary TB (see Table 24-5) than in other forms of the disease.

Nonspecific Hepatic Lesions

A high incidence of histologic abnormalities other than hepatic granulomas is often observed in pulmonary, extrapulmonary, and miliary TB (Table 24-6). Nearly 75% of patients with pulmonary involvement can be shown to have one or more nonspecific lesions, such as Kupffer cell hyperplasia, sinusoidal inflammation or dilatation, fatty metamorphosis, focal necrosis, periportal fibrosis, acidophilic bodies or amyloidosis,[32] and even peliosis hepatis.[12] In miliary TB, such changes receive

Table 24-2. Biopsy Incidence of Hepatic Granulomas in Pulmonary Tuberculosis

Series	Year	No. of Patients	Percentage with Granulomas
Van Buchem[23]	1949	9	0
Klatskin and Yesner[7]	1950	8	25
Seife et al.[24]	1951	70	13
Finkh et al.[6]	1953	25*	8
Ban[25]	1955	59	20
Haex and Van Beek[26]	1955	45	93
Mather et al.[27]	1955	34	3
Von Oldershausen et al.[28]	1955	248	19
Arora et al.[29]	1956	50†	12
Buckingham et al.[30]	1956	13	15
Salib et al.[31]	1961	39	0
Bowry et al.[32]	1970	32	25
Abdel et al.[33]	1997	29	45

*Received antituberculous therapy
†Included both pulmonary and extrapulmonary tuberculosis.

Table 24-3. Biopsy Incidence of Hepatic Granulomas in Extrapulomnary, Localized Hepatic, and Miliary Tuberculosis

Series	Year	No. of Patients	Percentage with Granulomas	Type of Tuberculosis
Haex and Van Beek[26]	1955	189	93	Extrapulmonary
Arora et al.[29]	1956	50	12	Extrapulmonary
Buckingham et al.[30]	1956	22	40	Extrapulmonary
Korn et al.[34]	1959	30	80	Extrapulmonary
Bowry et al.[32]	1970	5	80	Extrapulmonary
Klatskin and Yesner[7]	1950	4	100	Miliary
Mather et al.[27]	1955	22	68	Miliary and Meningeal
Von Oldershausen et al.[28]	1955	93	25.3	Miliary
Biehl[35]	1958	7	100	Miliary
Munt[22]	1971	9	67	Miliary
Gelb et al.[36]	1973	38	81.6	Miliary
Alvarez and Carpio[11]	1983	130	100	Localized hepatobiliary
Essop et al.[37]	1984	96	96	Localized hepatobiliary
Palmer et al.[38]	1985	90	9	Abdominal-peritoneal
Maharaj et al.[13]	1987	41	88	Localized hepatic
Al-Kawari et al.[39]	1995	130	14.6	Localized abdominal
Lundstedt et al.[40]	1996	112	10	Localized abdominal
Sinha et al.[41]	2003	143	102	Extrapulomnary

Table 24-4. Demonstration of Hepatic Acid-Fast Bacilli in Pulmonary Tuberculosis

Series	Year	No. with Granulomas with Caseation	Positive Ziehl-Neelsen Stain	Positive Culture
Seife et al.[24]	1951	13% (9 of 70)	0	
Buckingham et al.[30]	1956	23% (29 of 128)		
Guckian and Perry[42]	1966	29% (9 of 31)		
Bowry et al.[32]	1970	0% (0 of 32)	13% (4 of 31)	
Gelb et al.[36]	1970	37% (14 of 38)		
Munt[22]	1971	50% (3 of 6)		
Alexander and Galambos[43]	1973	Majority of 20	18% (2 of 11)	0% (0 of 10)

less attention, although Buckingham and associates[30] found "nonspecific reactive hepatitis" (i.e., focal and diffuse degenerative changes, Kupffer cell hypertrophy, and portal and periportal cellular infiltrates) in 45% of 32 patients with miliary TB.

Kupffer cell hyperplasia with stellate radiation into adjacent sinusoids has been variously called "retothelial" or "histiocytic" nodules. These cells in a rounded configuration have been regarded as an early lesion in the formation of microgranulomas.[34] Although not pathognomonic of TB, their presence has been reported in 80–91% of patients with pulmonary disease.[53,54]

Infiltration of the sinusoids with lymphocytes occurred in 44% of patients studied by Bowry and coworkers.[32] Such sinusoidal inflammation has been called "nonspecific reactive hepatitis" by Buckingham and colleagues.[30] It is usually observed only with moderate or severe pulmonary disease but may occur with miliary involvement. *Sinusoidal dilatation* is a nonspecific abnormality that also has been associated with neoplastic hepatic processes and hepatic congestion.

The incidence of *fatty metamorphosis* in pulmonary TB has ranged from 14–44%. It has generally been focal and mild. Alcoholism and malnutrition in patients with

Table 24-5. Caseating Granulomas in Hepatic Biopsy Material in Localized Hepatic and Miliary Tuberculosis

Series	Year	No. of Patients with Granulomas	No. with Caseating Granulomas	No. with Positive AFB Stain or culture
Korn et al.[34]	1959	6	6 (100%)	2 of 9
Klatskin and Yesner[7]	1950	4	3 (75%)	1 of 3
Munt[22]	1971	9	3 (33%)	3 of 3
Gelb et al.[36]	1973	38	14 (37%)	1 of 1
Biehl[35]	1958	7	7 (100%)	None
Hersch[44]	1964	200	86 of 114 (75%) at autopsy	5 of 6 at autopsy, 6 of 29 at autopsy
Guckian and Perry[42]	1966	33 of 34	30 of 34 (88%)	1 positive tuberculosis culture
Alexander and Galambos[43]	1973	39	Most of 39	61%
Alvarez and Carpio[11]	1983	130	97 (75%)	2 of 30
Essop et al.[37]	1984	92	77 (83%)	9%
Palmer et al.[38]	1985	8	0	1 of 8
Maharaj et al.[13]	1987	36	52%	59%
Huang et al.[45]	2003	5	4	1

AFB = acid-fast bacilli.

Table 24-6. Nonspecific Hepatic Lesions in Pulmonary Tuberculosis

Series	Year	Kupfer Cell-hyperplasia	Sinusoidal-dilation	Fatty Change	Focal Necrosis	Periportal Fibrosis	Acidophilic Bodies	Glycogen Nuclei	Amyloid	Peliosis	Siderosis
Ullom[1]	1909			35%					10%		
Torrey[4]	1916										
Saphir[3]	1929	80%		34%		67%					
Jones and Peck[51]	1944			42%							
Seife et al.[24]	1951			14%	62%	14%		3%			
Schaffner et al.[52]	1953	91%			70%			13%			
Ban (untreated)[25]	1955	0/34		35%	12	36%					
Arora et al.[29]	1956			36%							
Buckingham et al.[30]	1956								6%		
Hersch[44]	1964										28% at biopsy; 47% at autopsy
Bowry et al.[32]	1970	16%	44%	44%	16%	12%	6%				
Essop et al.[12]	1984			42%		20%			1%	2%	

TB, rather than the TB per se, are probably responsible for the steatosis. The rarity of fatty metamorphosis in modem biopsy series, despite its frequency in the former necropsy-based data, supports this view.

Focal necrosis of hepatocytes is common. It may be acute (poorly circumscribed foci of necrotic cells with polymorphonuclear infiltration) or subacute (more discrete foci with lymphocyte predominance).

Periportal fibrosis has been described in patients with pulmonary TB[53] and with predominantly hepatic involvement.[12] *Cirrhosis* may be present but probably precedes the TB lesions. Indeed, it had been previously suggested that cirrhosis might predispose toward the development of TB. There is, however, no convincing evidence that TB can lead to cirrhosis. Nevertheless, the possibility remains that fibrosis and architectural distortion secondary to hepatic involvement may result in a histologic picture similar to that of severe granulomatous involvement by sarcoidosis[7,55] or that attributed to the hepatic involvement of brucellosis.[56] In addition, radiocolloid scans of the liver in patients with hepatic TB may closely mimic the changes visible with cirrhosis.[57] Little attention, however, is given today to the earlier concept of "tuberculosis cirrhosis."[51]

Free acidophilic bodies were seen in 2 of 32 patients in the report of Bowry and colleagues[32] and in the studies of Korn and associates.[34] These rounded, deeply esosinophilic staining bodies are the remains of degenerating liver cells and are commonly visible in viral and drug-induced hepatitis.

A rare change occurring in miliary TB is the presence of giant hepatocytes, reported by Pintos and coauthors.[58] Such giant hepatocytes are more often characteristic of neonatal hepatitis.[59] *Glycogenated nuclei* were seen in 3% of patients in one series.[24] This change is also nonspecific and is more common in diabetic and in some patients receiving corticoteroids.

Amyloidosis was seen in 10% of one autopsy series[1] and in smaller number of patients with chronic untreated pulmonary TB in the reports by Ban[25] and Buckingham and coworkers.[30] Essop and colleagues[12] recorded a 1% prevalence among patients with predominanatly localized hepatic TB. Detectable by various special stains, amyloidosis most likely represents a response to the chronic infection.

Peliosis hepatitis, the presence of blood-filled lakes in the liver, is today a lesion seen predominantly in patients who have been taking anabolic or contraceptive steroids. Older reports have drawn attention to the association of peliosis with the terminal state of diseases characterized by "wasting," namely, TB and carcinomatosis.[60] In one series, the prevalence was recorded as 2%.[12]

Granulomatous hepatitis is a term that has been applied to the presence of multiple granulomas in the liver.[61,62] We think that a more exact use of the term would restrict it to granulomatous involvement accompanied by sinusoidal and other parenchymal cellular infiltrates and by parenchymal injury, including acidophilic bodies. Such lesions occur in miliary TB, brucellosis, histoplasmosis, Q fever, and other infections.[8] In sarcoidosis,[7] however, and in many of the patients with pulmonary TB, granulomas may be the only hepatic lesions present, in which case the histologic description would be better given as simply hepatic granulomas.

Although TB is a major cause of hepatic granulomas in most series, its frequency is highly variable and depends on the population studied. Sartin and Walker[54] reported only 3% incidence of TB in a series of 88 patients with granulomas at the Mayo Clinic. Other series reported higher frequencies ranging from 20–55% of patients (Table 24-7).

Table 24-7. Tuberculosis as Cause of Hepatic Granulomas

Series	Year	Country	No. of Cases	Percent with tuberculosis
Gilinsky et al.[63]	1981	S. Africa	116	50
Harrington et al.[64]	1982	Multiple	1129	20
Cunningham et al.[65]	1982	Scoteland	77	10
Anderson et al.[66]	1988	Australia	59	7
Sartin and Walker[54]	1991	USA	88	3
McCluggage and Sloan[67]	1994	Ireland	163	0.1
Sabharwal et al.[53]	1995	India	51	55
Mert et al.[68]	2001	Turkey	56	36
Gaya et al.[69]	2003	UK	63	8

In a review of granulomatous hepatitis by Harrington et al.[64] in 1982, TB accounted for approximately 20% of hepatic granulomas in 8 series totaling 1129 patients. In a series from India[53] tubercular cause of hepatic granulomas was found in 55% of 51 patients.

Biochemical Abnormalities in Tuberculosis

Biochemical evidence of hepatic dysfunction in TB has been observed in a large number of cases (Table 24-8), although in general the biochemical values themselves correlate poorly with the specific type of hepatobiliary TB and are considered of limited diagnostic value.[13]

Nevertheless, it remains useful to review the liver-related tests that have traditionally been used as potential markers of tuberculous involvement. The bromsulphalein (BSP) retention test was a popular one in years past and was the most common hepatic functional abnormality seen.[73] In contrast with extrapulmonary TB, in which impaired BSP excretion has been noted to be characteristic, pulmonary TB, even with the presence of hepatic granulomas, usually has not been accompanied by impaired liver function. There has been no correlation between serum alkaline phosphatase levels and hepatic granulomas in pulmonary or localized hepatic TB[13]; however, in immunocompromised patients with hepatic TB serum alkaline phosphatase level was significantly higher compared to immunocompetent patients.[74]

Abnormal serum protein levels are characteristic of TB. Hyperglobulinemia is frequent, occurring in up to 50% of patients with pulmonary TB and in up to 80% of patients with extrapulmonary and especially miliary disease. The elevation reflects the elevated Y-globulin fraction, a regular marker of chronic infection. Indeed, TB is one of the recognized causes of extreme hyperglobulinemia, and Schaffner and colleagues[52] have drawn attention to the usefulness of serum globulin level as a measure of intensity of nonspecific host reaction to the infection.

Serum cholesterol levels are variably affected. They are elevated in 10–20% and decreased in 21–40% of cases, as reported by Seife and associates[24] and Schaffner and coworkers.[52]

Hyperbilirubinemia in pulmonary TB is uncommon and is generally mild. Mild hyper-bilirubinemia (less than 3 mg/dL) was found in 13% of 123 miliary patients reported by Hersch[44] and in 5% of 63 patients with both miliary and pulmonary TB reported by Guckian and Perry.[42] Nearly one fourth of a group of patients with miliary TB reported by Munt[22] had elevations of serum bilirubin, all slight. Jaundice mimicking extrahepatic obstruction is an infrequent clinical presentation of localized tuberculous hepatitis, usually resulting from common bile duct obstruction due to compression by tuberculomas or enlarged lymph nodes at the porta.[11,12,75,76] Jaundice of this type, however, is rare outside of endemic areas.

Serum aminotransferases (SGOT, SGPT) are usually normal in patients with pulmonary TB in the absence of alcoholic liver disease or other drug toxicity. In acute miliary disease, transaminase levels are slightly increased. As a general rule, however, there is no correlation between the degree or incidence of biochemical abnormalities and the extent of histologic injury in pulmonary, localized hepatic, or miliary TB.[12,32,34]

Clinical Symptoms and Signs

No specific symptoms can be related to the hepatic abnormalities in pulmonary TB, although, of course, the constitutional symptoms associated with the underlying TB (fever, chills, fatigue, abdominal pain, and weight loss) are common.[42] Hepatomegaly occurs in approximately 50% of patients, and the spleen is enlarged in 25–40%. Physical manifestations of chronic alcoholism and malnutrition may be present. Patients with hepatic involvement due to granulomatous hepatitis may have fever of unknown origin.[77] In localized hepatic TB, as previously mentioned, the clinical presentation may simulate alcoholic or viral hepatitis,[12] amebic[78] or pyogenic liver abscess,[79,80] metastatic disease or primary hepatocellular carcinoma,[46,57,81–85] extrahepatic obstructive jaundice[11,12,75,86] and, rarely, an "acute abdomen."[87]

THE LIVER IN RELATION TO THE SITE OF TUBERCULOSIS

Pulmonary Tuberculosis

Tuberculosis confined to the lungs involves the liver less often than does miliary TB. Hepatic granulomas are found at biopsy in about 20% of patients, but tubercle bacilli are rarely demonstrable by strain or culture (see Table 24-5). A characteristic but nonspecific histologic manifestation of pulmonary TB is the presence of localized areas of Kupffer cell hyperplasia yielding lesions called retothelial or histiocytic nodules. Biochemical abnormalities in patients with pulmonary TB may include elevated levels of alkaline phosphatase and hyperglobulinemia. Jaundice is rare as a manifestation of hepatic involvement due to pulmonary TB alone.

Table 24-8. Hepatic Function Tests and Biochemical Abnormalities in Tuberculosis

Series	Year	No. of Patients	Abnormal BSP Retention	Elevated Alkaline Phosphatase	Bilirubin <3mg	Bilirubin >3 mg	Elevated SGOT/SGPT	Increased Globulin	Cholesterol High	Cholesterol Low	Tuberculosis Type
Hurst et al.[70]	1947	17	23%	55%							Pulmonary
Klatskin & Yesner[7]	1950	4	75%	67%	100%			67%			Miliary
Galen et al.[71]	1950	53	19%								Pulmonary
Seife et al.[24]	1951	70	14.30%	14.30%				50%	21.40%	10%	Pulmonary (treated)
Schaffner et al.[52]	1953	23						74%	40%	20%	Pulmonary (treated)
Ban[25]	1955	35	71%	0							Pulmonary (treated)
Ban[25]	1955	25	60%	0							Pulmonary (treated)
Korn et al.[34]	1959	50	85.70%	40.90%	26.7%			75%			Extrapulmonary
Hersch[44]	1964	123	100%	72% (18 of 25)		13%		50%	40%	20%	Miliary
Hersch[44]	1964	20	100%	87.5% (7 of 8)	14%	6%		43% (3 of 7)			Localized
Guckian and Perry[42]	1966	63		56%	50%		50% (slight)	60%			Hepatic
Bowry et al.[32]	1970	32	49%	16%	0	0	0	45%			Granulomatous Hepatitis
Munt[22]	1971	69	54.50%	34%	23%		93%				Pulmonary
Irani and Dobbins[72]	1979	9	12.50%	44%		0	12.50%	62.50%			Miliary
Essop et al.[12]	1984	96		Most (6 to 10-fold)							Combined
Alvarez and Carpio[11]	1983	130	55%	75%	65%	65%	35%/35%	81%			Localized
Maharaj et al.[13]	1987	41		87% (20% > 3x)	15%			78%			Localized

BSP = bromsulphalein; SGOT = serum glutamic-oxaloacetic transaminase; SGPT = serum glutamic-pyruvic transaminase.

Localized Extrapulmonary Tuberculosis

Korn and colleagues[34] described three patterns of hepatic dysfunction in 50 patients with extrapulmonary TB: (1) elevated alkaline phosphatase and BSP retention associated with space-occupying granulomas, (2) abnormal flocculation test results and hyperglobulinemia associated with chronic localized tuberculous infections such as osteomyelitis, and (3) a combination of the two, simulating intrinsic liver disease without overt jaundice. Hepatic granulomas were present in 80% of patients, and most (87.5%) had impaired BSP excretion. Large caseating granulomas were more frequent in patients with the greatest degree of hepatic dysfunction. They found granulomas in 14 of 15 patients with raised alkaline phosphatase levels; however, the biochemical abnormality was an insensitive measure of hepatic granulomas, because 10 of 15 patients without elevated alkaline phosphatase levels also had granulomas. Nonspecific abnormalities such as Kupffer cell hyperplasia and diffuse sinusoidal inflammation were common.

Abnormalities in one or more liver function or serum protein tests were present in all patients studied by Korn and colleagues.[34] Serum bilirubin was elevated in 26.7% (highest value 5.0 mg/dL), and slight jaundice was detected in three patients. Values for aminotransferases were only slightly elevated in most patients with extrapulmonary TB.

Palmer and associates[38] described 90 patients admitted to a London hospital with abdominal TB, most of whom were Asian immigrants. Liver biopsy often provided histologic confirmation in cases wherein the diagnosis was in doubt. Eight patients presented with fever and elevated alkaline phosphatase and had a histologic picture consistent with granulomatous hepatitis. The granulomas were noncaseating; tubercle bacilli were identified in biopsy tissue in only one patient.

Localized Hepatobiliary Tuberculosis

A subset of patients with extrapulmonary TB has the infection confined solely or predominantly to the liver or biliary tract. Terry and Bunnar[88] reported a dozen cases in 1957. They referred to this form of infection as *primary miliary tuberculosis* of the liver and defined it as "a condition in which there is hematogenous dissemination of tuberculosis of the liver with minimal involvement of other organs." Although inapparent sites of infection usually remained clinically silent, 4 of their 12 patients died with tuberculous spread to other organs. "Atypical tuberculosis of the liver" was the term proposed by Cleve and coworkers[89] to "designate exclusive or principal involvement of the liver by tuberculous infection leading to clinical manifestations of hepatic disease." Cinque and colleagues[90] suggested that tubercle bacilli reach the liver via the portal vein or hepatic artery. Indeed, in autopsy cases in which TB has been confined clinically to the liver, abdominal, and mediastinal lymph node involvement may be found and may result in miliary spread.

Although rare in the United States,[15] this form of localized hepatic TB is not infrequently encountered in areas with high rates of infection. For example, the prevalence of localized hepatic involvement in TB was 2.3% in 820 patients seen over an 8-year period in Saudi Arabia, the diagnosis being confirmed by endoscopic or laparoscopic biopsy in most cases.[39] Liver involvement was present in 14.6% of these persons overall with abdominal TB. Among 112 patients with abdominal symptoms due to TB, 10% had macronodular focal hepatic lesions, often associated with hepatomegaly as seen on abdominal imaging studies.[40] The report by Alvarez and Carpios[11] from the Philippines describes the clinical and histologic features of 130 patients with localized hepatobiliary TB seen over a 20-year period at the Santo Thomas University Hospital in Manila. In 82% of cases, the diagnosis was clinically suspected prior to histologic confirmation. The two major forms of presentation included (1) a hard nodular liver with fever and weight loss simulating cancer in 65% of patients and (2) chronic recurrent jaundice mimicking extrahepatic obstruction in 35%. A 2:1 male predominance was observed, and the majority of patients were in the 11–30-year-age range. Symptoms were generally present for 1–2 years prior to the diagnosis.

Percutaneous liver biopsy was performed in 71 persons and confirmed the diagnosis in 48 (67%). Laparoscopy yielded the correct diagnosis in 49 of 53 patients (92%), with the hepatic lesions appearing as cheesy, white, irregular nodules. In a few patients, however, what grossly appeared to be a tuberculoma was actually metastatic cancer on biopsy. Interestingly, a positive AFB stain was recorded in only 2 of 30 cases, although the mere presence of caseating granulomata was considered diagnostic by the authors.

Hepatic calcifications were efficient in 49% of patients. They appeared as rounded calcific densities with ill-defined margins scattered throughout the liver. Radiocolloid liver scan revealed filling defects in 52%. In three persons in whom hepatic arteriography was performed to exclude cancer, an avascular mass was seen, in contrast with the neovascularity usually expected with malignancy.

Hepatic enzyme abnormalities were seemingly dependent on whether or not jaundice was present; jaundice usually resulted from enlarged lymph nodes obstructing the common bile duct near the hepatoduodenal ligament or porta hepatis. Serum aminotransferase values were elevated in more than 90%, and alkaline phosphatase was raised in 100% of patients with jaundice. In contrast, only 5% of nonjaundiced patients had abnormal aminotransferase levels, and alkaline phosphatase values were elevated in only 60%. The presence or absence of jaundice also influenced the response to treatment. Seventy-five percent of nonjaundiced patients responded to conventional drug therapy, compared with only 25% with jaundice. Six of 45 jaundiced patients required surgical intervention for biliary decompression.

Overall, 12% of patients died, most owing to respiratory failure, a few secondary to tuberculous peritonitis, and approximately one third due to portal hypertension and variceal hemorrhage. All of these last patients had cirrhosis. Although fatal variceal hemorrhage has been linked to tuberculous hepatic involvement by others,[76] no causal relationship between TB and cirrhosis has been demonstrated.[91]

Essop and his colleagues in South Africa[12] reviewed the clinical features of 96 patients with what they called "tuberculous hepatitis," that is, a predominantly hepatic presentation during acute miliary TB or chronic hepatic presentation during acute miliary TB or chronic hepatic tuberculous secondary to reactivation of the disease. This form of TB represented 1.2% of all cases seen over a 6-year period. Physical signs and symptoms included tender hepatomegaly and fever in most patients. Splenomegaly was present in 45%. Right hypochondrial pain was common and led to exploratory laparotomy in two patients who presented with obstructive jaundice and an acute abdomen, respectively. Fourteen percent of the group had abdominal symptoms exclusively, 22% had respiratory symptoms, and 12% had only fever, sweats, malaise, and weight loss. Most patients had a combination of these three symptom complexes.

Granulomas were present on biopsy or at laparotomy or autopsy in 96% of patients and provided the first evidence of systemic granulomatous disease in 16 cases and helped diagnose pulmonary disease in another 13 patients. This high incidence of granulomas was largely due to the exclusion of cases with primary pulmonary or extra-abdominal TB with incidental hepatic involvement. Caseation was present in 83% of patients, but tubercle bacilli were demonstrable by stain in only 9% of cases (those with the greatest number of granulomas and highest degree of caseation).

Other histologic findings included fatty change in 42% and portal fibrosis in 20%. Peliosis hepatitis and amyloidosis were rare. Coexisting liver disease included cirrhosis in eight patients, alcoholic hepatitis in six, and hepatoma in one.

Serum alkaline phosphatase was moderately elevated (sixfold to tenfold) in the majority of patients, and hyperbilirubinemia was present in about 25%. Hyponatremia was a common presenting laboratory abnormality.

The cumulative mortality rate was 42% for the patients in this series; mortality was highest in those with acute miliary TB; age below 20 years; a predisposing factor such as steroid therapy, chronic renal failure, or diabetes mellitus; and the presence of coagulopathy. Hepatic enzymes were not useful in predicting patient survival.

Huang et al[45] described 5 patients with a local nodular form of hepatic TB from Taiwan over 4-year period. All 5 patients underwent surgery, and had a preoperative diagnosis of malignant hepatic neoplasm and a postoperative histological diagnosis of chronic granulomatous inflammation suggestive of TB. None of them had a known previous history of TB. All were positive for *M. tuberculosis* by polymerase chain reaction (PCR) analysis of the liver tissue. This report as well as others[85] highlights the difficulty in correctly diagnosing hepatic TB. It is often confused with primary or metastatic carcinoma of the liver. A high index of suspicion is required for diagnosis, which can be made by histology and bacterial studies as well as by PCR techniques.

Tuberculomas

Tuberculomas may occur as solitary or multiple nodules in patients with primary miliary TB of the liver or secondary to reactivation of hepatic foci of infection. As mentioned previously, lesions may have a diameter of up to 12 cm[49] and may undergo central caseation leading to abscess formation.[79,92–95] Symptoms of fever, malaise, and weight loss are common. Less often, abdominal pain and diarrhea occur. Hepatomegaly is frequent. Uncommon presenting signs have included portal hypertension, jaundice, and a palpable abdominal mass. Jaundice, when present, has been attributed to tuberculomas at the porta hepatis causing obstruction to bile flow.[12] Rarely, these lesions bleed, leading to a clinical presentation of an acute abdomen with progressive anemia.[87] Outside endemic areas, the diagnosis is often not suspected and is usually confirmed serendipitously with the finding of tuberculomas at laparotomy or at autopsy.

Biochemical parameters of hepatic injury are not prominently abnormal. Alkaline phosphatase levels are generally only slightly increased or normal, a pattern characteristic of space-occupying lesions of the liver.

Filling defects on liver scan or angiography may suggest primary or metastatic carcinoma. Indeed, there are several reports of tuberculous pseudotumors,[57,81,96,97] including at least one instance wherein hepatic tuberculomas resembled malignant disease arteriographically.[98] More commonly, tuberculomas are confused with an amebic or pyogenic liver abscess.[78–80] Blind percutaneous liver biopsy has generally not been helpful in confirming the diagnosis.[99,100] Bhargava and colleagues,[101] among others, reported the use of aspiration cytology at the time of laparoscopy to make the diagnosis in areas where the infection is common. Bacteriologic confirmation is difficult, and there are only a few reported instances of positive acid-fast stains or cultures.[80] Zipser and coworkers[49] suggest that because of the condition's resemblance to metastatic disease, culture is often not attempted. However, they note that with successful antituberculous therapy, complete resolution of tuberculomas can be expected within 6–9 months. In addition, percutaneous drainage of tubercular abscess has been shown as an effective alternative to surgery.[80] It should be pointed out that in regions where TB is endemic, the finding of caseating hepatic granulomata is generally sufficient to confirm the diagnosis, regardless of the results of AFB staining or cultures.[12]

Several reports describe the sonographic, computed tomographic (CT), and magnetic resonance imaging (MRI) appearance of macroscopic TB of the liver.[40,102–104] Ultrasonographic features that suggest a diagnosis of tuberculoma include a mass with irregular calcifications, the presence of ascites, splenomegaly with enlarged lymph nodes, and resolution of the lesion or lesions following antituberculous therapy.[102] Computed tomographic findings include low-density, solid, heterogeneous, and sometimes partially calcified lesions with a thickened wall and either no or minimal enhancement by contrast. Irregular calcifications are also characteristic. High-density ascites relating to high ascitic protein content is also a useful clue.[102] In children, single or multiple low attenuation intrahepatic lesions, hepatomegaly, ascites, and a positive tuberculin skin test result suggest the diagnosis of TB rather than disseminated malignancy.[103,105]

Murata and colleagues[106] described the MRI findings in one patient with surgically proven tuberculomas who had hypoechoic lesions in the lesion seen initially, as described by Kawamori and colleagues.[107] The lesions were hyperintense on weighted T2 images, indicating the tuberculomas can be of either increased or decreased signal intensity on MRI.

The role of endoscopic retrograde cholangio-pancreatography (ERCP) has been emphasized in patients with suspected tuberculous strictures of the common bile duct who present with obstructive jaundice[108] (see Tuberculosis of the Biliary Tract).

Miliary Tuberculosis

Hepatic involvement in disseminated TB is very common.[15,109–111] Granulomas have been demonstrated in 75–100% of patients with miliary disease (see Table 24-5). Characteristically, miliary lesions are small (1–2 mm), epithelioid granulomas. The proportion of patients with caseous necrosis has varied from 33–100%, depending on the series. Nonspecific hepatic lesions such as Kupffer cell hyperplasia and fatty metamorphosis also are common.

As with pulmonary and localized extrapulmonary disease, impaired BSP excretion is the most frequent biochemical abnormality in miliary TB. Alkaline phosphatase elevations occur in approximately 50% of cases. There is a poor correlation between hepatic function tests and liver histology in cases with miliary involvement. The clinical features of acute miliary infection localized predominantly to the liver have been reviewed by Essop and colleagues[12] and Alvarez and Carpio[11] (see Localized Hepatic Tuberculosis). Rarely has disseminated TB presented as hepatic failure. A case report described a Japanese patient who presented with jaundice, deteriorated rapidly, and died just 3 days after admission.[108]

Miliary Tuberculosis Presenting as Fulminant Hepatitis

Curry and Alcott[112] described fulminant hepatic failure caused by TB in 1955. Although deaths due to miliary TB are not infrequent, deaths specifically attributable to acute hepatic failure are unusual.[108,113,114] Hussain and colleagues[114] describe a 54-year-old woman who presented with a 5-day history of right-upper-quadrant pain, vomiting, and mild jaundice. Two months earlier, her hepatic enzyme levels had been normal. Twenty years earlier, she had been treated for active pulmonary TB with a 2-year drug regimen. On presentation, her bilirubin was elevated threefold, alkaline phosphatase twice normal, and aspartate aminotransferase (AST) five-times normal, along with hypoalbuminemia, hyponatremia, and hypoprothrombinemia. Acetaminophen levels were "negative," and all hepatitis viral serology was "negative." Her chest radiograph appeared normal, and an ultrasound scan showed an enlarged liver. She deteriorated clinically over the next 8 days with her AST peaking at 1790 IU/L and her serum sodium falling to a low of 114 mEq/L. A transjugular biopsy showed caseating granulomas, but AFB cultures remained negative. She was treated aggressively for TB but continued to deteriorate and experienced renal failure along with stage IV coma and she died 13 days after presentation. Autopsy revealed the presence of AFB in multiple organs, with the liver showing coagulative necrosis with more than 50% of the parenchyma destroyed by caseating necrosis. Culture of the liver grew *M. tuberculosis.*

Congenital Tuberculosis

Reports of congenital and neonatal TB are scant[115,116] but continue to appear.[96,117–120] Debre and colleagues[115] reported an infant who died with disseminated TB of the liver, spleen, lung, and hilar lymph nodes 7 weeks after being born to a mother with long-standing pulmonary TB. Although the child was separated from the mother immediately after delivery, jaundice was observed during the first week of the infant's life and it was concluded that there had been transplacental transmission of tubercle bacilli. When prompt treatment is initiated the prognosis is good, as has been illustrated by 2 cases.[117,120] Recently Berk et al[118] reported a neonate with congenital TB who presented with fulminant hepatic failure without respiratory compromise and was successfully treated with antitubercular therapy despite profound hepatic compromise.

Histologically, neonatal TB of the liver is characterized by diffuse, large, caseating granulomas containing numerous tubercle bacilli accompanied by fatty metamorphosis.[86] Hepatomegaly, jaundice, and failure to thrive in an infant born to a mother with active TB should alert the clinician to the diagnosis.

Atypical Mycobacterial Infection

Rarely is a mycobacterial organism other than *M. tuberculosis* isolated from the liver. McNutt and Fudenberg[121] have drawn attention to the fact that atypical mycobacteria most commonly cause localized pulmonary infection and generally do not result in disseminated disease. Stewart and Jackson[122] reported hepatic and splenic TB due to *Mycobacterium kansasii* diagnosed at autopsy in a patient with a myeloproliferative disease. In general, however, *M. kansasii* does not produce hepatic disease, even in HIV-infected persons.[17,105] Although *M. kansasii* can be cultured from the necrotic tuberculous lesions, no other gross pathologic or clinical features distinguish the infection from that due to *M. tuberculosis.*[105,123]

Mycobacterium avium is the most common organism associated with nontuberculous mycobacterial infection. Although rarely reported between 1940 and 1980, with only a few dozen cases in the literature, the advent of AIDS has brought a plethora of new cases to light[19,20] (see Hepatic Mycobacterial Infection in AIDS).

The portal of entry is thought to be the gastrointestinal tract and possibly the respiratory tree. Hematogenous dissemination is common, with fever, weight loss, local pain, cough, and night sweats being frequent presenting symptoms. Hepato-splenomegaly has been recorded in 35–45% of patients, and jaundice was noted in 8% of patients in the series reviewed by Horsburgh and associates.[19] The diagnosis can be achieved by several methods, but liver biopsy may be the most rapid and efficient as illustrated by case reports by.[124,125] Caseation was infrequent in all tissues examined, and AFBs were rarely visible. Culture was positive in only about 25% of cases.

In contrast with *M. avium* infection in association with AIDS, more than two thirds of patients without AIDS have responded to therapy (most having received cycloserine as part of the treatment regimen), although patients with large numbers of organisms were more likely to experience therapy failure.[19] Other atypical mycobacteria that may involve the liver include *Mycobacterium scrofulaceum,*[126] *Mycobacterium gordona,*[127] *Mycobacterium xenopi, Mycobacterium fortuitum,*[128] and *Mycobacterium chelonei.*[105]

Granulomatous Hepatitis Induced by Bacille Calmette-Guérin

Granulomatous involvement of the liver has been reported in 12–28% of patients receiving Bacille Calmette-Guérin (BCG) as immunotherapy for neoplastic disease.[69,129–133] Flippin and colleagues[130] reported that asymptomatic granulomatous hepatitis usually occurs within several months after the last BCG inoculation. The clinical appearance of constitutional symptoms, hepatomegaly, mildly elevated serum transaminase and bilirubin values, and moderately elevated alkaline phosphatase levels, focal defects, or non-homogeneous uptake on technetium liver scan plus the presence of granulomas, hepatocellular necrosis, lympho-histiocytic aggregates, and Kupffer cell hyperplasia represent the clinicopathologic spectrum of granulomatous hepatitis due to BCG.

The exact mechanism for the development of granulomatous disease.following BCG therapy is not known. A role for both viable BCG bacilli and hypersensitivity reaction has been proposed. O'Brien and Hyslop[134] note that an intense inflammatory reaction occurs at the site of vaccination, and BCG organisms often remain viable for weeks to months and may disseminate to various organs. The role that associated immunosuppressive chemotherapy plays in predisposing to systemic BCG infection is unclear. Rarely have acid-fast BCG bacilli been demonstrated in hepatic or lymph node tissue.[130] Hunt and associates[132] proposed that BCG preparations are antigenic and that granulomas develop as a result of the hypersensitivity response to these antigens.

Patients with symptomatic granulomatous hepatitis have a high rate of morbidity, and several fatalities have been reported.[130,135] O'Brien and Hyslop[134] warn that an early sign of BCG "overdose" may be the development of anergy to tuberculin purified protein derivative (PPD). Isoniazid (INH) and methanol extraction residue (MER) given concurrently during BCG inoculation have each been shown to protect against the development of granulomatous hepatitis.[136,137]

Severe and life threatening disseminated BCG infection with granulomatous hepatitis has been reported with local immunotherpay using BCG for urinary bladder cancer therapy.[131] This patient was successfully treated with empirical antituberalar therapy in combination with a short course of steroids.

Tuberculosis of the Hepato-Biliary-Pancreatic Tract

Tuberculosis of the Bile Ducts

Prior to 1900 biliary TB was commonly found at autopsy. Since the turn of the 20th century, however, the reported incidence has been low. Stemmerman[138] found only 45 instances in 1500 autopsies of patients with TB, yielding an incidence of approximately 3%. In that series the incidence of bile duct TB rose 7% in cases with miliary involvement. The distribution of periportal tubercles in those cases with bile duct involvement was not significantly different from cases having no bile duct involvement (47% vs. 43%), and there was no consistent relationship between the weight of the liver and either the size or the number of biliary abscesses.

The typical pathologic picture of bile duct (tubular) TB as reported by Stemmerman[138] is one of multiple small cavities (1–20 mm) containing greenish necrotic material. Rarely do these biliary abscesses reach large size (up to 12 cm) and rarely can a bile ductule be traced directly to the cavity. Microscopically, caseation and bile pigment are usually present within the cavity. Bile ductule and capillary remnants may be visible within the caseous process. The abscess capsule varies in thickness, being widest when bile duct proliferation and collagen bundles are present. AFBs, when found, are usually demonstrated at the junction of the outer capsule and the caseous inner wall.

Signs and symptoms attributable to bile duct TB are uncommon. Only three of the 45 patients reported by

Stemmerman had clinical jaundice (6.7%), and only one third had hepatomegaly. However, TB of other organs drained by the portal circulation was present in 41 of 45 cases, including caseous TB of mesenteric lymph nodes in 89%, tuberculous ulcerations of the intestinal tract in 73%, and tuberculous peritonitis in 27%.

The pathogenesis of bile duct TB has been linked to two possible mechanisms. Rosenkranz and Howard[139] showed that periportal tubercles could rupture into the walls of contiguous bile ductules, thereby giving rise to an abscess cavity. They thought that the excretion of AFB into the bile was always due to microscopic ruptures of this kind. Other workers postulated that the bile ducts may be infected primarily. Stemmerman[138] favored the theory that bile abscesses arise from tubercle bacilli, having gained entry into small bile ductules from the blood stream or lymphatics.

Jaundice Due to Hepatobiliary Tuberculosis

Jaundice is rare in TB.[32,34,140,141] Nevertheless, it has become axiomatic that visible jaundice, when present, may imply ductal obstruction in the absence of other hepatic or drug-induced injury. Patients with elevated bilirubin levels usually have cholestasis associated with the parenchymal damage due to tuberculous infection. Curry and Alcott[112] suggested that the intrahepatic type of jaundice was usually associated with acute, fulminating miliary disease, as illustrated by a case presenting as fulminant hepatitis.[108] The jaundice that has been occasionally noted in instances of chronic pulmonary TB generally has been attributed to the generalized dissemination of tubercle bacilli that occurs preterminally.

Jaundice due to intrahepatic cholestasis is usually mild (serum bilirubin levels being <5 to 6 fig/dL), and it is often clinically inapparent. In contrast, deep jaundice may occur when the larger biliary ducts are involved or when enlarged lymph nodes obstruct the porta hepatis.[12] There are several reports of tuberculous lymphadenitis involving the porta hepatis causing obstructive jaundice with bilirubin levels greater than 20 mg/dL.[11,89,109,142–147] Pineda and Dalmacio-Cruz[76] and Alvarez and Carpio[11] emphasized the potential complication of portal hypertension with ascites, splenomegaly, and ruptured esophageal varices that occurred in several of their patients with tuberculous involvement of the porta hepatis leading to biliary cirrhosis. Portal lymph nodes may be involved by direct contiguous spread from the gallbladder or by hematogenous or lymphatic spread from organs drained by these nodes.

Occasionally, jaundice has been reported secondary to a bile duct stricture in patients with known TB. Bearer and colleagues[148] described the ERCP findings in a Filipino immigrant with obstructive jaundice who was found to have a common bile duct stricture in the presence of granulomatous hepatitis. A diagnosis of TB was confirmed by aspirate and culture from the bile. The stricture persisted despite antituberculous therapy, and biliary cirrhosis developed, as was seen on follow-up liver biopsy. As a result, a biliary stent was inserted, which normalized the hepatic enzymes within a period of 2 months. Stanley and colleagues[146] have also reported the treatment of a tuberculous bile duct stricture using an endoprosthesis. Multiple intrahepatic biliary strictures, areas of dilation, beading, and ectasia resembling sclerosing cholangitis or cholangiocarcinoma are also described.[11,15,149] Biliary stricture may occur at hilar region or distal common bile duct with dilation of the intrahepatic ducts.

Tubercular cholangitis is extremely rare.[150] It is thought to occur as a result of rupture of a caseating granuloma from the portal tract into the bile duct. Clinical feature resemble bacterial cholangitis, with right upper quadrant pain, fever, and jaundice.

Tuberculosis of the Gallbladder

The gallbladder is an uncommon site of tuberculous infection. Leader,[93] in reviewing the literature in 1951, noted that few than 40 cases have been reported. The majority of cases were women over 30 years of age. Gallstones were present in more than one half of cases, and the most commonly reported symptoms and signs included epigastric pain made worse by eating and right upper quadrant tenderness.

Rarely has TB has been isolated to the gallbladder. Most cases occur in association with other organ involvement, including tuberculous peritonitis. Cholecystitis is the most frequent preoperative diagnosis, and cholangitis has also been reported. Miliary TB presenting as acute cholecystitis was reported by Garber and colleagues.[151]

Treatment usually requires cholecystectomy in combination with antituberculous therapy. Complications such as tuberculous abscess of the gallbladder requires prompt surgical attention.

Cryptic miliary TB clinically mimicking a case of cholecystitis with sepsis has been reported.[152] Pulmonay TB with gallbladder involvement presenting as acute cholecystitis and cholelithiasis was reported in a 14-year-old girl by Rozmanic et al.[153] A rare case of hepatobiliary TB presenting as a gall bladder tumor has also been described.[154]

Tuberculosis of the Pancreas

Tuberculosis of the pancreas or of the peripancreatic lymph nodes is infrequent compared to liver. We were able identify 115 cases reported in the literature from 1966 to 2004 (Table 24-9).

One explanation for the lower prevalence is that pancreatic enzymes destroy mycobacteria.[157] Pancreatic involvement can be isolated to the gland, a part of miliary TB or a site of reactivated disease. The most likely mechanism of spread is lymphohematogenous dissemination from an occult focus in the lungs.[156,159,164,188] Men and women are affected equally,[155,160] with a mean age of around 40 years. Reported cases of pancreatic TB are predominantly seen from northeast Asia or immigrants to Europe and the United States of America from countries where TB is endemic.[155] Patients with HIV infection have a greater incidence of atypical and extrapulmonary TB. Tubercular pancreatic abscess as an initial AIDS defining disorder in patients infected with HIV has been reported.[190]

The clinical manifestations of pancreatic TB depend on the type of involvement, acute or chronic pancreatitis, focal mass lesion mimicking carcinoma portal hypertension. Symptoms may include acute or chronic abdominal pain, weight loss, recurrent vomiting, obstructive jaundice, and occasionally fever of unknown origin. Most cases have a high sedimenation rate and tuberculin skin tests are positive in over 70% of cases.[155,160] The most frequent clinical presentation is a pancreatic mass mimicking carcinoma.[156,159,164,188] Less often acute or chronic pancreatitis is described.[156,160,164] Portal hypertension secondary to portal vein compression or thrombosis is rare.[157] A majority of cases involve the head and/or body of the pancreas; isolated involvement of the tail of the pancreas is uncommon.

Radiologic findings are often nonspecific. Focal pancreatic lesions in pancreatic TB are usually demonstrated by ultrasound or CT closely mimicking pancreatic carcinoma or mucinous tumors of the pancreas.[157] Occassionally the pancreatic mass is diagnosed on imaging as a pancreatic abscess.[158,160] Pombo et al[158] retrospectively reviewed the CT findings in 6 patients with pancreatic TB, 3 of whom had AIDS. Findings included focal mass lesions, multiple small low attenuation pancreatic nodules, or diffuse enlargement of gland in AIDS patients, whereas a nonspecific focal mass lesion was seen in HIV-seronegative patients. Low attenuation peripancreatic or periportal adenopathy with peripheral rim enhancement in conjunction with signs of disseminated TB were ancillary features that supported a diagnosis of pancreatic TB.

Table 24-9. Pancreatic Tuberculosis as Reported in the Literature

Reference	Year	No. of cases	Clinical Presentation	Imaging — Focal Mass	Type of involvement — Isolated	Type of involvement — Disseminated	Pancreatic pathology — Caseating Granuloma	Pancreatic pathology — Positive AFB Smear or M. Tuberculosis Culture	Outcome — Treated Successfully With ATT For 6–12 Months	Outcome — Mortality
Ladas et al.[155]	1966–97	41	Abdominal pain (60%), fever (40%), weight loss (37%), Jaundice (23%)	91%	100%		100%	38%		7%
Ladas et al.[155]	1997	2	Abdominal pain (1), fever (1), weight loss (2), anemia (1)	2	2		2	2	2	
Rezeig[156]	1998	4	Abdominal pain (4), fever (1), weight loss (2), Jaundice (1)	4	4		4	3	4	
Woodfield et al.[157]	2004	3	Abdominal pain (3), fever (1), weight loss (2), Jaundice (2)	3	3		3	2	3	
Pombo et al.[158]	1998	6	Abdominal pain (4), fever (3), weight loss (3), Jaundice (4), diarrhea (1), HIV + (3)	4	2	4	6	6	5	1
Demir et al.[159]	2001	2	Abdominal pain (2), fever (2), weight loss (2)	2	2		2		2	
Schneider et al.[160]	2002	2	Portal hypertension (1)	2	2		2	1	1	1
El Mansari et al.[161]	2003	2	Abdominal pain (1), weight loss (1), Jaundice (1)	2	2		2		1	1
Kumar et al.[162]	2003	2	Abdominal pain (1), fever (2), weight loss (2), Jaundice (1), HIV + (1)	2	2		2	1	1	1
Pramesh et al.[163]	2002	2							2	
Franco-Pardes et al.[164]	2002	2		2						
Xia et al.[165]	2002	16	Abdominal pain (75%), fever (50%), weight loss (69%), Jaundice (31%), back pain (38%)	100%	100%	Liver, spleen, bile duct involvement in 42%	75%	30%	100%	

Study	Year	No.	Clinical features						
Choudhary et al.[166]	2002	9	Mimicking pancreatic carcinoma (5), acute pseudocyst (1), pancreatic abscess (1), chronic pancreatitis (1), GIB (1)		9			8	1
Lo et al.[167]	1998	2		2				2	
Others*[168–189]	1998–2004	21	Abdominal pain (9), fever (6), weight loss (5), jaundice (7), duodenal stenosis with pancreatico-duodenal fistula(1), acute pancreatitis (2), recurrent pancreatitis (1), post-liver transplant (1), peri-ampullary mass (1)	16	21	14	8, PCR + (4)	17	

*Single case reports; AFB = acid fast bacillus; PCR = polymerase chain reaction; HIV = human immunodeficiency virus; ATT = antituberculosis therapy; GIB = gastrointestinal bleeding.

A definitive diagnosis of pancreatic TB is only achieved with histologic confirmation.[157] However, the success rate of image-guided fine needle aspiration cytology in diagnosing pancreatic TB is only approximately 50%.[160,176] In cases of pancreatic abscesses, clinical correlation and aspiration are necessary to differentiate between a pyogenic and tuberculous abscess. If TB is not confirmed by aspiration cytology or core biopsy then laparoscopy may prove to be helpful; however, even with the use of appropriate preoperative and intraoperative investigations, the diagnosis is often only made at the time of pancreatic resection.[159,188]

Hemobilia Secondary to Tuberculosis

Hemobilia (biliary tract hemorrhage) has been associated with various inflammatory and vascular lesions of the biliary tree, but only two cases of TB-related hemobilia have been described. Agarwal and associates[191] reported hemobilia following a percutaneous needle biopsy of the liver in a patient with disseminated TB. They argued that diffuse involvement of the liver was the primary cause of the hemobilia, postulating that one or more necrotic foci might have spontaneously eroded into a portal blood vessel and bile duct simultaneously. Nonetheless, percutaneous liver biopsy by itself has been associated with hemobilia[192–194] and there seems little reason to relate this extraordinarily rare event to the TB. Das et al.[195] reported hemobilia in a patient with disseminated TB presenting initially with non-localizable massive upper gastrointestinal bleeding but subsequently found to have pancreatitis, pleural effusion, and hemobilia, which was treated successfully. Hepatic artery mycotic aneurysm of tubercular etiology is also reported.[196]

Hepatic Mycobacterial Infection in AIDS

Histologic material obtained via liver biopsy or at autopsy in patients with AIDS has revealed hepatic pathology in the majority.[197–204] Although most lesions are nonspecific, the findings of hepatic granulomata has been relatively commonplace, and the diagnosis of *M. tuberculosis*, and *M. avium* infection is now being made with regularity.[17,18,20,183,205–207]

Mycobacterium Tuberculosis *in HIV and AIDS*

Persons infected with HIV are susceptible to infection with TB, both from reactivation of a latent disease and from newly acquired infections that can progress rapidly.[17] Infection rates upto 1000-fold higher have been reported in HIV positive persons compared with those not infected with HIV.[208] Selwyn and colleagues[206] found that 15% of HIV–positive intravenous drug users with a positive tuberculin test result developed active TB over a 2-year period, compared with none of the similar group of HIV-seronegative persons. Similarly, in a study of 1130 HIV-seropositive persons without AIDS followed for a median of 53 months, Markowitz and colleagues[208] found that patients with CD4 counts less than 200 cells/mm^3 and PPD-positive patients were at high risk for TB.

Although *M. tuberculosis* in an HIV infected patient is primarily a pulmonary infection, extra-pulmonary sites of disease are common. Between 25% and 70% of HIV-associated *M. tuberculosis* cases have extrapulmonary disease, a finding that fulfills current Centers for Disease Control (CDC) surveillance criteria for the diagnosis of AIDS.[17,162,209] Hepatosplenomegaly is frequently present in HIV-positive patients and thus is relatively nonspecific for the diagnosis of a mycobacterial infection. The most common extrapulmonary sites of involvement in patients with AIDS are lymph nodes, blood, bone marrow, the urinary tract, the liver, and the central nervous system. Extrapulmonary involvement is associated with poorer prognosis than in pulmonary TB alone in these patients because extrapulmonary disease is associated with a greater degree of immune deficiency.[17] Clinically and pathologically, generalized TB in the setting of AIDS is characterized by unusual features or the lack of typical features described for disseminated TB in patients who do not have AIDS. As a result many cases remain undiagnosed until postmortem examinations.[210]

A retrospective analysis of all patients with AIDS and TB in San Francisco between 1981 and 1988 by Small and coworkers[18] found a prevalence of *M. tuberculosis* at 2.2% (132 of 6103 AIDS cases). Patients with *M. tuberculosis* infection were more likely to be African American or Hispanic and to have intravenous drug abuse as a risk factor. Eighty percent were born in the United States. Fifty-nine percent of these patients developed TB prior to any other AIDS defining disease, and nearly 30% of this group had extrapulmonary involvement. Approximately one third had pulmonary TB, and the remaining one third had both pulmonary and extrapulmonary disease. Nearly 50% patients who experienced *M. tuberculosis* infection prior to any other infection had a positive tuberculin test result. Of those with extrapulmonary involvement liver biopsy was diagnostic in a number of patients. Although site specifics were not given in this review, the percentage of acid-fast stains from extrapulmonary sites that were positive was only 16% compared with 75% positivity for culture. In an autopsy series consisting of 29 patients with AIDS and a confirmed diagnosis of TB, hepatic involvement was seen in 45%.[33] African-American ethnicity is an independent risk factor for extrapulmonary TB. Mortality at 6 months correlates in part with dissemination of *M. tuberculosis* and the severity of underlying comorbidities.[211]

Vilaichone et al.[74] compared the clinical spectrum of hepatic TB between immunocompetent and immunocompromised patients. Fever, weight loss, hepatomegaly, disproportionate elevation of alkaline phosphatase, and reverse albumin: globulin ration were common in hepatic TB. Non-caseating granulomas without detection of AFB was a common finding in both groups; however, disproportionate elevation of alkaline phosphatase was significantly higher in the immunocompromised hosts. PCR techniques showed a sensitivity of 86% and the specificity of 100% in the diagnosis of hepatic TB.

Small and colleagues noted several atypical features of *M. tuberculosis* infection in HIV-positive persons in the series.[18] The first was that the 30% with extrapulmonary involvement was a substantially higher figure than the 13% reported in patients without AIDS from the San Francisco area. The other major difference was that although HIV-positive persons did not appear to respond any differently to antituberculous medication, they experienced a much higher incidence of adverse drug reactions (18%) compared with that reported for patients not infected with HIV (3.7%). Skin rashes accounted for 56% of adverse reactions, but hepatitis developed in 26%. Rifampin (RIF) was the most common drug associated with an adverse reaction, requiring its discontinuation. INH was withdrawn in 4% and ethambutol in 1%. Sixty percent of all adverse reactions occurred within the first month of treatment, and 95% were evident by the end of the second month. Of the 125 patients who received antituberculous therapy, eight (6.4%) died of tuberculosis-related causes (with six of eight deaths occurring in the first month of treatment). Overall, treatment failure occurred in just 1% and relapse in 5%, which was not different from patients without the AIDS.

Liberato et al.[212] compared characteristics of pulmonary TB in HIV seropositive and seronegative patients in a Northeastern region of Brazil. Patients with pulmonary TB and HIV infection were mostly male, showed higher frequency of weight loss (>10 kilos), had a higher rate of nonreaction result to the tuberculin skin test, a higher frequency of negative sputum smear examination for AFB and negative sputum culture for *M. tuberculosis*. Treatment failure was more common in those who were HIV positive. The association between extrapulmonary and pulmonary TB was more frequent in those who were seropositive for HIV compared to those without HIV infection (30% vs. 1.6%).

The higher incidence of adverse reactions to antituberculous medications in patients with AIDS has also been noted with other antimicrobials, such as trimethoprim-sulfamethoxazole and pentamidine, among others[213] (see below). As noted by Small and colleagues,[18] HIV-infected persons with AIDS appear to be at increased risk of hepatotoxicity from antituberculous therapy. Ozick and colleagues[214] observed that the combination of INH and RIF produced hepatocellular injury (defined as an alanine aminotransferase [ALT] >200 IU/L) in 11% of patients in New York City, several of whom were under the age of 35. Amarapurkar and colleagues[215] described a tuberculous abscess of the liver associated with HIV infection that had features similar to tuberculous abscesses that have developed in the non-HIV population.

Obstructive jaundice due to TB is usually seen in immunocompetent patients due to tubercular hilar adenoathy or biliary stricture. Recently, Probst et al.[216] reported a patient with obstructive jaundice in AIDS who was diagnosed by ERCP and endoscopic aspiration of bile. AFBs were detected in direct smears and identified as *M. tuberculosis* by PCR and by traditional culture. The patient was treated with antituberculous therapy with resolution of jaundice; however, she died after 4 weeks from suspected tuberculous sepsis.

Mycobacterium Avium Complex *in AIDS*

Disseminated infection with *Mycobacterium avium complex* (MAC) is the most common systemic bacterial infection complicating AIDS in the United States.[20] The annual incidence of MAC is up to 20% after an AIDS-defining illness has occurred.[217] Since the seminal report by Greene and colleagues[50] in 1982 first brought MAC to light as an opportunistic infection, numerous reports have followed. Although MAC is rarely reported as the initial opportunistic infection in AIDS, disseminated MAC has been present in up to 50% of patients with AIDS coming to autopsy, with the antemortem diagnosis being confirmed in 30–40%[218] (Table 24-10). According to Horsburgh,[19] this increased incidence is not only due to improved diagnostic methods but also reflects improved treatment regimens that may have influenced the decision to pursue the diagnosis. In addition, the introduction of zidovudine (AZT) and other retroviral therapies has increased survival among HIV-infected patients because *M. avium* typically occurs late in the course of AIDS. Such therapy also has permitted the diagnosis in increasing numbers of patients with *M. avium* disease.

Table 24-10. Hepatic Mycobacterium avium in AIDS

Author	Total No. Studied	No. with M. avium Infection	No. with Granulomas	No. with Positive AFB Stain	No. with Positive Culture	
				With Granuloma	Without Granuloma	
Greene et al.[50]	5	4	3	3	3	1
Glasgow et al.[198]	42	8	9	6		3 of 6
Reichert et al.[203]	9	3	0	3	2	
Lebovics et al.[200]	25	4	3	3	3	1
Lewis et al.[201]	9	2	1	2	1	1
Hawkins et al.[219]	366	67	NSR	NSR	6 of 6 (biopsy) 32 of 42 (autopsy)	
Orenstein et al.[202]	10	6	6	6	5	
Guarda et al.[199]	13	1	NSR	1 (bone marrow)	1 (bone marrow)	
Schneiderman et al.[204]	85	8 (biopsy) 6 (autopsy)	7 (biopsy) 1 (autopsy)	NSR		NSR
Chang et al.[220]	28	8	11	2		
Tarantino et al.[221]	12	5		12		

NSR = not specifically reported; AFB = acid-fast bacilli.

In contrast with *M. tuberculosis* in AIDS, which results largely from reactivation of a previous focus of infection, disseminated *M. avium* infection is usually the result of primary infection. The organism is ubiquitous in nature and is acquired by exposure to environmental sources such as food, water, soil, and house dust. The portal of entry is considered to be the gastrointestinal tract because local gastrointestinal infections are common. The organism disseminates hematogenously and has a predilection for parasitizing macrophages. As a result, reticuloendothelial system involvement is a hallmark of infection. Microscopically, the liver (and other organs) is filled with large numbers of distended histiocytes teeming with AFB as seen on Ziehl-Neelson staining (Fig. 24-5). Tissue loads are estimated to be as high as 10^9–10^{10} colony-forming units per gram with little evidence of granuloma formation or surrounding inflammatory response. Although phagocytosis of the organism appears to be normal, macrophages-mediated killing is apparently severely impaired. Histologically, the large numbers of organisms are present amid a minimal inflammatory response resembling that of lepromatous leprosy.[10,117] Caseation necrosis is rarely observed in the liver, being described more commonly in pulmonary *M. avium* infections.[19]

The most common clinical presentation of *M. avium* is persistent fever with or without night sweats and weight loss. The likelihood of disseminated disease is greater than 70% in febrile patients with AIDS in whom *Pneumocystis carinii*, cytomegalovirus (CMV), and other pathogens are excluded. Chronic diarrhea and abdominal pain suggest gastrointestinal involvement. Extrahepatic obstruction may produce a cholangitis or an acalculus cholecystitis picture. Severe anemia is another hallmark of *M. avium* infection, and frequent transfusions may be required. The diagnosis is confirmed by culture of peripheral blood, which has a sensitivity ranging from 86–96%. Bone marrow smear and culture are the best indicators for early dissemination. The liver as well as the bone marrow and lymph nodes remain important potential diagnostic biopsy sites. Tarantino et al.[221] evaluated fine needle aspiration biopsy in disseminated

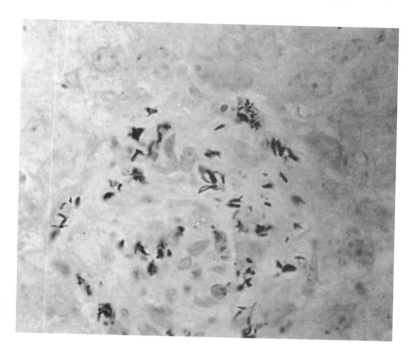

Fig. 24-5. *Mycobacterium avium* in a poorly formed granuloma in a patient with AIDS. (Courtesy of Dr. I. K. Ishak.)

mycobacterial infection in patients with HIV infection. Spleen and/or lymph node aspiration biopsy indicated the specific diagnosis in 100% of patients. Patients with disseminated *M. avium* infection have a significantly shortened survival (4.1 months) compared with a median survival of 1.1 months for patients without AIDS *M. avum* infection. At autopsy, however, death is seldom seen to be a direct result of the organism because causes of death are similar to those in patients with AIDS who do not have the infection. The shortened survival is presumably the result of severe malnutrition and weight loss associated with the organim.[19]

Jaundice due to hepatic involvement by *M. avium* is rare. Bilirubin values were normal in all cases of *M. avium* infection reported by Glasgow and colleagues[198] despite a florid granulomatous reaction involving about 40% of the hepatic parenchyma in one patient. Lewis and coworkers[201] described jaundice in one patient with disseminated *M. avium* infection involving the liver, but a concomitant CMV infection was also present. Serum alkaline phosphatase values have been elevated in nearly all cases of hepatic *M. avium*,[198] although the enzyme levels are not specific for *M. avium*, having been recorded in response to a hypersensitivity reaction to sulfonamide therapy as well as to other infectious agents such as histoplasmosis.[200]

One of the important differences between *M. tuberculosis*, and *M. avium* infection in AIDS is the relative lack of response of *M. avium* to conventional antituberculous therapy. Most early reports observed either a poor or absent response for most patients.[50,128,205,219,222–224] This lack of clinical responsiveness may have been a reflection of the severe immune dysfunction of these patients because *M. avium* typically occurs late in the course of AIDS when cell counts are at their lowest. CD4+ cell counts less than 60/mm^3 are typical of patients with disseminated *M. avium* infection, and the infection is rare in patients having more than 200 CD4+ cells. This explains why *M. avium* usually occurs *after* rather than concurrently *with* Kaposi's sarcoma or *P. carinii* pneumonia, which typically occurs in patients with greater than 100 CD4+ cells. With improvements in patient survival associated with the use of zidovudine and other agents, an improved response to multidrug regimens has been observed with *M. avium* infection.[19,225] In addition, alkaline phosphatase (reflective of hepatic involvement) may normalize following treatment.[19]

Other Mycobacteria

Although *M. avium* is the predominant nontuberculous mycobacterial infection in AIDS, a number of other atypical mycobacteria, including *M. fortuitum, M. gordonae,*

M. xenopi, and *M. chelonae*, have also caused disseminated disease in AIDS. *M. kansasii*, however, rarely if ever leads to liver disease or other extrapulmonary involvement. For example, in a study of 17 patients with pulmonary infection due to *M. kansasii*, none had laboratory evidence of hepatic dysfunction.[105] As with *M. avium*, a majority of patients infected with *M. kansasii* had lymphocyte counts less than 200/mm^3, indicating advanced immunosupression.

Tuberculosis Occurring in Liver Transplant Patients

The overall incidence of TB developing in solid organ transplant recipients around the world is estimated to be 1% to 4%, although the incidence of TB affecting the transplanted liver ranges from 0.9 to 2.3%.[226–228] Both adult and pediatric liver transplant recipients appear to be at risk for TB because of their immunocompromised state.[56,121] In a case series of 550 liver transplant patients followed for a 5-year period in New York City, Meyers and colleagues[229] diagnosed the new onset of TB in four persons for a prevalence of 0.7%. One person had evidence of miliary-TB in the peritoneum at the time of transplantation. The transplantation was performed, and the patient was treated successfully. In the other three patients, TB developed between 2 months and 57 months after transplantation, and one of these patients experienced a tuberculous liver abscess. The rate of infection with TB was similar to the 1.2% (5 of 462 cases) reported by Grauhan and colleagues[228] in Germany. Among 42 patients in San Francisco who underwent liver biopsy following liver transplantation and who were found to have granulomas, one patient had TB for a prevalence of 2.4%.[230] The majority of epithelioid granulomas or microgranulomas in the parenchyma (an overall prevalence of 50%) were associated with hepatocyte necrosis but without a specific infection being identified.

Recent data suggest an incidence of TB that is 8–100 fold higher in transplant recipients compared to the general population.[227,231] The majority of cases occur within the first 12 months after transplantation. Nonrenal transplantation, rejection within 6 months before the onset of TB, and type of primary immunosuppressive regimen are predictors of posttransplant TB.[227] Disseminated TB is common in the posttransplant setting. Receipt of OKT3 or anti-T cell antibodies is a significant predisposing factor.[227] The most likely cause of TB in organ transplant recipients is reactivation of old quiescent disease; however, nosocomial exposure and

transmission by cadaveric or living donors with TB is also responsible in some cases.[227]

Of greater concern than active TB developing post transplant is the risk of hepatotoxicity associated with INH prophylaxis, which is discussed later. Hepatic enzyme abnormalities associated with drug therapy can be confused with transplant rejection. The rationale for INH prophylaxis in liver transplant recipients is the fact that a majority of patients are anergic and on immuno-suppressive therapy, which places them at high risk for acquiring TB. The policy at many institutions is to treat active TB or patients who have evidence of old TB on chest radiograph as well as those who have a positive PPD result in the pretransplant period. Meyers and colleagues[229] also suggest that recipients of livers from donors with active TB should undergo treatment after transplantation. Because of the risk of INH hepato-toxicity in immunocompromised patients,[232] some institutions recommend that surveillance mycobacterial cultures and smears be obtained following liver trans-plantation as an alternative to the prophylactic use of INH. In a study conducted by Torre-Cisneros[233] in 100 liver transplant patients over the first 180 days after a transplant, only a single patient was identified by sputum or urine AFB smears and cultures as having active TB and was promptly treated. No patient who remained culture-negative experienced an active TB infection according to this approach.

Routine preoperative screening for TB via tuberculin skin testing and prophylactic treatment of patients with positive results is controversial because tuberculin skin test is an imperfect identifier of patients at risk of TB[231,234] and increased risk of INH hepatitis in liver transplant recepients, with a prophylactic treatment of patients with positive results. Nevertheless, a case control study demonstrated safety and efficacy of INH chemo-prophylaxis administered during liver transplant candidacy.[227] Aggressive management is required to prevent TB in transplant candidates. Based on retro-spective data,[234] patients that inadvertently undergo trans-plantation can be effectively treated when diagnosed early.

Clinically significant hepatotoxicity requiring discontinuation of INH was seen in 41–83.3% in postliver transplant patients,[227,235] but 8 of 15 liver biopsies in the series reported by Singh et al.[227] demonstrated acute or chronic rejection plus granulomas or only granulomas in patients receiving INH containing regimens. In the series by Meyers and colleagues from New York City liver biopsy revealed drug-induced hepatitis in 5 of 6 (88%) patients and rejection in 3 of 6 (50%) patients. Therefore, these data suggest that a presumptive diagnosis of INH hepatotoxicity may not be accurate for liver transplant recipients and liver biopsy should be considered for the evaluation of elevated liver enzymes levels since multiple etiologies could account for the occurrence of abnormal liver enzyme levels in these patients.

While managing patients with active TB in a post transplant setting, reduction of immunospression appears to be critical.[236] In addition, experience from a large transplant center in the United States reveals that liver transplant patients have poor tolerance for conventional therapy due to inherent toxicity of these agents and their concomitant bouts of organ rejection. Unconventional therapy consisting mainly of ethambutol and oflxoacin for a mean length 9 months yielded remarkably good results in six patients who developed drug induced hepatotoxicity with conventional agents.[235] However, active TB in posttransplant setting is associated with high moratlity. Singh et al.[227] reported mortality rate of 29% on the basis of compilation of published reports in the literature. Meyers et al.[235] and Verma et al.[237] also reported similar mortality rate from post liver transplant TB in adults and peditric transplant recipients in the United States. Disseminated infection, prior rejection, and receipt of OKT3 or anti-T-cell antibodies are significant predictors of mortality in patients with TB.[227]

ASSOCIATED AND COINCIDENTAL HEPATIC LESIONS IN TUBERCULOSIS

Alcoholic Hepatitis and Cirrhosis

Rolleston and McNee[91] found that nearly 30% of patients dying of cirrhosis had demonstrable TB infections, most commonly pulmonary and peritoneal. It was their contention that the cirrhosis was present prior to the TB and that the cirrhosis served to predispose to the infectious process. They supported their view by citing the lack of firm evidence that TB leads to cirrhosis in humans. To date, such evidence continues to be lacking, despite the earlier acceptance of the term "tuberculous cirrhosis."[238]

Alcoholism commonly has been associated with TB, having been recorded in up to 54% of patients with the infection.[22,24,44,239] Accordingly, the coexistence of histologic features of alcoholic liver disease (including steatosis and cirrhosis with hepatic granulomas) is to be expected. Indeed, Korn and colleagues[34] suggested that the fatty changes in the liver in patients with TB might be the result of concomitant alcohol ingestion. Alcohol also

increases the risk of hepatotoxicity from INH and other antituberculous therapy, as discussed later.

Viral Hepatitis

Tuberculosis does not appear to predispose to viral hepatitis, but outbreaks may occur in TB hospitals. Fitzgerald and associates[240] described an outbreak of hepatitis B involving 37 of 64 hospitalized TB patients that spread to both hospital staff members and close contacts of infected persons. Several patients experienced a carrier state for longer than 6 months. Petera and collegues, and McGlynn and coworkers have noted ahigh incidence of chronic hepatitis B surface antigen (HbsAg) carriage in TB patients.[241] Especially among persons from high-risk groups. There is little likelihood that coincidental chronic viral hepatitis might result in biochemical and clinical features that might be mistaken for tuberculous involvement of the liver, and histologic differences would, of course, clarify the situation. Hepatic steatosis due to concomitant non-A, non-B hepatitis may be an important cause of the macrovesicular fat in some patients with TB.[200] Chronic asymptomatic HbsAg carriers receiving INH therapy, although at one time considered to be at increased risk of hepatic injury, were not found to have higher SGOT levels than those not receiving INH in one study.[241]

Severe hepatotoxicity, however, was reported from the combination of INH and RIF in HbsAg-positive patients from Taiwan who were being treated for active TB.[242] The number of fatal cases led the authors to speculate that improved cellular immunity following successful antituberculous therapy may, in some patients, have precipitated a severe reactivation of hepatitis B with death due to viral injury rather than to drug toxicity.

Cirrhosis

Cirrhosis has been described as a possible risk factor for the development of drug-resistant TB.[243] In addition, patients with cirrhosis have been treated with ofloxacin for TB, which may be safer than traditional antituberculous therapy in patients with underlying liver disease.[25,244]

Other Hepatic lesions

Amyloidosis has been described in the livers of up to 10% of patients with hepatic TB.[1] In some patients the amyloid infiltration has been extensive, producing marked hepatomegaly. Most cases have occurred in patients with long-standing advanced disease, often involving the intestinal tract.[51] Currently available treatment for TB would make amyloidosis a rare complication today.

Nodular regenerative hyperplasia (NRH) of the liver is an uncommon lesion characterized by diffuse nodularity of the parenchyma with portal fibrosis. Hepatocyte atrophy may be present in some lobules and regenerative nodules in others. Although the pathogenesis is unknown, NRH has been described in a variety of disorders, including TB.[245–247] Whether or not the relationship to TB is fortuitous is not clear.

Hemosiderosis of the liver has been described in as many as 47% of autopsy cases and 28% of needle biopsy specimens in African patients with hepatic TB. It should be noted, however, that this high incidence occurred in a population containing a large proportion of Bantus, who are known to have a high incidence of hemosiderosis.[44] Tuberculosis by itself probably does not lead to hepatic iron deposition. An interesting report by Gordeuk and colleagues[248] reanalyzed an iron overload study originally conducted in 714 black South Africans in the 1920s to determine whether or not TB was related to the hepatic and splenic iron associated with hepatocellular carcinoma in these patients. They concluded that iron overload in these patients was probably a risk factor for death from hepatocellular carcinoma as well as from TB.

HEPATIC INJURY DUE TO ANTITUBERCULOUS THERAPY

Hepatic injury due to antituberculous drugs has a bearing on the liver disease associated with TB because it extends its spectrum. With the introduction of effective chemotherapy of TB after World War II came instances of drug-induced hepatic injury. Identification of the role of individual agents in the production of hepatic damage has been somewhat hampered by the use of several agents in combination for treatment. Nevertheless, a reasonably clear picture has emerged.[249]

Para-aminosalicylic acid (PAS) can lead to a syndrome of acute hepatocellular injury with jaundice accompanied by clinical manifestations that have led to the syndrome being dubbed "pseudo-mononucleosis," with fever rash, lymphadenopathy, eosinophilia, and lymphocytosis with "atypical" lymphocytes. The incidence has been estimated to approach 1%, and the mechanism can reasonably be deduced to be hypersensitivity.[250] In contrast with the case of INH, no age-relationship was apparent. The relative abandonment of this drug makes the hepatic injury of more historic and pathophysiologic interest than of clinical importance.

Isoniazid

INH causes acute hepatocellular jaundice in about 1% of all recipients, and at least 10% experience more trivial, anicteric hepatic injury. Clinical features are virtually indistinguishable from acute viral hepatitis, with malaise, anorexia, and nausea with or without vomiting, developing prior to the onset of jaundice. Fever and hepatomegaly are much less common. Biochemically, the condition also resembles acute viral hepatitis, with jaundice being a presenting feature in approximately 10% of patients. Case-fatality rates of approximately 10% occur in persons who experience jaundice with massive hepatic necrosis, leading to a fatal outcome.[251]

Susceptibility to INH hepatotoxicity seems importantly age-related, with children and adolescents under the age of 20 being far less susceptible than older persons. Young adults, aged 20–35 years, have shown an incidence of overt icteric liver damage of approximately 0.5%, whereas adults over the age of 35 show at least twice that incidence and those over 50 have an incidence that approaches 3%. Reports highlight the fact that young persons are indeed susceptible to INH injury, however, including the development of fatal hepatoxicity. Snider and Caras[252] reviewed the medical literature from 1965 to 1989 that dealt with INH hepatotoxicity. In addition, they searched Food and Drug Administration (FDA) files and a number of other databases and discovered a total of 177 deaths attributed to INH during this period. Of the 153 patients whose age was known, 9.2% were under the age of 20, 12.4% were aged 20–34, 17.6% were aged 35–49, 37.9% were aged 50–64, and 23% were over the age of 65. Women constituted nearly 70% of all the fatal cases. The racial mix was 40% non-Hispanic Caucasian, 38% African American, 15% Hispanic, 4% Native American, and only 1 % Asian. Among women aged 15–44 years in this series, 38% were within 1 year of having given birth. Others have also found an increased risk in postpartum females and in women in general.[63,252a] This series suggested that deaths from untreated TB were 25 times more likely than the risk of dying from INH hepatotoxicity based on the assumption that 5% of untreated infected persons experienced clinical TB. Chronic hepatitis C, B and HIV independently have been shown to increase the risk of INH induced hepatotoxicity.[253–256] Female sex and birthplace in Asia are additional risk factors for first line antitubercular agents induced hepatotoxicity.[256]

A number of reports have suggested that the risk of fulminant hepatitis from INH may be on the rise. The CDC as having experienced severe hepatitis from INH reported ten persons from New York City, several of whom required liver transplantation.[257] The median age of these persons was 33 years, with a range of 5–68 years. Three were under the age of 20 and six were women. The median duration of INH therapy given prophylactically was 57 days, and fulminant hepatic failure developed rapidly (a mean of 10 days) once symptoms developed. None of these individuals were alcoholic, but three were receiving phenytoin and one took acetaminophen that may have contributed to their toxicity. Meyers and his colleagues[258] reviewed the acute hepatic failure in several of these individuals. Five received a liver transplantation and one died postoperatively. Two others died awaiting liver transplantation, and one individual improved and did not require transplantation.

The mechanism of hepatic injury due to INH appears to be metabolic idiosyncrasy rather than hypersensitivity.[259] Although it was previously thought that susceptibility was increased among rapid acetylators,[260] more recent studies have failed to substantiate any relationship between hepatic toxicity and acetylator phenotype in children or adults.[261–264] Nevertheless, occasional dissenting reports continue to appear.[260,265] Alcoholics appear to be at increased risk of INH toxicity, most likely by inducing its metabolism. Similarly, INH has potentiated the toxicity of acetaminophen probably through the induction of the P4502E1 cytochrome pathway that is responsible for the toxic acetaminophen metabolite.[143,266] Cytochrome P450 2E1 genetic polymorphism may be associated with susceptibility to INH induced hepatitis.[83] The risk of hepatitis from INH is also seen in patients also taking other antituberculous drugs, especially RIF and pyrazinamide (PZA). Ozick and colleagues[214] found that the combination of INH and RIF in patients with AIDS led to an 11% incidence of hepatocellular injury, defined as ALT greater than 200 IU/L. Similarly, children receiving combination therapy appear to be at increased risk of hepatic injury from INH and RIF. In India, Parthasarathy and colleagues[145] found that the incidence of hepatic injury from daily regimens of INH and RIF was up to 39% in children being treated for tuberculous meningitis, 10% with spinal TB, and up to 8% of those being treated for pulmonary TB. The risk of hepatic injury was highest among those receiving daily therapy compared with twice-weekly regimens. In their series, there was no indication that PZA added to the hepatotoxic potential, as it appears to do in adults (as discussed further).

A report by Moulding and colleagues[267] from California that chronicles 20 deaths from INH over a 14-year period continues to highlight the need for careful monitoring in patients receiving chemoprophylaxis with INH. In this series of fatal cases, females outnumbered males by more than two to one, with the individual patients ranging in age from 15–55 years. Four deaths occurred in postpartum females who had started INH prophylaxis during pregnancy and continued it following delivery. Eight of the 20 deaths (40%) occurred in patients under the age of 35, which was considerably higher than expected. The authors made the important observation that in many of these patients, vomiting and abdominal pain were not considered specific symptoms of hepatitis, and this may have added to a delay in the diagnosis. In addition, management errors, such as not seeing patients on a monthly basis and providing several months worth of medication at a single visit for convenience, may also have contributed to a delay in diagnosing serious hepatic injury. When therapy is properly monitored, however, it is thought that the risk of INH injury is significantly reduced.[267]

Rifampin

RIF is no longer recommended for prophylaxis of latent TB in the absence of abnormal chest X-ray.[268] RIF is frequently used in combination with INH as well as other agents. Although RIF is thought to increase the likelihood that INH will lead to hepatic injury,[269,270] probably through induction of the cytochrome system that enhances conversion of INH to its toxic metabolite, RIF has also produced occasional instances of idiosyncratic, acute hepatocellular injury.[271] The clinical manifestations are those of acute viral hepatitis similar to the symptoms occurring with INH. However, these signs and symptoms generally occur within a month of initiating treatment with RIF, whereas INH injury usually does not occur until the second month (85% of cases). In addition to its ability to produce hepatocellular damage, RIF can also interfere with bilirubin uptake and excretion as a benign effect,[250,271] although marked hyperbilirubinemia can lead to anxiety on the part of both patient and physician.

Pyrazinamide

PZA may cause severe hepatitis when used as a single agent but, importantly, appears to increase the risk of fatal hepatotoxicity when used in combination with INH and RIF.[12,99] Durand and colleagues[272] reported 18 cases of fulminant or subfulminant hepatic failure secondary to antituberculous therapy. Nine patients received INH and RIF, and nine received the combination of INH plus RIF and PZA. Only two of the nine who received PZA survived, whereas eight of nine receiving only INH and RIF survived. These authors concluded that PZA potentiated the toxicity of INH and RIF. Survival in these cases was inversely related to the time to onset of jaundice, with survivors becoming jaundiced within the first 15 days of therapy. They recommend avoiding PZA in patients with abnormal hepatic or renal status and suggest that biochemical monitoring be performed on a weekly basis during the first 2 months of treatment. PZA should be discontinued if the ALT rises above threefold the upper limits of normal in these patients.

Mitchell and colleagues[273] from Kings College Hospital described four additional patients with acute liver failure from the combination of INH, RIF, and PZA, out of which two died. Rechallenge was performed in three of the patients and was noted to be positive.

Clarithromycin is currently being used to prevent and treat *M. avium* infections.[225,274] It has been described as causing a cholestatic illness in a patient being treated for *M. chelonae*. That patient was inadvertently rechallenged with clarithromycin and experienced a recurrence of cholestasis.[275] Macrolide antibiotics in general have long been known to cause cholestatic injury.[250,259]

Monitoring for Isoniazid and Combination Antituberculous Chemotherapy

With proper clinical and biochemical monitoring, it is thought that the risk of INH and combination chemotherapy-induced hepatic injury can be significantly reduced.[267] Data indicate that the incidence of clinical hepatitis is lower than was previously thought. Hepatitis occurred in only 0.1–0.15% of 11,141 persons receiving INH alone as treatment for latent TB infection in an urban TB control program.[276] Although recent guidelines of the American Thoracic Society, CDC and Infectious Diseases Society of North America[277] do not recommend routine monitoring for INH, RIF or PZA, unless the patient has baseline elevation of liver enzymes, clinical symptoms or is felt to be at higher risk due to chronic hepatitis B or C; our personal recommendation is for biochemical monitoring from the outset of therapy in all patients.

As a practical matter, we agree with the recommendations that if acute hepatitis occurs, INH, RIF, and/or PZA should be discontinued immediately, serologic tests for hepatitis A, B, and C (if not done at baseline) should be performed, and the patient should be questioned carefully regarding symptoms of biliary tract disease, exposure to other potential hepatotoxins, especially alcohol and hepatotoxic medications. Alternative antitubercular regimens should be used until the cause of the hepatitis is identified. Once AST level decrease <2 × ULN (upper limit of normal) and symptoms have significantly improved, the first line medications should be restarted in

sequential fashion at weekly intervals beginning with RIF and ending with PZA. However, if symptoms recur or ALT increases >2 × ULN or a significant increase in bilirubin/alkaline phosphatase levels occur, last drug added should be discontinued. If RIF and INH are tolerated, and the hepatitis was severe, PZA should be assumed to be responsible and should be discontinued.[278]

Support for our recommendations, however, is based on a number of reports of persons who despite not being in the traditional high-risk groups (especially patients under the age of 35) have developed severe and even fatal hepatic injury. For example, many of the patients reported by the CDC from New York City were young and did not drink alcohol.[258] Similarly, several of the fatal cases reported by Moulding and colleagues[267] were under the age of 35. Mitchell and colleagues[273] noted that even monthly monitoring would not have prevented two of their four fatalities, nor would it have prevented 11 of the 18 fatal cases described by Durand and colleagues[272] using these guidelines. These and other authors[279] have called for more frequent biochemical monitoring. In France, it has been recommended since 1993 that biochemical testing be performed weekly rather than monthly for the first month in patients receiving INH and for the first 2 months if PZA is used in combination.[272] If the ALT values rise above threefold or if serum bilirubin increases, then INH and PZA should be stopped. PZA should not be used for more than 2 months' duration in any case.[278] Mitchell and coworkers[273] called for African American and Hispanic females, postpartum females, and women on estrogen therapy to be monitored more closely because hepatic enzyme abnormalities are thought to occur well ahead of symptoms and therefore offer a window of opportunity to discontinue the antituberculous medications prior to the development of fulminant hepatic failure.

REFERENCES

1. Ullom JT. The Liver in tuberculosis. *Am J Med Sci.* 1909;137:694–699.
2. Rolleston HD. Tuberculosis of the liver and bile ducts. In: Disease of the Liver, Gallbladder and Bile Ducts. Philadelphia, PA: WB Saunders; 1905.
3. Saphir O. Changes in the liver and pancreas in chronic tuberculosis. *Arch Pathol.* 1929;7:1025–1039.
4. Torrey RG. The occurrence of miliary tuberculosis of the liver in the course of pulmonary tuberculosis. *Am J Med Sci.* 1916;151:549–556.
5. Gillman T, Gillman J. Modified liver aspiration biopsy apparatus and technique, with special reference to its clinical applications as assessed by 500 biopsies. *S Afr J Med Sci.* 1945;10:53–66.

6. Finkh ES, Baker SJ, Ryan MMP. The value of liver biopsy in the diagnosis of tuberculosis and sarcoidosis. *Med J Aust.* 1953;2:369–374.

7. Klatskin G, Yesner R. Hepatic manifestations of sarcoidosis and other granulomatous diseases: A study based on histologist examination of tissue obtained by needle biopsy of the liver. *Yale J Biol Med.* 1950;23:207–248.

8. Mansuy MM, Seiferth WJ. Miliary tuberculosis of the liver: Liver biopsy as an adjunct to diagnosis. *Am J Med Sci.* 1950;220:293–297.

9. Gold J, Widgerson A, Lehman E, et al. Tuberculosis hepatitis: Report of a case and review of the literature. *Gastroentology.* 1957;33:113–120.

10. Gulati PD, Vyas PB. Tuberculosis of the liver. *J Indian Med Assoc.* 1965;43:144–145.

11. Alverez SZ, Carpio R. Hepatobiliary tuberculosis. *Dig Dis Sci.* 1983;28:193–200.

12. Essop AR, Posen JA, Hodkinson Jo, et al. Tuberculosis hepatitis: A clinical review of 96 cases. *Q J Med.* 1984;53:465–477.

13. Maharaj B, Leary OP, Pudifin DJ. A prospective study of hepatic tuberculosis in 41 African-American patients. *Q J Med.* 1987;63:517–522.

14. Oliva A, Durate B, Jonasson O, et al. The nodular form of local hepatic tuberculosis: A review. *J Clin Gastroenterol.* 1990;12:166–173.

15. Bernhard JS, Bhatia G, Knauer MC. Gastrointestinal tuberculosis: an eighteen patient experience and review. *J Clin Gastroenterol.* 2000;30:397–402.

16. Snider GL. Tuberculosis then and now: A personal perspective on the last 50 years. *Ann Intern Med.* 1997;126:237–243.

17. Chaisson RE, Slutkin G. Tuberculosis and human immunodeficiency virus infection. *J Infect Dis.* 1989;159:96–100.

18. Small PM, Schecter GF, Goodman PC, et al. Treatment of tuberculosis in patients with advanced human immunodeficiency virus infection. *N Engl J Med.* 1991;324:289–294.

19. Horsburgh CR Jr. Mycobacterium avium complex infection in the acquired immunodeficiency syndrome. *N Engl J Med.* 1991;324:1332–1338.

20. Inderlied CB, Kemper CA, Bennudez LEM. The Mycobacterium avium complex. *Clin Microbiol Rev.* 1993;6:26–310.

21. Jacques J, Slan JM. The changing pattern of miliary tuberculosis. *Thorax.* 1970;25:237–240.

22. Munt PW. Miliary tuberculosis in the chemotherapy era: With a clinical review in 69 American adults. *Medicine.* 1971;51:139–155.

23. Van Buchem FSP. On morbid conditions of liver and diagnosis of disease of Besnier-Boeck-Shauman. *Acta Med Scand.* 1946;124:168.

24. Seife M, Messier BJ, Hoffman J, et al. A clinical, functional, and needle biopsy study of the liver in pulmonary tuberculosis. *Am Rev Tuberc.* 1951;63:202–209.

25. Ban B. Hepatic damage in chronic pulmonary tuberculosis. *Am Rev Tuberc.* 1955;72:71–90.

26. Haex AJC, Van Beek C. Tuberculosis and Aspiration Liver Biopsy. Haarlem: Bohn; 1955.

27. Mather G, Dawson J, Hoyle C. Liver biopsy in sarcoidosis. *Q J Med.* 1955;24:331–350.

28. Von Oldershausen HG, von Oldershausen R, Tellesz A. Zur Klinik und pathogenetischen Bedeutung der sogenannten "granulomatosen Hepatopathie" bei der Tuberculose. *Klin Wochenschz.* 1955;33:104.

29. Arora MM, Ali A, D'Souza AJ, et al. Clinical, functional and needle biopsy studies of the liver in tuberculosis. *J Indian Med Assoc.* 1956;26:341–344.

30. Buckingham WB, Turner GC, Knapp WB, et al. Liver biopsy in a tuberculosis hospital. *Dis Chest.* 1956;29:675–683.

31. Salib M, Legdvan PC, Arm Ha, et al. Clinical, histopathological and bacteriological study of the liver in chronic fibrocaseous pulmonary tuberculosis. *J Egypt Med Assoc.* 1961;44:226–232.

32. Bowry S, Chan CH, Weiss H, et al. Hepatic involvement in pulmonary tuberculosis: Histologic and functional characteristics. *Am Rev Respir Dis.* 1970;101:941–948.

33. Abdel-Dayem HM, Naddaf S, Aziz M, et al. Sites of tuberculous involvement in patients with AIDS: autopsy findings and evaluation of gallium imaging. *Clin Nucl Med.* 1997;22:310–314.

34. Korn RJ, Kellow WF, Heller P, et al. Hepatic involvement in extrapulmonary tuberculosis: Histologic and functional characteristics. *Am J Med.* 1959;27:60–71.

35. Biehl JP. Miliary tuberculosis: A review of sixty-eight adult patients admitted to a municipal general hospital. *Am Rev Tuberc.* 1958;77:605–624.

36. Gelb AF, Leffler C, Brewin A, et al. Miliary tuberculosis. *Am Rev Respir* Dis. 1973;108:1327–1333.

37. Essop AR, Hodkinson Jo, Posen J, et al. Simultaneous hepatic tuberculosis, cirrhosis and hepatoma: A case report. *S Afr Med J.* 1983;64:1102–1104.

38. Palmer KR, Patil DH, Basran AS, et al. Abdominal tuberculosis in Urban Britain: a common disease. *Gut.* 1985;26:1296–1305.

39. Al-Karawi MA, Mohamed AB, Yasawy MI, et al. Protean manifestations of gastrointestinal tuberculosis: Report on 130 patients. *J Clin Gastroenterol.* 1995;20:225–232.

40. Lundstedt C, Nyman R, Brismar J, et al. Imaging of tuberculosis: II. Abdominal manifestations in 112 patients. *Acta Radiol.* 1996;37:489–495.

41. Sinha SK, Chatterjee M, Bhattacharya S, et al. Diagnostic evaluation of extrapulmonary tuberculosis by fine needle aspiration (FNA) supplemented with AFB smear and culture. *J Indian Med Assoc.* 2003;101:588, 590–591.

42. Guckian JC, Perry JE. Granulomatous hepatitis: An analysis of 63 cases and review of the literature. *Ann Intern Med.* 1966;65:1081–1100.

43. Alexander IF, Galambos IT. Granulomatous hepatitis: The usefulness of liver biopsy in the diagnosis of tuberculosis and sarcoidosis. *Am J Gastroenterol.* 1973;59:23–30.

44. Hersch C. Tuberculosis of the liver: A study of 200 cases. *S Afr Med.* 1964;38:857–863.

45. Huang WT, Wang CC, Chen WJ, et al. The nodular form of hepatic tuberculosis: a review with 5 additional new cases. *J Clin Pathol.* 2003;56:835–839.

46. Yamaguchi BT, Braunstein H. Fluorescent stain for tubercle bacilli in histological sections: II. Diagnostic efficiency in granulomatous lesions of the liver. *Am J Clin Pathol.* 1965;43:184–187.

47. Okuda K, Kimura K, Takara K, et al. Resolution of diffuse granulomatous fibrosis of the liver with antituberculous chemotherapy. *Gastroenterology.* 1986;91:456–460.

48. Small MS. Tuberculosis of liver: Scan appearance before and after successful treatment. *J Nucl Med.* 1974;15:135–138.

49. Zipser RD, Rau IE, Ricketts RR, et al. Tuberculous pseudotumors of the liver. *Am J Med.* 1976;61:946–951.

50. Greene JB, Sidh GS, Lewin S, et al. Mycobacterium avium intracellulare: A cause of disseminated life threatening infection in homosexuals and drug abusers. *Ann Intern Med.* 1982;97:539–546.

51. Jones K, Peck WM. Incidence of fatty liver in tuberculosis with special reference to tuberculosis enteritis. *Arch Intern Med.* 1944;74:371–374.

52. Schaffner P, Turner GC, Eshbaugh DE, et al. Hypergammaglobulinemia in pulmonary tuberculosis. *Arch Intern Med.* 1953;92:490–493.

53. Sabharwal BD, Malhotra N, Garg R, et al. Granulomatous hepatitis: a retrospective study. *Indian J Pathol Microbiol.* 1995;38:413–416.

54. Sartin JS, Walker RC. Granulomatous hepatitis: a retrospective review of 88 cases at the Mayo Clinic. *Mayo Clin Proc.* 1991;66:914–918.

55. Rudzki C, Ishak IG, Zimmerman HJ. Chronic intrahepatic cholestasis of sarcoidosis. *Am J Med.* 1975;59:373–387.

56. McCullough NB, Eisele CW. Brucella leading to cirrhosis of the liver. *Arch Intern Med.* 1951;88:793–802.

57. Essop AR, Posen JA, Savitch I, et al. Radiocolloid liver imaging in tuberculous hepatitis. *Clin Nucl Med.* 1984;9:81–84.

58. Pintos JF, Rey LC, Boo JS, et al. Tuberculosis miliar hepatica combinada con una proliferacion de hepatocitos gigantes. *Rev Esp Enferm Apar Dig.* 1972;38:847–854.

59. Sherlock S. Diseases of the Liver and Biliary System, 6th ed. Oxford: Blackwell Scientific; 1981:395.

60. Steidl J, Heise FJ. Studies of liver function in advanced pulmonary tuberculosis. *Am J Med Sci.* 1933;186:631–640.

61. Ishak KG, Zimmerman HJ. Drug-induced and toxic granulomatous hepatitis. *Bailliéres Clin Gastroenterol.* 1988;2:463–480.

62. Valdez VA, Herrera NE. Granulomatous hepatitis: Spectrum of scintigraphic manifestations. *Clin Nucl Med.* 1978;3:392–396.

63. Gilinsky NH, Campbell JA, Kirsch RE. The Clinical spectrum of hepatic granulomas. *S Afr J Med Sci.* 1945;10:53–66.

64. Harrington PT, Gutierrez JJ, Ramirez-Ronda CH, et al. Granulomatous hepatitis. *Rev Infect Dis.* 1982;4:638–655.

65. Cunningham D, Mills PR, Quigley EM, et al. Hepatic granulomas: experience over a 10-year period in the West Scotland. *Q J Med.* 1982;51:162–170.

66. Anderson CS, Nicholls J, Rowland R, et al. Hepatic granulomas: a 15-year experience in the Royal Adelaide Hospital. *Med J Aust.* 1988;148:71–74.

67. McCluggage WG, Sloan JM. Hepatic granulomas in Northern Ireland: a thirteen year review. *Histopathology.* 1994;25:219–228.

68. Mert A, Ozaras R, Bilir M, et al. The etiology of hepatic granulomas. *J Clin Gastroenterol.* 2001;32:275–276.

69. Gaya DR, Thorburn D, Oien KA, et al. Hepatic granulomas: a 10 year single center experience. *J Clin Pathol.* 2003;56:850–853.

70. Hurst A, Maier HM, Lough SA. Studies of hepatic function in pulmonary tuberculosis. *Am J Med Sci.* 1947;214:431–435.

71. Galen RS, Weimer D, Hartmap SA. Functional hepatic impairment in pulmonary tuberculosis. *Dis Chest.* 1950;17:524–531.

72. Irani SK, Dobbins WO III. Hepatic granulomas: A review of 73 patients from one hospital and survey of the literature. *J Clin Gastroenterol.* 1979;1:131–143.

73. Steidl J, Heise FJ. Studies of liver function in advanced pulmonary tuberculosis. *Am J Med Sci.* 1933;186:631–640.

74. Vilaichone RK, Vilaichone W, Tumwasorn S, et al. Clinical spectrum of hepatic tuberculosis: comparison between immunocompromied and immunocompetent hosts. *J Med Assoc Thai.* 2003;86(suppl2):S432–S438.

75. Arrese M, Lopez F, Rossi R, et al. Extrahepatic cholestasis attributable to tuberculous adenitis. *Am J Gastroenterol.* 1997;92:912–913.

76. Pineda FM, Dalmacio-Cruz A. Tuberculosis of the liver and the porta hepatis: Report of 9 cases. *Acta Med Philipp.* 1966;2:128–139.

77. Simon HB, Wolff SM. Granulomatous hepatitis and prolonged fever of unknown origin: A study of 13 patients. *Medicine.* 1973;52:1–21.

78. Tahiliani RR, Parikh JA, Hedge AV, et al. Hepatic tuberculosis simulating hepatic amoebiasis. *J Assoc Physicians India.* 1983;31:697–680.

79. Essop AR, Segal I, Posen J, et al. Tuberculous abscess of the liver: A case report. *S Afr Med.* 1983;63:825–826.

80. Rahmatulla RH, Al-Mofleh IA, Al-Rashed RS, et al. Tuberculous liver abscess: a case report and review of literature. *Gastroenterol Hepatol.* 2001;13:437–440.

81. DeBray J, Krulik M, Bernard JF. La tuberculose pseudo. tumorale du foie: A propos dune observation personelle. *Semin Hop Paris.* 1972;48:3165–3167.

82. Fernandes JD, Nebesar RA, Wall Sa, et al. Report of tuberculous hepatitis presenting as metastatic disease. *Clin Nucl Med.* 1984;9:345–357.

83. Huang YS, Chern HD, Su WJ, et al. Cytochrome P450 2E1 genotype and the susceptibility to antituberculosis drug-induced hepatitis. *Hepatology.* 2003;37:924–930.

84. Hulnick DH, Megibow AJ, Naidich DP, et al. Abdominal tuberculosis: CT evaluation. *Radiology.* 1985;157:199–204.

85. Kok KY, Yapp Sk. Isolated hepatic tuberculosis: report of 5 cases and review of literature. *J Hepatobiliary Pancreat Surg.* 1999;6:195–198.

86. Petera V, Vesely V, Kulich V, et al. The clinical and morphological correlations in the Au/SH antigen carriers. *Digestion.* 1972;5:227–228.

87. Prochazka M, Vyhnanek F, Vorreith V, et al. Bleeding into solitary hepatic tuberculoma: Report of a case treated by resection. *Acta Chir Scand.* 1986;152:73–75.

88. Terry RB, Bunnar RM. Primary miliary tuberculosis of the liver. *JAMA.* 1957;164:150–157.

89. Cleve EA, Gibson JR, Webb WM. Atypical tuberculosis of the liver with jaundice. *Ann Intern Med.* 1954;41:251–260.

90. Cinque TJ, Gary NE, Palladino VS. "Primary" miliary tuberculosis of the liver. *Am J Gastroenterol.* 1964; 42:611–619.

91. Rolleston H, McNee JW. Diseases of the Liver, Gallbladder and Bile Ducts. London: Macmillan; 1929.

92. Hennan P, Pugliese V, Laurnio Neto R, et al. Nodular form of local hepatic tuberculosis: Case report. *J Trop Med Hyg.* 1995;98:141–142.

93. Leader SA. Tuberculosis of the liver and gallbladder with abscess formation: A review and case report. *Ann Intern Med.* 1951;37:594–605.

94. Rab SM, Zakaullah Beg M. Tuberculosis liver abscess. *Br J Clin Pract.* 1977;31:157–158.

95. Spegel CT, Tuazon CU. Tuberculous liver abscess. *Tubercle.* 1984;65:127–131.

96. Wissmer B. Tuberculosis of the liver. In: Bockus HL, ed. *Gastroenterology,* vol 3. Philadelphia, PA: WB Saunders; 1976:511–514.

97. Wee A, Nilsson B, Wang TL, et al. Tuberculous pseudotumor causing biliary obstruction: Report of a case with diagnosis by fine needle aspiration biopsy and bile cytology. *Acta Cytol.* 1995;39:559–562.

98. Dwek JH, Schechter LS, Grinberg ME. Hepatic angiography in a patient with tuberculosis of the liver. *Am J Gastroenterol.* 1981;75:307–308.

99. Bhargava SP, Sharma ML. Multiple tuberculoma of liver: A case report. *J Indian Med Assoc.* 1962;38:54–55.

100. Duckworth WC. Tuberculosis of the liver. *S Afr Med J.* 1964;38:945.

101. Bhargava DK, Venna K, Malaviya AN. Solitary tuberculoma of liver: Laparoscopic, histologic, and cytologic diagnosis. *Gastrointest Endosc.* 1983;29:329–330.

102. Brauner M, Buffard MD, Ieantils V, et al. Sonography and computed tomography of macroscopic tuberculosis of the liver. *J Clin Ultrasound.* 1989;17:563–568.

103. Moskovic E. Macronodular hepatic tuberculosis in a child: Computed tomographic appearances. *Br J Radiol.* 1990;63:656–658.

104. Nagai H, Shimizu S, Kawamoto H, et al. A case of solitary tuberculosis of the liver. *Jpn J Med.* 1989;28:251–255.

105. Levine V, Chaisson RE. Mycobacterium kansasii: A cause of treatable pulmonary disease associated with advanced human immunodeficiency virus (HIV) infection. *Ann Intern Med.* 1991;114:861–868.

106. Murata Y, Yamada I, Sumiya Y, et al. Abdominal macronodular tuberculomas: MR findings. *J Comput Assist Tomogr.* 1996;20:643–646.

107. Kawamori Y, Matsui 0, Kitagawa K, et al. Macronodular tuberculoma of the liver: CT and MR findings. *AJR Am J Roentgenol.* 1992;158:311–313.

108. Assada Y, Hayashi T, Sumiyoshi A, et al. Miliary tuberculosis presenting as fever and jaundice with hepatic failure. *Hum Pathol.* 1991;22:92–94.

109. Kohen MD, Altrnan KA. Jaundice due to a rare case: Tuberculous lymphadenitis. *Am J Gastroenterol.* 1973;59: 48–53.

110. Proudfoot AT, Akhtar AJ, Douglas AC, et al. Miliary tuberculosis in adults. *Br Med J.* 1992:273–276.

111. Shan SA, Neff TA. Miliary tuberculosis. *Am J Med.* 1974;56:495–505.

112. Curry FJ, Alcott D. Tuberculosis hepatitis with jaundice: Report of 2 cases. *Gastroenterology.* 1955;28:1037–1042.

113. Godwin JE, Coleman AA, Sahn SA. Miliary tuberculosis presenting as hepatic and renal failure. *Chest.* 1991;99: 752–754.

114. Hussain W, Mutimer D, Harrison R, et al. Fulminant hepatic failure caused by tuberculosis. *Gut.* 1995;36:792–794.

115. Debre R, Furiet-Laforet M, Royer P. Congenital transplacental tuberculosis of icteric form. *Arch Fr Pediatr.* 1948;5:225–231.

116. Tobias H, Sherman A. Hepatobiliary tuberculosis. In: Rom WN, Garay SM, eds. *Tuberculosis,* 2nd ed. Phildelphia, PA: Lippincott, Williams & Wilkins; 2002:537–547.

117. Ariede KI. Congenital miliary tuberculosis. *Ann Trop Paediatr.* 1990;10:363–368.

118. Berk DR, Sylvester KG. Congenital tuberculosis presenting as progressive liver dysfunction. *Pediatr Infect Dis J.* 2004;23:78–80.

119. Chen HJ, Chiu NC, Kao HA, et al. Perinatal tuberculosis in a three-month-old infant. *J Formos Med Assoc.* 2004;103:144–147.

120. Chou YH. Congenital tuberculosis proven by percutaneous liver biopsy: report of a case. *J Perinatal Medicine.* 2002;30:423–425.

121. McNutt DR, Fudenberg HH. Disseminated scotochromogen infection and unusual myeloproliferative disorder. *Ann Intern Med.* 1971;75:737–744.

122. Stewart C, Jackson L. Spleno-hepatic tuberculosis due to Mycobacterium kansasii. *Med J Aust.* 1976;2:99–101.

123. Smith ER, Penman Ha. Histological diagnosis of M. kansasii lung infection. *Pathology.* 1971;3:93.

124. Hsieh SM, Hung CC, Chen MY, et al. The role of tissue studies in facilitating early inititation of antimycobacterial treatment in AIDS patients with diseeminated tuberculosis disease. *Int J Tub Lung Dis.* 1999;3:521–527.

125. Shah SR, Rastegar DA, Nicol TL. Case report. Diagnosis of disseminated mycobacterium avium complex infection by liver biopsy. *AIDS Read.* 2000;10:669–672.

126. Patel KM. Granulomatous hepatitis due to Mycobacterium scrofulaceum: Report of a case. *Gastroenterology.* 1981;81: 156–158.

127. Kurnik PB, Padmanabh U, Bonatosos C, et al. Case report: Mycobacterium gordonae as a human hepatoperitoneal pathogen, with a review of the literature. *Am J Med Sci.* 1983;285:45–48.

128. Minamoto G, Armstrong D. Combating infections in patients with AIDS: Update on the evolving epidemiology, issues in screening, and therapy. *J Crit Illness.* 1986;1: 37–48.

129. Bodurtha A, Kin YH, Laucius IF, et al. Hepatic granulomas and other hepatic lesions associated with BCG immunotherapy for cancer. *Am J Clin Pathol.* 1974;6:727–752.

130. Flippin T, Mukherji B, Dayal Y. Granulomatous hepatitis as a late complication of BCG immunotherapy. *Cancer.* 1980;46:1759–1762.

131. Gottke MU, Wong P, Muhn C, et al. Hepatitis in disseminated bacillus Calmette-Guérin infection. *Can J Gastroenterol.* 2000;14:333–336.

132. Hunt JS, Silverstein MJ, Sparks FC, et al. Granulomatous hepatitis: A complication of BCG immunotherapy. *Lancet.* 1973;2:820–821.

133. Ozbakkaloglu B, Tunger O, Surucuoglu S, et al. Granulomatous hepatitis following bacillus Calmette-Guérin therapy. *Int Urol Nephrol.* 1999;31:49–53.

134. O'Brien TF, Hyslop NE Jr. Case records of the Massachusetts General Hospital, case 34-1975. *N Engl J Med.* 1975;293:443–448.

135. McKhann CF, Hendrickson CG, Spitler LE, et al. Immunotherapy of melanoma with BCG: two fatalities following intralesional injection. *Cancer.* 1975;35:514–520.

136. Krown SE, Hilal EY, Pinsky CM. Intralesional injection of methanol extraction residue of bacille Calmette-Guérin (MER) into cutaneous metastasis of malignant melanoma. *Cancer.* 1978;42:2648–2660.

137. Sparks FC, Albert NE, Breeding JH. Effect on isonicotinic acid hydrazide on the intratumor injection of BCG. *J Natl Cancer Inst.* 1977;58:367–368.

138. Stemmerman M. Bile duct tuberculosis. *Q Bull Sea View Hosp.* 1941;6:316–324.

139. Rosenkranz K, Howard LD. Tubular tuberculosis of the liver. Arch Pathol. 1936;22:743–754.

140. Cruice JM. Jaundice in tuberculosis. *Am J Med Sci.* 1914;147:720–726.

141. Frank BB, Raffensperger EC. Hepatic granulomata: Report of a case with jaundice improving on antituberculosis therapy and review of the literature. *Arch Intern Med.* 1965;115:223–234.

142. Abascal I, Martin F, Abreu L, et al. Atypical hepatic tuberculosis presenting as obstructive jaundice. *Am J Gastroenterol.* 1988;83:1183–1186.

143. Murphy R, Swartz R, Watkins PB. Severe acetaminophen toxicity in a patient receiving isoniazid. *Ann Intern Med.* 1990;113:799–800.

144. Murphy TF, Gray GF. Biliary tract obstruction due to tuberculous adenitis. *Am J Med.* 1980;68:452–454.

145. Parthasarathy R, Sarma GR, Janardhanam B, et al. Hepatic toxicity in South Indian patients during treatment of tuberculosis with short course regimens containing isoniazid, rifampicin and pyrazinamide. *Tubercle.* 1986;67:99–108.

146. Stanley HJ, Yantis PL, Marsh WH. Periportal tuberculous adenitis: A rare cause of obstructive jaundice. *Gastrointest Radiol.* 1984;9:227–229.

147. Yeh TS, Chen NH, Jan YY, et al. Obstructive jaundice caused by biliary tuberculosis: spectrum of the diagnosis and management. *Gastrointest Endosc.* 1999;50:105–108.

148. Bearer ED, Savides TJ, McCutchan JA. Endoscopic diagnosis and management of hepatobiliary tuberculosis. *Am J Gastroenterol.* 1996;91:2602–2604.

149. Hickey N, McNulty JG, Osborne H, et al. Acute hepatobiliary tuberculosis: a report of two cases and review of the literature. *Eur Radiol.* 1999;9:886–889.

150. Sherlock S. The liver in infections. In: Sherlock S, ed. *Diseases of the liver and biliary system,* 7th edition. Oxford: Blackwell Science; 1985:460–461.

151. Garber HI, Mason GR, Bouchelle WH. "Primary" miliary tuberculosis of the liver presenting as acute cholecystitis. *Md State Med J.* 1981;3:73–74.

152. Siemann M, Rabenhorst G, Bramann A, et al. A case of cryptic miliary tuberculosis mimicking cholecystitis with sepsis. *Infection.* 1999;27:44–45.

153. Rozmanic V, Kilvain S, Ahel V, et al. Pulomary tuberculosis with gall bladder involvement: a review and case report. *Peditrics International.* 2001;43:511–513.

154. Ben RJ, Young T, Lee HS. Hepatobiliary tuberculosis presenting as a gallbladder tumor. *Scand J Infect Dis.* 1995;27:415–417.

155. Ladas SD, Vaidakis E, Lariou C, et al. Pancreatic tuberculosis in non-immunocompromised patients: report of two cases and a literature review. *Eur J Gastroenterol Hepatol.* 1998;10:973–976.

156. Rezeig MA. Pancreatic tuberculosis mimicking pancreatic carcinoma: four case reports and review of the literature. *Dig Dis Sci.* 1998;43:329–331.

157. Woodfield JC, Windsor JA, Godfrey CC, et al. Diagnosis and management of isolated pancreatic tuberculosis. *ANZ J Surg.* 2004;74:368–371.

158. Pombo F, Diaz Candamio MJ, Rodriguez E, et al. Pancreatic tuberculosis: CT findings. Abdominal imaging. 1998;23:394–397.

159. Demir K, Kaymakoglu S, Besisik F, et al. Solitary pancreatic tuberculosis in immunocompetent patients mimicking pancreatic carcinoma. *J Gastroenterol Hepatol.* 2001;16: 1071–1074.

160. Schneider A, von Birgelen C, Duhrsen U, et al. Two cases of pancreatic tuberculosis in nonimmunocompromised patients. A diagnostic challenge and a rare cause of portal hypertension. *Pancreatology.* 2002;2:69–73.

161. El Mansari O, Tajdine MT, Mikou I, et al. Pancreatic tuberculosis: report of two cases. *Gastroenterol Clin Biol.* 2003;27:548–550.

162. Kumar R, Kapoor D, Singh J, et al. Isolated tuberculosis of the pancreas: a report of two cases and review of the literature. *Trop Gastroenterol.* 2003;24:76–78.

163. Pramesh CS, Heroor AA, Shukla PJ, et al. Pancreatic tuberculosis. *Trop Gastroenterol.* 2002;23:142–143.

164. Franco-Pardes C, Leonardo M, Jurado R, et al. Tuberculosis of the pancreas: report of 2 cases and review of the literature. *Am J Med Sci.* 2002;323:54–58.

165. Xia F, Poon R T-P, Wang S-G, et al. Tuberculosis of pancreas and peripancreatic lymph nodes in immunocompetent patients: experience from China. *World J Gastroenterol.* 2003;9:1361–1364.

166. Chaudhary A, Negi SS, sachdev, AK, et al. Pancreatic tuberculosis: still a histopathological diagnosis. Dig Surg. 2002;19:389–392.

167. Lo SF, Ahchong AK, Tang CN, at al. Pancreatic tuberculosis: case reports and review of the literature. *J R Coll Surg Edinb.* 1998;43:65–68.

168. Babu RK, John V. Pancreatic tuberculosis: case report and review of the literature. *Trop Gastroenterol.* 2001;22:213–214.

169. Baraboutis I, Skoutelis A. Isolated tuberculosis of the pancreas. *JOP.* 2004;5:155–158.

170. Beaulieu S, Chouillard E, Petit-Jean B, et al. Pancreatic tuberculosis: a rare cause of pseudoneoplastic obstrucutive jaundice. *Gastroenterol Clin Biol.* 2004;28:295–298.

171. Brugge WR, Mueller PR, Misdraji J. Case 8-2004: A 28-year-old man with abdominal pain, fever, and mass in the region of pancreas. *N Engl J Med.* 2004;350:1131–1138.

172. Chen CH, Yang CC, Yeh YH, et al. Pancreatic tuberculosis with obstructive jaundice—a case report. *Am J Gastroenterol.* 1999;94:2534–2536.

173. Coelho JC, Wiederkehr JC, Parolin MB, et al. Isolated tuberculosis of the pancreas after orthotopic liver transplantation. *Liver Transpl Surg.* 1999;5:153–155.

174. D'Cruz S, Sachdev A, Kaur L, et al. Fine needle aspiration diagnosis of isolated pancreatic tuberculosis. A case report and review of the literature. *JOP.* 2003;4:158–162.

175. Desai CS, Lala M, Joshi A, et al. Co-existance of peri-ampullary carcinoma with peripancreatic tuberculous lymphadenopathy. *J Pancreas* (online). 2000;5:145–147.

176. Jenney AW, Pickles RW, Hellard ME, et al. Tuberculous pancreatic abscess in an HIV antibody-negative patient: case report and review. *Scand J Infect.* 1998;30:99–104.

177. Kouraklis G, Glinavou A, Karayiannakis A, et al. Primary tuberculosis of the pancreas mimicking a pancreatic tumor. *Int J Pancreatol.* 2001;29:151–153.

178. Liu Q, Zhenping H, Ping B. Solitary pancreatic tuberculous abscess mimicking pancreatic cystadenocarcinoma: a case report. *BMC Gastroenterology.* 2003;3:16.

179. Ozick LA, Jacob L, Comer GM, et al. Hepatotoxicity from isoniazid and rifampin in inner-city AIDS patients. *Am J Gastroenterol.* 1995;90:1978–1980.

180. Panzuto F, D'Amato A, Laghi A, et al. Abdominal tuberculosis with pancreatic involvement: case report. *Dig Liver Dis.* 2003;35:283–287.

181. Redha S, Suresh RL, Subramaniam J, et al. Pancreatic tuberculosis presenting as recurrent acute pancreatitis. *Med J Malaysia.* 2001;56:95–97.

182. Riaz AA, Singh P, Robshaw P, et al. Tuberculosis of the pancreas diagnosed with needle aspiration. *Scand J Infect Dis.* 2001;34:303–304.

183. Sanabe N, Ikematsu Y, Nishiwaki Y, et al. Pancreatic tuberculosis. *J Hepatobiliary Pancreat Surg.* 2002;9:515–518.

184. Sekikawa A, Indad M, Tsuyuoka K, et al. A case of pancreatic tuberculosis resembling pancreatic serous cystadenoma. *Jpn J Gastroenterol.* 2001;98:1298–1303.

185. Shan Y-S, Sy ED, Lin P-W. Surgical resection of isolated pancreatic tuberculosis presenting as obstructive jaundice. *Pancreas.* 2000;21:100–101.

186. Singh B, Moodley J, Batitiang S, et al. Isolated pancreatic tuberculosis and obstructive jaundice. *S Afr Med J.* 2002;92:357–359.

187. Small G, Wilks D. Pancreatic mass caused by Mycobacterium tuberculosis with reduced drug sensitivity. *J Infect.* 2001;42:201–202.

188. Turan M, Sen M, Koyuncu A, Aydin C, et al. Pancreatic pseudotumor due to peripancreatic tuberculous lymphadenitis. *Pancreatology.* 2002;2:561–564.

189. Yokoyama T, Miyagawa S, Noike T, et al. Isolated pancreatic tuberculosis. *Hepatogastroenterology.* 1999;46:2011–2014.

190. Jaber B, Gleckman R. Tuberculous pancreatic abscess as an initial AIDS-defining disorder in a patient infected with the human immunodeficiency virus: a case report and review. *Clin Infect Dis.* 1995;20:890–894.

191. Agarwal HS, Benson JW, Major JJ. An unusual case of hemobilia: Hepatic tuberculosis with hemorrhage. *Arch Surg.* 1967;95:202–206.

192. Elfe PM, van Aken WG, Agenant DM, et al. Hemobilia after liver biopsy. *Arch Intern Med.* 1980;140:839–840.

193. Levinson JD, Olsen G, Terman JW, et al. Hemobilia secondary to percutaneous liver biopsy. *Arch Intern Med.* 1972;120:396–400.

194. Lewis J, Varma V, Tice H, et al. Hepatobiliary scanning in hemobilia-induced acute cholecystitis. *Gastrointest Radiol.* 1982;7:168–171.

195. Das D, Mandal Sk, Majumdar D, et al. Disseminated tuberculosis presenting as hemobilia, successfully treated with arterial embolization. *J Assoc Physicians India.* 2003;51:229–231.

196. Beeresha, Ghotekar LH, Dutta, TK, et al. Hepatic artery aneurysm of tubercular etiology. J Assoc Phys India. 2000;48:247–248.

197. Devars du Mayne JF, Marche C, Penalba C, et al. Liver disease in acquired immune deficiency syndrome: Study of 20 cases. *Presse Med.* 1985;14:1177–1180.

198. Glasgow BJ, Anders K, Layfield LF, et al. Clinical and pathologic findings of the liver in the acquired immune deficiency syndrome (AIDS). *Am J Clin Pathol.* 1985;83:582–588.

199. Guarda LA, Luna MA, Smith JL, et al. Acquired immune deficiency syndrome: Postmortem findings. *Am J Clin Pathol.* 1984;81:549–557.

200. Lebovics E, Thung SN, Schafner F, et al. The liver in the acquired immunodeficiency syndrome: A clinical and histologic study. *Hepatology.* 1985;5:293–298.

201. Lewis JH, Winston BJ, Garone MA, et al. The liver in AIDS: A clinicopathologic correlation. *Gastroenterology.* 1985;88:1675.

202. Orenstein MS, Tavitian A, Yonk B, et al. Granulomatous involvement of the liver in patients with AIDS. *Gut.* 1985;26:1220–1225.

203. Reichert CM, O'Leary TJ, Levens DL, et al. Autopsy pathology in the acquired immune deficiency syndrome. *Am J Pathol.* 1983;112:357–382.

204. Schneiderman DJ, Arenson DM, Cello JP. Hepatic disease in patients with the acquired immune deficiency syndrome. *Gastroenterology.* 1986;90:1620.

205. Armstrong D, Gold JWN, Dryjanski J, et al. Treatment of infections in patients with the acquired immunodeficiency syndrome. *Ann Intern Med.* 1985;103:738–745.

206. Selwyn PA, Lewis VA, Schoenbaum EE, et al. HIV infection and tuberculosis in intravenous drug users in a methadone program [Abstract 7549]. In: Proceedings of the IVth International Conference on AIDS: Stockholm; 1988.

207. Sunderam G, McDonald RJ, Maniatis T, et al. Tuberculosis as a manifestation of the acquired immunodeficiency syndrome (AIDS). *JAMA.* 1986;256:362–366.

208. Markowitz N, Hansen NI, Hopewell PC, et al. Incidence of tuberculosis in the United States among HIV-infected persons. *Ann Intern Med.* 1997;126:123–132.

209. Poprawski D, Pitisuttitum P, Transuphasawadikul S. Clinical presentation and outcomes of tuberculosis among HIV-positive patients. *Southeast Asian J Trop Med Public Health.* 2000;31(suppl 1):140–142.

210. Smith MB, Boyars MC, Veasey S, et al. Generalized tuberculosis in the acquired immunodeficiency syndrome. *Arch Pathol Lab Med.* 2000;124:1267–1274.

211. Gonzalez OY, Adams G, Teeter LD, et al. Extra-pulmonary manifestations in a large metropolitan area with a low incidence of tuberculosis. *Int J Tuberc Lung Dis.* 2003;7:1178–1185.

212. Liberato IR, de Albuquerque Mde F, Campelo AR, et al. Characteristics of pulmonary tuberculosis in HIV seropositive and seronegative patients in a Northeastern region of Brazil. *Rev Soc Bras Med Trop.* 2004;37:46–50.

213. Satter FR, Cowan R, Nielsen DM, et al. Trimethoprim-sulfamethoxazole compared with pentamidine for treatment of Pneumocystis carinii pneumonia in the acquired immunodeficiency syndrome: A prospective, noncross-over study. *Ann Intern Med.* 1988;109:280–287.

214. Ozick LA, Jacob L, Comer GM, et al. Hepatotoxicity from isoniazid and rifampin in inner-city AIDS patients. *Am J Gastroenterol.* 1995;90:1978–1980.

215. Amarapurkar DN, Chopra KB, Phadke AY, et al. Tuberculous abscess of the liver associated with HIV infection. *Indian J Gastroenterol.* 1995;1421–1422.

216. Probst A, Schmidbaur W, Jechart G, et al. Obstructive jaundice in AIDS: Diagnosis of biliary tuberculosis by ERCP. *Gastrointest Endosc.* 2004;60:145–148.

217. Horsburgh CR Jr, Metchock B, Gordon SM, et al. Predictors of survival in patients with AIDS and disseminated mycobacterium avium complex disease. *J Infect Dis.* 1994;170:573–577.

218. Chaisson RE, Moore RD, Richman DD, et al. Incidence and natural history of Mycobacterium avium-complex infections in patients with advanced human immunodeficiency virus disease treated with zidovudine. *Am Rev Respir Dis.* 1992;146:285–289.

219. Hawkins CC, Gold JWM, Whimbey E, et al. Mycobacterium avium complex infections in patients with the acquired immunodeficiency syndrome. *Ann Intern Med.* 1986;105:184–188.

220. Chang YG, Chen PJ, Hung CC, et al. Opportunistic hepatic infections in AIDS patients with fever of unknown origin. *J Formos Med Assoc.* 1999;98:5–10.

221. Tarantino L, Giorgio A, de Dtefano G, et al. Disseminated mycobacterial infection in AIDS patients: abdnominal US features and value of fine-needle aspiration biopsy of lymph nodes and spleen. *Abdom Imaging.* 2003;28:602–608.

222. Kiehn TE, Edwards FF, Brannon P, et al. Infections caused by Mycobacterium avium complex in immunocompromised patients: Diagnosis by blood culture and fecal examination, antimicrobial susceptibility test, and morphological and seroagglutination characteristics. *J Clin Microbiol.* 1985;21:168–173.

223. O'Brien RJ, Lyle MA, Johnson MW, et al. Ansamycin LM427 therapy in AIDS patients with Mycobacterium avium (MAI) complex infection: A preliminary report. In: *Abstracts from the International Conference on Acquired Immunodeficiency Syndrome.* Philadelphia, PA: American College of Physicians; 1985:47.

224. Wong B, Edwards FF, Kiehn TE, et al. Continuous high-grade Mycobacterium a.vium-intracellulare bacteremia in patients with the acquired immune deficiency syndrome. *Am J Med.* 1985;78:35–40.

225. Shafran SD, Singer J, Zarowny DP, et al. A comparison of two regimens for the treatment of Mycobacterium avium complex bacteremia in AIDS: Rifabutin, ethambutol, and clarithromycin versus rifampin, ethambutol, clofazimine, and ciprofloxacin. *N Engl J Med.* 1996;335:377–383.

226. Aguada JM, Herrero JA, Gavalda J, et al. Clinical presentation and outcome of tuberculosis in kidney, liver and heart transplant recipients in Spain. *Transplantation.* 1997;63:1278.

227. Singh N, Wagener MM, Gayowski T. Safety and efficacy of isoniazid chemoprophylaxis administered during liver transplant candidacy for the prevention of posttransplant tuberculosis. *Transplantation.* 2002;74:892–895.

228. Grauhan O, Lohmann R, Lemmens T, et al. Mycobacterial infection after liver transplantation. *Langenbecks Arch Chir.* 1995;380:171–175.

229. Meyers BR, Halpern M, Sheiner P, et al. Tuberculosis in liver transplant patients. *Transplantation.* 1994;58:301–306.

230. Ferrell LD, Lee R, Brixko C, et al. Hepatic granulomas following liver transplantation: Clinical-pathologic features in 42 patients. *Transplantation.* 1995;60:926–933.

231. Benito N, Sued O, Moreno A, et al. Diagnosis and treatment of latent tuberculosis infection in liver transplant recipients in an endemic area. *Transplantation.* 2002;74:1381–1386.

232. Schluger LK, Sheiner PA, Jonas M, et al. Isoniazid hepatotoxicity after orthotopic liver transplantation. *Mt Sinai J Med.* 1996;63:364–369.

233. Torre-Cisneros J, Caston JJ, Moreno J, et al. Tuberculosis in the transplant candidate: importance of early diagnosis and treatment. *Transplantation.* 2004;77:1376–1380.

234. Torre-Cisneros J, de la Mataivl, Rufian S, et al. Importance of surveillance of mycobacterial cultures after liver transplantation. *Transplantation.* 1995;60:1054–1055.

235. Meyers BR, Papanicolau GA, Sheiner P, et al. Tuberculosis in orthotopic liver transplantation patients: increased toxicity of recommended agents; cure of disseminated infection with nonconventional regimens. *Transplantation.* 2000;69:74.

236. Thora S, Chansoria M, Kaul KK. Congenital tuberculosis: A case with unusual features. *Indian J Pediatr.* 1985;52: 425–427.

237. Verma A, Dhawan A, Wade JJ, et al. Mycobacterium tuberculosis infection in peditric liver transplant recipients. *Pediatr Infect Dis.* 2000;19:625–630.

238. Karsner HT. Morphology and pathogenesis of hepatic cirrhosis. *Am J Clin Pathol.* 1943;13:569–606.

239. Gelb AM, Brazenas N, Sussman H, et al. Acute granulomatous disease of the liver. *Digest Dis.* 1970;15:842–847.

240. Fitzgerald GR, Grimes H, Reynolds M, et al. Hepatatitis-associated-antigen positive hepatitis in a tuberculosis unit. *Crut.* 1975;16:421–428.

241. McGlynn KA, Lustbader ED, London WT. Immune responses to hepatitis B virus and tuberculosis infections in Southeast Asian refugees. *Am J Epidemiol.* 1985;122:1032–1036.

242. Wu J-C, Lee S-D, Yeh P-F, et al. Isoniazid-rifampin-induced hepatitis in hepatitis B carriers. *Gastroenterology.* 1990;98:502–504.

243. Nishioka SA. Cirrhosis as a risk factor to drug-resistant tuberculosis. *Eur Respir J.* 1996;9:2188–2189.

244. Bagnato GF, DiCesare E, Gulli S, et al. Long-term treatment of pulmonary tuberculosis with ofloxacin in a subject with liver cirrhosis. *Monaldi Arch Chest Dis* 1995;50:279–281.

245. Rougier P, Degott C, Rueff B, et al. Nodular regenerative hyperplasia of the liver: Report of six cases and review of the literature. *Gastroenterology.* 1978;75:169–172.

246. Steiner PE. Nodular regenerative hyperplasia of the liver. *Am J Pathol.* 1959;35:943–953.

247. Wanless IR, Solt LC, Kortan P, et al. Nodular regenerative hyperplasia of the liver associated with macroglobulinemia. *Am J Med.* 1981;70:1203–1209.

248. Gordeuk VR, McLaren CE, MacPhail AP, et al. Associations of iron overload in Africa with hepteocellular carcinoma and tuberculosis: Strachan's 1929 thesis revisited. *Blood.* 1996;87:3470–3476.

249. Zimmennan HJ, Lewis JH. Hepatic toxicity of antimicrobial agents. In: Root RK, Sande MA, eds. *New Dimensions in Antimicrobial Therapy.* New York, NY: Churchill Livingstone; 1984:153–201.

250. Zimmerman HJ. Hepatotoxicity: The Adverse Effects of Drugs and Other Chemicals on the Liver. New York, NY: Appleton-Century-Crofts; 1978:485–495.

251. Mitchell JR, Ishak KG, Snodgrass WR. Isoniazid liver injury: Clinical spectrum, pathology and probable pathogenesis. *Ann Intern Med.* 1976;84:181–192.

252. Snider DE, Caras GJ. Isoniazid associated hepatitis: A review of available information. *Am Rev Respir Dis.* 1992;145:494–497.

252a. Franks AL, Binkin NJ, Snider DE, et al. Isoniazid hepatitis among pregnant and postpartum Hispanic patients. *Public Health Rep.* 1989;104:151–155.

253. Fernandez-Villar A, Sopena B, Vazquez R, et al. Isoniazid hepatotoxicity among drug users: the role of hepatitis C virus. *Clin Infect Dis.* 2003;36:293–298.

254. Ungo JR, Jones D, Ashkin D, et al. Antituberculosis drug-induced hepatotoxicity. The role of hepatitis C virus and the human immunodeficiency virus. *Am J Respir Crit care Med.* 1998;157(6Pt1):1871–1876.

255. Wong WM, Wu PC, Yuen MF, et al. Antituberculosis drug-related liver dysfunction in chronic hepatitis B infection. *Hepatology.* 2000;31:201–206.

256. Yee D, Valiquette C, Pelletier M, et al. Incidence of serious side effects from first line antituberculosis drugs among patients treated for active tuberculosis. *Am J Respir Crit Care Med.* 2003;167:1472–1477.

257. Centers for Disease Control and Prevention. Severe isoniazid-associated hepatitis: New York, 1991–1993. *MMWR Morb Mortal Wkly Rep.* 1993;42:545–547.

258. Meyers BR, Halpem M, Sheiner P, et al. Acute hepatic failure in seven patients after prophylaxis and therapy with antituberculous agents: Successful treatment with orthotopic liver transplantation. *Transplantation.* 1994;58:372–377.

259. Lewis JH, Zimmerman HJ. Drug-induced liver disease. *Med Clin North Am.* 1989;73:775–792.

260. Mitchell JR, Thorgeirsson UP, Black M, et al. Increased incidence of isoniazid hepatitis in rapid acetylators: Possible relation to hydrazine metabolites. *Clin Pharmacol Ther.* 1975;18:70–79.

261. Dickinson DS, Bailey WC, Hirschowitz BI. Risk factors for isoniazid (INH)-induced liver dysfunction. *J Clin Gastroenterol.* 1981;3:271–279.

262. Gurumurthy P, Kirshnamurthy MS, Nazareth O, et al. Lack of relationship between hepatic toxicity and acetylator phenotype in three thousand South Indian patients during treatment with isoniazid for tuberculosis. *Am Rev Respir Dis.* 1984;129:58–61.

263. Martinezroig A, Carni J, LIorens-Terol J, et al. Acetylation phenotype and hepatotxicity in the treatment of tuberculosis in children. *Pediatrics.* 1986;77:912–915.

264. Seth V, Beotra A. Hepatic function in relation to acetylator phenotype in children treated with antitubercular drugs. *Indian J Med Res.* 1989;89:306–309.

265. Karnamoto T, Suou T, Hirayama C. Elevated serum aminotransferase induced by isoniazid in relation to isoniazid acetylator phenotype. *Hepatology*. 1986;6:295–298.

266. Nolan CM, Sandblom RE, Thummel KE, et al. Hepatoxicity associated with acetaminophen usage in patients receiving multiple drug therapy for tuberculosis. *Chest*. 1994;105:408–411.

267. Moulding TS, Redeker AG, Kanel GC. Twenty isoniazid-associated deaths in one state. *Am Rev Respir Dis*. 1989;140:700–705.

268. Update. Adverse event data and revised American Thoracic Society/CDC recommendations against the use of rifampin and pyrazinamide for treatment of latent tuberculosis infection- United States, 2003. *MMWR Morb Mortal Wkly Rep*. 2003;52:735–738.

269. Akaard DS, Wilcke T, Dossing M. Hepatotoxicity caused by the combined action of isoniazid and rifampicin. *Thorax*. 1995;50:213–214.

270. Steele MA, Burk RF, DesPrez RM. Toxic hepatitis with isoniazid and rifampin: A meta-analysis. *Chest*. 1991;99:465–471.

271. Scheuer P, Surnmerfield JA, Lal S, et al. Rifampicin hepatitis: A clinical histological study. *Lancet*. 1974;1: 421–425.

272. Durand F, Bernuau J, Passayre D, et al. Deleterious influence of pyrazinamide on the outcome of patients with fulminant or sub-fulminant liver failure during antituberculous treatment including isoniazid. *Hepatology*. 1995;21:929–932.

273. Mitchell I, Wendon J, Fitt S, Williams R. Antituberculous therapy and acute liver failure. *Lancet*. 1995;345:555–556.

274. Pierce M, Crampton S, Henry D, et al. A randomized trial of clarithromycin as prophylaxis against disseminated *Mycobacterium Avium* complex infection in patients with advanced acquired immunodeficiency syndrome. *N Engl J Med*. 1996;335:384–391.

275. Wai-Yew W, Hung-Chau C, Lee I, et al. Cholestatic hepatitis in a patient who received clarithromycin therapy for a *Mycobacterium chelonae* lung infection. *Clin Infect Dis*. 1994;1025:18.

276. Nolan CM, Goldberg SV, Buskin SE, et al. Hepatotoxicity associated with isoniazid preventive therapy. *JAMA*. 1999;281:1014–1018.

277. American Thoracic Society, CDC, Infectious Diseases Society of America: Treatment of tuberculosis. *Am J Respir Crit Care Med*. 2003;167:603–662.

278. Lewis JH. The rational use of potentially hepatotoxic medications in patients with underlying liver disease. *Exper Opin Drug Saf*. 2002;1(2):159–72.

279. Noble A: Antituberculous therapy and acute liver failure [Letter].*Lancet*. 1995;345:867.

25

Cutaneous Tuberculosis

Michael K. Hill
Charles V. Sanders

Cutaneous tuberculosis (TB) is not a well-defined entity but comprises a wide spectrum of clinical manifestations. In the past, much of the confusion regarding cutaneous TB has resulted from misleading, redundant nomenclature and cumber-some, nonclinically oriented classifications of cutaneous disease. These classifications have been based on various criteria, including chronic versus labile disease, localizing versus hematogenous disease, histologic forms of disease, immunologic status of the patient, primary disease versus reinfection, and listing of the various types of cutaneous mycobacteriosis.[1–3] A more clinically relevant classification has been developed that uses three criteria: pathogenesis, clinical presentation, and histologic evaluation (Table 25-1).[1]

Skin involvement may occur as a result of exogenous inoculation (in previously nonsensitized hosts, regional adenopathy occurs) by contagious spread from a focus underlying the skin, particularly from osteomyelitis, epididymitis, or lymphadenitis, and by hematogenous spread from a distant focus or as a part of a generalized hematogenous dissemination.[4,5] Although it is rare in the United States and accounts for less than 1% of cases in European dermatologic clinics, there has been an increase in the incidence of cutaneous TB.[5,6] Contrary to earlier claims that cutaneous TB is uncommon in the tropics, reports from India, Southeast Asia, and Africa prove otherwise.[7]

INOCULATION CUTANEOUS TUBERCULOSIS FROM AN EXOGENOUS SOURCE

Primary inoculation TB results from the entry of mycobacteria into the skin or, less frequently, the mucosa of a person who has not previously been infected or who has no natural or artificial immunity to *Mycobacterium tuberculosis*. Because the acid-fast bacilli (AFB) cannot penetrate the normal intact skin barrier, some form of injury is required to initiate the infection. The entry point for AFB is usually through minor skin abrasions, hangnail wounds, impetigo, or furuncles.

Although inoculation can occur in a variety of ways, most reports have involved persons working in medically related professions (Fig. 25-1). Laennec described his own "prosector's wart" in 1826. Tuberculous lesions have followed mouth-to-mouth resuscitation, inoculation of laboratory guinea pigs, injection with poorly sterilized needles, ear piercing, intramuscular injections given by a nurse with active TB, tattooing, insect bites, sexual intercourse leading to venereal inoculation TB, and venipuncture in an infant.[8–21] Historically, ritualistic circumcision performed by a practitioner with active pulmonary TB has resulted in miliary disease in the infant.[13]

Mucocutaneous involvement may account for one third of the total primary cutaneous TB cases and includes infection of the conjunctiva or of the oral cavity after tooth extraction or after drinking nonpasteurized milk infected with *Mycobacterium bovis*.[4,5,7,22]

The pathogenesis of cutaneous TB from an exogenous source is similar to that of other primary diseases. Over 2–4 weeks, as the organism multiplies in the skin, a tuberculous chancre slowly develops, initially appearing as a nodule that evolves into an indolent, firm, nontender, sharply delineated ulcer. It also may develop into impetigenous or ichthymotic forms. Lymphatic extension occurs, and lymphadenopathy occurs 3–8 weeks after skin inoculation. The purified protein derivative (PPD) skin test result becomes positive, and enlarged lymph nodes may become fluctuant and drain spontaneously. The complex of the tuberculous chancre and regional adenopathy is the cutaneous analog of the primary tubercular infection of the lung, the Gohn complex. Within 2–3 years, calcification can be found in draining nodes.

The early histologic picture is an acute neutrophilic reaction with embedded areas of necrosis associated with numerous AFB. Three to six weeks later, the infiltrate becomes granulomatous and caseation necrosis becomes evident. In some instances, the dermal infiltrate is nonspecific. AFB may or may not be present.[5]

In patients with preexisting immunity to TB, postprimary cutaneous inoculation usually results in development of a hyperkeratotic papule—the "prosector's wart"—which eventually becomes verrucous. The lesion progresses centrifugally in an annular or a serpiginous fashion. Spontaneous resolution is common in the center of the lesion. Unlike the primary lesion no associated adenopathy occurs. The postprimary lesion also rarely ulcerates, and spontaneous involution may occur over months to years.[5,16]

Table 25-1. Classification of Cutaneous TB and Synonymous Terms Used Previously

Classification of Cutaneous TB	Clinical Appearance	Histology	Associated Finding	Terms Previously Used in Literature
Cutaneous TB from Exogenous Source				
Primary inoculation	Ulcer, nodule, local disease, lymphatic extension	Chronic inflammation, granulomatous inflammation	History of trauma	Primary inoculation Tuberculosis chancre Tuberculosis primary complex
Post-primary inoculation	Hyperkeratotic papule, "wart"	Hyperkeratosis	History of trauma	Tuberculosis verrucosa cutis Warty TB Verruca necrogenica Prosector's wart Tuberculosis cutis verrucosa
Cutaneous TB from Endogenous Source				
Contiguous spread	Sinus tract, abscess	Granulomatous inflammation, sinus tract	Underlying infected source	Scrofuloderma TB colliquativa cutis
Autoinoculation	Ulcer at body orifice	Ulceration, granulomatous inflammation	Widespread TB	Orificial TB Tuberculosis cutis orificialis Tuberculosis ulcerosa cutis et mucosae
Cutaneous TB from Hematogenous Spread				
Lupus vulgaris	Multiple nodules and plaques on face, neck	Granulomatous inflammation	May develop carcinoma	Lupus vulgaris Tuberculosis luposa cutis
Acute hematogenous dissemination	Multiple papules and pustules	Nonspecific inflammation	Acute presentation	Acute miliary TB of the skin Tuberculosis cutis miliaris disseminate Tuberculosis cutis acuta generalisata
Nodules or abscesses	Multiple soft tissue abscesses	Granulomatous inflammation	May arise at site of trauma	Tuberculosis gumma Metastatic tuberculous abscess

Source: Adapted from Beyt BE Jr, Ortbals DW, Santa Cruz DJ, et al. Cutaneous mycobacteriosis: Analysis of 34 cases with a new classification of the disease. Medicine 1981;60:95.

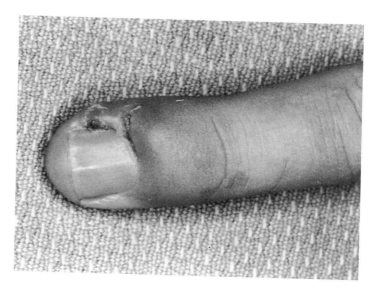

Fig. 25-1. Paronychia in a pathology resident after performing an autopsy on a patient with unsuspected TB. (From Goette DK, Jacobsen KW, Doty DR. Primary inoculation TB of the skin. *Arch Dermatol.* 1978;114:567)

CUTANEOUS TUBERCULOSIS FROM AN ENDOGENOUS SOURCE

Cutaneous infection with TB may result from contiguous involvement of the skin overlying a subcutaneous focus (most commonly tuberculous lymphadenitis), TB of the bones and joints, or secondary to tuberculous epididymitis (Fig. 25-2). In the past, the term *scrofuloderma* was used to describe this condition. Cervical lymph nodes are affected most often, and children are afflicted more frequently than are adults.[23]

The initial lesion is typically a firm subcutaneous swelling or nodule that, although initially mobile, soon firmly attaches to the overlying skin. It then suppurates, and eventually an indolent chronic draining sinus tract or cutaneous abscess develops. Multiple ulcers may form; these are arranged linearly. Watery, purulent, or caseous discharge may occur from the sinus. Spontaneous healing, if it does occur, may take years to complete.

Histopathologically, caseation necrosis and granuloma formation occur; AFB are demonstrated on special stains. As the lesion ages, granuloma formation may be replaced

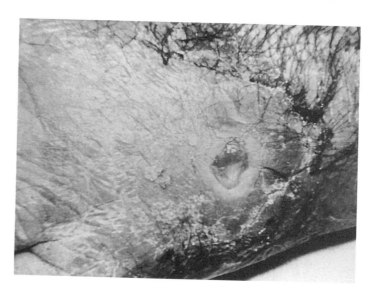

Fig. 25-2. Draining ulcerative lesion over dorsum of the left hand associated with tuberculous osteomyelitis of the fourth and fifth metacarpal. (From Beyt BE Jr, Ortbals DW, Santa Cruz DJ, et al. Cutaneous mycobacteriosis: Analysis of 34 cases with a new classification of the disease. *Medicine.* 1981;60:95, 1981.)

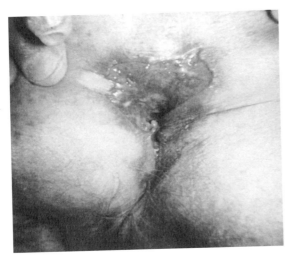

Fig. 25-3. Shallow 10-cm draining ulcer extending from the anorectal line in a patient with external pulmonary TB. (From Beyt BE Jr, Ortbals DW, Santa Cruz DJ, et al. Cutaneous mycobacteriosis: Analysis of 34 cases with a new classification of the disease. *Medicine.* 1981;60:95.)

by a nonspecific chronic inflammatory infiltrate and AFB may become scarce.[5,16] The PPD test result is usually positive, and concurrent pulmonary TB occurs frequently.

Occasionally, cutaneous TB results from the auto-inoculation of the mucous membrane and adjoining skin of the orifices that occurs when viable organisms are either expectorated or passed in patients without significant immunity[7,24] (Fig. 25-3). The organisms invade tissue that is normally resistant to infection. In the past, the term *orifacial tuberculosis* was used to describe this condition. The typical patient with this condition is older, lacks PPD reactivity, and has far-advanced pulmonary, intestinal, or genitourinary TB.[5,25] AFB shed from these primary foci are inoculated into the mucocutaneous areas of the orifices at previously traumatized sites. Lesions occur in the oral cavity or perineal/perirectal skin[7,26,27]; they are ulcerative and painful and do not heal spontaneously. Nonspecific ulceration and lymphedema occur superficially.[7,16] In most cases, granuloma formation and caseation necrosis are found deep in the dermis. AFB are usually present.

CUTANEOUS TUBERCULOSIS FROM A HEMATOGENOUS SOURCE

Lupus vulgaris is a particular type of chronic cutaneous TB in a previously sensitized person with a high degree of TB sensitivity. Hematogenous or lymphatic seeding accounts for the majority of cases. Occasionally, lupus vulgaris appears over a primary inoculation site, in a scar of scrofuloderma or after recurrent Bacille Calmette-Guérin vaccinations.[28–31] These lesions are usually solitary plaques or nodules with some ulceration and scarring; they typically appear as "apple jelly" nodules on diascopy and are most commonly located on the face or neck (Fig. 25-4). Several diverse presentations of lupus vulgaris have been reported and include psoriasiform lesions, nasal ulcerations, and eventual destruction of the cartilagenous part of the nasal septum, as well as widespread systemic dissemination.[24,32–34] Because of the broad range of clinical presentations, many cases are mis-diagnosed for years.[35–38] The tuberculin skin test result is frequently positive. Malignancy develops in up to 8% of patients with long-standing lupus vulgaris. Squamous cell carcinoma is most common, although basal cell carcinoma and sarcoma occur occasionally.[39–41] An instance of Hodgkin's disease complicating lupus vulgaris also has been described.[42,43] The histopathologic picture of lupus vulgaris is diverse and not always diagnostic. When caseation necrosis is present, it is minimal, and AFB are difficult to demonstrate.[44]

An uncommon fulminant form of cutaneous TB, previously known as TB cutis miliaris disseminata, occurs in infants or children after acute hematogenous dissemination of *M. tuberculosis*.[4,45,46] The initial focus of infection is either pulmonary or meningeal, and it may be preceded by an exanthematous disease such as measles.[47] Lesions occur most commonly on the trunk, thigh, buttocks, and genitalia, beginning as papules capped by minute vesicles that eventually rupture and crust.[5,45,48,49]

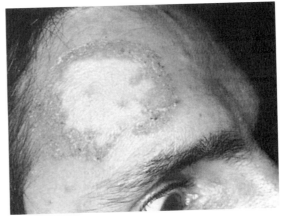

Fig. 25-4. Typical lesion of lupus vulgaris on a patient whose skin biopsy grew *Mycobacterium tuberculosis.*

Histologic examination of these lesions reveals a non-specific inflammatory cellular infiltrate with focal areas of necrotizing vasculitis, and vascular thrombi containing numerous bacilli have been reported.[5,46,50] The disease is usually fatal, although a few cases of improvement after antituberculous chemotherapy have occurred.[5,51]

Cutaneous hematogenous dissemination of *M. tuberculosis* may present subacutely as soft tissue abscesses or nodules.[51–55] Occasionally the abscess develops at the site of previous trauma, suggesting localization of blood-borne organisms in the injured tissue. Multiple cold abscesses and chronic recurrent perirectal abscesses have been reported in patients with AIDS, and multiple skin nodules from disseminated TB have also occurred in these patients.[56–59] The multiple skin nodules can be nondescript in the patient with AIDS, necessitating a high degree of suspicion on the clinician's part, especially in patients with CD4 counts under 200/mm.[3] In some cases these isolates develop multidrug resistance and become rapidly fatal.[60–62]

TUBERCULOUS MASTITIS

Tuberculosis of the breast—tuberculous mastitis—is difficult to recognize and is frequently misdiagnosed as breast cancer. It occurs most often in women 20 to 50 years of age who present with a hard, nontender nodule or mass in the breast along with axillary adenopathy.[34, 63–66] The inflammatory lesion may suppurate and drain. Breast involvement is a result of retrograde lymphatic extensions from underlying mediastinal, parasternal, axillary, or cervical lymph nodes. Histologically, granulomatous inflammation and caseation may be found.

TUBERCULIDS

Tuberculids are a group of cutaneous conditions occurring in the presence of TB but containing no stainable or culturable AFB; based on histopathology, then, they were previously regarded as an allergic reaction to the infection. These conditions have included erythema induratum, papulonecrotic tuberculids, and lichen scrofulosorum. Many of these lesions are now thought to be secondary to nontuberculous processes. A possible exception to this is erythema nodosum, which has been attributed to primary TB.

DIAGNOSIS

Because of the varied clinical spectrum and rarity of cutaneous TB, a high index of suspicion is needed to identify skin lesions that may be tubercular in origin and will therefore require biopsy for histopathology purposes

as well as an AFB stain and culture. In some cases, histopathology shows nonspecific inflammation without granuloma formation. Fluorescent staining with auramine or rhodamine may be useful.[67,68] Enzyme-linked immunosorbent assay (ELISA) for antibodies to PPD and to *M. tuberculosis* antigen 5 also may be helpful.[48,69–71] Monoclonal antibody assays and the polymerase chain reaction (PCR) technique have become increasingly useful clinically.[72,73] Recently, for example, PCR amplification has proven to be a rapid and accurate means of identifying *M. tuberculosis* from patients with cutaneous TB.[74–76]

THERAPY

The mainstay of therapy is chemotherapy. Treatment of lupus vulgaris with isoniazid alone has resulted in high cure rates.[77,78] Combination chemotherapy is recommended for patients with extracutaneous disease and multiple skin lesions and for those with profound immunosuppression. The reader is referred to Chap. 6 for a detailed discussion. Surgery, which can include excisional biopsy and debridement, also may play a minor adjuvant role in treatment. With the exception of TB cutis miliaris disseminata (discussed earlier in this chapter), most forms of cutaneous TB respond to chemotherapy and carry a good prognosis.

A paradoxical skin reaction sometimes occurs in patients undergoing anti-tuberculous therapy, particularly in anergic patients treated for miliary TB: Weeks or months into therapy, fluctuant swellings appear that on aspiration yield pus. Smear and culture for *M. tuberculosis* are often positive, and the isolate usually retains its susceptibility to the patient's treatment regimen. This paradoxical response is thought to represent an immunologic phenomenon—not resistance—and typically responds to continued chemotherapy.

REFERENCES

1. Beyt BE Jr, Ortbals DW, Santa Cruz DJ, et al. Cutaneous mycobacteriosis: Analysis of 34 cases with a new classification of the disease. *Medicine.* 1981;60:95.
2. Lenzini L, Rottoli P, Rottoli L. The spectrum of human tuberculosis. *Clin Exp Immunol.* 1977;27:230.
3. Michelson HE, Laymon CW. Classification of tuberculosis of the skin. *Arch Dermatol.* 1945;52:108.
4. Dinning WJ, Marston S. Cutaneous and ocular tuberculosis: A review. *J R Soc Med.* 1985;78:576.
5. Sehgal VN, Wagh SA. Cutaneous tuberculosis: Current concept. *Int J Dermatol.* 1990;29:237.
6. Sehgal VN, Jani MK, Srivastavia G. Changing patterns of cutaneous tuberculosis. *Int J Dermatol.* 1989;28:231.

7. Shengold MA, Sheingold H. Oral tuberculosis. *Oral Surg.* 1951;4:239.

8. Bjornstad R. Tubercular primary infection of genitalia: Two case reports of venereal genital tuberculosis. *Acta Dermatol Venereol.* 1947;27:106.

9. Fisher I, Orkin M. Primary tuberculosis of the skin. *JAMA.* 1966;195:314.

10. Goette DK, Jacobson KW, Doty DR. Primary inoculation tuberculosis of the skin. *Arch Dermatol.* 1978;114:567.

11. Heilman KM, Muschenheim C. Primary cutaneous tuberculosis resulting from mouth-to-mouth respirations. *N Engl J Med.* 1965;273:1035.

12. Heycock JB, Noble TC. Four cases of syringe-transmitted tuberculosis. *Tubercle.* 1961;42:25.

13. Hole LE. Tuberculosis acquired through ritual circumcision. *JAMA.* 1913;61:99.

14. Hoyt EM. Primary inoculation tuberculosis. *JAMA.* 1981;245:1556.

15. Minkowitz S, Brandt IJ, Rapp Y, et al. "Prosector's Wart" (cutaneous tuberculosis) in a medical student. *Am J Clin Pathol.* 1969;51:260.

16. Montgomery H. Histopathology of various types of cutaneous tuberculosis. *Arch Dermatol.* 1961;35:698.

17. O'Donnell TF, Jurgenson PF, Weyerich NF. An occupational hazard—tuberculosis paronychia. *Arch Surg.* 1971;103:757.

18. Pereira CA, Webber B, Orson JM. Primary tuberculous complex of the skin. *JAMA.* 1976;235:942.

19. Rytel MW, Davis ES, Prebil KJ. Primary cutaneous inoculation tuberculosis. *Am Rev Respir Dis.* 1970;102:264.

20. Sahn SA, Pierson DJ. Primary cutaneous inoculation drug-resistant tuberculosis. *Am J Med.* 1974;57:676.

21. Strand S. Tubercular primary lesion on penis-cancer, penis venereal tuberculosis. *Acta Dermatol Venereol.* 1946;26:462.

22. Weaver RA. Tuberculosis of the tongue. *JAMA.* 1978;235:2418.

23. Michelson HE. Scrofuloderma gummosa (tuberculosis colliquativa). *Arch Dermatol.* 1924;10:565.

24. Fisher JR. Miliary tuberculosis with unusual cutaneous manifestations. *JAMA.* 1977;238:241.

25. McAndrew PG, Adekeye ZO, Ajdukiewicz AB. Miliary tuberculosis presenting with multifocal oral lesions. *Br Med J.* 1976;1:1320.

26. Engleman WR, Putney FJ. Tuberculosis of the tongue. *Trans Am Acad Ophthalmol Otolaryngol.* 1972;76:1384.

27. Nepomuceno OR, O'Grady JF, Eisenberg SW, et al. Tuberculosis of the anal canal: Report of a case. *Dis Colon Rectum.* 1971;14:313.

28. Izumi AK, Matsunaga J. BCG vaccine-induced lupus vulgaris. *Arch Dermatol.* 1982;118:171.

29. Maguire A. Lupus marinus: The discovery, diagnosis and treatment of seventeen cases of lupus marinus. *Br J Dermatol.* 1968;80:419.

30. Caplan SE, Kauffman CL. Primary inoculation tuberculosis after immunotherapy for malignant melanoma with BCG vaccine. *J Am Acad Dermatol.* 1996;35:783.

31. Lee SM, Hann SK, Chun SI, et al. An unusual form of skin tuberculosis following B.C.G. vaccination. *J Dermatol.* 1994;21:106.

32. Bateman DE, Makepeace W, Lensa M. Miliary tuberculosis in association with chronic cutaneous tuberculosis. *Br J Dermatol.* 1980;103:557.

33. Fine RM, Meltzer HD. Psoriasiform lupus vulgaris: A case report. *Int J Dermatol.* 1970;9:273.

34. Warin AP, Jones EW. Cutaneous tuberculosis of the nose with unusual clinical and histologic features leading to a delay in the diagnosis. *Clin Exp Dermatol.* 1977;2:235.

35. Case 43–1972. *N Engl J Med.* 1972;287:872.

36. Duncan WC. Cutaneous mycobacterial infections. *Tex Med.* 1968;64:66.

37. Schmidt CL, Ho M, Pomeranz JR. Lupus vulgaris: recovery of living tubercle bacilli 35 years after onset. *Cutis.* 1976;18:221.

38. Stevens CS, Ploeg DEV. Lupus vulgaris: A case that escaped diagnosis for twenty-eight years. *Cutis.* 1981;27:510.

39. Forstrom L. Carcinomatous changes in lupus vulgaris. *Ann Clin Res.* 1969;1:213.

40. Gueli F. Neoplasms originating in areas affected by lupus vulgaris. *JAMA.* 1952;148:152.

41. Nyfors A. Lupus vulgaris, isoniazid and cancer. *Scand J Respir Dis.* 1968;49:264.

42. Harrison PV, Marks JM. Lupus vulgaris and cutaneous lymphoma. *Clin Exp Dermatol.* 1980;5:73.

43. Schein PS, Vickers HR. Lupus vulgaris and Hodgkins disease. *Arch Dermatol.* 1972;105:244.

44. Seghal VN, Srivastavia G, Khurana VK, et al. An appraisal of epidermologic, clinical, bacteriologic, histopathologic, and immunologic parameters in cutaneous tuberculosis. *Int J Dermatol.* 1987;26:521.

45. Platou RV, Lennox RA. Tuberculous cutaneous complexes in children. *Am Rev Tuberc.* 1950;74:160.

46. Yamauchi T, Klein JD, Fanell WF. Tuberculosis of the skin. *Am J Dis Child.* 1973;125:855.

47. Sundt H. A case of lupus disseminatus (post exanthematic miliary tuberculosis cutis). *Br J Dermatol.* 1925;37:316.

48. Braunstein H, Adriano SM. Fluorescent stain of tubercle bacilli in histologic sections. *Am J Clin Pathol.* 1961;36:37.

49. McCray MK, Esterly NB. Cutaneous eruption in congenital tuberculosis. *Arch Dermatol.* 1981;117:460.

50. Lipper S, Watkins DL, Kahn LB. Nongranulomatous septic vasculitis due to miliary tuberculosis. *Am J Dermatopathol.* 1980;2:71.

51. Kennedy C, Knowles GK. Miliary tuberculosis presenting with skin lesions. *Br Med J.* 1975;3:356.

52. Munt PW. Miliary tuberculosis in the chemotherapy era: With a clinical review of 69 American adults. *Medicine.* 1971;51:139.

53. Reitbrock RC, Dahlmans RPM, Smedts F, et al. Tuberculous cutis miliaris dissemination as a manifestation of miliary tuberculosis: A literature review and report of a case of recurrent skin lesions. *Rev Infect Dis.* 1991;13:265.

54. Shaw NM, Basu AK. Unusual cold abscesses. *Br J Surg.* 1970;57:418.

55. Ward AS. Superficial abscess formation: An unusual presenting feature of tuberculosis. *Br J Surg.* 1971;58:540.

56. Handwerger S, Mildvan D, Senie R, et al. Tuberculosis and the acquired immunodeficiency syndrome at a New York City Hospital: 1978–1985. *Chest.* 1987;91:176.

57. Sunderam G, McDonald RJ, Maniatis T, et al. Tuberculosis as a manifestation of the acquired immunodeficiency syndrome (AIDS). *JAMA.* 1986;256:362.

58. Sunderam G, Mongura BT, Lombardo JM, et al. Failure of "optimal" four-drug short course tuberculosis chemotherapy in a compliant patient with human immunodeficiency virus. *Am Rev Respir Dis.* 1987;136:1475.

59. Daikos GL, Uttamchandani RB, Tuda C, et al. Disseminated miliary tuberculosis of the skin in patients with AIDS: Report of four cases. *Clin Infect Dis.* 1998;27:205.

60. Antinori S, Galimberti L, Tadini GL, et al. Tuberculosis cutis miliaris disseminata due to multidrug-resistant *Mycobacterium tuberculosis* in AIDS patients. *Eur J Clin Microbiol Infect Dis.* 1995;14:911.

61. Corbett EL, Crossley I, DeCock KM, et al. Disseminated cutaneous *Mycobacterium tuberculosis* infection in a patient with AIDS. *Genitourin Med.* 1995;71:308.

62. Libraty DH, Byrd TF. Cutaneous miliary tuberculosis in the AIDS era: Case report and review. *Clin Infect Dis.* 1996; 23:706.

63. Cohen C. Tuberculous mastitis. *S Afr Med.* 1977;52:12.

64. Mukerjee P, Cohen RV, Niden AH. Tuberculosis of the breast. *Am Rev Respir Dis.* 1971;104:601.

65. Schaefer G. Tuberculosis of the breast, a review with the additional presentation of ten cases. *Am Rev Tuberc.* 1955;72:810.

66. Vaishnar P, Muthuswamy P. Tuberculosis of the breast. *Am Rev Respir Dis.* 1982;125(S):181.

67. Koch ML, Cote RH. Comparison of fluorescence microscopy with Ziehl-Neelsen stain for demonstration of acid-fast bacilli in smear preparations and tissue sections. *Am Rev Respir Dis.* 1965;91:283.

68. Wilner G, Nassar SA, Siket A, Azar HA. Fluorescent staining for mycobacteria in sarcoid and tubercular granuloma. *Am J Clin Pathol.* 1969;51:584.

69. Benjamin RG, Daniel TM. Serodiagnosis of tuberculosis using the enzyme-linked immunoabsorbent assay (ELISA) of antibody to *Mycobacteria tuberculosis* antigen-5. *Am Rev Respir Dis.* 1982;126:1013.

70. Daniel TM, Benjamin RG, Debanne SM, et al. ELISA of IgG antibody to *M. tuberculosis* antigen 5 for serodiagnosis of tuberculosis. *Indian J Pediatr.* 1985;52:349.

71. Nassau E, Parsons ER, Johnson GD. The detection of antibodies to *Mycobacterium tuberculosis* by microplate enzyme-linked immunosorbent assay (ELISA). *Tubercle.* 1976;57:67.

72. Senturk N, Sahin S, Kocagoz T. Polymerase chain reaction in certain tuberculosis: is it a reliable diagnostic method in paraffin-embedded tissue. *Int J Dermatol.* 2002;41:863.

73. Tan SH, Tan BH, Goh CL, et al. Detection of *Mycobacterium tuberculosis* DNA using polymerase chain reaction in cutaneous tuberculosis. *Int J Dermatol.* 1999;38:122.

74. Baselga E, Barnadas MA, Margall N, et al. Detection of *M. tuberculosis* complex DNA in a lesion resembling sarcoidosis. *Clin Exp Dermatol.* 1996;21:235.

75. Margall N, Baselga E, Coll P, et al. Detection of *Mycobacterium tuberculosis* complex DNA by the polymerase chain reaction for rapid diagnosis of cutaneous tuberculosis. *Br J Dermatol.* 1996;135:231.

76. Quiros E, Maroto MC, Bettinardi A, et al. Diagnosis of cutaneous tuberculosis in biopsy specimens by PCR and southern blotting. *J Clin Pathol.* 1996;49:889.

77. Bruck C, Carlson AW. Treatment of lupus vulgaris with INH exclusively. *Acta Dermatol Venereol.* 1964;44:223.

78. Forstrom L. Isoniazid treatment of lupus vulgaris. *Ann Clin Res.* 1969;1:36.

26

Miliary Tuberculosis

Daniel W. Fitzgerald

INTRODUCTION

Miliary tuberculosis (TB) is defined as progressive disseminated hematogenous TB. The term *miliary* describes the presence of innumerable, 1–2 mm, discrete tuberculous lesions in the lungs and other organs owing to the seeding of these tissues by blood-borne tubercle bacilli. John Jacob Manget used the word "miliary" originally in 1700 to describe the resemblance of the pathologic lesions to millet seeds.

A number of variables affect the pathogenesis and clinical manifestations of miliary TB, and various classification schemes have attempted to divide miliary TB accordingly. The variables and their impact on disease are briefly described below, but no classification scheme is attempted in this chapter.

Young versus Old Age

Classically, miliary TB was a disease of young children; however, in the last thirty years miliary TB is increasingly reported in immunocompromised adults and in the elderly.

Primary Infection versus Reactivation

Miliary TB may result from progression of primary TB infection or from reactivation of latent TB years after primary infection (Fig. 26-1). The former is more typical in children and the latter in the elderly. In immunocompromised hosts, including HIV infected adults, either may occur.

Brisk versus Nonreactive Immune Response

The immune response to the hematogenously disseminated tubercles may run the spectrum from brisk with histologically typical tissue reaction to nonreactive with huge numbers of organisms and little organized tissue response. HIV infected adults pass from a well developed to a nonreactive immune response as their CD4 T cell count decreases and immune compromise worsens.

Acute versus Chronic

Symptoms of miliary TB may start abruptly and progress with rapid hematogenous dissemination or the disease may start from a chronic active tuberculous lesion with intermittent hematogenous dissemination and a more prolonged disease course.

Cryptic versus Overt

The diagnosis of miliary TB may be overt with a history of TB exposure, signs, and symptoms suggestive of TB, classic miliary pattern on chest radiograph, and a positive sputum smear for acid-fast bacilli. Alternatively, the disease may be cryptic presenting in an elderly person with multiple complicating illnesses, no history of TB, nonspecific clinical findings, normal chest radiograph, and a negative sputum exam.

PATHOGENESIS

Miliary TB results from a massive hematogenous spread of tubercle bacilli, which may occur either at the time of primary infection or at a time remote from the primary infection. The quantity of the tuberculous bacillemia and the immunologic competence of the host are important factors that determine the outcome of such dissemination. The bacilli may gain access to the blood stream via the lymphatics or via direct discharge from a tuberculous lesion into the blood stream.

Lymphohematogenous dissemination designates the entry of tubercle bacilli, usually from a parenchymal pulmonary focus, into the lymphatics, lymph nodes, and ducts, with ultimate drainage into the bloodstream, producing bacillemia. Lymphohematogenous dissemination following primary infection is the usual mechanism causing miliary TB in infants and children.

Miliary dissemination may also occur when an older tuberculous lesion in the lung or in an extra-pulmonary site reactivates and discharges tubercle bacilli directly into the bloodstream. This is believed to be the mechanism of most miliary TB in the older population. Slavin and his coworkers reviewed 100 postmortem examinations of patients who had died from disseminated TB in the period from 1937 to 1959.[1] In 46 cases the lungs could be identified as the source of miliary dissemination. There was, however, a striking difference in the role of extrapulmonary sites as a source of dissemination between the pre and postchemotherapeutic era. Prior to 1948, nonpulmonary sources were identified in 40% of cases, but these increased to 75% in the postchemotherapeutic era. This may, in part, explain the more common appearance of cryptic disease in the postchemotherapeutic era.

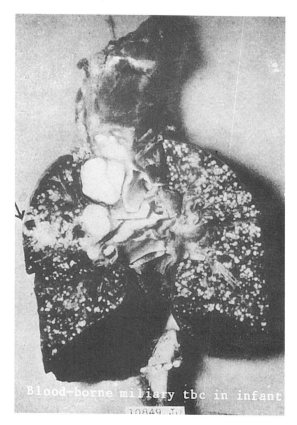

Fig. 26-1. Miliary tuberculosis in an 11-month-old infant. Most of the caseous areas are of hematogenous origin. *Arrow* indicates the primary lesions. (From the collection of the late A. R. Rich and W. G. MacCallum, Department of Pathology, School of Medicine, Johns Hopkins University. Courtesy of Dr. Arthur M. Dannenberg, Jr.)

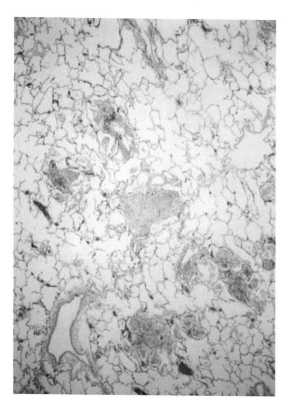

Fig. 26-2. The cut surface of a portion of inflated lung parenchyma. The small, rounded, dark lesions are miliary tubercles subsequent to hematogenous dissemination. Original magnification × 2. (Courtesy: Dr. Yale Rosen, Department of Pathology, Brookdale Hospital Medical Center.)

PATHOLOGY

Grossly, the lungs or other affected organs have small, punctate, rounded lesions of more or less uniform size. The term miliary is descriptive of the small seed like appearance on gross inspection. The lesions vary in color from yellow to gray to reddish-brown, depending on the organ examined and their stage of development (Figs. 26-2, 26-3, and 26-4).

Miliary foci lead to the classic changes described as *tubercles.* Lymphocytes and macrophages are intermixed with epithelioid cells arranged in roughly spherical dimensions. When caseation necrosis affects the central core, the lesions are described as soft or exudative.

When there is no caseation, the lesions are described as hard or proliferative. With appropriate staining, acid-fast bacilli may be found within macrophages or epithelioid cells or in the central caseum.

The pathology may shed light on the mechanism and timing of hematogenous dissemination. In persons in whom a large caseous lesion can be demonstrated to involve a large blood vessel or the thoracic duct, it is hypothesized that the large lesion served as the source of a massive tuberculous bacillemia via direct seeding of the vessel. The organisms disseminate in accord with the blood flow, and lesions can be demonstrated in the lungs, liver, bone marrow, spleen, kidneys, adrenals, meninges, and eyes. Much less commonly, they seed the thyroid, breast, pancreas, heart, prostate, testes, and pituitary (Table 26-1).

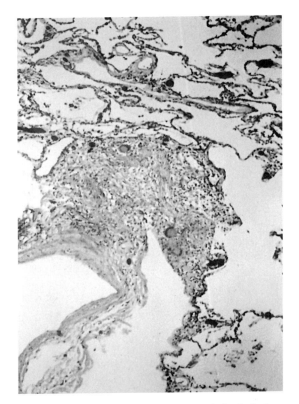

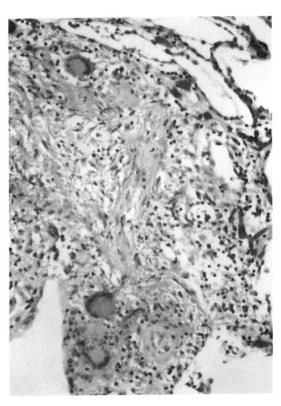

Fig. 26-3. Histologic appearance of a miliary lesion in the lung. Original magnification × 100. (Courtesy: Dr. Yale Rosen, Department of Pathology, Brookdale Hospital Medical Center.)

Fig. 26-4. Higher magnification of miliary lesion shown in Figure 26-3. Note the elongated epithelioid cells and multinucleated giant cells. Original magnification × 250. (Courtesy: Dr. Yale Rosen, Department of Pathology, Brookdale Hospital Medical Center.)

Table 26-1. Organ Involvement in Miliary Tuberculosis at Necropsy

	Slavin et al.[1]	Gelb et al.[2]	Prout and Benatar[3]
No. of cases	100	21	34
Organ (% involved):			
Spleen	100%	86%	79%
Liver	97	91	85
Lungs	86	100	91
Bone marrow	77	24	47
Kidneys	64	62	56
Adrenals	53	14	29
Eye	50		
Thyroid	14	19	7

Often no blood vessel invasion is detected, but one or several large caseous lesions are found in the lungs, other organs, or lymph nodes and are presumed to be the source of dissemination. Rich described a situation in which careful dissection failed to demonstrate a macroscopic focus involving a large blood vessel and postulated that bacilli may be discharged into microscopic vessels within caseous lesions, which in turn seeded large vessels.[4]

The miliary lesions may be of uniform histology or mixed. If the miliary lesions are of a similar histology, a single massive episode of dissemination is suggested. If soft caseous lesions are admixed with hard tubercles with cellular organization and fibrosis, then intermittent showering of bacilli over time is suggested.

Miliary lesions in HIV-positive patients may present the same pathologic features as in HIV-negative subjects. In general, however, the lesions demonstrate more necrosis and less cellular reaction. Acid-fast bacilli are usually more numerous than in lesions from HIV-negative cases. Granulomas tend to be poorly formed and giant cells infrequent. In advanced AIDS cases, miliary lesions may consist of foci of necrosis teeming with tubercle bacilli but with little or no surrounding cellular reaction. Entry into the bloodstream in HIV infected adults appears to occur principally from heavily infected necrotic lymph nodes in the hilum, in the mediastinum, or from extrathoracic sites.

EPIDEMIOLOGY

In years past, the incidence of miliary TB was greatest in children, with more than one third of the cases occurring in children under 3 years of age.[5] Measles, whooping cough, and other childhood exanthems were believed to predispose to lymphohematogenous dissemination. A classic description of childhood disseminated TB was supplied by Dr. Edith Lincoln at Bellevue Hospital in 1935.[6]

In developing countries with a high prevalence rate of infectious TB and where chemoprophylaxis is not employed, miliary TB remains a major problem during childhood. Bacille Calmette-Guérin (BCG) vaccination is widely employed in such countries in an effort to protect against miliary and meningeal TB; however, case series demonstrate that children vaccinated with BCG may still develop miliary TB. Hussey and colleagues in 1991 reported a retrospective review of 94 cases of childhood miliary TB between 1985 and 1989 in South Africa.[7] Fifty-two percent of these patients were less than 1 year of age, and the median age was 10.5 months. A history of BCG vaccination was documented in 88% of these

children. Miliary TB accounted for 8.3% of all childhood admissions for TB.

At the Hospital Albert Schweitzer in rural Haiti, which serves a population of 200,000 people, 100 children are diagnosed each year with TB and of these, 20 have miliary TB. The mortality for miliary TB in children approaches 50%. Limited tools for the diagnosis of TB in children likely results in a gross underestimation of the true impact of miliary TB in our population and in other resource-poor settings.[8]

Over the last thirty years miliary TB is increasingly reported in immunocompromised adults and in the elderly. Immunologic disorders in adults, congenital or acquired, whether related to coexisting disease or to immunosuppressive therapy, underlie many cases of disseminated TB today.

The worldwide presence of HIV infection has greatly influenced the epidemiology and significance of TB, including miliary TB. HIV infected people are at increased risk for active TB, and the risk increases with advanced immune suppression.[9–11] The risk of progressive hematogenous dissemination also increases with advanced immune suppression. In our experience in Haiti, miliary dissemination is clinically recognizable in at least 10% of HIV-related TB.[12,13]

Among HIV-negative subjects in the United States, miliary TB is most likely to occur in older patients, in minority racial groups, and in patients with underlying conditions such as malignancy, malnutrition, pregnancy, rheumatologic disease, renal failure, or alcoholism or with treatment with immunosuppressive medication including steroids, chemotherapy, or tumor necrosis factor (TNF) inhibitors.[14,15] The largest study of TB complicating malignancy was reported at the New York Memorial Sloan-Kettering Hospital by Kaplan and coworkers, who reviewed the records of 201 patients in whom TB developed as a complication of neoplastic disease or its therapy.[16] Thirty-four cases of disseminated TB were found (17% of all cases), and 29 of the 34 had received cancer therapy, often a combination of chemotherapy, radiation, and steroids. Disseminated TB was most common in patients with lymphoma or hematogenous malignancy; in these patients it was more common than isolated pulmonary involvement.

The role of chronic renal failure as a risk factor in TB is somewhat less certain. Pradhan and associates reported the incidence of TB in dialyzed patients to be 15 times higher than that of the general population, which has been confirmed by others.[17,18] Freeman and colleagues, however, were able to document only one case of TB in more than 300 patients in their dialysis program.[19] It is certain, however, that the incidence of extrapulmonary and miliary disease in dialysis patients who develop TB is extremely high, approaching 50% in some series.

Proudfoot and coworkers coined the term *cryptic* to describe the difficulty of diagnosing miliary TB in older patients with underlying chronic disease or immune suppression, in whom clinical presentation may be atypical.[20] Perhaps in consequence, the number of cases of disseminated TB diagnosed first at postmortem examination also appears to be increasing. Jacques and Sloan, in a retrospective study in Belfast, compared all autopsy records for the 3-year period 1946 through 1949 with those during 1966 through 1969.[21] A similar number of autopsies were performed: Although the incidence of miliary TB at autopsy dropped from 1.7% in the early period to 0.47% in the later period, the percentage of cases unsuspected prior to death doubled. In the latter period, patients were older and appeared to lack some of the characteristic features of the disease. In addition, their more advanced age prompted physicians to attribute their generalized debility and progression of symptoms to an undiagnosed carcinoma.

More recent cases of miliary TB continue to show a shift in the demographics of this disease, with older persons having a significant number of underlying medical conditions. Sime and associates from Edinburgh compared cases of miliary TB from the periods of 1954–1967 and 1984–1992 and showed an increase in the mean age of presentation from 59.5 in the earlier period to 73.5 in the later period.[22] In another series from North Carolina, the average age at presentation was 60 years.[23] These reports also document the frequent atypical presentation of the disease, the cryptic form and that the diagnosis of disseminated TB is made only at necropsy in many instances.

SYMPTOMS

The clinical presentation of miliary TB may vary significantly. Common symptoms are listed in Table 26-2 and include fever, weakness, anorexia, weight loss, and cough. Fever may be continuous but is often low-grade and intermittent.

Fever is common even among patients with underlying malignancy and in those immunosuppressed from cancer chemotherapy or other causes. Less common symptoms include headache, abdominal pain, and dyspnea. Headache is ominous and often signifies the presence of tuberculous meningitis.[25] Abdominal pain is less specific but has been associated with involvement of the peritoneum or partial intestinal obstruction secondary to lymph node or omental involvement. Dyspnea, when present, may be the result of underlying lung disease or of decreased diffusing capacity secondary to extensive interstitial tubercles.[26] The symptoms are usually protracted, averaging between 3 and 15 weeks except in immunosuppressed patients or those with serious coexisting disease in whom the onset may be more abrupt.

PHYSICAL SIGNS

The signs most often present on physical examination include fever, tachycardia, tachypnea, and adventitious sounds on pulmonary examination (Table 26-3).

Table 26-2. Presenting Symptoms in Patients with Miliary Tuberculosis

	Prout and Benatar[3]	Sharma et al.[24]	Kim et al.[23]
No. of patients	62	100	38
Symptoms (% patients):			
Fever	44%	89%	89%
Anorexia	51	79	78
Weight loss	59	84	66
Weakness	42	52	53
Cough	63	71	55
Hemoptysis	8.5	6	10
Abdominal pain	30		13
Dyspnea	37	34	50
Headache	17		5
Chest pain	15	3	3

Table 26-3. Physical Findings in Patients with Miliary Tuberculosis

	Prout and Benatar[3]	Sharma et al.[24]	Kim et al.[23]
No. of patients	62	100	38
Signs (% of patients):			
Febrile	95%	89%	90%
Inanition	57	59	13
Adventitious pulmonary sounds	33	50	50
Tachypnea	33		47
Tachycardia	39		
Hepatomegaly	62	70	16
Splenomegaly	12	31	13
Lymphadenopathy	28	26	16
Nuchal rigidity	16	10	3

Splenomegaly and lymphadenopathy, although common in children, are less frequent findings in adults. Hepatomegaly is common; studies from Groote Shur Hospital in South Africa documented hepatomegaly in 50–65% of patients, most of whom were adults.[27] Nuchal rigidity is present in about 15–20% of cases and usually signifies the coexistence of tuberculous meningitis.

Choroidal tubercles are gray or yellowish lesions usually less than one quarter the size of the optic disc and appearing within 2 mm of the optic nerve. They are usually multiple and bilateral, with one to five found in the choroid of both eyes. Reports vary widely on the frequency of their occurrence ranging from rates of 10–30% in adults and 15–60 % in children.[28–30] The use of mydriatics may increase the sensitivity of this sign. It should be noted that choroidal tubercles are not pathognomonic for miliary TB and have been reported in cases of isolated pulmonary TB as well.

LABORATORY FINDINGS

Anemia occurs in up to two thirds of patients.[31] Leukopenia is less common but more frequent than leukocytosis. Monocytosis and an elevated sedimentation rate are common. Rarely, disseminated TB may lead to pancytopenia, aplastic anemia, or leukemoid reaction that may easily be confused with acute leukemia. Coagulopathies may occur, including a full-blown disseminated intravascular coagulation (DIC) syndrome, and this may be the underlying mechanism for the adult respiratory distress syndrome that has been reported to complicate miliary TB.[32] It is not always possible to prove that the hematologic abnormalities are secondary to disseminated TB and not the result of a coexisting primary hematologic disorder.[33]

Sharma and colleagues measured lymphocyte subsets in 10 patients with miliary TB.[24] As compared with normal controls, their blood absolute lymphocyte counts were significantly lower. Lymphocyte subpopulations CD3, CD4, CD8, and B cells were likewise decreased. Bronchoalveolar lavage (BAL) was also performed on these patients and showed an increase in the lymphocyte subpopulations. This suggested compartmentalization of lymphocytes at the site of inflammation causing their depletion in the peripheral blood. These findings mimic the BAL findings of patients with sarcoidosis.

Hyponatremia with the laboratory features of inappropriate secretion of antidiuretic hormone is commonly reported in almost all series of miliary TB. Seventy-eight percent of patients had a serum sodium level of less than 135 mmol/L in the series by Maartens and associates, and 67% of patients had hyponatremia in the series reported by Sharma and coworkers. Addison's disease should be considered as a cause of hyponatremia, especially if corticosteroid treatment is anticipated.

A higher proportion of patients with miliary TB fail to react to tuberculin than do those with localized pulmonary or extrapulmonary TB (Table 26-4).

At least two factors contribute to the cause of fewer tuberculin reactors. First, more patients with miliary TB have an underlying immunosuppressive disorder such as severe malnutrition, malignancy, renal failure, or HIV

Table 26-4. Tuberculin Skin Test (5-TU) in Miliary Tuberculosis

Study (First Author)	No. of Patients Tested	% with Positive Result
Munt[25]	57	52
Grieco and Chmel[34]	28	36
Gelb et al.[2]	2	56
Prout and Benatar[3]	21	38
Maartens et al.[27]	47	43
Kim et al.[23]	38	21

infection as a cause for anergy and as a predisposing cause for disseminated TB. Second, the presence of extensive generalized tuberculous infection and antigen excess may divert cellular immune responses so as to blunt the host reaction to intradermal antigen. Some patients who are nonreactive to tuberculin when first discovered to have miliary TB experience a positive reaction after their disease has been successfully treated. Regardless of the underlying cause, a negative tuberculin reaction does not exclude the diagnosis of miliary TB, and a positive PPD reaction only signifies that miliary TB is a possibility.

CHEST RADIOGRAPHS

The chest radiograph is the single most important means for detecting miliary TB. The classic pattern is diffuse, bilateral, symmetrical, discrete, pinpoint 2 mm densities.

At first the tiny nodules may have faint, hazy outlines, but they sharpen, as they grow larger. Often they appear more numerous at the central and basal areas of the film because of the greater thickness of the lung at these sites. The nodules are usually most apparent where the lung shadow is superimposed over a radiodense structure such as the heart or diaphragm (Figs. 26-5 and 26-6).

The size of the nodules visualized in the initial chest film varies with their age. When symptoms or other clinical evidence raises suspicion of miliary TB, it is important to realize that a normal-appearing chest film, especially early in the illness, does not exclude this diagnosis. In this circumstance, repeated chest x-ray studies should be obtained every few days in order to detect lesions when they appear. It is also useful to examine the chest film before a bright light, which provides better visualization of the tiny nodules, especially in over-penetrated dark films.

In a retrospective study by Kwong and colleagues of 71 patients with proven miliary TB, chest radiographs allowed identification of miliary lesions in 59–69% of cases when reviewed by three independent radiologists.[35]

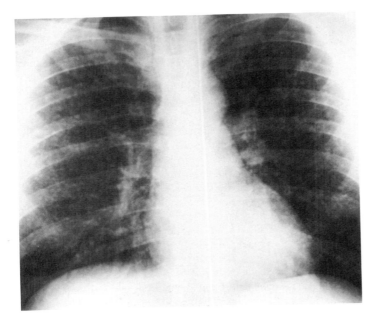

Fig. 26-5. Chest radiograph of a patient with military tuberculosis. Note the extensive, symmetrical distribution of 2- to 3-mm lesions throughout both lungs. (Courtesy: Dr. Dorothy McCauley, Department of Radiology, New York University School of Medicine.)

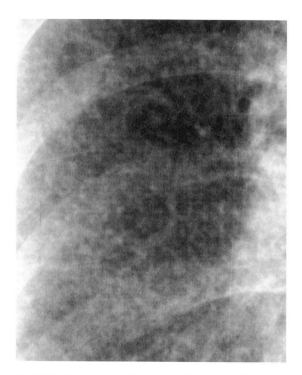

Fig. 26-6. Close-up view of the chest radiograph in Figure 26-5. Note the uniform distribution of nodules throughout the lung parenchyma. (Courtesy: Dr. Dorothy McCauley, Department of Radiology, New York University of Medicine.)

Among cases that were misdiagnosed, the appearance of chest radiographs was atypical for the disease, ranging from focal consolidation to pleural effusion. In the series of Sharma and colleagues, chest radiographs of 88% of the patients showed the typical miliary pattern. A series from Edinburgh in 1994 showed that 61% of patients had a miliary pattern on chest radiograph. Hill and associates reported a series of 51 patients with HIV infection who also had miliary TB and found a miliary pattern on chest radiographs in only 43% of the patients; Fourteen percent had normal-appearing chest radiographs.[36]

The chest radiograph may also demonstrate evidences of other tuberculous infection in addition to miliary lesions. The most common are the focal parenchymal lesions of pulmonary TB, including confluent infiltrates, nodules, and cavities. In addition, hilar or mediastinal lymphadenopathy may be found, especially in patients with recent tuberculous infection or with coexisting HIV infection. Pleural effusions are not common; however,

tuberculous pleural effusions occurring concomitantly in both pleural cavities may indicate the presence of miliary dissemination. Rarely, pneumothorax and pneumomediastinum occur in the course of miliary TB.[37]

Tuberculosis is not the exclusive cause of a miliary pattern on chest radiograph. Other clinical entities cause a similar appearance that may closely resemble miliary TB, such as sarcoidosis, disseminated carcinoma, various infections, hypersensitivity pneumonitis, and others. Disseminated *Mycobacterium avium* complex (MAC) and disseminated BCG can have similar radiographic and histologic manifestations; the latter entity has been reported in cases wherein BCG has been used in the treatment of carcinoma of the bladder.[38]

Computed tomography (CT) often is useful to demonstrate tiny miliary lesions that are too small to be visualized on a conventional radiograph (Fig. 26-7).[39] This is especially important in the early stages of the disease when chest radiographs can be read as normal.

DIAGNOSIS

The diagnostic investigation of a suspected case of miliary TB should aim to obtain proof of tuberculous infection as rapidly as possible as mortality from miliary TB is often due to delays in treatment. Rapid diagnostic tests for the diagnosis of miliary TB include staining for acid-fast bacilli, nucleic acid amplification assays, and biopsy. Despite the availability of newer broth-based culture media like the BACTEC and MGIT systems, which have shortened the time required for mycobacterial growth, these culture techniques still require 1–3 weeks and often more rapid diagnostic tests are required.

Sputum smears are positive in most published experience in the range from 25–36%. See Table 26-5. Series reporting the highest percentages of positive sputum acid-fast bacillus smears contain a larger proportion of cases with coexisting infiltrative or cavitary pulmonary TB. Organisms may also be found in acid-fast stains of the cerebrospinal fluid (CSF) from patients with coexisting tuberculous meningitis. The presence of saprophytic acid-fast organisms in urine and gastric contents lessens the diagnostic value of acid-fast smears of these specimens.

Nucleic acid amplification assays offer another rapid technique for the direct detection of *Mycobacterium tuberculosis* in clinical specimens. The sensitivity of nucleic acid amplification is intermediate between acid-fast staining and culture, and amplification provides results within two days. In sputum acid-fast smear-positive cases, positive nucleic acid amplification

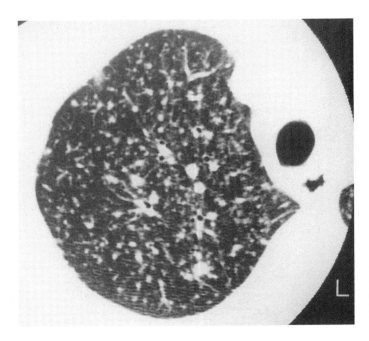

Fig. 26-7. High-resolution computed tomography of lung showing numerous, widespread military foci of tuberculosis. (Courtesy: Dr. Georgeann McGuinness, Department of Radiology, New York University Medical Center.)

indicates the presence of *M. tuberculosis* complex and confirms active TB. When there is a high clinical index of suspicion for TB but with a negative acid-fast smear, a positive nucleic acid amplification test is highly predictive of TB and allows early initiation of therapy.[40] For sputum smear-positive specimens, the sensitivity and specificity of nucleic acid amplification exceeds 95%. For smear-negative sputum specimens sensitivity has ranged from 40–77% and the specificity remains over 95%.[41,42] Case series of suspected disseminated TB suggest that nucleic acid amplification of nonrespiratory specimens (pleural fluid, urine, CSF, tissue, bone marrow, liver, etc.) may expedite diagnosis.[43–46]

In spite of the delay imposed by cultures for mycobacteria, specimens such as sputum, CSF, urine, and bone marrow aspirate should always be cultured, and biopsy specimens should also be cultured for mycobacteria as well as examined histologically. Efforts should be made at the time of biopsy to ensure that some tissue is saved for culture and not all placed in fixative. Patients in whom AIDS is suspected, blood cultures for acid-fast organisms and stool cultures should also be obtained (Fig. 26-8). Isolation of the organism is important not only to prove mycobacterial infection but to identify the species and to provide colonies for drug susceptibility tests as well. Culture confirmation is reported in 50–75% of military TB cases.

Table 26-5. Results of Smears and Mycobacterial Cultures among Patients with Miliary Tuberculosis

	Kim et al.[23]	Munt[25]	Maartens et al.[27]	Prout and Benatar[3]
No. of patients	33	68	64	62
% positive				
Smear	36%	31%	33%	25%
Culture	76%	63%	62%	31%

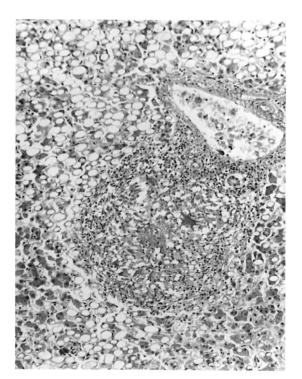

Fig. 26-8. Tuberculous lesion in the liver of a patient with AIDS and military tuberculosis. The predominant cells are polymorphonuclear leukocytes. Acid-fast bacillus (AFB) stain showed numerous organisms. Original magnification × 200. (Courtesy: Dr. Roger Schinella, Department of Pathology, Bellevue Hospital, New York University School of Medicine.)

Histologic confirmation of disseminated TB is best sought by biopsy of the lung, liver, bone marrow, or specific tissue that clinically appears involved, such as lymph nodes, skin, and pleura. The finding of caseating granulomas or acid-fast bacilli is highly suggestive of TB.

Fiberoptic bronchoscopy and transbronchial biopsy of the lung is presently the most useful technique to diagnose miliary TB.[47] This method was first reported by Sahn and Levin in 1975.[48] The sensitivity of transbronchial biopsy is probably due to the fact that miliary lesions are both extensively and uniformly distributed in the lungs. In the absence of acid-fast organisms or positive cultures, the etiology of such granulomas must be interpreted in light of the clinical setting, and other diseases should be considered as well as miliary TB.

Percutaneous needle biopsy of the liver was used extensively in the past; such biopsies demonstrated granuloma in the liver in up to 90% of cases in various clinical series. Autopsy examination revealed nearly 100% involvement of the liver. Noncaseating granulomas are more common than caseating granulomas, and AFB are detected in liver sections in less than 25% of patients. Except for biopsies from HIV-positive cases, visible organisms are most likely to be associated with caseating granulomas.[49] In a minority of cases, cultures of liver tissue may be positive for tubercle bacilli, occasionally in the absence of demonstrable granulomas.

Bone marrow examination has yielded positive results for granuloma in 30–70% of cases of miliary TB. The yield is higher with bone marrow biopsy than aspirate and is improved by culture of the marrow. The marrow is most likely to be involved in patients with abnormalities in the peripheral blood such as anemia, leukopenia, or thrombocytopenia.[50]

Unfortunately, histologic examination of liver or bone marrow may reveal granulomata that are not specific for TB but may be seen in a variety of other diseases. Among the most common causes for granuloma of the liver besides TB are sarcoidosis and histoplasmosis. A similar differential diagnosis is applicable when granulomata are obtained from bone marrow biopsies.[51] Although caseation is more suggestive of TB, its presence does not exclude the presence of other infectious causes, including histoplasmosis and coccidioidomycosis. It should be noted that caseating granuloma and AFB may also be visible in liver biopsy specimens in patients with pulmonary TB who do not have miliary TB. Such granuloma were present in 25% of biopsies and in 65% of postmortem specimens.[51,52]

Before the advent of transbronchial biopsy, thoracotomy and surgical biopsy of the lung tissue were sometimes required in order to establish the diagnosis. This procedure is rarely required in miliary TB today.

TREATMENT

The principles underlying antituberculous chemotherapy are equally applicable to TB systemically disseminated. When tuberculous meningitis accompanies miliary TB, therapy must be designed specifically for this more serious manifestation.

Based on these principles, the therapy for miliary TB in an individual with no past history of TB treatment is an initial intensive phase of chemotherapy with four drugs of isoniazid (INH), rifampin (RIF), pyrazinamide (PZA), and ethambutol (EMB).[53] In children, ethambutol is not routinely used unless there is high suspicion of isoniazid resistance. Streptomycin may also be added as a fourth drug in children.

The optimal length of therapy in miliary TB has never been tested in large controlled trials as has been done with pulmonary and focal extrapulmonary TB infections. The multitude of infected foci throughout the body and the likelihood of seeding the central nervous system and meninges, even in the absence of signs, prompts a conservative approach of 9–12 months of therapy, 2 months with the four drugs indicated earlier followed by 7–10 months of INH and RIF.

As patients with advanced HIV disease are at increased risk of recurrent TB,[54] HIV infected patients with miliary TB should receive a minimum of 12 months of TB therapy. As extrapulmonary TB is an AIDS defining illness, patients with HIV also require antiretroviral therapy.[55] Tuberculosis therapy must be started immediately; however, the optimal time to start antiretroviral therapy, either at the initiation of TB therapy, after the intensive phase, or after the completion of the continuation phase is still not certain, but in general depends upon the stage of immune suppression and risk of delaying ART.

Cases should receive an appropriate retreatment regimen when there is a history of prior treatment of TB and organisms are suspected or proved to be resistant to one or more antitubercubus drugs. The design of the retreatment regimen depends on the history of antituberculous agents previously used and on the results of drug-susceptibility tests.

The role of corticosteroids in miliary TB remains controversial, in part because controlled clinical trials have not been conducted in this type of tuberculous infection. Placebo controlled trials have shown benefit of corticosteroids in pericardial and meningeal TB,[56–58] and when military TB is complicated by infection in these sites, corticosteroids should be strongly considered.

With treatment, the patient usually improves promptly, with reduction of fever and night sweats within 10–14 days and gradual improvement of appetite, strength, and a sense of well being over several weeks. The lesions visible in the chest radiograph usually diminish in size within 2–3 weeks after effective chemotherapy is begun. Some patients, possibly with older, more caseous lesions, show a slower resolution of lesions as assessed by serial chest films. In our experience, virtually all successfully treated cases demonstrate complete disappearance of the lesions, with no radiologic evidence of fibrotic or cascous residuals at the sites of miliary foci.

The mortality for miliary TB ranges from 20–30% in reported case series. Generally, the prognosis is much better for patients with miliary TB who undergo early diagnosis and prompt treatment. Second episodes of miliary TB rarely occur. Patients who discontinue therapy prematurely are at risk of exacerbation of infection in a pulmonary or extrapulmonary site in the future. The life expectancy of HIV-positive patients who are successfully treated for miliary TB depends largely on the course of their HIV related disease and the availability of antiretroviral therapy rather than on the risk of exacerbation of active TB.

ACKNOWLEDGMENT

This is a revision of the chapter by Ruth Divinangracia and H William Harris in the 4th edition.

REFERENCES

1. Slavin RE, Walsh TJ, Pollack AD. Late generalized tuberculosis: A clinical pathological analysis and comparison of 100 cases in the preantibiotic and antibiotic eras. *Medicine.* 1980;59:352.
2. Gelb AF, Leffler C, Brewin A, et al. Miliary tuberculosis. *Am Rev Respir Dis.* 1973;108:1327.
3. Prout S, Benatar SR, Disseminated tuberculosis. *S Afr Med J.* 1980;58:835.
4. Rich AR. The Pathogenesis of Tuberculosis, 2nd ed. Springfield, IL: Charles C Thomas; 1951.
5. Debre R. *Miliary tuberculosis in children.* 1952;2:545.
6. Lincoln EM. Hemarogenous tuberculosis in children. *Am J Dis Child.* l935;50:84.
7. Hussey G, Chisholm T, Kibel M. Miliary tuberculosis in children: A review of 94 cases. *Pediatr Infect Dis J.* 1991;10:832.
8. Perkins M. New Diagnostic Tests for Tuberculosis. *Int J Tuberc Lung Dis.* 2000;4:S182–S188.
9. De Kock KM, Soro B, Coulibaly IM, et al. Tuberculosis and HIV infection in sub-Saharan Africa. *JAMA.* 1992;268: 1581–1587.
10. Advisory Committee for the Elimination of Tuberculosis (ACET). Tuberculosis and Human Immunodeficiency Virus Infection. *MMWR Morb Mortal Wkly Rep.* 1998;47RR20: 18–42.
11. Dye C, Scheele S, Dolin P, et al. Consensus statement. Global burden of tuberculosis: estimated incidence, prevalence, and mortality by country. WHO Global Surveillance and Monitoring Project. *JAMA.* 1999;282:677–686.
12. Pape JW, Liautaud B, Thomas F, et al. Characteristics of the acquired immunodeficiency syndrome (AIDS) in Haiti. *N Engl J Med.* 1983;309:945–950.
13. Deschamps MM, Fitzgerald DW, Pape JW, et al. HIV infection in Haiti: natural history and disease progression. *AIDS.* 2000;14:2515–2521.
14. Sorrentino D, Avellini C, Zearo E. Colonic sarcoidosis, infliximab, and tuberculosis: a cautionary tale. *Inflamm Bowel Dis.* 2004;10:438–440.
15. Keane J, Gershon S, Wise RP, et al. Tuberculosis associated with infliximab, a tumor necrosis factor alpha-neutralizing agent. *N Engl J Med.* 2001;345:1098–1104.
16. Kaplan MH, Annstrong D, Rosen P, et al. Tuberculosis complicating neoplastic disease. i. 1974;33:850.

17. Pradhan RP, Katz LA, Nidus BD, et al. Tuberculosis in dialysis. *JAMA*. 1974;229:798.

18. Sasaki S, Akiba T, Suenaga M, et al. Ten years' survey of dialysis-associated tuberculosis. *Nephron*. 1979;24:141.

19. Freeman RM, Newhousc CE, Rawton RL. Absence of tuberculosis in dialyzed patients. *JAMA*. 1975;233:1356.

20. Proudfoot AT, Akhtar AJ, Douglas AC, et al. Miliary tuberculosis in adults. *Br Med J*. 1969;2:273.

21. Jacques J, Sloan, JM. The changing pattern of miliary tuberculosis. *Thorax*. 1970;25:237.

22. Sime PJ. Chilvers ER, Leitch AG. Miliary tuberculosis in Edinburgh—a comparison between 1984–1992 and 1954–1967. *Respir Med*. 1994;88:609.

23. Kim JH, Langston AA, Gallis HA. Miliary tuberculosis: Epidemiology, clinical manifestations, diagnosis and outcome. *Rev Infect Dis*. 1990:12:583.

24. Sharma SK, Pande JN, Singh YN, et al. Pulmonary function and immunologic abnormalities in miliary tuberculosis. *Am Rev Respir Dis*. 1992;145:1167.

25. Munt PW. Miliary tuberculosis in the chemotherapy era: With a clinical review in 69 American adults. *Medicine*. 1971;51:139.

26. McClement JH, Renzetti AD Jr, Carroll O, et al. Cardiopulmonary functions in hematogenous pulmonary tuberculosis in patients receiving streptomycin. *Am Rev Tuberc*. 1951;64:583.

27. Maartens G, Willcox PA, Benatar SR. Miliary tuberculosis: Rapid diagnosis, hensatologic abnormalities, and outcome in 109 treated adults. *Am J Med*. 1990:89:291.

28. Massaro 0, Katz S, Sachs M: Choroidal TB. a clue to hematogenous tuberculosis. *Ann Intern Med*. 1964;60:231.

29. Illingsworth RS, Lorbar J. Tuhercles of the choroid. *Arch Dis Child*. 1956;32:467.

30. Lincoln EM, Sewell EM. *Tuberculosis in Children*. New York, NY: McGraw-Hill; 1963.

31. Hussain SF, Irfan M, Abbasi M, et al. Clinical characteristics of 110 miliary tuberculosis patients from a low HIV prevalence country. *Int J Tuberc Lung Dis*. 2004;8:493–499.

32. Murray HW, Tuazon CU, Kirmani N, et al. The adult respiratory distress syndrome associated ith miliary tuberculosis. *Chest*. 1978;73:37.

33. Coburn RJ, England JM, Samson DM, et al. Tuberculosis and blood disorders. *Br J Haematol*. 1973;25:793.

34. Grieco MH, Chmel H. Acute disseminated tuberculosis as a diagnostic problem. *Am Rev Respir Dis*. 1974;109:554–560.

35. Kwong JS, Carignan S, Kang EY, et al. Miliary tuberculosis—diagnostic accuracy of chest radiography. *Chest*. 1996;110:339.

36. Hill AR, Premkumar S. Brustein S. et al. Disseminated tuberculosis in the acquired immunodeficiency syndrome era. *Am Rev Respir Dis*. 1991;144:1164.

37. Narang RK, Kumar 5, Gupta A. Pneurnothorax and pneumomediastinum complicating acute miliary tuberculosis. *Tubercle*. 1977;58:79.

38. McParland C, Cotton DJ, Gowda KS, et al. Miliary *Mycobacterium bovis* induced by intravesical Bacille Calmette-Guérin immunotherapy. *Am Rev Respir Dis*. 1992;146:1330.

39. Tanoue LT, Mark EJ. Case records of the Massachusetts General Hospital. Weekly clinicopathological exercises. Case 1-2003. A 43-year-old man with fever and night sweats. *N Engl J Med*. 2003;348:151–161.

40. Catanzaro A, Perry S, Clarridge JE et al. The role of clinical suspicion in evaluating a new diagnostic test for active tuberculosis: results of a multicenter prospective trial. *JAMA*. 2000;283:639–645.

41. Barnes PF. Rapid diagnostic tests for tuberculosis—progress but no gold standard. *Am J Respir Crit Care Med*. 1997;155:1497–1498.

42. Centers for Disease Control and Prevention. Nucleic acid amplification tests for tuberculosis. *MMWR Morb Mortal Wkly Rep*. 1996;45:951.

43. Pfyffer GE, Kissling P, Jahn EM, et al. Diagnostic performance of amplified *Mycobacterium tuberculosis* direct test with cerebrospinal fluid, other nonrespiratory, and respiratory specimens. *J Clin Micro*. 1996;34:834–841.

44. O'Sullivan CE, Miller DR, Schneider PS, etal. Evaluation of Gen-Probe amplified mycobacterium tuberculosis direct test by using respiratory and nonrespiratory specimens in a tertiary care center laboratory. *J Clin Micro*. 2002;40: 1723–1727.

45. Piersimoni C, Scarparo C, Piccoli P et al. Performance assessment of two commercial amplification assays for direct detection of *Mycobacterium tuberculosis* complex from respiratory and extrapulmonary specimens. *J Clin Micro*. 2002;40:4138–4142.

46. Escobedo-Jaimes L, Cicero-Sabido R, Criales-Cortez JL, et al. Evaluation of the polymerase chain reaction in the diagnosis of miliary tuberculosis in bone marrow smear. *Int J Tuberc Lung Dis*. 2003 Jun;7(6):580–586.

47. Willcox PA, Potgieter PD, Bateman ED, et al. Rapid diagnosis of sputum negative miliary tuberculosis using the flexible fiberoptic bronchoscope. *Thorax*. 1986;41: 681–684.

48. Sahn SA, Levin DC. Diagnosis of miliary tuberculosis by transbronchial biopsy. *Am Med J*. 1975;2:667.

49. Guckian JC, Perry JE. Granulomatous hepatitis: An analysis of 63 cases and review of the literature. *Ann Intern Med*. 1966;65:1081.

50. Cucin RL, Coleman M, Eckardt JJ, et al. The diagnosis of miliary tuberculosis: utility of peripheral blood abnormalities, bone marrow and liver needle biopsy. *J Chronic Dis*. 1973;26:355.

51. Bowry S, Chan Cl-I, Weiss I-I, et al. Hepatic involvement in pulmonary tuberculosis: Histologic and functional characteristics. *Am Rev Respir Dis*. 1970;101:941.

52. Seife M, Kessler BJ, Hoffman J. et al. A clinical, functional and needle biopsy study of the liver in pulmonary tuberculosis. *Am Rev Tuberc*. 1951;63:202.

53. American Thoracic Society, Centers for Disease Control, Infectious Disease Society of America, Treatment of Tuberculosis. *MMWR Morb Mortal Wkly Rep*. 2003;52:36–42.

54. Fitzgerald DW, Desvarieux M, Severe P, et al. Effect of post-treatment isoniazid on prevention of recurrent tuberculosis in HIV-1-infected individuals: a randomised trial. *Lancet.* 2000;356:1470–1474.

55. Panel on Clinical Practices for treatment of HIV infection. Guidelines for the use of antriretroviral agents in HIV-Infected Adults and adolescents. U.S. Department of Health and Human Services (DHHS); March 23, 2004.

56. Thwaites GE, Nguyen DB, Nguyen HD, et al. Dexamethasone for the treatment of tuberculous meningitis in adolescents and adults. *N Engl J Med.* 2004;351:1741–1751.

57. Strang JIG, Kakaza HHS, Gibson DG, et al. Controlled clinical trial of complete open surgical drainage and of prednisolone in treatment of tuberculous pericardial effusion in Transkei. *Lancet.* 1988;2:759–764.

58. Hakim JG, Ternmouth I, Mushangi E, Siziya S, Robertson V, Malin A. Double blind randomised placebo controlled trial of adjunctive prednisolone in the treatment of effusive tuberculous pericarditis in HIV seropositive patients. *Heart.* 2000;84:183–188.

27

Endocrine and Metabolic Aspects of Tuberculosis

Emily A. Blumberg
Elias Abrutyn

Endocrinologic and metabolic derangements are infrequent in patients with tuberculosis (TB), but are important when they occur. The basis for these abnormalities is complex. *Mycobacterium tuberculosis* has been described to infect virtually every endocrine gland; however, the incidence of endocrine gland involvement is low, especially in the era of effective antimycobacterial chemotherapy. Furthermore, endocrine and metabolic abnormalities do not always reflect direct infection of the gland and sometimes result from physiologic response to active infection or even as a consequence of chemotherapy. In some instances, hormonal therapy is necessary, but in many cases the infection-related complications do not require therapeutic intervention other than antimycobacterial chemotherapy.

ADRENAL GLAND MANIFESTATIONS

The incidence of *M. tuberculosis* infection of the adrenal gland is unknown. One large series from Hong Kong, an area with endemic TB, reported that 6% of patients with active TB at autopsy had adrenal infection.[1] Not all of these patients had adrenal insufficiency.

In the preantibiotic era, TB was the most common cause of adrenal insufficiency, accounting for 70–80% of reported cases of Addison's disease.[2,3] With the advent of effective therapy for the treatment of TB, the incidence of TB-related adrenal insufficiency decreased dramatically. In the developed world, the estimated proportion of Addison's disease attributed to TB is approximately 20%; developing nations with substantial endemic TB and less well-developed systems for delivering medical care appear to have a higher rate of this complication.[2]

Adrenal TB results from early lymphohematogenous spread; consequently, it is often associated with other extra-adrenal foci of infection. Isolated adrenal TB was noted in only 3% of Guttman's[3] large case series of Addison's disease and of a more recent Boston survey[4] and 1.5% in the autopsy series.[1] The most frequently noted associations include pulmonary and genitourinary TB.[5]

In most cases, both adrenal glands are involved; however, they may not be equally affected.[5–7]

The histopathologic findings of adrenal TB vary with the stage of the illness. There are four classic patterns of involvement: caseating or non-caseating granulomas, glandular enlargement with adrenal destruction by inflammatory granulomas, mass lesions secondary to the development of cold abscesses, and adrenal atrophy from fibrosis related to chronic infection.[5] Epithelioid granulomas occur less frequently in the adrenals as compared with extra-adrenal foci, possibly reflecting the local production of anti-inflammatory steroids.[8] Calcification of the gland is a common but not specific finding. Although descriptions of adrenal TB often focus on cortical involvement, it is important to note that the medulla may also be involved. Signs and symptoms of adrenal insufficiency appear after >90% of the gland has been destroyed.

The effects of TB on adrenocortical function are complex, with adrenal insufficiency resulting from direct glandular involvement, from extra-adrenal infection, or as a byproduct of antituberculous chemotherapy. Several patterns of direct adrenal gland involvement have been described. Most commonly, Addison's disease results from chronic infection of the adrenal gland, with clinical manifestations becoming apparent years after the initial presentation with TB. Adrenocortical insufficiency related to adrenal infection with *M. tuberculosis* may also occur as an isolated presenting manifestation of early or reactivation disease; however, with or without concurrent extra-adrenal TB.[3,9,10]

Most patients present with progressive symptoms; these may include weakness, hyponatremia, hyperkalemia, hyperpigmentation, and relative hypotension. There have been rare reports of patients presenting with the acute onset of life-threatening adrenal insufficiency.[10,11] In cases of adrenal infection with resulting adrenal insufficiency, patients typically have diminished baseline and adrenocorticotropic hormone (ACTH)—stimulated cortisol levels. The administration of rifampin, an inducer of the cytochrome P450 microsomal enzymes responsible for glucocorticoid metabolism, can exacerbate adrenal impairment.[12] There are no data on the impact of rifabutin when this drug is used in place of rifampin.

Relative impairment of adrenal function secondary to extra-adrenal, notably pulmonary, infection has been studied. Initial reports suggested that a majority of patients with active pulmonary TB had suboptimal cortisol responses to infusions of ACTH and its analogs.[13,14] Further study has demonstrated that although some patients with extensive active pulmonary TB lose their diurnal variation in cortisol secretion and manifest impaired response to exogenous ACTH stimulation, baseline cortisol levels are generally higher than those found in normal persons.[15,16] Thus, these patients appear to be maximally stimulated secondary to active extra-adrenal TB, demonstrating that they do have intact adrenal function. Other studies of adrenal function in patients with pulmonary TB noted an accentuated response to low dose (1μg) ACTH administration, suggesting activation of the hypothalamic-pituitary-adrenal axis.[17] HIV coinfection did not affect adrenal responses to low dose ACTH.[18] Although the adrenal response may be normal, glucocorticoid metabolism may be peripherally altered in patients with active pulmonary TB. Preliminary investigation has demonstrated an increased conversion of exogenously administered cortisone to the active metabolite, cortisol, in plasma and bronchoalveolar lavage fluid in patients with acute pulmonary infection.[19] Whether this promotes reactivation of infection or occurs in response to infection is unknown.

The possibility of adrenal involvement with *M. tuberculosis* should be considered when patients with a history of active TB or a positive tuberculin skin test present with the classic manifestations of adrenal insufficiency, including malaise, anorexia, orthostatic hypotension, and hyperpigmentation. Laboratory abnormalities may include anemia and electrolyte abnormalities, including hyponatremia and hyperkalemia. Adrenal insufficiency should be verified by demonstrating depressed morning plasma cortisol levels with a diminished response to synthetic ACTH. Computed tomography (CT) is currently a useful noninvasive adjunct to diagnosis; there is no significant experience with magnetic resonance imaging (MRI) in this condition. During the first two years of illness, the most common CT findings include non-calcified, enlarged adrenal glands with areas of lucency secondary to necrosis.[20–22] Typically there is bilateral enlargement, although unilateral involvement has also been noted. It is important to recognize that the differential diagnosis for adrenal enlargement also includes malignancy, hemorrhage, fungal infection, amyloidosis, sarcoidosis, adenomas, hemangiomas, and hyperplasia. With more chronic infection (i.e., >2 years in duration), the typical CT appearance is of shrunken adrenal glands, often with associated calcifications. The incidence of calcifications increases with the duration of illness, and their presence increases the likelihood of a diagnosis of TB. Nevertheless, it is important to note that calcifications are not a pathognomonic finding. Occasionally the adrenal glands have a normal CT appearance. In the event of

adrenal enlargement, the diagnostic possibilities are numerous. Whenever possible, tissue specimens should be obtained for microbiologic and pathologic analysis, especially in cases in which adrenal involvement is the only evidence of TB. CT-guided needle aspirate of the adrenal gland has been used successfully to obtain adequate tissue specimens for diagnosis.[7,21]

Treatment recommendations for adrenal TB are similar to those outlined for pulmonary TB in all cases, except for children with miliary TB for whom prolonged treatment in excess of the standard 6-month regimen is recommended.[23] As previously noted, rifampin induces the hepatic enzymes responsible for the metabolism of steroids, thereby potentially increasing the metabolism of glucocorticoids; aldosterone is less likely to be affected.[24–27] Consequently, patients at risk for adrenal insufficiency, including those on rifampin therapy and patients with autoimmune disease, metastatic malignancy, sarcoidosis, amyloidosis, HIV infection, or concurrent treatment with other potential adrenal suppressants, should be monitored closely and given replacement therapy in the event of hypoadrenalism. In the absence of documented adrenal insufficiency, adjuvant corticosteroid therapy is only recommended for individuals with TB pericarditis or infection of the central nervous system.[23] With chronic disease, adrenal gland destruction is usually substantial and treatment is unlikely to result in recovery of adrenal function. There are several reports of adrenal recovery; however, when patients receive antituberculous therapy early in the course of the infection, prior to the destruction of the adrenal gland.[12,28–30] Similarly patients with extra-adrenal infection and blunted adrenal responses to ACTH have experienced improvement in adrenal function in response to antimycobacterial therapy.[14]

CORTICOSTEROID ADMINISTRATION AND TUBERCULOSIS

The exact impact of corticosteroid administration on the development and diagnosis of TB remains somewhat controversial and the critical dose and duration of corticosteroid exposure associated with TB reactivation is unknown. The American Thoracic Society recommends that all patients with positive tuberculin skin tests results (reaction ≥5 mm of induration) who receive >15 mg of prednisone (or its equivalent) on a daily basis for a minimum of 1 month should receive prophylactic therapy to prevent the development of active TB.[31] Whether or not some patients receiving smaller doses of long-term steroids should also receive preventive therapy is unclear. There are data to suggest that at risk patients receiving chronic low dose corticosteroid therapy for treatment of systemic rheumatologic diseases do not experience reactivation of TB.[32] Higher corticosteroid doses have been associated with reactivation in patients with rheumatic diseases but the critical dose threshold is unknown.[33] Steroid-dependent asthmatics with a history of positive tuberculin skin tests may not be at increased risk for the development of active infection.[34] In addition, there does not appear to be any increased risk for patients with acquired immunodeficiency syndrome (AIDS) who are receiving steroids as adjunctive therapy for *Pneumocystis carinii* pneumonia.[35,36] There is no contraindication to continuing steroid administration in patients with active TB who require steroid therapy for other indications, including select manifestations of TB, as long as these patients are undergoing antituberculous chemotherapy.[37] Although reactivation of TB coincident with inhaled corticosteroid therapy has been reported,[38] high dose inhaled corticosteroids have not been associated with reactivation in tuberculin positive pediatric patients with prior BCG vaccination.[39]

The impact of steroid administration on the reliability of tuberculin skin test results has been explored in detail. Healthy patients who receive corticosteroid therapy do experience inhibition of the delayed type hypersensitivity response to intradermal purified protein derivative (PPD) administration. Bovornkitti and colleagues[40] gave healthy adult volunteers who were known to be PPD-positive 40 mg of prednisone per day for 1 month. In their study, the inhibition of the response to PPD began at a mean of 13.6 ± 10.1 days and ended 6.0 ± 3.3 days after suspension of steroid therapy. It is unknown whether or not their data can be generalized to the population at large. Smaller steroid doses affect skin test responses unpredictably.[34,41] Patients who receive alternate-day steroid therapy generally have preserved responses to tuberculin skin testing.[34,42] Of note, patients who are given corticosteroids to treat underlying immunologic disorders may actually experience augmented responses to tuberculin skin testing.[41]

THYROID GLAND TUBERCULOSIS

Tuberculosis rarely involves the thyroid gland. In a series of selected patients with late generalized TB occurring in pre- and post-antibiotic eras, 14% of patients had evidence of thyroid seeding.[43] Most series cite a substantially lower rate of thyroid involvement, however, with histologically documented disease occurring in 0.1% to 1.15% of patients in whom thyroid tissue has been sampled for any indication.[1,44–46]

Tuberculosis of the thyroid can result from hematogenous dissemination or by direct extension from an active laryngeal or lymph node focus.[47] Five distinct presentations have been described. These are a solitary cold abscess, diffuse goiter (often with caseation), acute abscess, multiple lesions from miliary spread, and chronic fibrosing TB.[48] Of these, miliary disease and cold abscesses mimicking the presentation of thyroid carcinoma are most common.[49] Acute tuberculous abscess is least common.[50] Pathologically, TB causes the formation of epithelioid granulomas, usually with central caseation necrosis, Langerhans' giant cells, and peripheral lymphocyte cuffing.[51] Acid-fast stains are often, but not consistently positive.

When mycobacterial thyroiditis is compared with acute bacterial thyroiditis, distinct presentations have been reported.[52] Patients with tuberculous thyroiditis are less likely to note pain, thyroid tenderness, and fever than are patients with acute bacterial infection. Consequently, the duration of symptoms tends to be greater in the patient with TB. In one comparative series, the mean duration of symptoms prior to diagnosis was 105 days for patients with TB as compared with 18 days for patients with acute bacterial thyroiditis.[52] Patients with TB report a history of prior thyroid disease less frequently and are more likely to have normal leukocyte counts at the time of diagnosis. Both groups of patients may develop dysphagia, dysphonia, or even recurrent laryngeal nerve palsy related to compression of adjacent structures or fibrosis. These local extrathyroidal findings may be more common in patients with acute bacterial infection.[52,53]

Thyroid function tests are usually normal in patients with tuberculous thyroiditis, but thyrotoxicosis due to rapid release of stored thyroid hormone from the thyroid gland and myxedema caused by thyroid gland destruction have been reported.[46,49,51,54] The ultrasonographic appearance varies, ranging from solid masses, often with heterogeneous echo appearances, to cystic or hypoechoic lesions.[45] Radionuclide thyroid scans typically reveal diminished uptake in the affected tissue.[46] Consequently, tuberculous thyroiditis should be considered in patients with a solitary cold thyroid nodule after customary causes have been excluded, especially in the tuberculin positive patient with normal thyroid function studies.

Fine-needle aspiration for cytology and microbiology is the preferred diagnostic tool for the differentiation of tuberculous thyroiditis from carcinoma and other granulomatous entities, including sarcoid, syphilis, and Hashimoto's thyroiditis.[45,46] The definitive diagnosis of TB depends upon the demonstration of consistent cytopathologic changes with either a positive acid-fast stain or culture for *M. tuberculosis*. In countries with a high incidence of TB, the diagnosis should be suspected and treatment started if epithelioid granulomas with caseation are found, even in the absence of confirmatory acid-fast studies.[45] Although early definitions of thyroid TB required the demonstration of an extrathyroidal focus of infection, this requirement has been suspended in view of the more recent recognition of isolated involvement of the thyroid gland.

Many cases of thyroid TB have been treated with a combination of surgical and antimicrobial therapy. In most cases, surgery has been performed because the prevailing preoperative diagnosis was malignancy. In cases in which thyroidal TB was treated solely with standard antimicrobial therapy, the response has been favorable, often with resolution of any abnormal results of thyroid function studies.[52,54] Treatment regimens are identical to those outlined for adrenal TB.

Thyroid abnormalities may be noted in patients with active TB who do not have associated infection of the thyroid gland. Pulmonary TB is not typically associated with significant alterations in thyroid function, although elevations of free tri-iodothyronine and total tri-iodothyronine have been reported in response to therapy.[55] In patients who are hospitalized with TB, the incidence of euthyroid sick syndrome has been substantial, ranging from 63–92%.[56,57] The presence of the euthyroid sick syndrome may serve as an indicator of severity of illness. Not only has it been described more frequently in hospitalized patients but Chow and colleagues[56] noted a strong association between mortality and diminished T_3 levels at the time of presentation. Within 1 month of therapy, the results of all thyroid studies were normal in survivors.

Anti-tuberculous therapy may also have some effect on thyroid appearance and function. Munkner[58] reported an association between the administration of para-aminosalicylic acid (PAS) and the development of goiters. In addition, rifampin induction of hepatic microsomal enzymes may enhance the extrathyroidal metabolism of thyroid hormones, specifically decreasing levels of serum free T_4 and possibly reverse T_3.[59,60] Practically, these fluctuations are unlikely to significantly affect the patient's clinical course, and there are no reports of thyroid hormone supplementation being required for patients receiving rifampin.

PITUITARY GLAND TUBERCULOSIS

Pituitary gland TB is an extremely rare entity, occurring in less than 1% of persons with TB. In the select group of patients with late generalized TB, Slavin and colleagues[43] noted a 4% incidence of pituitary involvement. In an 11-year preantibiotic era autopsy series involving 14,160 specimens from Cook County Hospital, only two specimens yielded evidence of anterior pituitary involvement.[61] This series included 652 cases of pulmonary TB and 368 cases of tuberculous meningitis. It is important to note that in many cases tuberculous involvement of the pituitary is diagnosed purely on pathologic grounds, often in the absence of confirmatory microbiology or even of positive acid-fast stains. Consequently, in a 1986 literature review of infections involving the sella turcica, Berger and coworkers[62] were only able to document nine cases in which there was adequate evidence to diagnose TB definitively.

It has been postulated that pituitary TB can arise from hematogenous seeding, either in the presence or absence of miliary disease, or from direct extension from the sphenoid sinus, brain, or meninges.[61] Depending on the pathogenesis, infection can involve the pituitary gland alone or be associated with TB in an adjacent or distant site.

The clinical presentation of pituitary TB can vary significantly. Compared with acute bacterial infection, the presentation is typically more indolent.[62] Fever is often present. Patients may experience symptoms related to pituitary enlargement, including headache and visual complaints, with or without selective hypopituitarism.[62–64] Sometimes, the selective hypopituitarism occurs in the absence of other symptoms.[65] Patients may be relatively asymptomatic, and the endocrinologic abnormalities may be subtle and noted only on detailed investigation. Any portion of the pituitary (including anterior, posterior, and the stalk) or the hypothalamus can be involved; consequently, presentations can vary and have included growth retardation, hypogonadism, galactorrhea-amenorrhea related to excess prolactin secretion, diabetes insipidus, and even panhypopituitarism.[61,63–66] Because of the small numbers of cases reported and the incomplete documentation of many of the reported cases, there does not appear to be a pathognomonic endocrinologic presentation associated with TB of the pituitary.

Although hypopituitarism may result from direct involvement of the pituitary gland, it may also occur in association with tuberculous meningitis.[67–69] The pathogenesis of this has not been clearly delineated. According to MRI performed on a small group of patients with abnormal pituitary function following tuberculous meningitis, the pituitary often appeared normal; in some cases, third ventricle dilatation, pituitary atrophy, or enhancement of a portion of the gland or hypothalmus was noted.[69] Skull radiographs may reveal calcifications in the vicinity of the sella.[68,69] It has been presumed that meningitis may lead to scarring of the hypothalamus, adjacent basal cisterns, or both and that this may then play a role in the endocrinologic dysregulation. As with pituitary infection, the endocrinologic manifestations can be variable, are often selective, and may become apparent within months to years after recovery from meningitis.

The true incidence of pituitary dysfunction following tuberculous meningitis is unknown but historically was assumed to be low. In the only detailed assessment of this phenomenon, Lam and colleagues[69] attempted to study all available patients who experienced tuberculous meningitis prior to the age of 21 years at a single hospital in Hong Kong. The investigators were only able to locate 49 of 246 eligible patients. Of these 49 patients, 10 had evidence of abnormal pituitary function; growth hormone deficiency occurred most frequently in their cohort. Consequently, it appears that pituitary dysfunction after childhood tuberculous meningitis may be more common than was previously presumed.

Infection of the pituitary itself should be suspected when patients with TB elsewhere present with any signs or symptoms of hypopituitarism. In addition to assessing endocrinologic function, radiologic studies are a useful adjunct to diagnosis. Skull films may demonstrate calcifications in the region of the sella turcica, and the CT or MRI appearance is suggestive of intrasellar tumor; angiography results are normal.[62,64,70] In some cases, thickening of the pituitary stalk with or without pituitary involvement or extension into the sphenoid sinus may be noted on CT or MRI.[71,72] Because of the association with tuberculous meningitis, lumbar puncture should be considered in patients who have symptoms suggestive of tuberculous meningitis. Definitive diagnosis rests on the pathologic demonstration of characteristic caseating granuloma with documentation of the organism. Acid-fast stains are often negative; consequently, the diagnosis must also be considered if the patient has a positive tuberculin skin test result or evidence of TB in another location. Whenever possible, confirmatory cultures should be obtained. The differential diagnosis includes other granulomatous diseases of the pituitary, notably sarcoid, histiocytosis X, lymphocytic adenohypophysitis, syphilis, and giant cell granuloma.[62]

There are no specific treatment recommendations for pituitary TB. Given the association with central nervous system infection, it seems advisable to apply the guidelines for the treatment of tuberculous meningitis to pituitary infection. In those few instances in which the diagnosis has been made premortem and the patients treated with standard therapy for TB, follow-up imaging studies have demonstrated good response with resolution of compressive symptoms and often of the endocrinologic abnormalities.[64,70]

HYPONATREMIA AND THE SYNDROME OF INAPPROPRIATE ANTIDIURETIC HORMONE PRODUCTION

Disorders of sodium have long been associated with TB. Infrequently, hypernatremia secondary to diabetes insipidus has been recognized in patients with either pituitary TB or tuberculous meningitis.[63,67] Hyponatremia is a much more frequent occurrence in active TB, with reported incidences of 10.7% and 43% in two large series.[73,74] *Harrison's Principles of Internal Medicine* lists pulmonary TB as a significant cause of the syndrome of inappropriate antidiuretic hormone (SIADH) production.[75]

Although the association of TB and hyponatremia has long been recognized, Weiss and Katz[76] were the first to note the association with SIADH. Although they did not measure vasopressin levels, they did follow the effects of salt and fluid restriction on the serum and urine sodium levels in four patients with active pulmonary TB who presented with hyponatremia in whom they excluded dehydration and adrenal insufficiency. They noted excessive urinary sodium excretion in the presence of hyponatremia; with marked fluid restriction, the patients experienced an increase in the serum sodium and decrease in urinary sodium excretion. With antituberculous therapy, the three surviving patients all experienced normalization of their serum sodium levels.

Vorherr and colleagues[77] were the first to demonstrate elevated vasopressin levels in a patient with pulmonary TB and hyponatremia. They measured vasopressin levels in a suspension of *M. tuberculosis*, as well as infected and uninfected lung tissue, urine, and serum in a patient who died from active pulmonary TB. Arginine vasopressin was detected in affected lung tissue and urine but not in uninvolved lung tissue, serum, or the *M. tuberculosis* suspension, leading these authors to conclude that there was a direct relationship between the presence of active pulmonary TB and the production of excessive antidiuretic hormone.

More recent studies have demonstrated the presence of circulating arginine vasopressin in living patients with active pulmonary or miliary TB. In a study of 28 hyponatremic patients with tuberculous meningitis, Hill, et al.[78] excluded all other causes of SIADH and then measured free water clearance after water loading. Despite the presence of hyponatremia, patients were noted to have measurable circulating vasopressin, the levels of which decreased somewhat in response to water loading.

The pathogenic mechanism for vasopressin secretion in the presence of hyponatremia and the incomplete response to water loading is unknown, but may reflect dysregulation of osmoreceptor control or a response to nonosmotic stimulation of vasopressin secretion.

Although SIADH is most commonly linked to pulmonary TB, it has also been described in patients with tuberculous meningitis, miliary TB, and tuberculous epididymo-orchitis.[79–82] Most significant among these is the association with tuberculous meningitis. In a pediatric population with tuberculous meningitis, SIADH was noted in 71% of patients and appeared to be a predictor of increased mortality.[79] One case series noted that children with tuberculous meningitis and SIADH were more likely to have increased intracranial pressure.[80]

Vasopressin may not be the only hormone contributing to hyponatremia in patients with tuberculous meningitis. A recent report evaluated a group of critically ill patients with tuberculous meningitis, all of whom had hydrocephalus.[83] In this very select group, plasma atrial natriuretic peptide was universally elevated. Because only three percent of these patients had elevated vasopressin levels, the authors concluded that atrial natriuretic peptide was the likely cause of the hyponatremia in this group of patients.

The degree of hyponatremia is generally quite variable in patients with TB and most patients are asymptomatic.[78] The vast majority of patients correct their hyponatremia concurrently with their response to treatment of their TB. After ruling out volume depletion as the cause of hyponatremia, water restriction should be considered only in those patients with severe or symptomatic hyponatremia. Additional pharmacological interventions are generally not required.

Although the majority of patients with TB and hyponatremia have SIADH, there have been a few case reports of patients with hyponatremia secondary to severe volume depletion caused by cerebral salt wasting.[84,85] These patients are presumed to have defective renal absorption of sodium mediated by the central nervous system release of a natriuretic hormone. They can be differentiated from patients with SIADH by their evidence of hypovolemia in the presence of elevated urine sodium. Successful treatment requires volume repletion and salt.

Diabetes Mellitus

Patients with diabetes mellitus appear to be at increased risk for the development of TB. This observation was initially noted in studies from the pretreatment era, including a 1946 survey from Philadelphia in which the incidence of radiographically demonstrated TB was nearly twofold higher in patients with diabetes.[86] More recent studies from New Guinea and Korea support this observation, noting that the risk of developing active pulmonary TB was three to eleven times greater in diabetics than in nondiabetics.[87,88] Tuberculosis risk does not appear to be linked to the duration of diabetes.[89] Some investigators argue that diabetes mellitus may not be an independent risk factor for the development of active TB, noting that more recent studies exhibit selection and/or detection bias.[90] Nevertheless, there may be a physiologic basis for the increased incidence of pulmonary TB in diabetic patients.[91]

In their review of pulmonary infections in patients with diabetes mellitus, Koziel and Koziel[91] note that the results of immunologic studies in diabetic patients suggest that there may be some significant abnormalities that predispose them to the development of chronic pulmonary infections. In particular, patients with diabetes, especially those with hyperglycemia, have impaired granulocyte chemotaxis, phagocytosis, bactericidal activity, and superoxide production. Furthermore, monocyte-macrophage function may also be impaired. Reduced numbers of circulating peripheral monocytes, decreased phagocytosis, and alterations in surface receptors may all contribute to enhanced diabetic susceptibility to infections with intracellular pathogens.[92,93] Impaired *in vitro* lymphocyte responses have also been reported in patients with poorly controlled diabetes.[94] Koziel and Koziel[91] caution that immunologic studies in diabetic patients may not adequately assess the impact of age or the pathophysiologic differences between insulin dependent and noninsulin dependent diabetes. Moreover peripheral blood cell studies may not accurately reflect the immunologic function of the alveolar macrophage. Nevertheless, there appears to be some basis for the reports of increased susceptibility to TB in diabetic patients.

Commonly, the presentation of TB in diabetic patients resembles that of nondiabetics; however, some differences have been noted with regard to radiographic findings in these patients. Both early and later reports suggested that diabetics were more likely to have involvement of lower lobes or unusual segments of the middle and upper lobes and/or multilobar disease, and that pleural effusions occurred more frequently in this population.[95–100] Ikezoe and colleagues[101] evaluated the CT appearance of pulmonary TB, comparing diabetic patients with other immunocompromised patients and those with no prior history of immunologic impairment. They failed to find any difference in the distribution of pulmonary infection; however, they did note that diabetic and immunocompromised subjects were more likely to have multiple cavities within any single lesion and that nonsegmental distribution occurred more commonly in these two patient groups. Additional radiologic reviews have failed to substantiate a link between diabetes mellitus and multilobar involvement.[102]

Hyperglycemia is a common occurrence in patients with TB and individuals who have no prior history of diabetes mellitus may present with glucose intolerance at the time of diagnosis. In one study of 506 consecutive patients with active pulmonary TB, 9 had a history of diabetes mellitus, 25 were found to be newly diabetic, and 82 (16.2%) had impaired glucose tolerance tests.[103] Additional studies have supported the association between active pulmonary infection and glucose intolerance, noting that impaired glucose tolerance resolved with effective antituberculous treatment.[104,105] This suggests that similar to other serious infections, active TB is also associated with transient hyperglycemia.

Because diabetics are considered to be at increased risk for the development of active TB, the Advisory Committee for Elimination of Tuberculosis included diabetics in the group of high-risk patients who should be screened routinely for TB.[31] Pozilli and colleagues have demonstrated that well-controlled diabetics do respond to standard intradermal testing.[106] Intradermal testing results in poorly controlled diabetics have not been evaluated; consequently routine recommendations for skin testing should be followed. In the event that a diabetic patient is found to have a positive tuberculin skin test (i.e., ≥10 mm), the American Thoracic Society recommends preventive therapy with isoniazid for a minimum of 6 months, even for those patients who are older than 35 years.[31]

In general, treatment recommendations for active TB are identical for diabetic and nondiabetic patients. There has been a single study reporting a higher incidence of relapse in diabetics treated with a 9-month regimen but this observation needs to be confirmed.[107] Bashar and colleagues[108] noted an increased incidence in multidrug-resistant TB in their center; however, this observation has not been more generally reported. It is important to remember that the high rate of peripheral neuropathy in diabetics may increase their risk of neuropathy associated with isoniazid.[91] Consequently diabetics should be given pyridoxine and closely followed for development of this common adverse event.

Hypercalcemia

Tuberculosis is a well-described cause of hypercalcemia. In one large series of patients from Hong Kong, 6% of patients with confirmed hypercalcemia had TB.[109] The actual prevalence of hypercalcemia is difficult to estimate, as concurrent serum albumin levels are not always reported. Moreover, the reported rates vary considerably, depending on the geographic conditions. Surveys from India, Hong Kong, the United States, Malaysia, and Greece report prevalence rates between 11% and 48% with the highest rates occurring in the sunniest climates and in patients receiving supplemental calcium and/or vitamin D.[110–115] In contrast, surveys from countries like Great Britain and Belgium, where sunshine is less plentiful, reveal a much lower prevalence of hypercalcemia.[116,117] Although most reports focus on infection related hypercalcemia, hypocalcemia has also been described.[118]

The majority of the reports of hypercalcemia are associated with pulmonary TB, perhaps reflecting the preponderance of pulmonary infection over other sites of infection. However, hypercalcemia has been less frequently noted in conjunction with extrapulmonary disease, including miliary infection, peritonitis, and osteomyelitis.[119–121] Recently there have been several reports of unexplained hypercalcemia as a presenting manifestation of TB in patients on peritoneal or hemodialysis.[122,123] Often patients with hypercalcemia and pulmonary infection will have more extensive lung involvement than do infected normocalcemic patients; but the association with more severe infection is not consistently predictable.[109,113,124] Frequently hypercalcemia is not noted at the time of diagnosis but occurs early in the course of treatment.[109,124] Initial assessments may fail to take into account disease-related hypoalbuminemia; as the serum albumin increases in response to treatment of the infection, hypercalcemia may become apparent. The later detection of hypercalcemia may not reflect its later onset, but rather enhanced detection following improvement in nutritional status with treatment.[125]

The cause of hypercalcemia in TB has been a topic of significant controversy. Multiple studies have excluded the common causes of hypercalcemia in these patients, including coexisting hyperparathyroidism, malignancy, adrenal insufficiency, milk-alkali syndrome and hyper thyroidism.[110] Currently, as noted with other granulomatous diseases, hypercalcemia has been most frequently attributed to abnormal vitamin D production.[126]

Support for Vitamin D as an important cofactor causing hypercalcemia in TB includes both clinical and *in vitro* observations. It has long been recognized that TB-associated hypercalcemia occurs more frequently in climates where sunshine is more plentiful. Presumably individuals residing in sunnier locales have a greater likelihood of exposure to vitamin D. Abbasi and colleagues[110] noted that patients who received supplemental vitamin D were more likely to develop hypercalcemia than those who did not receive vitamin D supplements. Because administration of similar amounts of vitamin D to patients with COPD failed to result in hypercalcemia, the authors concluded that the development of hypercalcemia was in some way directly related to active TB. Multiple investigators have reported elevated 1,25-dihydroxyvitamin D levels and low to normal 25-hydroxy D levels in patients with hypercalcemia.[127–131] This phenomenon has been described repeatedly in anephric patients; consequently the site of conversion of 1,25-dihydroxyvitamin D is presumed to be extrarenal.[128–130] In one case report, alveolar macrophages recovered from a patient with active pulmonary TB were demonstrated to synthesize 1,25-dihydroxyvitamin D *in vitro*.[132] *In vitro* studies suggest that macrophage production of 1,25-dihydroxyvitamin D may serve to enhance the antimycobacterial activity of the monocyte, either as a direct effect or by enhancing cellular responses to gamma interferon.[133] Thus, enhanced production of 1,25-dihydroxyvitamin D may occur as part of the normal host defense mechanism. An incidental by-product of this response would be increased intestinal absorption of calcium, thereby explaining the resulting hypercalcemia noted in patients with active TB.

Although the vitamin D hypotheses serve as a rational explanation for the development of hypercalcemia, there are also data to refute the importance of vitamin D in the pathogenesis of TB-associated hypercalcemia. Clinical trials of patients with active TB from the United States, Africa, and Belgium have failed to demonstrate a correlation between 1,25-dihydroxyvitamin D levels and serum calcium measurements.[116,134,135] The authors did not measure ionized calcium values, but did correct for hypoalbuminemia. Their observations are supported by the work of Cadranel and colleagues[132] who studied in detail a single patient with active pulmonary TB and hypercalcemia. Although these authors were able to document production of 1,25-dihydroxyvitamin D by pulmonary macrophages, they also noted an inverse relationship between plasma 1,25-dihydroxyvitamin D levels and serum calcium levels. They proposed that an alternative mechanism to explain the hypercalcemia might need to be explored and suggested that other inflammatory mediators could play an important role.

Antituberculous therapy may also have some impact on calcium homeostasis. In normal individuals, both isoniazid and rifampin have been demonstrated to reduce circulating levels of 25-hydroxyvitamin D and 1-25-dihydroxyvitamin D.[135,136] Although long term administration of both drugs to patients with TB did affect 25-hydroxyvitamin D levels, especially in slow acetylators, the effect of the combination was less than anticipated. Levels of 1-25-dihydroxyvitamin D were not affected with long-term administration and the overall clinical impact appears to have been insignificant. In most cases, hypercalcemia associated with TB is mild and the patients are asymptomatic; however, when hypercalcemia is marked, patients may develop any of the symptoms characteristically associated with hypercalcemia, including lethargy and even metastatic calcifications.[119]

Most patients with hypercalcemia are asymptomatic and specific treatment for this syndrome is required only when patients are overtly symptomatic.[114,115] Otherwise, patients typically experience complete resolution within one to seven months of antituberculous therapy and require no additional intervention.[111] Patients who are receiving vitamin D and/or calcium supplements should have these discontinued if hypercalcemia is detected.

SUMMARY

The endocrine and metabolic manifestations of TB are protean. Infection of actual endocrine glands is only one way in which TB can affect hormonal and metabolic function. Indirect effects of infection and the impact of treatment on hormonal function must also be considered. Ultimately, treatment plans should be tailored which take into account both the direct and indirect impact of *M. tuberculosis* infection.

REFERENCES

1. Lam KY, Lo CY. A critical examination of adrenal tuberculosis and a 28-year autopsy experience of active tuberculosis. *Clin Endocrinol*. 2001;54:633–639.
2. Miller W, Chrousos GP. The adrenal cortex. In: Felig P, Frohman LA eds. *Endocrinology and Metabolism*, 4th ed. New York, NY: McGraw-Hill; 2001:387–524.
3. Guttman PH. Addison's disease: a statistical analysis of 566 cases and a study of pathology. *Arch Pathol*. 1930;10:742–785, 895–935.
4. Alvarez S, McCabe WR. Extrapulmonary tuberculosis revisited: A review of experience at Boston City and other hospitals. *Medicine*. 1984;63:25–55.
5. Kannan, CR. *The adrenal gland. Clinical surveys in endocrinology*, vol II. New York, NY: Plenum Medical Book Company; 1988.
6. Kelestimur F, Özbakir Ö, Saglam A, et al. Acute adrenocortical failure due to tuberculosis. *J Endocrinol Invest*. 1993;16:281–284.

7. Benini F, Savarin T, Senna GE, et al. Diagnostic and therapeutic problems in a case of adrenal tuberculosis and acute Addison's disease. *J Endocrinol Invest.* 1990;13:597–600.

8. Lack EE, Kozakewich HPW. Embryology, developmental anatomy, and selected aspects of non-neoplastic pathology. In: Lack EE, ed. *Pathology of the adrenal glands. Contemporary issues in surgical pathology,* vol IV. New York, NY: Churchill Livingstone; 1990:52–53.

9. Sanford JP, Favour CB. The interrelationsips between Addison's disease and active Tuberculosis: A review of 125 cases of Addison's disease. *Ann Intern Med.* 1956;45:56–72.

10. Ward S, Evans CC. Sudden death due to isolated adrenal tuberculosis. *Postgrad Med J.* 1985;61:635–636.

11. Osborne TM, Sage MJ. Disseminated tuberculosis causing acute adrenal failure, C.T. findings with post mortem correlation. *Australas Radiol.* 1988;32:394–397.

12. Wilkins EG, Hnizdo E, Cope A. Addisonian crisis induced by treatment with rifampicin. *Tubercle.* 1989;70:69–73.

13. Ellis ME, Tayoub F. Adrenal function in tuberculosis. *Br J Dis Chest.* 1986;80:7–12.

14. Prasad GA, Sharma A, Mohan N, et al. Adrenocortical reserve and morphology in tuberculosis. *Indian J Chest Dis Allied Sci.* 2000;42:83–93.

15. Sarma GR, Immanuel C, Ramachandran G, et al. Adrenocortical function in patients with pulmonary tuberculosis. *Tubercle.* 1990;71:277–282.

16. York EL, Enarson DA, Nobert EJ, et al. Adrenocortical function in patients investigated for active tuberculosis. *Chest.* 1992;101:1338–1341.

17. Kelestimur F, Goktas Z, Gulmez J, et al. Low dose (1mg) adrenocorticotropin stimulation test in the evaluation of the hypothalamo-pituitary-adrenal axis in patients with active pulmonary tuberculosis. *J Endocrinol Invest.* 2000;23:235–239.

18. Kaplan FJL, Levitt NS, Soule SG. Primary hypoadrenalism assessed by the Img ACTH test in hospitalized patients with active pulmonary tuberculosis. *QJ Med.* 2000;93:603–609.

19. Baker RW, Walker BR, Shaw RJ, et al. Increased cortisol cortisone ratio in active pulmonary tuberculosis. *Am J Resp Crit Care Med.* 2000;162:1641–1647.

20. Vita JA, Silverberg SJ, Goland RS et al. Clinical clues to the cause of Addison's disease. *Am J Med.* 1985;78:461–466.

21. Buxi TBS, Vohra RB, Sujatha, et al. CT in adrenal enlargement due to tuberculosis: A review of literature with five new cases. *Clin Imaging.* 1992;16:102–108.

22. Doppman JL, Gill JR, Nienhuis AW, et al. CT findings in Addison's disease. *J Comput Assist Tomogr.* 1982;6:757–761.

23. American Thoracic Society: Centers for Disease Control and Prevention/Infectious Diseases Society of America. Treatment of Tuberculosis, *Am J Resp Crit Care Med.* 2003;167:603–662.

24. Edwards OM, Courtenay-Evans RJ, Galley JM, et al. Changes in cortisol metabolism following rifampicin therapy. *Lancet.* 1974;2:549–551.

25. Schulte HM, Mönig H, Benker G, et al. Pharmacokinetics of aldosterone in patients with Addison's disease: Effect of rifampicin treatment on glucocorticoid and mineralocorticoid metabolism. *Clin Endocrinol.* 1987;27:655–662.

26. Kyriazopoulou V, Parparousi O, Vagenakis AG. Rifampicin-induced adrenal crisis in Addisonian patients receiving corticosteroid replacement therapy. *J Clin Endocrinol Metab.* 1984;59:1204–1206.

27. Keven K, Uysal AR, Erdogan G. Adrenal function during tuberculous infection and effects of antituberculous treatment on endogenous and exogenous steroids. *Int J Tuberc Lung Dis.* 1998;2:419–424.

28. Annear TD, Baker GP. Tuberculous Addison's disease: A case apparently cured by chemotherapy. *Lancet.* 1961;1:577–578.

29. Coleman EN, Arneil GC. Acute tuberculous adrenocortical failure with clinical recovery. *Lancet.* 1962;1:886–888.

30. Nordin BEC. Addison's disease with partial recovery. *Proc R Soc Med.* 1955;48:1024–1026.

31. American Thoracic Society. Targeted tuberculin testing and treatment of latent tuberculosis infection. *Am J Resp Crit Care Med.* 2000;161:S221–S247.

32. Andonopoulos AP, Safridi C, Karokis D, et al.. Is a purified protein derivative skin test and subsequent antituberculous chemoprophylaxis really necessary in systemic rheumatic disease patients receiving corticosteroids? *Clin Rheumatol.* 1998;17:181–185.

33. Kim HA, Yoo CD, Back HJ, et al. *Mycobacterium tuberculosis* infection in a cortico- steroid-treated rheumatic disease patient population. *Clin ExpRheumatol.* 1998;16:9–13.

34. Schatz M, Patterson R, Kloner R, et al. The prevalence of tuberculosis and positive tuberculin skin tests in a steroid-treated asthmatic population. *Ann Intern Med.* 1976;84:261–265.

35. Martos A, Podzamczer D, Martinez-Lacasa J, et al. Steroids do not enhance the risk of developing tuberculosis or other AIDS-related diseases in HIV-infected patients treated for *Pneumocystis carinii* pneumonia. *AIDS.* 1995;9:1037–1041.

36. Jones BE, Taikwel EK, Mercado AL, et al. Tuberculosis in patients with HIV infection who receive corticoids for presumed *Pneumocystis carinii* pneumonia. *Am J Respir Crit Care Med.* 1994;149:1686–1688.

37. The Committee on Therapy: Adrenal corticosteroids and tuberculosis. *Am Rev Respir Dis.* 1968;97:484–485.

38. Shaikh WA. Pulmonary tuberculosis in patients treated with inhaled beclomethasone. *Allergy.* 1992;47:327–330.

39. Bahceciler NN, Nuhoglu Y, Nursoy MA, et al. Inhaled corticosteroid therapy is safe in tuberculin-positive asthmatic children. *Pediatric Infect Dis J.* 2000;19:215–218.

40. Bovornkitti S, Kangsdal P, Sathirapat P, et al. Reversion and reconversion rate of tuberculin skin test reactions in correlation with the use of prednisone. *Dis Chest.* 1960;38:51–55.

41. Truelove LH. Enhancement of Mantoux reaction coincident with treatment with cortisone and prednisolone. *Br Med J.* 1957;2:1135–1137.

42. MacGregor RR, Sheagren JN, Lipsett MB, et al. Alternate-day prednisone therapy: evaluation of delayed hypersensitivity responses, control of disease and steroid side effects. *N Engl J Med.* 1969;280:1427–1431.

43. Slavin RE, Walsh TJ, Pollack AD. Late generalized tuberculosis: A clinical pathologic analysis and comparison of 100 cases in the preantibiotic and antibiotic eras. *Medicine.* 1980;59:352–366.

44. Rankin FW, Graham AS. Tuberculosis of the thyroid gland. *Ann Surg.* 1932;96:625–648.

45. Das DK, Pant CS, Chachra KL, et al. Fine needle aspiration cytology diagnosis of tuberculous thyroiditis. A report of eight cases. *Acta Cytol.* 1992;36:517–522.

46. Mondal A, Patra DK. Efficacy of fine needle aspiration cytology in the diagnosis of tuberculosis of the thyroid gland: a study of 18 cases. *J Laryngol Otol.* 1995;109:36–38.

47. Groen JN, Wolffenbuttel RHR, Baggen MGA, et al. Tuberculosis of the thyroid gland. *Neth J Med.* 1988;32:199–203.

48. Khan EM, Haque I, Pandey R, et al. Tuberculosis of the thyroid gland: A clinicopathological profile of four cases and review of the literature. *Aust N Z J Surg.* 1993;63:807–810.

49. Barnes P, Weatherstone R. Tuberculosis of the thyroid: Two case reports. *Br J Dis Chest.* 1979;73:187–191.

50. Johanson AG, Phillips ME, Thomas RJS. Acute tuberculous abscess of the thyroid gland. *Br J Surg.* 1973;60:668–669.

51. Kapoor VK, Subramani K, Das SK, et al. Tuberculosis of the thyroid gland associated with thyrotoxicosis. *Postgrad Med J.* 1985;61:339–340.

52. Berger SA, Zonszein J, Villamena P, et al. Infectious diseases of the thyroid gland. *Rev Infect Dis.* 1983;5:108–122.

53. Emery P: Tuberculous abscess of the thyroid with recurrent laryngeal nerve palsy: a case report and review of the literature. *J Laryngol Otol.* 1980;94:553–558.

54. Nieuwland Y, Tan KY, Elte JWF. Miliary tuberculosis presenting with thyrotoxicosis. *Postgrad Med J.* 1992;68:677–679.

55. Ilias I, Tseleb A, Boufas A, et al. Pulmonary tuberculosis and its therapy do not significantly affect thyroid function tests. *Int J Clini Pract.* 1998;52:227–228.

56. Chow CC, Mak TWL, Chan CHS, et al. Euthyroid sick syndrome in pulmonary tuberculosis before and after treatment. *Ann Clin Biochem.* 1995;32:385–391.

57. Post FA, Soule SG, Willcox PA, et al. The spectrum of endocrine dysfunction in active pulmonary tuberculosis. *Clin Endocrinol.* 1994;40:367–371.

58. Munkner T. Studies on goitre due to para-aminosalicylic acid. *Scand J Respir Dis.* 1969;50:212–226.

59. Christensen HR, Simonsen K, Hegedüs L, et al. Influence of rifampicin on thyroid gland volume, thyroid hormones, and antipyrine metabolism. *Acta Endocrinol.* 1989;121:406–410.

60. Ohnhaus EE, Studer H. A link between liver microsomal enzyme activity and thyroid hormone metabolism in man. *Br J Clin Pharmacol.* 1983;15:71–76.

61. Kirshbaum JD, Levy HA. Tuberculoma of hypophysis with insufficiency of anterior lobe: a clinical and pathological study of two cases. *Arch Intern Med.* 1941;68:1095–1104.

62. Berger SA, Edberg SC, David G. Infectious disease in the sella turcica. *Rev Infect Dis.* 1986;8:747–755.

63. Rickards AG, Harvey PW. Giant-cell granuloma and the other pituitary granulomata. *Q J Med.* 1954;92:425–435.

64. Ranjan A, Chandy MJ. Intrasellar tuberculoma. *Br J Neurosurg.* 1994;8:179–185.

65. Delsedime M, Aguggia M, Cantello R, et al. Isolated hypophyseal tuberculoma: case report. *Clin Neuropathol.* 1988;7:311–313.

66. Brooks MH, Dumlao JS, Bronsky D, et al. Hypophyseal tuberculoma with hypopituitarism. *Am J Med.* 1973;54:777–781.

67. Haslam RHA, Winternitz WW, Howieson J. Selective hypopituitarism following tuberculous meningitis. *Am J Dis Child.* 1969;118:903–908.

68. Sherman BM, Gorden P,di Chiro G. Postmeningitic selective hypopituitarism with suprasellar calcification. *Arch Intern Med.* 1971;128:600–604.

69. Lam KSL, Sham MMK, Tam SCF, et al. Hypopituitarism after tuberculous meningitis in childhood. *Ann Intern Med.* 1993;118:701–706.

70. Flannery MT, Pattani S, Wallach PM, et al. Case Report: Hypothalamic tuberculoma associated with secondary panhypopituitarism. *Am J Med Sci.* 1993;306:101–103.

71. Sharma MC, Arora R, Mahapatra AK, et al. Intrasellar tuberculoma—an enigmatic pituitary infection: a series of 18 cases. *Clin Neurol Neurosurg.* 2000;102:72–77.

72. Stalldecker G, Diez S, Carabelli A, et al. Pituitary stalk tuberculoma. *Pituitary.* 5;2002:155–162.

73. Chung DK, Hubbard, WW. Hyponatremia in untreated active pulmonary tuberculosis. *Am Rev Respir Dis.* 1969;99:595–602.

74. Morris CDW, Bird AR, Nell H. The haemotological and biochemical changes in severe pulmonary tuberculosis. *Q J Med.* 1989;73:1151–1159.

75. Singer GG, Brenner BM. Fluid and elctrolyte disturbances. In: Braunwald E, Hauser SL, Fauci AS, Longo DL, Kasper DL, Jameson JL, eds. *Harrison's Principles of Internal Medicine, 15th ed.* New York, NY: McGraw-Hill; 2001:271–283.

76. Weiss H Katz S. Hyponatremia resulting from apparently inappropriate secretion of antidiuretic hormone in patients with pulmonary tuberculosis. *Am Rev Resp Dis.* 1965;92:609–616.

77. Vorherr H, Massry SG, Fallet R, et al. Antidiuretic principle in tuberculous lung tissue of a patient with pulmonary tuberculosis and hyponatremia. *Ann Intern Med.* 1970;72:383–387.

78. Hill AR, Uribarri J, Mann J. Altered water metabolism in tuberculosis: role of vasopressin. *Am J Med.* 1990;88:357–364.

79. Cotton MF, Donald PR, Schoeman JF, et al. Plasma arginine vasopressin and the syndrome of inappropriate

antidiuretic hormone secretion in tuberculous meningitis. *Pediatr Infect Dis J.* 1991;10:831–842.

80. Cotton MF, Donald PR, Schoeman JF, et al. Raised intracranial pressure, the syndrome of inappropriate antidiuretic homone secretion, and arginine vasopressin in tuberculous meningitis. *Childs Nerv Syst.* 1993;9:10–16.

81. Cockcroft DW, Donevan RE, Copland GM, et al. Miliary tuberculosis presenting with hyponatremia and thrombocytopenia. *Can Med Assoc J.* 1976;115:871–873.

82. Motiwala HG, Sanghvi NP, Barjatiya MK, et al. Syndrome of inappropriate antidiuretic hormone following tuberculous epididymo-orchitis in renal transplant recipient: case report. *J Urol.* 1991;146:1366–1367.

83. Narotam PK, Kemp M, Buck R, et al. Hyponatremic natriuretic syndrome in tuberculous meningitis: The probable role of atrial natriuretic peptide. *Neurosurgery.* 1994;34:982–988.

84. Ti LK, Kang SC, Cheong KF. Acute hyponatraemia secondary to cerebral salt wasting syndrome in a patient with tuberculous meningitis. *Anaesth Intensive Care.* 1998;26:420–423.

85. Dass R, Nagaraj R, Murlidharan J, et al. Hyponatraemia and hypovolemic shock with tuberculous meningitis. *Indian J Pediatr.* 2003;70:995–997.

86. Boucot K, Cooper P, Dillon E, et al. Tuberculosis among diabetics. The Philadelphia Survey. *Am Rev Tuberc.* 1952;65(suppl 1):1.

87. Patel MS, Phillips CB, Cabaron Y. Frequent hospital admissions for bacterial infections among aboriginal people with diabetes in central Australia. *Med J Aust.* 1991;155: 218–222.

88. Kim SJ, Hong YP, Lew WJ, et al. Incidence of pulmonary tuberculosis among diabetics. *Tuberc Lung Dis.* 1995;76: 529–533.

89. Ezung T, Devi NT, Singh NT, et al. Pulmonary tuberculosis and diabetes mellitus—a study. *J Indian Med Assoc.* 2002;100:377–379.

90. Ellenberg M, Rifkin H. Diabetes mellitus: theory and practice. New York, NY: McGraw-Hill; 1970:740.

91. Koziel H, Koziel MJ. Pulmonary complications of diabetes mellitus: pneumonia. *Inf Dis Clin North Am.* 1995;9:65–96.

92. Geisler G, Almdal T, Bennedsen J, et al. Monocyte functions in diabetes mellitus. *Acta Pathol Microbiol Immunol Scand.* 1982;90:33–37.

93. Glass EJ, Stewart J, Matthews DM, et al. Impairment of monocyte "lectin-like" receptor activity in Type I (insulin dependent) diabetic patients. *Diabetologia.* 1987;30: 228–231.

94. Casey JI, Heeter BJ, Klyshevich KA. Impaired response of lymphocytes of diabetic subjects to antigen of Staphylococcus aureus. *J Infect Dis.* 1987;136:495–501.

95. Hadlock FP, Park SK, Awe RJ, et al. Unusual radiographic findings in adult pulmonary tuberculosis. *Am J Roentgenol.* 1980;134:1015–1018.

96. Berger HW, Granada MG. Lower lung field tuberculosis. *Chest.* 1974;65:522–526.

97. Sosman MC, Steidl JH. Diabetic tuberculosis. *Am J Roentgenol.* 1927;17:625–629.

98. Boucot KR. Diabetes mellitus and pulmonary tuberculosis. *J Chronic Dis.* 1957:6:256–279.

99. Perez-Guzman C, Torres-Cruz A, Villareal-Velarde H, et al. Progressive age-related changes in pulmonary tuberculosis images and the effect of diabetes. *Am J Resp Crit Care Med.* 2000;162:1738–1740.

100. Bacakoglu F, Basoglu OK, Cok G, et al. Pulmonary tuberculosis in patients with diabetes mellitus. *Respiration.* 2001;68:595–600.

101. Ikezoe J, Takeuchi N, Johkoh T, et al. CT appearance of pulmonary tuberculosis in diabetic and immunocompromised patients: Comparison with patients who had no underlying disease. *Am J Roentgenol.* 1992;159:1175–1179.

102. Morris JT, Seaworth BJ, McAllister CK. Pulmonary tuberculosis in diabetics. *Chest.* 1992;102:539–541.

103. Mugusi F, Swai ABM, Alberti KGMM, et al. Increased prevalence of diabetes mellitus in patients with pulmonary tuberculosis in Tanzania. *Tubercle.* 1990;71:271–276.

104. Oluboyo PO, Erasmus RT. The significance of glucose intolerance in pulmonary tuberculosis. *Tubercle.* 1990;71: 135–138.

105. Gülbas Z, Erdogan Y, Balci S. Impaired glucose tolerance in pulmonary tuberculosis. *Eur J Respir Dis.* 1987;71: 345–347.

106. Pozilli P, Pagani S, Aruduini P, et al. *In vivo* determination of cell mediated immune response in diabetic patients using a multiple intradermal antigen dispenser. *Diabetes Res.* 1987;6:5–8.

107. Kameda K, Kawabata S, Masuda N. Follow-up study of short-course chemotherapy of pulmonary tuberculosis complicated with diabetes mellitus. *Kekkaku.* 1990;65:791–803.

108. Bashar M, Alcabes P, Rom WN, et al. Increased incidence of multidrug-resistant tuberculosis in diabetic patients on the Bellevue Chest Service, 1987 to 1997. *Chest.* 2001;120: 1514–1519.

109. Shek CC, Natkunam A, Tsang V, et al. Incidence, causes and mechanism of hypercalcemia in a hospital population in Hong Kong. *Q J Med.* 1990;77:1277–1285.

110. Abbasi AA, Chemplavil JK, Farah S, et al. Hypercalcemia in active pulmonary tuberculosis. *Ann Intern Med.* 1979;90:324–328.

111. Sharma SC. Serum calcium in pulmonary tuberculosis. *Postgrad Med J.* 1981;57:694–696.

112. Chan TYK, Chan CHS, Shek CC. The prevalence of hypercalcemia in pulmonary and miliary tuberculosis—a longitudinal study. *Singapore Med J.* 1994;35:613–615.

113. Kitrou MP, Phytou-Pallikari A, Tzannes SE, et al. Hypercalcemia in active pulmonary tuberculosis. *Ann Intern Med.* 1982;96:255.

114. Liam CK, Lim KH, Srinivas P, et al. Hypercalcemia in patients with newly diagnosed tuberculosis in Malaysia. *Int J Tuberc Lung Dis.* 1998;2:818–823.

115. Roussos A, Lagogianni I, Gonis A, et al. Hypercalcaemia in Greek patients with tuberculosis before the initiation of anti-tuberculous treatment. *Respir Med.* 2001;95:187–190.

116. Fuss M, Karmali R, Pepersack T, et al. Are tuberculous patients at a great risk from hypercalcemia? *Q J Med.* 1988;69:869–878.

117. Subcommittee of the Research Committee of the British Thoracic Association: A controlled trial of six months chemotherapy in pulmonary tuberculosis. *Br J Dis Chest.* 1981;75:141–153.

118. Ali-Gombe A, Ornadeko BO. Serum calcium levels in patients with active pulmonary tuberculosis. *Afr J Med Med Sci.* 1997;26:67–68.

119. Wyllie JP, Chippindale AJ, Cant AJ. Miliary tuberculosis and symptomatic hypercalcemia. *Pediatr Infect Dis.* 1993;12:780–782.

120. Lin S-M, Tsai S-L, Chan C-S. Hypercalcemia in tuberculous peritonitis without active pulmonary tuberculosis. *Am J Gastroenterol.* 1994;89:2249–2250.

121. Braman SS, Goldman AL, Schwarz MI. Steroid responsive hypercalcemia in disseminated bone tuberculosis. *Arch Intern Med.* 1973;132:269–271.

122. Lee C-T, Hung K-H, Lee C-H, et al. Chronic hypercalcemia as the presenting feature of tuberculous peritonitis in a hemodialysis patient. *Am J Nephrol.* 2002;22:555–559.

123. Hung Y-M, Chan H-H, Chung H-M. Tuberculous peritonitis in different dialysis patients in southern Taiwan. *Am J Trop Med Hyg.* 2004;70:532–535.

124. Shai F, Baker RK, Addrizzo JR, et al. Hypercalcemia in mycobacterial infection. *J Clin Endocrinol.* 1972;34:251–256.

125. Need AD, Phillips PJ. Pulmonary tuberculosis and hypercalcemia. *Ann Intern Med.* 1979;91:652–653.

126. Haviv YS, Silver J. Hypercalcemia. In: Wass JAH, Shalet SM, eds. *Oxford Textbook of Endocrinology and Diabetes.* New York, NY: Oxford University Press; 2002:614.

127. Saggese G, Bertelloni S, Baroncelli GI, et al. Ketoconazole decreases the serum ionized calcium and 1,25-dihydroxyvitamin D levels in tuberculosis-associated hypercalcemia. *Am J Dis Child.* 1993;147:270–273.

128. Felsenfeld AJ, Drezner MK, Llach F. Hypercalcemia and elevated calcitriol in a maintenance dialysis patient with tuberculosis. *Arch Intern Med.* 1986;146:1941–1945.

129. Peces R, Alvarez J. Hypercalcemia and elevated 1,25(OH)$_2$D$_3$ levels in a dialysis patient with disseminated tuberculosis. *Nephron.* 1987;46:377–379.

130. Gkonos PJ, London R, Hendler ED. Hypercalcemia and elevated 1,25-dihydroxyvitamin D levels in a patient with end-stage renal disease and active tuberculosis. *N Engl J Med.* 1984;311:1683–1685.

131. Isaacs RD, Nicholson GI, Holdaway IM. Miliary tuberculosis with hypercalcemia and raised vitamin D concentrations. *Thorax.* 1987;42:555–556.

132. Cadranel J, Hance AJ, Milleron B, et al. Vitamin D metabolism in tuberculosis. Production of 1,25(OH)$_2$D$_3$ by cells recovered by bronchoalveolar lavage and the role of this metabolite in calcium homeostasis. *Am Rev Respir Dis.* 1988;138:984–989.

133. Rook GAW, Steele J, Fraher L, et al. Vitamin D$_3$, gamma interferon, and control of proliferation of *Mycobacterium tuberculosis* by human monocytes. *Immunology.* 1986;57:159–163.

134. Sullivan JN, Salmon WD. Hypercalcemia in active pulmonary tuberculosis. *South Med J.* 1987;80:572–576.

135. Davies PDO, Church HA, Brown RC, et al. Raised serum calcium in tuberculosis patients in Africa. *Eur J Respir Dis.* 1987;71:341–344.

136. Brodie MJ, Boobis AR, Hillyard CJ, et al. Effect of rifampicin and isoniazid on vitamin D metabolism. *Clin Pharmacol Ther.* 1982;32:525.

28

Hematologic Changes in Tuberculosis

Randall A. Oyer
David Schlossberg

Tuberculosis (TB) exerts a dazzling variety of hematologic effects (Table 28-1). These abnormalities involve both cell lines and plasma components. Antituberculous therapy has its own spectrum of hematologic toxicity also. This chapter reviews and summarizes the known hematologic effects of TB and its therapy.

ERYTHROCYTES

Tuberculosis has profound effects on hemoglobin and hematocrit. Either anemia or polycythemia can occur. Anemia is much more common, effecting greater than 90% of patients actively infected with TB.[1]

Usually, the anemia in TB results from anemia of chronic disease, most often described as normochromic normocytic anemia.[2] In this situation, the anemia is associated with a low or normal mean cell volume[3] (MCV); this in turn reflects a shortened red blood cell (RBC) lifespan without a compensatory marrow response.[4]

Accompanying this change is a decrease in serum iron, total iron binding capacity, and transferrin saturation, as well as an increase in serum ferritin, C-reactive protein, and erythrocyte sedimentation rate (ESR). These abnormalities result from a redistribution of iron as an acute-phase reaction. Total body stores may be normal, but iron is unavailable for normal hematopoiesis, and excess nonhemic iron is visible in the marrow.[5]

New information suggests that *Mycobacterium tuberculosis* must acquire iron from the extracellular environment at sites of replication in order to multiply and cause disease in its host. The bacterium releases high-affinity iron-binding siderophores called exochelins. These exochelins bind iron and deprive the host of available iron and undoubtedly add to the pathogenesis of what we currently understand as the anemia of chronic disease.[6]

The anemia of chronic disease is known to entail a blockade in reticuloendothelial transfer of iron to the nucleus of the developing red cell. Inflammation is known to activate reticuloendothelial cells, which in turn,

sequester iron, causing hypoferremia and iron-limited erythropoiesis. This reticuloendothelial activation may accelerate red cell destruction and promote an exacerbated erythropoietin response. Additionally, there may be a defective marrow response to erythropoietin with abnormal erythroid colony growth. Finally, lactoferrin, which is present in normal white cell granules, is released during phagocytosis. It then binds iron, preventing attachment of iron to transferrin, an attachment necessary for normal iron transfer. This results in anemia and can also limit use of iron by invading microorganisms.[7]

Recently described is a blunted erythropoietin response to anemia in untreated TB. It is postulated that the release of tumor necrosis factor alpha or other cytokines by TB-activated monocytes suppresses the erythropoietin production that normally occurs in the setting of the anemia of chronic disease.[8]

A macrocytic anemia can result from folate or B_{12} deficiency. The former is a consequence of poor intake or increased use of folate in the course of active TB. Much less common is the B_{12} deficiency due to malabsorption in patients with ilial TB.[9] An elevated MCV can also be seen in the course of treatment for active TB due to the acceleration of the normal resumption of hematopoiesis when the anemia of acute inflammation subsides and iron becomes, once again, available for normal hematopoiesis.[10]

Also reported is a transient autoimmune hemolytic anemia, which is Coombs positive.[11] This hemolysis occurs while the patient is actively infected and resolves with successful antituberculosis treatment. The Coombs test then becomes negative. It may, however, cause folate deficiency.[12]

Abnormal B6 metabolism may promote sideroblastic anemia. This is rare and may represent a genetic tendency to form ring sideroblasts.[13]

Bone marrow effects of TB are protean. All hematologic lines may be affected. Bone marrow fibrosis may result from proliferation of macrophages (which are abundant in normal marrow) after they engulf mycobacteria. In addition, TB may directly stimulate a secondary fibrotic reaction.[14] This proliferation damages the marrow microenvironment with a resultant diminution in cell lines; this is called myelophthisis.[15]

Myelofibrosis with myelophthisis can accompany miliary TB, cavitary pulmonary TB, and granulomatous involvement of the spleen, lymph nodes, and liver.[16] Myelophthisic anemias are characterized by the presence of teardrop erythrocytes, nucleated red cells, and early granulocytes on the peripheral blood smear. Bone marrow hypoplasia and aplasia may complicate miliary TB. The anemia or pancytopenia in this setting is usually secondary

Table 28-1. Cell Lines Affected by Tuberculosis

Erythrocytes
Decrease because of:
   Anemia of chronic disease
   Folate deficiency secondary to anorexia
     or increased use
   Folate and B_{12} malabsorption with or without
     ileal involvement
   Autoimmune hemolysis
   Sideroblastic anemia secondary to abnormal
     B_6 metabolism
   Bone marrow fibrosis
   Bone marrow aplasia
   Bone marrow necrosis
   Amyloid infiltration of marrow
   Hypersplenism
   Iron deficiency
Increase because of:
   Renal tuberculosis causing increased erythropoietin

Granulocytes
Decrease (neutrophils or basophils or eosinophils)
because of:
   Folate deficiency secondary to anorexia
     or increased use
   Bone marrow fibrosis
   Bone marrow aplasia
   Bone marrow necrosis
   Amyloid infiltration of marrow
   Chronic infection
   Hypersplenism
Increase (neutrophils or basophils or eosinophils or
monocytes) because of:
   Inflammatory response

Platelets
Decrease because of:
   Immunologic mechanisms
   Disseminated intravascular coagulation
   TTP
   Bone marrow fibrosis
   Bone marrow aplasia
   Bone marrow necrosis
   Hypersplenism
   Shortened platelet survival
Increase because of:
   Acute phase reaction

Lymphocytes
Decrease because of:
   Tuberculous infection
Increase because of:
   Inflammatory response

to marrow dysfunction rather than aplasia, however.[17] Marrow and peripheral blood counts return to normal after successful antituberculous treatment.[18] Additional mechanisms causing anemia include direct marrow infiltration with granulomata, development of amyloidosis of the marrow and bone marrow necrosis.[19–22] Bone marrow necrosis is accompanied not only by anemia but also by leucopenia, thrombocytopenia, elevated LDH, and elevated alkaline phosphatase. Bone marrow necrosis is also accompanied by an increased reticulin and subsequent fibrosis.[22]

A rare effect of tuberculous involvement of the kidney is an increase in erythropoietin level sufficient to cause polycythemia.[23]

GRANULOCYTES

Granulocytes may be affected in several ways during the course of TB. Chronic neutrophilia is well known, occurring in greater than 45% of patients.[1] In the past, macrophages have been considered a major immune defense in mycobacterial infection. Newer data show the importance of neutrophils, however; neutrophilia is T-cell-mediated and resolves with treatment.[24] In the extreme, some patients experience leukemoid reactions, an outpouring of mature and immature granulocytes in peripheral blood; however, there are insufficient marrow blasts to support a diagnosis of acute leukemia. Additionally, flow cytometry identifies these immature granulocytes as polyclonal, indicating that they are reactive rather than malignant. Leukemoid reactions occur only in patients who are extremely ill from their TB. Although classic leukemia has been reported in patients with TB, the leukemia in these patients does not resolve with antituberculous therapy and therefore cannot be considered a complication of TB.[25] The Pelger-Huet anomaly, which is most often associated with leukemia, does occur in TB and is reversible. In this condition, granulocytes appear abnormal with a disturbance of nuclear segmentation, displaying a dumbbell-shaped nucleus, two nuclear lobes connected by a thin strand of chromatin. There is an underlying defect in chromatin synthesis and decreased chemotaxis may result. Originally described by Pelger in 1928, the Pelger-Huet anomaly, which can be acquired during active TB infection, responds to appropriate antituberculous therapy.[26,27] The importance of the Pelger-Huet anomaly is equivocal. Some researchers have indicated an association with a severity of the TB infection in the affected individual. The presence of the Pelger-Huet anomaly should prompt a search for its cause and TB should be included in the differential diagnosis.

Neutropenia is a consequence of many of the same factors causing anemia, which include bone marrow fibrosis, marrow dysfunction, and splenic sequestration. Additionally, experiments have shown the suppression of granulopoiesis by activated T cells, which are part of the inflammatory response.[19] Severe folate deficiency and B[12] deficiency may cause neutropenia as well. Aplastic anemia increases susceptibility to TB and is more likely a factor in the development of the disease, rather than an effect of it.[28,29]

Basophilia and eosinophilia are both described in TB.[30] They also occur in patients with marked inflammatory responses of other causes, although basophilia and eosinophilia are rare in the course of pyogenic bacterial infection.

The monocyte/macrophage line plays an essential role in the immune response to tuberculous infection.[31] True monocytosis is well documented as a consequence of chronic inflammation.[32] There may be a significant quantitative increase in monocytes as well as morphologic changes. Circulating monocytes may be large and vacuolated and may, in fact, be circulating macrophages. It is the monocyte/macrophage line that is responsible for the formation of granulomata.[33] The macrophage serves as the initial habitat for mycobacteria after activation by T-lymphocytes. These macrophages become effectors against the engulfed pathogens.[34] *M. tuberculosis* may enter the host macrophage and cause maturation arrest.[35] This maturation arrest leads to impaired phagosomal capability.[36,37] At least three pathogenic events occur. These include decreased phagolysosome activity,[36] apoptosis, and abnormal interleukin-12 production.[38,39]

Another complication of activated macrophage production is the hemophagocytic syndrome (HPS). This syndrome includes febrile hepatosplenomegaly, pancytopenia, hypofibrinemia, and liver dysfunction. This syndrome is well described in the setting of TB and other inflammatory conditions. The hematologic sequelae may be primarily anemia, neutropenia, thrombocytopenia, or a combination of these. Hemophagocytic syndrome usually responds to treatment of the underlying cause, in this case antituberculous treatment. Therapeutic plasma exchange has been suggested as a therapeutic tool for HPS refractory to conventional therapy.[40–47]

PLATELETS

Thrombocytopenia in TB is usually a complication of therapy; however, many mechanisms specific to the disease itself can cause thrombocytopenia. First, marrow effects such as fibrosis, granulomatosis, amyloidosis, and necrosis cause thrombocytopenia just as they cause a decrease in other cell lines.[48] In these instances, thrombocytopenia is less common than neutropenia or anemia. Second, hypersplenism complicating TB may be associated with thrombocytopenia.[49] Disseminated intravascular coagulation (DIC) is a known complication of TB.[50,51] A form of thrombocytopenia not attributable to DIC (without marrow or spleen involvement) is also described. This is similar to the non-DIC thrombocytopenia which occurs in a variety of viral infections.[52]

There continue to be additional reports of immune thrombocytopenia in association with or as a pressing feature of TB.[53,54] It is postulated that the tubercle bacilli stimulates suppressor monocytes and decreases T-lymphocytes. The reduction in T-cell suppression then permits development and expression of an antiplatelet antibody. In these patients, the thrombocytopenia occurs before antituberculous therapy.[55] New cases suggest the development of an antiplatelet antibody directed against cryptic antigens which become exposed during infection. Supportive evidence includes immunofluorescence showing an increase in binding of circulating cytotoxic immunoglobins to autologous platelets.[56,57] Unlike the usual pattern in ITP, there are no circulating antiplatelet antibodies that react with normal donor platelets.[34] It has been reported that therapy with intravenous immunoglobins, which would be expected to bind destructive antibodies, rapidly reverses thrombocytopenia.[58]

Thrombocytopenia is a prominent feature of the pentad of manifestations known as thrombocytopenic purpura (TTP). The disorder also includes microangiopathic hemolytic anemia, renal and neurologic dysfunction, and fever. This complex has occurred in association with many types of infection, but rarely with TB. Two cases document the association with untreated TB and remission of the TTP with successful antituberculous treatment.[59] The production of interleukin-1, which is a procoagulant, is postulated to lead to the vasculitic damage that is responsible for this syndrome.[60] Additionally Henoch-Schonlein purpura, a syndrome similar to TTP but including only thrombocytopenia and transient renal dysfunction, has been seen with pulmonary TB.[61]

Thrombocytosis is a well-known response to inflammation and is common in TB, occurring in a reported 12.9% in one series.[1,62] For unknown reasons, patients with tuberculous pneumonia have higher platelet counts than similarly ill patients with nontuberculous pneumonia.[63]

The degree of thrombocytosis corresponds with the degree of inflammatory response as measured by the erythrocyte sedimentation rate. The inflammatory process leads to production of a plasma-platelet stimulating factor; this factor parallels the inflammatory phase of the illness and resolves as the patient improves. Platelet survival is decreased, and there is an increase in small megakaryo-cytes in the marrow, some of which show decreased nuclear ploidy. These platelets may exhibit increased *in vitro* aggregation, which is not the usual observation in inflammatory thrombocytosis.[64]

The lymphoid system is also widely affected by tuberculous infection. Both lymphocytosis[65] and lympho-cytopenia are reported. Active TB causes a decrease in total T-cells secondary to a decrease in T4 cells.[66] The CD4 count may fall transiently to fewer than 200/ml^3, even in human immunodeficiency virus (HIV)-negative patients. Initially described in patients older than 60 years, the marked T-lymphocytopenia was recently described in a 47-year-old HIV-negative patient.[67,68] As with other infections that may result in a transient fall in CD4 count in HIV-negative patients, TB is usually associated with a CD4:CD8 ratio greater than 1.0.[69] In addition, T cells in TB patients have been shown to be less functional with lower production of interleukin-2 and interferon gamma as compared to normal healthy controls.[70] Total B cells are also decreased. Multiple cytokines, including interleukin and tumor necrosis factor, are activated.[71] Successful anti-tuberculous treatment restores these values to normal.[72] Lymphocytosis is not unexpected because this is a normal immune response, both in blood and in the secondary lymphoid organs. Localized and generalized lym-phadenopathy, splenomegaly, and increased circulating lymphocytes occur as related phenomena.[73] Secondary increases in IgG, IgA, and IgM are detected. Decreased levels of interferon-gamma are not uncommon.[74]

An interesting case of a patient with active pulmonary TB and secondary cryoglobulinemia has been reported. The patient had secondary proteinuria, an elevated sedi-mentation rate, and anemia. All manifestations resolved with successful treatment of TB.[75]

COAGULATION SYSTEM

We have already mentioned the hypercoagulable state associated with TTP occurring in association with untreated TB. Other inflammatory responses leading to hypercoagulability demonstrated *in vitro* include pro-duction of fibrinogen, fibrin degradation products, and tissue plasminogen activator.[76,77] In one study, the activated macrophages in patients with TB were shown to have pro-coagulant activity due to elaboration of thromboplastin, which is involved in the formation of fibrin.[76] Other proco-agulant changes include disrupted vascular endothelium due to cytokines released by activated monocytes,[78] cytokine-mediated platelet hyperreactivity, and DIC with its combination of endothelial damage and consumption

of naturally occurring anticoagulants.[79] Other hemostatic changes which result in hypercoagulability include elevated factor VIII, depressed antithrombin III, consumption of protein C, and increased platelet activation.[80,81]

DIC in association with TB is well described and additional cases have been reported.[82] The manifestations of DIC vary. Evidence of hypocoagulability is frequent as evidenced clinically by abnormality bleeding, con-sumption of clotting factors, and consumption or dys-function of platelets. Additionally, acquired factor V dysfunction due to presence of an inhibitor or an IgG or IgM inflammatory response has been described. One of four cases has been associated with hemorrhage.[83] Others have been associated with serologic abnormalities but no clinical bleeding. Recently described is a patient with active TB who developed a high titer of factor VIII inhibitor leading to active bleeding. This patient had an elevated activated partial thromboplastin time (APTT). His clinical bleeding and elevated APTT improved gradually as his factor VIII inhibitor levels declined in response to treatment of his TB.[84]

EFFECTS OF ANTITUBERCULOUS MEDICATIONS

Antituberculous medications have significant hematologic effects (Fig 28-1). For example, isoniazid may cause sider-oblastic anemia due to abnormal B$_6$ metabolism. Supplementation of isoniazid therapy with pyridoxine 200 mg daily can prevent this sideroblastic anemia.[85] Sideroblastic anemia can also occur with cycloserine and pyrazinamide.[86] Sometimes ringed sideroblasts persist after an offending drug has been discontinued or, alternatively, they may appear during treatment in patients who do not develop anemia. Para-amino salicylic acid (PAS) can produce B$_{12}$-deficient megaloblastic anemia.[87] PAS and rifampin can both induce hemolytic anemia. The rifampin-induced anemia has been associated with strongly positive direct antiglobulin tests for IgG and C3d. Specific testing for rifampin-dependent antibodies have been positive. It is thought that rifampin stimulates the production of autoan-tibodies and/or drug-dependent antibodies.[88] Rifampin can be associated with a flu-like syndrome that may herald the onset of hemolysis during treatment.[89] This flu-like syndrome has been described with and without con-comitant TTP.[18] Isoniazid has been reported to cause pure red cell aplasia.[90] Rifampin is well known as a cause of thrombocytopenia.[91–93] Rifampin has been shown to be a cause of direct drug-dependent binding of antibody to the platelet glycoprotein Ib/IX complex.[93] This complication is more commonly noted with intermittent rifampin

	Ethionamide	Rifapentine	Levofloxacin	Capreomycin	Ciprofloxacin	Cycloserine	Ethambutol	Isoniazid	Ofloxacin	PAS	Pyrazinamide	Rifabutin	Rifampin	Streptomycin	Thiacetazone
ERYTHROCYTE															
Red cell aplasia															
Sideroblastic anemia								X							X
B$_{12}$ deficient megaloblastosis						X		X		X					
Immune hemolysis								X	X						
G-6-PD hemolysis	X	X						X	X	X		X	X	X	X
Aplastic anemia														X	
Folate deficiency	X	X						X	X	X		X	X	X	
Methemoglobinemia									X						
Acute porphyria	X												X		
GRANULOCYTE															
Leukopenia	X	X	X	X			X	X	X	X		X	X	X	
Eosinophilia			X	X											
Agranulocytosis	X							X		X		X	X		
Leukemoid reaction	X									X			X		X
THROMBOCYTE															
Thrombocytopenia	X	X	X	X	X		X	X	X	X	X	X	X		X
Thrombotic thrombocytopenic purpura		X	X										X		
Thrombocytosis								X							

Fig. 28-1. Hematologic complications of antituberculous medications. (Adapted from Huxley HM, Knox-Macaulay HM. Tuberculosis and the haemopoietic system. *Bailliere's Clin Haematol.* 1992;5:101–129. Copyright 1992 Elsevier Ltd. Reprinted with permission from Elsevier.)

administration because daily rifampin appears to provide immune desensitization, and the thrombocytopenia from rifampin correlates with the presence of rifampin-dependent antibodies.[94] A description of the safe reintroduction of rifampin in a patient who had rifampin-associated thrombocytopenia challenges the standard proscription against use of rifampin once there has been a decrease in platelets regardless of whether this has occurred with continuous or interrupted treatment. Care should be used in the interpretation of this single-case report.[95] Thrombocytopenia is also a prominent feature of rifampin-induced TTP. This syndrome is reversible upon cessation of rifampin.[96] Both ethambutol and pyrazinamide have been reported to cause thrombocytopenia.[97,98]

Neutropenia is reported as a consequent of PAS, isoniazid, rifampin, and streptomycin. The proposed mechanisms include marrow toxicity and immune destruction.[99]

Decreased myelopoiesis has been documented in a patient with rifampin-induced neutropenia.[100]

Streptomycin has been reported to cause a drug rash with eosinophilia and systemic symptoms (DRES).[101] Isoniazid has been reported to cause a lupus syndrome which includes hematologic effects and arthralgia.[102]

Finally, a reversible inhibitor of factor XIII has been attributed to isoniazid in a patient with Waldenstrom macroglobulinemia.[103]

CONCLUSION

These hematologic consequences of TB are varied and complex. They may provide a valuable clue to a perplexing diagnosis, indicate a complication of underlying infection requiring specific therapy, or warn the clinician of drug toxicity or allergy. Taken as a whole, they remind us that the blood is yet another organ seriously affected by tuberculous infection.

REFERENCES

1. Olaniyi JA, Aken'Ova YA. Haematologic profile of patients with pulmonary tuberculosis in Ibadan, Nigeria. *A J Med Sci.* 2003 September;32(3):239–242.

2. Singh KJ, Ahluwalia G, Sharma SK, et al. Significance of haematological manifestations in patients with tuberculosis. *J Assoc Physicians India* 2001;49,788: 790–794.

3. Baynes RD, Flax H, Bothwell TH, et al. Red blood cell distribution width in the anemia secondary to tuberculosis. *Am J Clin Pathol.* 1986:226–229.

4. Douglas SW, Adamson JW. The anemia of chronic disorders: studies of marrow regulation and iron metabolism. *Blood.* 1990;45(1):55–65.

5. Baynes RD, Flax H, Bothwell TH, et al. Haematological and iron-related measurements in active pulmonary tuberculosis. *Scand J Haematol.* 1986;36(3):280–287. *Am J Clin Pathol.* 1986;85(2):226–229.

6. Gobin J, Horwitz MA. Exochelins of *Mycobacterium tuberculosis* remove iron from human iron-binding proteins and donate iron to mycobactins in the *M. tuberculosis* cell wall. *J Exp Med.*, 1996;183(4):1527–1532.

7. Boeser HP. Iron metabolism in inflammation and malignant disease. In: Jacobs A, Worwood M, eds. *Iron in Biochemistry and Medicine, II.* London: Academic Press; 1974:605–640.

8. Ebrahim O, Folb PI, Robson SC, et al. Blunted erythropoietin response to anaemia in tuberculosis. *Eur J Haematol.* 1995;55(4):251–254.

9. O'Connor NJ, Hotfbrand AV. Anaemia in systemic disease. In: Delamore IW, Liu Yin JA, eds. *Haematologic Aspects of Systemic Disease.* London: Bailliere Tindall; 1998:38.

10. Das BS, Devi U, Mohan Rao C, et al. Effect of iron supplementation on mild to moderate anaemia in pulmonary tuberculosis. *Br J Nutr* 2003;90(3):541–550.

11. Kuo PH, Yang PC, Kuo SS, et al. Severe immune hemolytic anemia in disseminated tuberculosis with response to antituberculosis therapy. *Chest.* 2001;119(6):1961–1963.

12. Murray HW. Transient autoimmune hemolytic anemia and pulmonary tuberculosis. *N Engl J Med.* 1978;299(9):488.

13. Nusbaum NJ: Concise review: Genetic bases for sideroblastic anemia. *Am J Hematol.* 1990;37:41–44.

14. Viallard JF, Parrens M, Boiron JM, et al. Reversible myelofibrosis induced by tuberculosis. *Clin Infect Dis,* 2002;34(12):1641–1643.

15. Laszlo J, Huang AT. Anemia associated with marrow infiltration. In: William WJ, Beutler E, Erslev AJ, et al., eds. *Hematology*, 4th ed. New York, NY: McGraw-Hill;1990: 546–548.

16. Andre J, Schwartz R, Dameshek W. Tuberculosis and myelosclerosis with myeloid metaplasia; report of three cases. *JAMA.* 1961;178:1169–1174.

17. Adamson JW, Ersley AJ. Aplastic anemia. In: Williams WJ, Beutler E, Ersley AJ, et al., eds. *Hematology*, 4th ed. New York, NY: McGraw-Hill; 1990:158–174.

18. Ip M, Cheng KP, Cheung WC. Disseminated intravascular coagulopathy associated with rifampicin. *Tubercle.* 1991; Dec;72(4):291–293.

19. Huxley HM, Knox-Macaulay HM. Tuberculosis and the haemopoietic system. *Bailliere's Clin Haematol.* 1992;5: 101–129.

20. Sunga MN Jr, Reyes CV, Zvetina J, et al. Resolution of secondary amyloidosis 14 years after adequate chemotherapy for skeletal tuberculosis. *South Med J.* 1989;82(1):92–93.

21. Singh R, Singh MM, Lahiri VL, et al. Tuberculosis as a continuing cause of secondary amyloidosis in northern India. *J Indian Med Assoc.* 1987;85(11):328–332.

22. Paydas S, Ergin M, Baslamisli F, et al. Bone marrow necrosis: clinicopathologic analysis of 20 cases and review of the literature. *Br J Haematol.* 2002;70(4):300–305.

23. Gallagher NI, Donati RM. Inappropriate erythropoietin elaboration. *Ann N Y Acad Sci.* 1968;149(1):528–538.

24. Appleberg R, Silva MT. T-cell-dependent chronic neutrophilia during mycobacterial infections. *Clin Exp Immunol.* 1989;78:478–483.

25. Twomey JJ, Leavell BS: Leukemoid reactions to tuberculosis. *Arch Intern Med.* 1965;116:21–28.

26. Savage PJ, Dellinger RP, Barnes JV, et al. Pelger-Huet anomaly of granulocytes in a patient with tuberculosis. *Chest.* 1984;85(1):131–132.

27. Cicchitto G, Parravicini M, De Lorenzo S, et al. Tuberculosis and Pelger-Huet anomaly. Case report. *Panminerva Med.* 1999;41(4):367–369.

28. Glasser RM, Walker RI, Herion JC. The significance of hematologic abnormalities in patients with tuberculosis. *Arch Intern Med.* 1970;125(4):691–695.

29. Coburn RJ, England JM, Samson DM, et al. Tuberculosis and blood disorders. *Br J Haematol.* 1973;25(6):793–799.

30. Juhlin L. Basophil and eosinophil leukocytes in various internal disorders. *Acta Med Scand.* 1963;174:249–254.

31. Ina Y, Takada K, Yamamoto M, et al. Antigen-presenting capacity of alveolar macrophages and monocytes in pulmonary tuberculosis. *Eur Respir J.* 1991;4(1):88–93.

32. Kelsey PR. Blood film and marrow. In: Delamore IW, Liu Yin JA, eds, *Haematologic Aspects of Systemic Disease.* London: Bailliere Tindall; 1990:3.

33. Sewell RL. Lymphocyte abnormalities in myeloma. *Br J Haematol.* 1977;36(4):545–551.

34. Kaufmann SH. The macrophage in tuberculosis: sinner or saint? The T-cell decides. *Pathobiology.* 1991;59(3):153–155.

35. Vergne I, Chua J, Deretic V. *Mycobacterium tuberculosis* phagosome maturation arrest: selective targeting of PI3P-dependent membrane trafficking. *Traffic.* 2003; 4(9): 600–606.

36. Vergne I, Chua J, Deretic V. Tuberculosis toxin blocking phagosome maturation inhibits a novel Ca2+/calmodulin-PI3K hVPS34 cascade. *J Exp Med.* 2003;198(4): 653–659.

37. Malik ZA, Thompson CR, Hashimi S, et al. Cutting edge: *Mycobacterium tuberculosis* blocks Ca2+ signaling and

phagosome maturation in human macrophages via specific inhibition of sphingosine kinase. *J Immunol.* 2003; 170(6): 2811–2815.

38. Dao DN, Kremer L, Guerardel Y, et al. *Mycobacterium tuberculosis* lipomannan induces apoptosis and interleukin-12 production in macrophages. *Infect Immun,* 2004; 72(4): 2067–2074.

39. Gil DP, Leon LG, Correa LI, et al. Differential induction of apoptosis and necrosis in monocytes from patients with tuberculosis and healthy control subjects. *J Infect Dis.* 2004;189(11):2120–2128.

40. Chandra P, Chaudhery SA, Rosner F, et al. Transient histiocytosis with striking phagocytosis of platelets, leukocytes, and erythrocytes. *Arch Intern Med.* 1975;135(7):989–991.

41. Risdall RJ, Brunning RD, Hernandez JI, et al. Bacteria-associated hemophagocytic syndrome. *Cancer.* 1984; 54(12):2968–2972.

42. Weintraub M, Siegman-Igra Y, Josiphov J, et al. Histiocytic hemophagocytosis in miliary tuberculosis. *Arch Intern Med.* 1984;144(10):2055–2056.

43. Satomi A, Nagai S, Nagai T, et al. Effect of plasma exchange on refractory hemophagocytic syndrome complicated with myelodysplastic syndrome. *Ther Apher.* 1999;3(4):317–319.

44. Dhote R, Simon J, Papo T, et al. Reactive hemophagocytic syndrome in adult systemic disease: report of twenty-six cases and literature review. *Arthritis Rheum.* 2003;49(5); 633–639.

45. Karras A, Thervet E, Legendre C. Hemophagocytic syndrome in renal transplant recipients: report of 17 cases and review of literature. *Transplantation.* 2004; 77(2): 238–243.

46. Yang WK, Fu LS, Lan JL, et al. *Mycobacterium avium complex*-associated hemophagocytic syndrome in systemic lupus erythematosus patient: report of one case. *Lupus.* 2003;12(4):312–316.

47. Mariani F, Goletti D, Ciaramella A, et al. Macrophage response to *Mycobacterium tuberculosis* during HIV infection: relationships between macrophage activation and apoptosis. *Current Molecular Medicine.* 2001;1(2): 209–216.

48. Finch SC, Castleman B. Case records of the Massachusetts General Hospital. *N Engl J Med.* 1963;268:378.

49. Ersley AJ. Hypersplenism and hyposplenism. In: Williams WJ, Beutler E, Ersley AJ. et al., eds. *Hematology,* 4th ed. New York, NY: McGraw-Hill; 1990:695.

50. Rosenberg MJ, Rumans LW. Survival of a patient with pancytopenia and disseminated coagulation associated with miliary tuberculosis. *Chest.* 1978;73(4):536–539.

51. Murray HW, Tuazon CU, Kirmani N, et al. The adult respiratory distress syndrome associated with miliary tuberculosis. *Chest.* 1978;73(1):37–43.

52. Chia YC, Machin SJ. Tuberculosis and severe thrombocytopaenia. *Br J Clin Pract.* 1979;33(2):55–56, 58.

53. Ghobrial MW, Albornoz MA. Immune thrombocytopenia: a rare presenting manifestation of tuberculosis. *Am J Hematol.* 2001;67(2):139–143.

54. Spedini P. Tuberculosis presenting as immune thrombocytopenic purpura. *Haematologica.* 2002;87(2):ELT09.

55. Jurak SS, Aster R, Sawaf H. Immune thrombocytopenia associated with tuberculosis. *Clin Pediatr (Phila).* 1983; 22(4):318–319.

56. Richards EM, Shneerson JM, Baglin TP. Thrombocytopenia responding to empirical antituberculous therapy. *Clin Lab Haematol.* 1994;16(1):89–90.

57. Al-Majed SA, Al-Momen AK, Al-Kassimi FA, et al. Tuberculosis presenting as immune thrombocytopenic purpura. Acta Haematol. 1995;94(3):135–138.

58. Boots RJ, Roberts AW, McEvoy D. Immune thrombocytopenia complicating pulmonary tuberculosis: case report and investigation of mechanisms. *Thorax.* 1992;47(5): 396–397.

59. Pavithran K, Vijayalekshmi N. Thrombocytopenic purpura with tuberculous adenitis. *Indian J Med Sci.* 1993;47(10): 239–240.

60. Toscano V, Bontadini A, Falsone G, et al. Thrombotic thrombocytopenic purpura associated with primary tuberculosis. *Infection.* 1995;23(1):58–59.

61. Islek I, Muslu A, Totan M, et al. Henoch-Schonlein purpura and pulmonary tuberculosis. *Pediatr Int.* 2002;44(5): 545–546.

62. Baynes RD, Bothwell TH, Flax H, et al. Reactive thrombocytosis in pulmonary tuberculosis. *J Clin Pathol.* 1987; 40(6):676–679.

63. Hui KP, Chin NK, Chan TB, et al. Platelet count as an independent predictor differentiating between tuberculosis and non-tuberculosis pneumonia. *Tuber Lung Dis.* 1994; 75(2):157.

64. Marchasin S, Wallerstein RO, Aggeler PM. Variations of the platelet count in disease. *Calif Med.* 1964;101: 95–100.

65. Hamblin TJ, Kruger A. Lypmphocyte abnormalities. In: Delamore IW, Liu Yin JA, eds: *Haematologic Aspects of Systemic Disease.* London: Bailliere Tindall; 1990:155.

66. Onwubalili JK, Edwards AJ, Palmer L. T4 lymphopenia in human tuberculosis. *Tubercle.* 1987;68(3):195–200.

67. Fantin B, Joly V, Elbim C, et al. Lymphocyte subset counts during the course of community-acquired pneumonia: evolution according to age, human immunodeficiency virus status, and etiologic microorganisms. *Clin Infect Dis.* 1996;22(6):1096–1098.

68. Zaharatos GJ, Behr MA, Libman MD. Profound T-lymphocytopenia and cryptococcemia in a human immunodeficiency virus-seronegative patient with disseminated tuberculosis. *Clin Infect Dis.* 2001;33(11): E125–E128.

69. Laurence J. T-cell subsets in health, infectious disease, and idiopathic CD4+ T-lymphocytopenia. *Ann Intern Med.* 1993;119(1):55–62.

70. Talreja J, Bhatnagar A, Jindal SK, et al. Influence of *Mycobacterium tuberculosis* on differential activation of helper T-cells. *Clin Exp Immunol.* 2003;131(2); 292–298.

71. Law K, Weiden M, Harkin T, et al. Increased release of interleukin-1 beta, interleukin-6, and tumor necrosis factor-alpha by bronchoalveolar cells lavaged from

involved sites in pulmonary tuberculosis. *Am J Respir Crit Care Med.* 1996;153(2):799–804.

72. Singhal M, Banavalikar JN, Sharma S, et al. Peripheral blood T-lymphocyte subpopulations in patients with tuberculosis and the effect of chemotherapy. *Tubercle.* 1989; 70(3):171–178.

73. Williams WJ. Lymph node enlargement. In Williams WJ, Beutler E, Ersley AJ. et al., eds. *Hematology*, 4th ed. New York, NY: McGraw-Hill; 1990:954–955.

74. Kyle RA.: Monoclonal gammopathy of undetermined significance (MGUS): a review. *Clin Haematol.* 1982; 1(1):123–150.

75. Teruel JL, Matesanz R, Mampaso F, et al. Pulmonary tuberculosis, cryoglobulinemia and immune complex glomerulonephritis. *Clin Nephrol.* 1987 Jan;27(1):48–49.

76. Robson SC, White NW, Aronson I, et al. Acute-phase response and the hypercoagulable state in pulmonary tuberculosis. *Br J Haematol.* 1996;93(4):943–949.

77. Selvaraj P, Venkataprasad N, Vijayan VK, et al. Procoagulant activity of bronchoalveolar lavage fluids taken from the site of tuberculous lesions. *Eur Respir J.* 1994;7(7):1227–1232.

78. Sarode R, Bhasin D, Marwaha N, et al. Hyperaggregation of platelets in intestinal tuberculosis: role of platelets in chronic inflammation. *Am J Hematol.* 1995;48(1):52–54.

79. Manzella JP, Kellogg J, Sanstead JK. *Mycobacterium tuberculosis* bacteremia and disseminated coagulation. *JAMA.* 1985;254(19):2741.

80. Turken O, Kunter E, Sezer M, et al. Hemostatic changes in active pulmonary tuberculosis. *Int J Tuberc Lung Dis.* 2002;6(10):927–932.

81. Casanova-Roman MM, Rios J, Sanchez-Porto A, et al. Deep venous thrombosis associated with pulmonary tuberculosis and transient protein S deficiency. *Am J Hematol.* 2004;75(2):118–119.

82. Stein DS, Libertin CR. Disseminated intravascular coagulation in association with cavitary tuberculosis. *South Med J.* 1990;83(1):60–63.

83. Aliaga JL, de Gracia J, Vidal R, et al. Acquired factor V deficiency in a patient with pulmonary tuberculosis. *Eur Respir J.* 1990;3(1):109–110.

84. Ogata H, Sakai S, Koiwa F, et al. Plasma exchange for acquired hemophilia: a case report. *Ther Apher.* 1999;3(4): 320–322.

85. Demiroglu H, Dundar S. Vitamin B6 response of sideroblastic anaemia in a patient with tuberculosis. *Br J Clin Pract.* 1999;51(3):146.

86. Sharp RA, Lowe JG, Johnston RN. Anti-tuberculous drugs and sideroblastic anaemia. *Br J Clin Pract.* 1990; 44(12): 706–707.

87. Cameron SJ. Tuberculosis and the blood—a special relationship? *Tubercle.* 1974;55(1):55–72.

88. Ahrens N, Genth R, Salama A. Belated diagnosis in three patients with rifampicin-induced immune haemolytic anaemia. *Br J Haematol.* 2002;117(2):441–443.

89. Yeo CT, Wang YT, Poh SC. Mild haemolysis associated with flu-syndrome during daily rifampicin treatment—a case report. *Singapore Med J.* 1989;30(2):215–216.

90. Claiborne RA, Dutt AK. Isoniazid-induced pure red cell aplasia. *Am Rev Respir Dis.* 1985 Jun;131(6):947–949.

91. Aquinas M, Allan WG, Horsfall PA, et al. Adverse reactions to daily and intermittent rifampicin regimens for pulmonary tuberculosis in Hong Kong. *Br Med J.* 1972; 1(803):765–771.

92. Prasad R, Kant S, Pandey DK. Rifampicin induced thrombocytopenia. *J Assoc Physicians India.* 1999;47(2): 252.

93. Pereira J, Hidalgo P, Ocqueteau M, et al. Glycoprotein Ib/IX complex is the target in rifampicin-induced immune thrombocytopenia. *Br J Haematol.* 2000;110(4): 907–910.

94. Lee CH, Lee CJ. Thrombocytopenia—a rare but potentially serious side effect of initial daily and interrupted use of rifampicin. *Chest.* 1989;96(1):202–203.

95. Bhasin DK, Sarode R, Puri S. Can rifampicin be restarted in patients with rifampicin-induced thrombocytopenia? *Tubercle.* 1991;72(4):306–307.

96. Fahal IH, Williams PS, Clark RE, et al. Thrombotic thrombocytopenic purpura due to rifampicin. *BMJ.* 1992; 304(6831):882.

97. Prasad R, Mukerji PK. Ethambutol-induced thrombocytopaenia. *Tubercle.* 1989;70(3):211–212.

98. Malik GH, Al-Harbi AS, Al-Mohaya S, et al. Eleven years of experience with dialysis associated tuberculosis. *Clin Nephrol.* 2002;58(5):356–362.

99. Mandell GL, Sande MA. Drugs used in the chemotherapy of tuberculosis and leprosy. In: Goodman LS, Gilman A, eds. *Pharmacologic Basis of Therapeutics*, 8th ed. New York: Pergamon Press; 1990:1146–1164.

100. Van Assendelft AH. Leukopenia in rifampicin chemotherapy. *J Antimicrob Chemother.* 1985;16(3):407–408.

101. Passeron T, Ndir MC, Aubron C, et al. Drug rash with eosinophilia and systemic symptoms (DRESS) due to streptomycin. *Acta Derm Venereol.* 2004;84(1):92–93.

102. Siddiqui MA, Khan IA. Isoniazid-induced lupus erythematosus presenting with cardiac tamponade. *Am J Ther.* 2002;9(2):163–165.

103. Krumdieck R, Shaw DR, Huang ST, et al. Hemorrhagic disorder due to an isoniazid-associated acquired factor XIII inhibitor in a patient with Waldenstrom's macroglobulinemia. *Am J Med.* 1991;90(5):639–645.

29

Tuberculosis in Infants and Children

Jeffrey R. Starke

The clinical expression of disease caused by *Mycobacterium tuberculosis* is greatly different in infants, children and adolescents from what it is in adults. Much adult pulmonary tuberculosis (TB) is caused by a reactivation of dormant organisms, which are lodged in the apices of the lungs during hematogenous dissemination at the time of infection. Childhood TB is usually a complication of the pathophysiologic events surrounding the initial infection. The time interval between infection and disease is usually years to decades long in adults, but is often only weeks to months long in small children. Children are more prone to developing extrapulmonary TB, but rarely infectious pulmonary disease. As a result of the basic differences in pathophysiology of TB between adults and children, the approach to diagnosis, treatment and prevention of infection and disease in children are necessarily different.

Many aspects of the various forms of childhood TB have been discussed briefly in other chapters of this book. This chapter will focus on the fundamental nature of exposure, infection and disease in children, emphasizing how and why children are approached differently from adults. The effects of these differences on the public health approach to TB control in children also will be explained.

TERMINOLOGY

The terminology used to describe various stages and presentation of childhood TB often has been a source of confusion for physicians. It follows the pathophysiology, but the stages are sometimes not completely distinct in children.

Exposure means that the child has had significant contact with an adult or adolescent with infectious pulmonary TB. The contact investigation—examining those individuals close to a suspected case of TB with a tuberculin skin test, chest radiograph, and physical examination—is the most important activity in a community to prevent cases of TB in children.[1] The most frequent setting for exposure of a child is the household, but it can occur in school, daycare center, or any other closed setting. In this stage, the tuberculin skin test is negative, the chest radiograph is normal, and the child lacks signs or symptoms of disease. Some exposed children may have inhaled droplet nuclei infected with *M. tuberculosis* and have early infection, but the clinician cannot know it because it takes up to 3 months for delayed hypersensitivity to tuberculin, a positive skin test, to develop. The World Health Organization recommends that children younger than 5 years of age in the exposure stage should be treated to prevent the rapid development of disseminated or meningeal TB, which can occur before the skin test becomes reactive.

Infection occurs when the individual inhales droplet nuclei containing *M. tuberculosis*, which becomes established intracellularly within the lung and associated lymphoid tissue. The hallmark of TB infection is a reactive tuberculin skin test. In this stage, the child has no signs or symptoms and the chest radiograph is either normal or reveals only granuloma or calcifications in the lung parenchyma and/or regional lymph nodes. In developed countries, all children with TB infection should receive treatment, usually with isoniazid (INH), to prevent the development of disease in the near or distant future. Disease occurs when signs or symptoms, or radiographic manifestations caused by *M. tuberculosis* become apparent.

The word *tuberculosis* refers to disease. Not all infected individuals have the same risk of developing disease. An immunocompetent adult with untreated TB infection has approximately a 5–10 percent lifetime risk of developing disease; half of the risk occurs in the first 2–3 years after infection. Historical studies have shown that up to 40% of immunocompetent infants with untreated TB infection develop disease, often serious, life-threatening forms, within 1–2 years.

The phrase "primary tuberculosis" has been used to describe childhood pulmonary disease that arises as a complication of the initial infection. Unfortunately, this phase also has been used to describe the initial infection even in the absence of radiographic or clinical manifestations. Infection and the onset of disease are separated by time, in adults and are usually fairly distinct events. In children, disease complicates the initial infection so the two stages are on a continuum, often with indistinct borders.[2] This lack of clarity can cause confusion when deciding which treatment regimen—how many drugs—to use. The current consensus is to consider disease to be present if adenopathy or other chest radiograph manifestations of infection by *M. tuberculosis* can be seen.

EPIDEMIOLOGY

Disease and Infection

Because most children with TB infection and disease acquired the organism from an adult in their environment, the epidemiology of childhood TB tends to follow that in adults. The risk of a child acquiring TB infection is environmental, determined by the likelihood she will be in contact with an adult with contagious TB. In contrast, the risk of a child developing TB disease depends more on host immunologic and genetic factors.

It is estimated that the worldwide annual burden of TB on children is 1.5 million cases and 500,000 deaths.[3] Adult TB case numbers have increased over the past decade in every region of the world except Western Europe. There are no comparable data, but it is likely that childhood TB has grown in numbers as well.

Between 1953 and 1980, childhood TB rates in the United States declined about 6% per year. Between 1980 and 1987, the case rates remained relatively flat, but they began to increase in 1988. With improvements in TB control, rates of childhood TB started to decline in 1993 and have continued on a downward trend (Fig. 29-1).[4] In 2003, there were 992 cases in children less than 15 years old.[5] About 60% of cases occur among infants and children less than 5 years of age. Between the ages of 5 and 14, often called the "favored age", children usually have the lowest rates of TB disease in any population. The clinical expression of TB in childhood differs by age (Table 29-1). Other than meningitis or lymph node disease, other forms of extrapulmonary TB are more common in older children and adolescents. The gender ratio for TB in children is about 1:1 in contrast to adults, in whom males predominate.

Table 29-1. Median Age of Children (less than 20 years old) with Tuberculosis by Predominant Site, United States, 1988*

Site	Case Number (%)	Median Age (Years)
Pulmonary	1,213 (77.5)	6
Lymphatic	209 (13.3)	5
Pleural	49 (3.1)	16
Meningeal	29 (1.9)	2
Bone/Joint	19 (1.2)	8
Miliary	14 (0.9)	1
Genitourinary	13 (0.8)	16
Peritoneal	4 (0.3)	13
Other	16 (1.1)	12
Total	1,566 (100)	6

*Provided by the Centers for Disease Control and Prevention.

Tuberculosis case rates historically have been the highest between January and June in the Northern Hemisphere, possibly because of more extensive indoor contact with infectious adults during the colder months. Childhood TB is geographically focal in the United States, with 8 states—California, Florida, Georgia, Illinois, New York, New Jersey, Pennsylvania, and Texas—accounting for 70% of reported cases among children less than 5 years of age.[4] As expected, disease rates are highest in cities with more than 250,000 residents.

Childhood TB case rates in the United States are strikingly higher among ethnic and racial minority groups

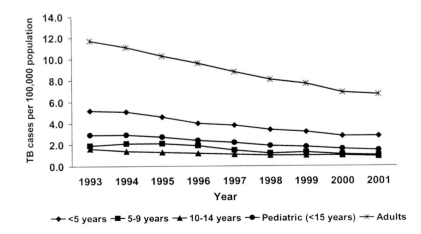

Fig. 29-1. Tuberculosis case rates by age group for children, 1993–2001. (Data in the public domain, courtesy of the Centers for Disease Control and Prevention).

and the foreign-born than in Whites. Approximately 88% of cases occur among African American, Hispanic, Asian and Native American children; this reflects the risk of transmission within the living conditions of these children.[4,6] Although most of these children were born in the United States, from 1986 to 2001 the proportion of foreign-born children with TB rose from 13% to 28%. Most cases occur within 5 years of immigration. Foreign-born adoptee children also have high rates of TB.[7]

Most children are infected with *M. tuberculosis* in the home but outbreaks of childhood TB centered in elementary and high schools, nursery schools, family day-care homes, churches, school buses, and stores still occur. A high-risk adult working in the area has been the source of the outbreak in most cases.

The recent epidemic of HIV infection has had a profound effect on the epidemiology of TB among children as a result of two major mechanisms: (1) HIV-infected adults with TB may transmit *M. tuberculosis* to children, some of whom will develop TB disease,[8] and (2) children with HIV infection may be at increased risk of progressing from TB infection to disease.[9] Several studies of childhood TB have demonstrated that increased case rates have been associated with a simultaneous increase among HIV-infected adults in the community. In general, HIV-infected children may be more likely to have contact with HIV-infected adults who are at high risk for TB. Tuberculosis is probably under-diagnosed among HIV-infected children for two reasons: (1) because of the similarity of its clinical presentation to other opportunistic infections and acquired immunodeficiency syndrome (AIDS)-related conditions and (2) the difficulty in confirming the diagnosis with positive cultures. Children with TB disease should have HIV serotesting because the two infections are linked epidemiologically.

Although data on TB disease in children are readily available, data concerning TB infection without disease (positive skin test) are lacking. Tuberculosis infection is a reportable condition in only four states, and national surveys were discontinued in 1971. The most efficient method of finding children infected with *M. tuberculosis* is through contact investigations of adults with infectious pulmonary TB.[1] On average, 30–50% of all household contacts of an index case have a reactive skin test.

In developing countries, TB infection rates among the young population average 20–50%. In most US children, the risk is less than 1%, but in some urban populations the risk is much higher. In a 1990 study of Boston public schools, 5.1% of seventh graders and 8.9% of tenth graders were tuberculin skin test-positive.[10] In Los Angeles and Houston public schools, 2–5% of elementary school children are infected. In these and other surveys, the majority of children with reactive skin tests were foreign-born. The upward trend in reported childhood TB cases among foreign-born children in the United States and the results from these skin test surveys in urban areas imply that the pool of infected children and young adults in the United States is growing in some areas.

Transmission

Children usually are infected by an adult or adolescent in the immediate household, most often a parent, grandparent, older sibling or boarder. Casual extrafamilial contact is the source of infection much less often, but babysitters, school-teachers, music teachers, school-bus drivers, parishioners, nurses, gardeners and candy-store keepers have been implicated in individual cases and in hundreds of miniepidemics within limited population groups.[11] Within the household of an infectious adult, the infants and toddlers almost always are infected. Also at high risk are the older children and teenagers who help the ailing adult, whereas children between 6 and 12 years of age often escape infection. Adults with pulmonary disease who are receiving regular, appropriate chemotherapy probably rarely infect children; much more dangerous are those with chronic TB disease that is unrecognized, inadequately treated, or in relapse because of development of resistance.

Wallgren,[12] based on studies in orphanages, was the first to point out that children with TB rarely, if ever, infect other children. Those few children who have transmitted *M. tuberculosis* have the characteristics typical of adult type TB.[13] Many children with TB have tuberculin-negative siblings and parents. Children with TB often have been cared for by their families or in hospitals and institutions without infecting their contacts.[14] When transmission of *M. tuberculosis* has been documented in children's hospitals, it almost invariably has come from an adult with undiagnosed pulmonary TB.[15] In tuberculous chidren, tubercle bacilli in endobrachial secretions are relatively sparse, and productive cough is not at all characteristic of endothoracic TB or of miliary disease.[16] When young children cough, they lack the tussive force of adults. Guidelines issued by the Centers for Disease Control and Prevention (CDC) state that most children with typical childhood TB do not require isolation in the hospital unless they have an uncontrolled productive cough, a cavitary lesion or acid-fast organism-positive sputum smears.[17] Adolescents with typical reactivation-type pulmonary TB may be as infectious as adults. Children nevertheless play an extremely important role in the transmission of TB, not so much because they are likely to contaminate their immediate environment, but rather because they harbor a partially healed infection that lies dormant, only to reactivate as infectious pulmonary TB many years later under the social, emotional, and physiologic stresses arising during adolescence, pregnancy or old age. Thus, children infected with *M. tuberculosis* constitute a long-lasting reservoir of TB in the population.

The risk of infection for child contacts of adults receiving antituberculosis chemotherapy often is a matter of practical concern. Several studies have revealed that most childhood contacts are infected by the index case before diagnosis and the start of treatment. Although it is not possible to carry out a definitive clinical study, evidence indicates that patients on effective chemotherapy rarely transmit *M. tuberculosis*. Nevertheless, it seems prudent to avoid exposing additional children to adults with positive sputum smears or positive cultures and to assume that adults positive by smear or culture remain infectious for at least two weeks after the start of chemotherapy.

PATHOGENESIS IN CHILDREN

The primary complex of TB consists of local disease at the portal of entry and the regional lymph nodes that drain the area of the primary focus. The portal of entry is the lung in more than 95% of cases. Tubercle bacilli within particles larger than 10 µm usually are caught by the mucociliary mechanisms of the bronchial tree and are expelled. Small particles are inhaled beyond these clearance mechanisms. However, primary infection may occur anywhere in the body. Ingestion of milk infected with bovine TB can lead to a gastrointestinal primary lesion. Infection of the skin or mucous membrane can occur through an abrasion, cut or an insect bite. The number of tubercle bacilli required to establish infection in children is unknown, but only several organisms are probably necessary.

The incubation period in children between the time the tubercle bacilli enter the body and the development of cutaneous hypersensitivity is usually 2–12 weeks, most often 4–8 weeks. The onset of hypersensitivity may be accompanied by a febrile reaction that lasts from 1–3 weeks. During this phase of intensified tissue reaction, the primary complex may become visible on chest radiograph. The primary focus grows larger during this time but does not yet become encapsulated. As hypersensitivity develops, the inflammatory response becomes more intense and the regional lymph nodes often enlarge.

The parenchymal portion of the primary complex often heals completely by fibrosis or calcification after undergoing caseous necrosis and encapsulation. The parenchymal lesion occasionally enlarges, resulting in focal pneumonitis and thickening of the underlying pleura. If caseation is intense the center of the lesion may liquefy, empty into the associated bronchus, and leave a residual primary tuberculous cavity.

Tubercle bacilli from the primary complex spread via the bloodstream and lymphatics to many parts of the body during the development of the parenchymal lesion and the accelerated caseation brought on by the development of hypersensitivity. The areas most commonly seeded are the apices of the lungs, liver, spleen, meninges, peritoneum, lymph nodes, pleura, and bone. This dissemination can involve either large numbers of bacilli, which leads to disseminated TB disease, or small numbers of bacilli that leave microscopic tuberculous foci scattered in various tissues. These metastatic foci are clinically inapparent initially, but they are the origin of both extrapulmonary TB and reactivation pulmonary TB in some children and many adults.

The tubercle foci in the regional lymph nodes develop some fibrosis and encapsulation, but healing is usually less complete than in the parenchymal lesions. Viable *M. tuberculosis* may persist for decades after calcification of the nodes. The lymph nodes remain normal in size in most cases of primary TB infection; however, because of their location, hilar and paratracheal lymph nodes that become enlarged by the host inflammatory reaction may encroach upon the regional bronchus. Partial obstruction caused by external compression leads at first to hyperinflation in the distal lung segment. Such compression may occasionally cause complete obstruction of the bronchus, resulting in atelectasis of the lung segment.[18,19] More often inflamed caseous nodes attach to the bronchial wall and erode through it, leading to endobronchial TB or a fistulous tract. The extrusion of infected caseous material into the bronchus can transmit infection to the lung parenchyma and cause bronchial obstruction and atelectasis. The resultant lesion is a combination of pneumonia and atelectasis. The radiographic findings of this process have been referred to as "epituberculosis," "collapse-consolidation," and "segmental" TB. Rarely, TB intrathoracic lymph nodes invade other adjacent structures such as the pericardium or esophagus.

A fairly predictable time table for primary TB infection and its complications in infants and children is apparent.[20] Massive lymphohematogenous dissemination leading to meningitis, miliary or disseminated disease occurs in 0.5–2% of infected children, usually no later than 2–6 months after infection. Clinically significant lymph node or endobronchial TB usually appears within 3–9 months. Lesions of the bones and joints usually take at least a year to develop; renal lesions may be evident 5–25 years after infection. In general, complications of the primary infection occur within the first year.

Tuberculosis disease that occurs more than a year after the primary infection is thought to be secondary to endogenous regrowth of persistent bacilli from the primary infection and subclinical dissemination. Exogenous reinfection may result in TB disease, in rare cases, but most cases of postprimary or reactivation TB in adolescents are believed to be secondary to endogenous organisms. Reactivation TB is rare in infants and young children. Reactivation TB among adolescents affects females twice as often as males for unknown reasons. The most common form of reactivation TB is an infiltrate or cavity in the apex of the lung where oxygen tension is high and there is a heavy concentration of tubercle bacilli deposited during the primary subclinical dissemination of organisms. Dissemination during reactivation TB is rare among immunocompetent adolescents.

The age of the child at acquisition of TB infection seems to have a great effect on the occurrence of both primary and reactivation TB. Hilar lymphadenopathy and subsequent segmental disease complicating the primary infection occur most often in younger children. Approximately 40% of untreated children less than 1 year of age develop radiographically significant lymphadenopathy or segmental lesions, compared with 24% of children 1–10 years of age and 16% of children 11–15 years of age.[21] Nevertheless, if young children do not suffer early complications, their risk of developing reactivation TB later in life appears to be quite low. Conversely, older children and adolescents rarely experience complications of the primary infection but have a much higher risk of developing reactivation pulmonary TB as an adolescent or adult.

CLINICAL MANIFESTATIONS

How Children with Tuberculosis are Discovered

In the developing world, the only way children with TB disease are discovered is when they present with a profound illness that is consistent with TB.[22] Having an ill adult contact is an obvious clue to the correct diagnosis. The only available laboratory test usually is an acid-fast smear of sputum, which the child rarely produces. Chest radiography is not available in many high burden countries. To aid in diagnosis, a variety of scoring systems have been devised based on available tests, clinical signs

and symptoms, and known exposures; however, the sensitivity and specificity of these systems can be very low, leading to both over- and under-diagnosis of TB.[23] No clinical scoring system has been validated in a clinical trial.

In industrial countries, children with TB usually are discovered in one of three ways.[24] Obviously, one way is consideration of TB as the cause of a symptomatic pulmonary or extrapulmonary illness. Discovering an adult contact with infectious TB is an invaluable aid to diagnosis; the "yield" from contact investigation usually is higher than that from cultures from the child. The second way is discovery of a child with pulmonary TB during the contact investigation of an adult with TB. The affected child typically has few or no symptoms, but investigation reveals a positive tuberculin skin test and an abnormal chest radiograph. Up to 50 percent of children with pulmonary TB are discovered in this manner in some areas of the United States, before significant symptoms have begun. A smaller number of children with TB disease are found as the result of a community— or school-based tuberculin skin testing program.

Pulmonary Disease

The symptoms and physical signs of intrathoracic TB in children are surprisingly meager considering the degree of radiographic changes often seen. The physical manifestation of disease tends to differ by the age of onset. Young infants are more likely to have significant signs or symptoms.[25]

More than one half of infants and children with radiographically moderate to severe pulmonary TB, have no physical findings and are discovered only via contact tracing of an adult with TB. The chest radiograph typically is "sicker" than the child. Infants are more likely to experience signs and symptoms, probably because of their small airway diameters relative to the parenchymal and lymph node changes in primary TB (Table 29-2). Nonproductive cough and mild dyspnea are the most common symptoms. Systemic complaints such as fever, night sweats, anorexia, and decreased activity (malaise) occur less often. Some infants have difficulty gaining weight and develop a failure-to-thrive presentation that often does not improve significantly until after several months of treatment.

Pulmonary signs are even less common. Some infants and young children with bronchial obstruction show signs of air trapping, such as localized wheezing or decreased breath sounds that may be accompanied by tachypnea or frank respiratory distress. Antibiotics occasionally alleviate these nonspecific symptoms and signs.

Table 29-2. Symptoms and Signs of Childhood Pulmonary TB

Symptom	Infants & Young Children	Older Children & Adolescents
Fever	Common	Uncommon
Night Sweats	Rare	Uncommon
Cough	Common	Common
Productive Cough	Rare	Common
Sign		
Hemoptysis	Never	Rare
Dyspnea	Common	Rare
Rales	Common	Uncommon
Wheezing	Common	Uncommon
Dullness	Rare	Uncommon
Diminished Breath Sounds	Common	Uncommon

This suggests that bacterial superinfection distal to the focus of tuberculous bronchial obstruction contributes to the clinical presentation of disease.

A rare but serious complication of primary TB in children occurs when the parenchymal focus enlarges and develops a caseous center. The radiographic and clinical picture of progressive primary TB is that of bronchopneumonia with high fever, moderate to severe cough, night sweats, dullness to percussion, rales, and decreased breath sounds. Liquefaction in the center may result in formation of a thin-walled cavity.[26] The enlarging focus may slough debris into adjacent bronchi leading to intrapulmonary dissemination. Rupture of the cavity into the pleural space may cause a bronchopleural fistula or pyopneumothorax; rupture into the pericardium can cause acute pericarditis with constriction. Before the advent of antituberculosis chemotherapy, the mortality rate of progressive primary pulmonary TB was 30–50%. Currently, with effective treatment, the prognosis is excellent.

Older children and adolescents, especially those with reactivation-type TB, are more likely to experience fever, anorexia, malaise, weight loss, night sweats, productive cough, chest pain, and hemoptysis than children with primary pulmonary TB.[27] Nonetheless, findings on physical examination are usually minor or absent even when cavities or large infiltrates are present. Most signs and symptoms improve within several weeks of starting effective treatment although cough may last for several months.

As expected, the radiographic findings in childhood TB reflect the pathophysiology, and are quite different from findings in adults (Table 29-3). The hallmark of primary pulmonary TB is the relatively large size and importance of the lymphadenitis compared with the less significant size of the initial parenchymal focus. Because of the usual pattern of lymphatic circulation within the lungs, a left-sided parenchymal focus often leads to bilateral hilar adenopathy, while a right-sided focus is associated only with right-sided lymphadenitis. Hilar and/or mediastinal lymphadenopathy is invariably present with childhood TB, but may not be distinct (from the atelectasis and infiltrate) or may be too small to be seen clearly on a plain radiograph.

Table 29-3. Comparison of Chest Radiographs of Pulmonary TB in Adults and Children

Characteristic	Adults	Children
Location	Apical	Anywhere (25% multilobar)
Adenopathy	Rare (except HIV-related)	Usual
Cavitation	Common	Rare (except adolescents)
Signs & Symptoms	Consistent	Relative paucity

Computed tomography (CT) may reveal small lymph nodes when the chest radiograph is normal, but this finding appears to have no clinical implications.[28] It can, however, create a dilemma in deciding on a treatment regimen, and reinforces the idea that, in children, infection and disease are on a continuum with often indistinct borders.[2]

In most cases of TB infection in children, the initial mild parenchymal infiltrate and lymphadenitis resolve spontaneously and the chest radiograph is normal. In some children, the hilar or mediastinal lymph nodes continue to enlarge. Partial airway obstruction caused by external compression from the enlarging nodes causes air trapping and hyperinflation. As the nodes attach to and infiltrate the airway, caesium filling the lumen causes complete obstruction, resulting in atelectasis that involves the lobar segment distal to the obstructed lumen (Fig. 29-2). The resulting radiographic shadows are called collapse-consolidation or segmental lesions (Figs. 29-3 and 29-4). These findings resemble those in foreign body aspiration; in the case of TB, the lymph node is acting as the foreign body. Multiple segmental lesions in different lobes may appear simultaneously, as can atelectasis and hyperinflation.

Other radiographic findings are noted in some children. Occasional children have a lobar pneumonia without distinct hilar adenopathy. In infants and young children, the radiographic appearance can resemble exudative

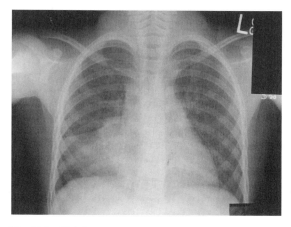

Fig. 29-3. Slightly more extensive right-sided adenopathy with atelectasis in a 2-year old with TB.

pneumonia, similar to that caused by *Klebsiella pneumonia* or *Staphylococcus aureus*. (Fig. 29-5). A secondary bacterial pneumonia may contribute to this appearance. When TB infection is progressively destructive, liquefaction of lung parenchyma leads to formation of a thin-walled primary TB cavity. Peripheral bullous lesions occur rarely and can lead to pneumothorax.[29] Enlargement of subcarinal nodes causes compression of the esophagus, difficulty swallowing, and rarely, a bronchoesophageal fistula.

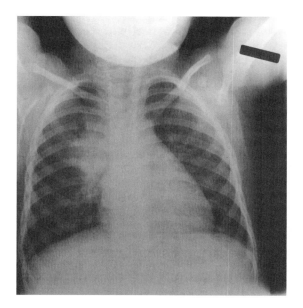

Fig. 29-2. Early collapse—consolidation lesion in a child with TB. Mediastinal adenopathy also is present on the right side.

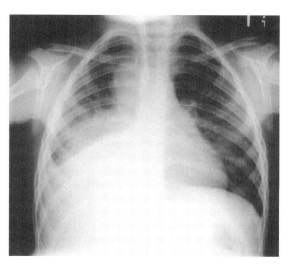

Fig. 29-4. Well-formed collapse-consolidation lesion on the right, with large mediastinal and hilar adenopathy and atelectasis.

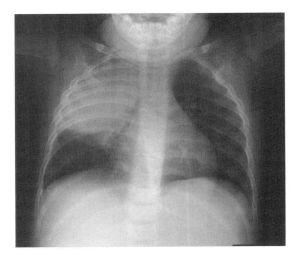

Fig. 29-5. Tuberculous pneumonia with bowing of the horizontal fissure. Children with this finding may have an associated bacterial infection.

One sign of early subcarinal TB is horizontal splaying of the mainstem bronchi.

Adolescents with pulmonary TB may develop segmental lesions with associated adenopathy, but more often they develop the infiltrates with or without cavitation that are typical of adult reactivation TB (Fig. 29-6). The lesions are often smaller in adolescents than in adults, and lordotic views, tomograms or even a CT scan may be necessary to demonstrate small apical foci of disease.

The course of thoracic lymphadenopathy and bronchial obstruction can follow several paths. The segment of lobe re-expands in most cases and the radiographic abnormalities resolve completely. The resolution occurs slowly, over months to several years, and is not affected greatly by antituberculosis therapy. Of course, children still have infection with *M. tuberculosis* and are at high risk of reactivation TB in subsequent years if chemotherapy has not been taken. In some cases, the segmental lesion resolves but residual calcification occurs in the primary parenchymal focus or regional lymph nodes. The calcification usually occurs in fine particles creating a stippling effect. Calcification begins 6 months or more after infection. Even with chemotherapy, the enlarged lymph nodes and endobronchial lesions may persist for many months, occasionally resulting in severe airway obstruction. Surgical or endoscopic removal of intraluminal lesions is rarely necessary. Finally, bronchial obstruction may cause scarring and progressive contraction of the lobe or segment, which is often associated

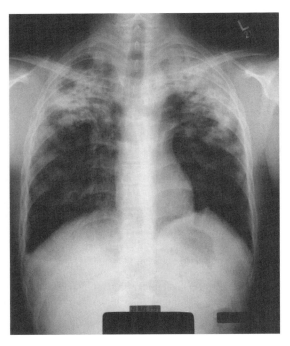

Fig. 29-6. Reactivation-type TB in an adolescent boy.

with cylindrical bronchiectasis. Complete radiographic and clinical resolution without calcification occurs in the vast majority of cases with early institution of adequate treatment for collapse-consolidation lesions.

Pleural Disease

Tuberculous pleural effusions, which can be local or general, usually originate in the discharge of bacilli into the pleural space from a subpleural pulmonary focus or caseated subpleural lymph nodes.[30] Asymptomatic local pleural effusion is so frequent in primary TB that it is basically a component of the primary complex. Most large and clinically significant effusions occur months to years after the primary infection (Fig. 29-7). Tuberculous pleural effusion is infrequent in children younger than 6 years of age and rare in those below 2 years of age. Such effusions are usually unilateral but can be bilateral. They are virtually never associated with a segmental pulmonary lesion and are rare in miliary TB.

The clinical onset of tuberculous pleurisy in children is usually fairly sudden, with low to high fever, shortness of breath, chest pain especially on deep inspiration, dullness to percussion, and diminished breath sounds on the affected side. The presentation is similar to that of

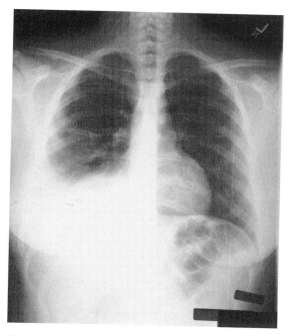

Fig. 29-7. A tuberculous pleural effusion in an adolescent girl.

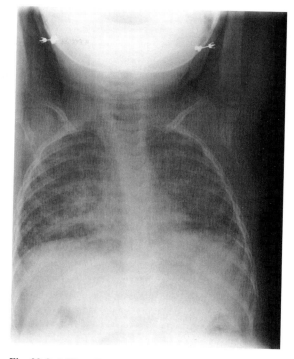

Fig. 29-8. Miliary TB in an infant. The child presented with fever and respiratory distress.

pyogenic pleurisy. The fever and other symptoms may last for several weeks after the start of antituberculosis chemotherapy. Although corticosteroids may reduce the clinical symptoms, they have little effect on the ultimate outcome. The tuberculin skin test is positive in only 70–80% of cases. The prognosis is excellent; radiographic resolution takes months, however. Scoliosis rarely complicates recovery of a long-standing effusion.

Extrathoracic Tuberculosis

The various forms of extrapulmonary TB are reviewed in detail in other chapters. Up to 25–35% of childhood TB cases are extrapulmonary (Table 29-1), and a careful physical examination is an essential component of the evaluation of a child with TB exposure or infection.

The two forms of extrapulmonary TB that receive the most attention, because of their life-threatening nature, are disseminated (miliary) disease (Fig. 29-8) and meningitis. Both forms of disease occur early, often within 2–6 months of initial infection. Correct diagnosis requires a high index of suspicion because it is difficult to confirm these diseases microbiologically. Acid-fast stains of body fluids are almost always negative; cultures for *M. tuberculosis* are positive in only 50% or less of cases

and they often take weeks to grow because the initial inoculum of organisms is so low.[31–33] In addition, the tuberculin skin test may be nonreactive initially in up to 50% of pediatric patients, and the chest radiograph in both diseases may be normal early on. The key element to correctly diagnose each condition is an epidemiologic history, a search for the adult from whom the child acquired *M. tuberculosis*. Unfortunately, an initial negative history for exposure does not really help. In a recent study of 31 consecutive infants and children with central nervous system TB in Houston, Texas, the initial family history was negative for TB in 30 cases, although the adult source case was ultimately identified in over 60% of cases.[33] The ill adult often has not yet been diagnosed correctly because the incubation period of disseminated TB and meningitis in children may be short. An evaluation of the family and other adults and adolescents in close contact with the child should be considered a public health emergency when serious TB disease is suspected in a child.

The most feared complication of TB in children is meningitis. Although the clinical onset of tuberculous meningitis in children may occur gradually over several weeks, recent studies describe more rapid progression over several days. Early on, the clinical presentation may be similar to that of viral or pyogenic meningitis; however, tuberculous meningitis in children is more likely to be complicated by cranial nerve involvement, basalar leptomeningeal involvement, hydrocephalus and infarct caused by vasculitis. These findings in any child with meningitis, when no other cause is readily apparent, should prompt immediate initiation of antituberculosis chemotherapy while diagnostic studies and investigation of close contacts for TB are carried out as quickly as possible.

The widespread use of improved cranial imaging such as CT scan and magnetic resonance imaging have shown that tuberculoma is more common than previously realized, and the distinction in children between tuberculous meningitis and tuberculoma is not as clear as once thought. Tuberculomas account for up to 40% of brain tumors in children in some developing countries. They often occur in children less than 10 years of age, may be single or multiple, and are often located at the base of the brain, near the cerebellum. On the other hand, a recently recognized phenomenon is the paradoxical development of intracranial tuberculomas appearing or enlarging during treatment of meningeal, disseminated, and even pulmonary TB.[34] This phenomenon appears to be similar to the well-described worsening of intrathoracic adenopathy seen in many children during the first few months of ultimately successful chemotherapy for TB. The tuberculomas seem to be mediated immunologically; they respond (slowly) to corticosteroid therapy and a change in antituberculosis therapy is not required. Some infants with pulmonary TB and very subtle neurologic signs or symptoms will have one or several tuberculomas, even with a normal cerebrospinal fluid evaluation. Any neurologic abnormality in a child with suspected TB should be evaluated with a neuroimaging study, when feasible.[33]

Tuberculosis in HIV-infected Children

In adults infected with both HIV and *M. tuberculosis*, the rate of progression from asymptomatic infection to disease is increased greatly.[9,35,36] The clinical manifestations of TB in HIV-infected adults tend to be typical when the CD4+ cell count is more than 500 per mm[3], but become "atypical" as the CD4+ cell count falls. Similar correlations have not been reported for dually-infected children, though there is some epidemiologic evidence that TB rates are higher in HIV-infected children in the United States than in the general population. When HIV-infected children develop TB, the clinical features tend to be fairly typical of disease in immunocompetent children, although the disease often progresses more rapidly and clinical manifestations are more severe. There may be an increased tendency for extrapulmonary disease, but the trend is not as dramatic as it is in HIV-infected adults.[9] The diagnosis of TB in an HIV-infected child can be difficult to establish as skin test reactivity may be absent, culture confirmation is slow and difficult, and the clinical presentation may be similar to other HIV-related infections and conditions. A diligent search for an infectious adult in the child's environment often yields the strongest clue to the correct diagnosis.

DIAGNOSIS

Tuberculin Skin Test

The tuberculin skin test has been reviewed extensively in a previous chapter. The placement of the Mantoux intradermal skin test, while fairly simple and routine in a cooperative adult, can be a challenge in a squirming, scared child. The technique shown in Fig. 29-9 allows for better control during placement. The skin tester anchors her hand along the longitudinal axis of the child's arm, which enhances stability and allows the last two fingers to become a fulcrum to guide inoculation of the solution. The tuberculin is injected laterally across the arm. As with adults, a wheal of 6–10 mm should be raised after injection. The test is interpreted at 48–72 hours after placement. Although recent formal studies are lacking, most experts believe the time course of the reaction and amount of induration produced is similar in children and adults. Infants may make slightly less induration, on average, when infected.

The interpretation of the Mantoux skin test should be similar in children and adults (Table 29-4)[37–39]; however, most of the "risk factors" for children are actually the risk factors of the adults in their environment—the likelihood that the child has had significant contact with an adult with contagious pulmonary TB. Correctly classifying a child's reaction supposes that the risk factors of the adults around the child have been considered. The American Academy of Pediatrics (AAP) has suggested that 10 mm should be the cutpoint for all children less than 4 years of age.[40] This recommendation is not based on diminished ability to make an induration reaction in children; it was made to minimize false negative reactions in small children who are at increased risk of developing life-threatening forms of TB once infected.

The same factors that influence the accuracy of tuberculin skin testing in adults also affect children.

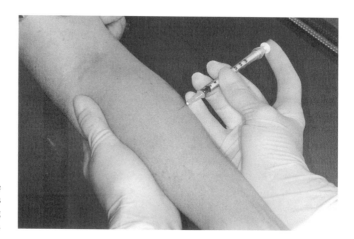

Fig. 29-9. A helpful technique for applying the Mantoux tuberculin skin test on a child. The hand is anchored on the side of the child's arm, providing stability. The tuberculin is injected in a lateral direction.

About 10–20% of children with TB disease initially have a negative reaction to tuberculin.[41] The lack of reactivity may be global or may occur only for tuberculin, so "control" skin tests may be of limited usefulness in children. In most cases (other than those with advanced HIV infection or other ongoing immunosuppression) the reaction becomes positive as the child recovers on chemotherapy. Incubating or manifest viral infections are a frequent cause of false-negative results in children.

Previous inoculation with a Bacille Calmette-Guérin (BCG) vaccination can pose problems with interpretation of a subsequent tuberculin skin test. Although many infants who receive a BCG vaccine never develop a skin test reaction to tuberculin, about 50% will. The reactivity fades over time, but can be boosted in children with repeated skin testing.[42] Most experts agree that skin test interpretation in children who received a BCG vaccine more than 3 years previously should be the same as if they had never received vaccine. When skin testing is done sooner after vaccination, interpretation is more difficult. The clinician should have a clear understanding of why the test was placed and realize that a positive reaction most likely represents infection with *M. tuberculosis* if the child had a specific exposure to an infectious adult or adolescent.

Diagnostic Mycobacteriology in Children

The demonstration of acid-fast bacilli in stained smears of sputum is presumptive evidence of pulmonary TB in most patients; however, in children, tubercle bacilli usually are relatively few in number, and sputum cannot be obtained

Table 29-4. Amount of Induration from a Mantoux Tuberculin Skin Test Considered Positive in Children

Reaction Size	Factor
≥5 mm	• Contact with an infectious case • Abnormal x-ray or clinical finding • HIV infection or immune suppression
≥10 mm	• Birth or previous residence in a high prevalence country • Residence in a long-term care facility • Contact with high risk adults (when a specific source is not known) • Age <4 years
≥15 mm	• Absence of risk factors

spontaneously from children younger than about 10 years of age. Gastric washings, which often are used in lieu of sputum, can be contaminated with acid-fast organisms from the mouth. Nevertheless, fluorescence microscopy of gastric washing has been found useful, though the yield is less than 10%.[43] Tubercle bacilli in cerebrospinal fluid, pleural fluid, lymph node aspirate, and urine are sparse; thus, only rarely are direct-stained smears for tubercle bacilli positive in pediatric practice. Cultures for tubercle bacilli are of great importance, not only to confirm the diagnosis, but also increasingly to permit testing for drug susceptibility. Nonetheless, if culture and drug susceptibility data are available from the associated adult case and the child has a classic presentation of TB (positive skin test, consistent abnormal chest radiograph, exposure to an adult case), obtaining cultures from the child adds little to the management.

Painstaking collection of specimens is essential for culture diagnosis in children because fewer organisms usually are present then in adults. Gastric lavage should be performed in the very early morning, when the patient has had nothing to eat or drink for 8 hours and before the patient has a chance to wake up and start swallowing saliva, which dilutes the bronchial secretions that were brought up during the night and made their way into the stomach. Inhalation of superheated nebulized saline prior to gastric lavage has been reported to increase the bacteriologic yield.[44] The stomach contents should be aspirated first. No more than 50–75 ml of sterile distilled water (not saline) should be injected through the stomach tube and the aspirate added to the first collection. The gastric acidity (poorly tolerated by tubercle bacilli) should be neutralized immediately. Concentration and culture should be performed as soon as possible after collection. Even with optimal, in-hospital collection of three early-morning gastric aspirate samples, *M. tuberculosis* can be isolated from only 30–40% of children and 70% of infants with pulmonary TB.[25,39] The yield from random outpatient gastric aspirate samples is exceedingly low.

Bronchial secretions obtained by stimulating cough with an aerosol solution of propylene glycol in 10 percent sodium chloride can be used in older children.[45] The aerosol is heated in a nebulizer at 46°C–52°C (114.8°F–125.6°F) and administered to the patient for 15–30 minutes. This method gives good results and may be superior to gastric lavage both in yield of positive cultures and patient acceptance. Bronchial aspirate obtained at bronchoscopy is often thick, and the laboratory will process it using a mucolytic agent, as such as N-acetyl-L-cysteine. The yield of *M. tuberculosis* from bronchoscopy specimens has been lower in most studies than from properly obtained gastric aspirates.[46,47]

Nucleic Acid Amplification

The main form of nucleic acid amplification studied in children with TB is the polymerase chain reaction (PCR), which uses specific DNA sequences as markers for micro-organisms. Various PCR techniques, most using the mycobacterial insertion element IS6110 as the DNA marker for *M. tuberculosis* complex organisms, have sensitivity and specificity of more than 90 percent compared with sputum culture for detecting pulmonary TB in adults. Then again, test performance varies even among reference laboratories.[48] The test is relatively expensive, requires fairly sophisticated equipment, and requires scrupulous technique to avoid cross-contamination of specimens.

Use of PCR in childhood TB has been limited. Compared with a clinical diagnosis of pulmonary TB in children, sensitivity of PCR has varied from 25–83 % and specificity has varied from 80–100%.[49–52] The PCR of gastric aspirates may be positive in a recently infected child even when the chest radiograph is normal, demonstrating the occasional arbitrariness of the distinction between TB infection and disease in children. The PCR may have a useful but limited role in evaluating children for TB. A negative PCR never eliminates TB as a diagnostic possibility, and a positive result does not confirm it. The major use of PCR is, evaluating children with significant pulmonary disease, when clinical or epidemiologic grounds do not establish the diagnosis readily. PCR may be helpful in evaluating immunocompromised children with pulmonary disease, especially in children with HIV infection, although published reports of its performance in such children are lacking. PCR also may aid in confirming the diagnosis of extrapulmonary TB.

MANAGEMENT

The first line drugs, their formulations and pediatric doses are listed in Table 29-5.

Exposure

Children exposed to potentially infectious adults with pulmonary TB should be started on treatment, usually isoniazid (INH) only, if the child is younger than 5 years of age or has other risk factors for the rapid development of TB disease, such as immunocompromise of some kind.[53] Failure to do so may result in development of

Table 29-5. Commonly Used Drugs for the Treatment of TB in Children

Drug	Dosage Forms	Daily Dose (mg/kg/day)	Twice Weekly Dose (mg/kg/dose)	Maximum Daily Dose
Ethambutol	Tablets: 100 mg 400 mg	15–25	50	2.5 mg
Isoniazid*,†	Scored tablets: 100 mg 300 mg Syrup:‡ 10 mg/mL	10–15†	20–30	Daily: 300 mg. Twice weekly: 900 mg
Pyrazinamide	Scored tablets: 500 mg	20–40	50	2 g
Rifampin*	Capsules: 150 mg 300 mg Syrup: formulated in syrup from capsules	10–20	10–20	Daily: 600 mg Twice weekly: 600 mg
Streptomycin (IM administration)	Vials: 1 g	20–40 4 g	20–40	

*Rifamate is a capsule containing 150 mg of isoniazid and 300 mg of rifampin. Two capsules provide the usual adult (>50 kg body weight) daily doses of each drug.

†When isoniazid is used in combination with rifampin, the incidence of hepatotoxicity increases if the isoniazid dose exceeds 10 mg/kg/day.

‡Most experts advise against the use of isoniazid syrup due to instability and a high rate of gastrointestinal adverse reaction (diarrhea, cramps) when more than 5 cc is given.

severe TB disease even before the tuberculin skin test becomes reactive; the "incubation period" of disease may be shorter than that for the skin test. The child is treated for a minimum of 3 months after contact when the infectious case is broken (by physical separation or effective treatment of the case). After 3 months, the tuberculin skin test is repeated. If the second test is positive, infection is documented and INH should be continued for a total duration of 9 months; if the second test is negative, the treatment can be stopped. If the exposure was to a case with an INH-resistant but rifampin (RIF)-susceptible isolate, RIF is the recommended treatment.

Two circumstances of exposure deserve special attention. A difficult situation arises when the exposed child is anergic because of immune compromise. These children are particularly vulnerable to rapid progression of TB, and it will not be possible to tell if infection has

occurred. In general, these children should be treated as if they have TB infection.

The second situation is exposure of a newborn to a mother (or other adult) with a positive tuberculin skin test, or rarely, a nursery worker with contagious TB. The management is based on further evaluation of the mother.

1. *Mother has a normal chest radiograph.* No separation of the infant and mother is required. Although the mother should receive treatment for TB infection and other household members should be evaluated for TB infection or disease, the infant needs no further work-up or treatment unless a case of disease is found.

2. *Mother has an abnormal chest radiograph.* The mother and child should be separated until the mother has been evaluated thoroughly. If the radiograph, history, physical examination, and analysis of sputum reveal no evidence of active pulmonary TB in the

mother, it is reasonable to assume the infant is at low risk of infection. Nevertheless, if the mother remains untreated, she may later develop contagious TB and expose her infant. Both mother and infant should receive appropriate follow-up care, but the infant does not need treatment. If the radiograph and clinical history are suggestive of pulmonary TB in the mother, the child and mother should remain separated until both have begun appropriate chemotherapy. The infant should be evaluated for congenital TB. The placenta should be examined. If the mother has no risk factors for drug-resistant TB, the infant should receive INH and close follow-up care. The infant should have a tuberculin skin test at 3 or 4 months after the mother is judged no longer to be contagious; evaluation of the infant at this time follows the guidelines for other exposures of children. If no infection is documented at this time, it would be prudent to repeat the tuberculin skin test in 6–12 months. If the mother has TB caused by a multidrug-resistant isolate of *M. tuberculosis* or she has poor adherence to therapy, the child should remain separated from her until she no longer is contagious or the infant can be given a BCG vaccine and be kept separated until the vaccine "takes" (marked by a reactive tuberculin skin test).

Infection

The recommendation for treatment of asymptomatic tuberculin-positive individuals is based on data from several well-controlled studies; it applies particularly to children and adolescents who are at high risk for the development of overt disease but at very low risk for the development of the main toxic manifestation of INH therapy, which is hepatitis.[54–57] The large, carefully controlled U.S. Public Health Study of 1955, followed by others, demonstrated the favorable effect of 12 months of INH on the incidence of complications due to progression of TB infection. The younger the tuberculin reactor, the greater the benefit.[58]

The American Thoracic Society and the CDC[59] recommend that INH treatment of TB infection be given to all positive tuberculin reactors at risk for developing disease. The question arises as to how long the protective effect can be expected to last. Comstock and associates,[60] in their final report on INH prophylaxis in Alaska, demonstrated the protective effect of 1 year of chemoprophylaxis to be at least 19 years. Hsu[56] reported on 2494 children followed for up to 30 years and showed that adequate drug treatment prevented reactivation of

TB during adolescence and into young adulthood. It is likely that the decreased risk of TB after INH therapy may be life-long in children infected with INH-susceptible tubercle bacilli. Failure of INH after exposure to INH-resistant *M. tuberculosis* has been documented. No controlled study of an alternative regimen has been reported. RIF alone is recommended and widely used.

The dosage of INH to be used has had little study. Most investigators have used a regimen based on 4–8 mg/kg of body weight/day, usually taken all at once, for a period of 6–12 months. A dose of 5 mg/kg/day was found satisfactory in one study.[61] Most clinicians prescribe a dose of 10–15 mg/kg/day to a total of 300 mg/day for treatment of infection to be sure of achieving therapeutic levels even among patients who inactivate the drug rapidly by acetylation.

The duration of INH treatment initially was set arbitrarily at 12 months. A large trial was conducted on adults in Eastern Europe with old fibrotic lesions caused by TB, comparing regimens of daily INH taken for 12, 24 and 52 weeks with a placebo for their ability to prevent TB disease.[62] Therapy for 1 year was most effective, especially if patients were adherent; however, therapy for 24 weeks afforded a fairly high level of protection. A subsequent analysis concluded that the 24-week duration of preventive therapy was more cost-effective for adults than the 52-week duration.[63] Subsequently, many health departments accepted 6 months of INH therapy as their standard regimen for adults. Nonetheless, the cost-effectiveness analysis does not apply to children. For many years, the AAP and CDC have recommended a duration of 9 months for children. INH is taken daily under self-supervision or can be taken twice weekly under directly observed therapy.[53] When the child is infected with an INH-resistant but RIF-susceptible strain of *M. tuberculosis*, 6 months of RIF should be substituted for INH. If the infecting strain is resistant to both INH and RIF, usually two other drugs are used. No combination of drugs is known to be superior to the others; usually two from among pyrazinamide (PZA), ethambutol, ethionamide, cycloserine, or a fluoroquinolone are chosen.

Disease

Clinical trials of antituberculosis drugs in children are difficult to perform, mostly because of the difficulty in obtaining positive cultures at diagnosis or relapse and the need for long-term follow-up.[64] Recommendations for treating children with TB were extrapolated historically from clinical trials of adults with pulmonary TB. On the other hand, during the past 25 years, a large number of clinical trials involving only children has been reported. In 1983, Abernathy and colleagues[65] reported successful treatment of 50 children with TB in Arkansas using INH and RIF daily for 1 month, then twice weekly for 8 months. Most pulmonary infiltrates cleared by the end of therapy, but hilar adenopathy usually still was present radiographically, then gradually cleared over 2–3 years. Patients with only hilar adenopathy can be treated successfully with INH and RIF for 6 months.[66,67]

Several major studies of 6-month therapy in children using at least three drugs in the initial phase have been reported.[68–75] The most commonly used regimen was 6 months of INH and RIF supplemented during the first 2 months with PZA. The overall success rate has been greater than 98 % and the incidence of clinically significant adverse reactions <2%. Regimens not using streptomycin were as successful as those that included it. Using twice-weekly medications (under directly observed therapy) during the continuation phase was as effective and safe as daily administration. Three studies used twice-weekly therapy throughout the treatment regimen with excellent success,[71,73,75] and one used daily therapy for only the first 2 weeks.[74] The 6-month, three-drug regimen was successful, tolerated well, and less expensive than the 9-month regimen.[76] It also effects a cure faster, so that there is a greater likelihood of successful treatment if the child becomes nonadherent later in therapy.

Controlled treatment trials for various forms of extrapulmonary TB are rare. Several of the 6-month, three-drug trials in children included extrapulmonary cases,[69,71] Most non-life-threatening forms of extrapulmonary TB respond well to a 9-month course of INH and RIF or to a 6-month regimen including INH, RIF, and PZA.[77] One exception may be bone and joint TB, which may have a high failure rate when 6-month chemotherapy is used, especially when surgical intervention has not taken place.

Tuberculous meningitis usually is not included in trials of extrapulmonary TB therapy because of its serious nature and low incidence. Treatment with INH and RIF for 12 months generally is effective.[78] Kendig[79] reported 15 children who absconded from therapy for tuberculous meningitis between 4 and 9 months of therapy; only 2 children died, and the majority of survivors had a good outcome. A more recent study from Thailand showed that a 6-month regimen including PZA for serious tuberculous meningitis led to fewer deaths and better outcomes than did longer regimens that did not contain PZA.[80] Most children are treated initially with four drugs (INH, RIF, PZA and ethionamide or streptomycin). The PZA and fourth drug are stopped after 2 months, and INH and RIF are continued for a total of 7–12 months.

Drug Resistance

Patterns of drug resistance in children tend to mirror those found in adult patients in the population.[81–84] Outbreaks of drug-resistant TB in children occurring at schools have been reported.[85] The key to determining drug resistance in childhood TB usually comes from the drug susceptibility results of the infectious adult contact case's isolate.

Therapy for drug-resistant TB is successful only when at least two bactericidal drugs to which the infecting strain of *M. tuberculosis* is susceptible are given.[86,87] When INH resistance is considered a possibility, on the basis of epidemiologic risk factors or the identification of an INH-resistance source case isolate, an additional drug—usually ethambutol or streptomycin—should be given initially to the child until the exact susceptibility pattern is determined and a more specific regimen can be designed. Exact treatment regimens must be tailored to the specific pattern of drug resistance. Duration of therapy usually is extended to at least 9–12 months if either INH or RIF can be used, and to at least 18–24 months if resistance to both drugs is present. Surgical resection of a diseased lung or lobe is rarely required in children. An expert in TB always should be involved in the management of children with drug-resistant TB infection or disease.

Adherence and Directly Observed Therapy (DOT)

For many families with a child with TB, the disease is but one of many social and other problems in the family's life, and at certain times, other problems may supersede the perceived importance of TB. To combat this problem of nonadherence with treatment, most health departments have developed programs of directly observed therapy (DOT) in which a third party, usually but not always a health care worker is present during the administration of each dose of medication. DOT should be considered standard therapy for children with TB disease. The clinician should coordinate this treatment with the local health department. In the author's clinic, all children with TB are treated exclusively with directly observed therapy, which can be given at an office, clinic, home, school, work, or any other setting. It is highly effective and safe, and the patient satisfaction is high if it is offered as a special service to treat TB. High-risk children with TB infection are being treated with DOT at schools or in other locations to ensure completion of therapy. DOT also should be considered for all child contacts of adult TB patients, especially when the adult also is receiving DOT. Although specific controlled studies are lacking, twice weekly DOT appears to be effective for treating TB exposure and infection in children and adolescents.

Follow-Up

Follow-up of children treated with antituberculosis drugs has become more streamlined in recent years. The patient should be seen monthly while receiving chemotherapy, both to encourage regular taking of the prescribed drugs and to check, by a few simple questions (concerning appetite, well-being) and a few observations (weight gain; appearance of skin and sclerae; palpation of liver, spleen and lymph nodes) that the disease is not spreading and that toxic effects of the drugs are not appearing. Routine biochemical monitoring for hepatitis is not necessary in children, unless they have liver disease or are taking other hepatotoxic drugs. Repeat chest radiographs should be obtained 1–2 months after the onset of chemotherapy to ascertain the maximal extent of disease before chemotherapy takes effect; therafter, they rarely are necessary. Chemotherapy has been so successful that follow-up beyond its termination is not necessary, except for children with serious disease, such as tuberculous meningitis, or those with extensive residual chest radiographic findings at the end of chemotherapy. Chest radiograph findings resolve slowly; it is typical that enlarged lymph nodes take 2–3 years to resolve, well beyond the completion of ultimately successful chemotherapy. A normal chest radiograph is not a necessary criterion for stopping therapy.

PUBLIC HEALTH ASPECTS OF PEDIATRIC TUBERCULOSIS

Hopefully, it has become obvious that the control of TB in children—for a community and for individuals—depends on close cooperation between the clinician and the local health department. It is critically important that clinicians report cases of TB to the health department as soon as possible. Public health law in all U.S. states requires that the *suspicion* of TB disease in an adult or child to be reported immediately to the health department. The clinician should not wait for microbiologic confirmation of the diagnosis because it is this reporting that leads to the initiation of the contact investigation that may find infected children and allow them to be treated before disease occurs. The child may progress from infection to disease before intervention can occur if the clinician waits for confirmatory laboratory results. The clinician should always feel free to contact the local health department about special issues involving TB exposure, infection, or disease

in a child. Not every clinical situation can be anticipated by normal guidelines and, in some cases, an unusual intervention may be warranted.

It is estimated that about 1 million children in the United States have infection by *M. tuberculosis*. The major purpose of finding and treating these children is to prevent future cases of TB. Frequent or periodic skin testing of children; however, will prevent few cases of childhood TB, especially if the screening is centered on school-aged children (who rarely develop primary disease).[88,89] The major purpose of testing children is to prevent future cases of TB in adults. The infection rates are low among young children even in very high-risk groups in the United States. The incubation period for childhood TB is weeks to months, so even annual testing will not prevent many cases. The best way to prevent childhood TB is via prompt contact investigation centered on adults with suspected contagious TB.[90] This investigation has a high yield—on average, 30–50% of childhood household contacts are infected—but also finds the most important individuals, those most recently infected who are in the period of their lives when they are most likely to develop TB disease. The most important activity in a community to prevent cases of childhood TB is the contact investigation activity of the public health department.

If perfect contact investigations were performed and foreign-born children coming to the United States received tuberculin skin tests, there would be virtually no reason to perform the skin-test on any other child, simply because all infected children would be found. Obviously, these two activities do not occur in a perfect fashion, and testing of certain selected individuals is appropriate. The CDC and AAP have changed and refined their recommendations for tuberculin skin testing of children several times in the past decade. The AAP continues to emphasize that routine tuberculin skin testing of all children, including school-based programs that include populations at low risk, has a low yield of positive results or a large number of false-positive results, representing an inefficient use of limited health care resources.[53] Children without specific risk factors who reside in areas with a low prevalence of TB, therefore, do not need to have any routine tuberculin skin testing. School-based testing may be appropriate only for children with specific risk factors. A child should be considered at increased risk if: the child was born in, has resided in, or has traveled (non-tourist) to a country with high TB rates (Central and South America, Africa, Asia, Eastern Europe); there is a family history of TB infection or disease; the child is in foster care; or the child is a member of a group identified locally to be at increased risk for TB infection (examples may include migrant worker families, the homeless, certain census tracts or neighborhoods).

Much of the focus on tuberculin skin-testing should be placed on identification of risk factors for a child being in a group with a high prevalence of infection. Although some risk factors may apply across the country, local health departments must identify those risk factors that are germane to their area. Clinicians and their organizations must work closely with local health departments to establish which child should be tested and which should not. Health departments should advise school districts as to whether any type of school-based skin testing is appropriate and what nature it should take. Social and political problems can occur when selective testing is suggested. What is correct from a public health point of view may not be easy to translate into a workable and generally acceptable policy. Local clinicians can be extremely helpful to health departments in advancing prudent and reasonable TB control policies, particularly when other government or public agencies are involved.

REFERENCES

1. Kimmerling M, Barker J, Bruce F, et al. Preventable childhood tuberculosis in Alabama: implications and opportunity. *Pediatrics.* 2000;105:e53.
2. Khan EA, Starke JR. Diagnosis of tuberculosis in children. Increased need for better methods. *Emerg Infect Dis.* 1995;1:115.
3. Kochi A. The global tuberculosis situation and the new control strategy of the World Health Organization. (Leading Article). *Tubercle.* 1991;72:1.
4. Nelson LJ, Schneider E, Wells CD, et al. Epidemiology of childhood tuberculosis in the United States, 1993–2001: the need for continued vigilance. *Pediatrics.* 2004;114:333.
5. Centers for Disease Control and Prevention. Reported tuberculosis in the United States, 2003. U.S. Department of Health and Human Services; 2004.
6. Ussery XT, Valway SE, McKenna M, et al. Epidemiology of tuberculosis among children in the United States. *Pediatr Infect Dis J.* 1996;15:697.
7. Saiman L, Aronson J, Zhou J, et al. Prevalence of infectious diseases among internationally adopted children. *Pediatrics.* 2001;109:608.
8. Jones D, Malecki J, Bigler W, et al. Pediatric tuberculosis and human immunodeficiency virus infection in Palm Beach County, Florida. *Am J Dis Child.* 1992;146:1166.
9. Blusse van Oud-Alblas HJ, van Vliet ME, Kimpen JL, et al. Human immunodeficiency virus infection in children hospitalized with tuberculosis. *Ann Trop Paediatr.* 2002;22:115.
10. Barry MA, Shirley L, Grady MT, et al. Tuberculosis infection in urban adolescents: results of a school-based testing program. *Am J Public Health.* 1990;80:439.
11. Lincoln EM. Epidemics of tuberculosis. *Adv Tuberc Res.* 1965;14:159.
12. Wallgren A. On contagiousness of childhood tuberculosis. *Acta Paediatr.* 1937;22:229.
13. Curtis A, Ridzon R, Vogel R, et al. Extensive transmission of *Mycobacterium tuberculosis* from a child. *N Engl J Med.* 1999;341:1491.
14. Munoz FM, Ong LT, Seary D, et al. Tuberculosis among adult visitors of children with suspected tuberculosis and employees at a children's hospital. *Infect Cont Hosp Epidemiol.* 2002;23:568.
15. Weinstein J, Barrett C, Baltimore R, et al. Nosocomial transmission of tuberculosis from a hospital visitor on a pediatrics ward. *Pediatr Infect Dis J.* 1995;14:232.
16. Starke JR. Transmission of *Mycobacterium tuberculosis* to and from children and adolescents. *Semin Pediatr Infect Dis.* 2001;12:115.
17. Centers for Disease Control and Prevention. Guidelines for preventing the transmission of *Mycobacterium tuberculosis* in health-care facilities. 1994. *MMWR Morb Mortal Wkly Rep.* 1994;43 (RR-13);1.
18. Marais BJ, Gie RP, Schaaf HS, et al. The natural history of childhood intra-thoracic tuberculosis is a critical review of literature from the prechemotherapy era. *Int J Tuberc Lung Dis.* 2004;8:392.
19. Marais BJ, Gie PR, Schaaf HS, et al. The clinical epidemiology of childhood pulmonary tuberculosis: in a critical review of literature from the pre-chemotherapy era. *Int J Tuberc Lung Dis.* 2004;8:278.
20. Wallgren A. The time-table of tuberculosis. *Tubercle.* 1948; 29:245.
21. Miller FJ W, Seale RME, Taylor MD. *Tuberculosis in Children.* Boston, MA: Little Brown; 1963:214.
22. Salazar GE, Schmitz TL, Cama R, et al. Pulmonary tuberculosis in children in a developing country. *Pediatrics.* 2001;108:448.
23. Hesseling A, Schaaf H, Gie R, et al. A critical review of diagnostic approaches used in the diagnosis of childhood tuberculosis. *Int J Tuberc Lung Dis.* 2002;6:1038.
24. American Thoracic Society. Diagnostic standards and classification of tuberculosis in adults and children. *Am J Respir Crit Care Med.* 2000;161:1376.
25. Vallejo J, Ong L, Starke J. Clinical features, diagnosis and treatment of tuberculosis in infants. *Pediatrics.* 1994; 94:1.
26. Teeratkulpisarn J, Lumbigagnon P, Pairojkul S, et al. Cavitary tuberculosis in a young infant. *Pediatr Infect Dis J.* 1994; 13:545.
27. Nemir RL, Krasinski K. Tuberculosis in children and adolescents in the 1980s. *Pediatr Infect Dis J.* 1988;7:375.
28. Delacourt C, Mani TM, Bonnerot V, et al. Computed tomography with normal chest radiograph in tuberculous infection. *Arch Dis Child.* 1993;69:430.
29. Matsaniotis N, Kattanis C, Economou-Mavrou C, et al. Bullous emphysema in childhood tuberculosis. *J Pediatr.* 1967;71:703.

30. Lincoln EM, Davies PA, Bovornkitti S. Tuberculous pleurisy with effusion in children. *Am Rev Tuberc.* 1958;77:271.

31. Hussey G, Chisolm T, Kibel M: Miliary tuberculosis in children. a review of 94 cases. *Pediatr Infect Dis J.* 1991; 10:832.

32. Schuit KE. Miliary tuberculosis in children. *Am J Dis Child.* 1979;133:583.

33. Doerr CA, Starke JR, Ong LT. Clinical and public health aspects of tuberculous meningitis in children. *J Pediatr.* 1995;127:27.

34. Afghani B, Lieberman JM. Paradoxical enlargement or development of intracranial tuberculomas during therapy: case Report and review. *Clin Infect Dis.* 1994;19:1092.

35. Chan SP, Birnbaum J, Rao M. Clinical manifestations and outcome of tuberculosis in children with acquired immunodeficiency syndrome. *Pediatr Infect Dis J.* 1996;15:443.

36. Khouri Y, Mastrucci M, Hutto C, et al. *Mycobacterium tuberculosis* in children with human immunodeficiency virus type 1 infection. *Pediatr Infect Dis J.* 1992;11:950.

37. Huebner RE, Schein MF, Bass JB. The tuberculin skin test. *Clin Infect Dis.* 1993;17:968.

38. Eamranond P, Jaramillo E. Tuberculosis in children: reassessing the need for improved diagnosis in global control strategies. *Int J Tuberc Lung Dis.* 2001;5:594.

39. Shingadia D, Novelli V. Diagnosis and treatment of tuberculosis in children. *Lancet Infect Dis.* 2003;3:624.

40. American Academy of Pediatrics. Red Book, Report of the Committee on Infectious Disease, 2003.

41. Steiner P, Rao M, Victoria MS, et al. Persistently negative tuberculin reactions: their presence among children culture positive for *Mycobacterium tuberculosis. Am J Dis Child.* 1980;134:747.

42. Sepulveda RL, Burr C, Ferrer X, et al. Booster effect of tuberculosis testing in healthy 6-year-old school children vaccinated with Bacilli Calmette-Guérin at birth in Santiago, Chile. *Pediatr Infect Dis J.* 1988;7:578.

43. Laven GI. Diagnosis of tuberculosis in children using fluorescence microscopic examination of gastric washings. *Am Rev Respir Dis.* 1977;115:743.

44. Giammona ST, Zelkowitz PS. The use of superheated nebulized saline and gastric lavage to obtain bacterial cultures in primary pulmonary tuberculosis in children. *Am J Dis Child.* 1969;117:198.

45. Zar H, Tannenbaum E, Apolles P, et al. Sputum induction for the diagnosis of pulmonary tuberculosis in infants and young children in an urban setting in South Africa. *Arch Dis Child.* 2000;82:305.

46. Abadco D, Steiner P. Gastric lavage is better than bronchoalveolar lavage for isolation of *Mycobacterium tuberculosis* in childhood pulmonary tuberculosis. *Pediatr Infect Dis J.* 1992;11:735.

47. Chan S, Abadco D, Steiner P. Role of flexible fiberoptic bronchoscopy in the diagnosis of childhood endobronchial tuberculosis. *Pediatr Infect Dis J.* 1994;13:506.

48. Noordhoek G, Kolk A, Bjune G, et al. Sensitivity and specificity of PCR for detection of *Mycobacterium tuberculosis*: a blind comparison study among seven laboratories. J Clin Microbiol. 1994;32:277.

49. Delacourt C, Poveda JD, Churean C, et al. Use of polymerase chain reaction for improved diagnosis of tuberculosis in children. *J Pediatr.* 1995;126:703.

50. Pierre C, Olivier C, Lecossier D, et al. Diagnosis of primary tuberculosis in children by amplification and detection of mycobacterial DNA. *Am Rev Respir Dis.* 1993;147:420.

51. Smith KC, Starke JR, Eisenach K, et al. Detection of *Mycobacterium tuberculosis* in clinical specimens from children using a polymerase chain reaction. *Pediatrics.* 1996;97:155.

52. Pastrana DG, Torronteras R, Caro P, et al. Comparison of Amplicor, in-house polymerase chain reactions and conventional culture for the diagnosis of tuberculosis in children. *Clin Infect Dis.* 2001;32:17.

53. Pediatric Tuberculosis Collaborative Group. Diagnosis and Treatment of latent tuberculosis infection in children and adolescents. *Pediatrics*: 2004;114:1175.

54. Dormer BA, Harrison I, Swart JA, et al. Prophylactic isoniazid protection of infants in a tuberculosis hospital. *Lancet.* 1959;2:902.

55. Ferrebee SH. Controlled chemoprophylaxis trials in tuberculosis: A general review: *Adv Tuberc Res.* 1969;17:28.

56. Hsu KHK. Thirty years after isoniazid: its impact on tuberculosis in children and adolescents. *JAMA.* 1984;251:1283.

57. O'Brien RJ, Long MW, Cross FS, et al. Hepatoxicity from isoniazid and rifampin among children treated for tuberculosis. *Pediatrics.* 1983;72:491.

58. Comstock GW, Livesay VT, Woopert SF. Prognosis of a positive tuberculin reaction in childhood and adolescence. *Am J Epidemiol.* 1974;99:131.

59. American Thoracic Society/Centers for Disease Control and Prevention/Infectious Diseases Society of America. Treatment of tuberculosis. *Am J Respir Crit Care Med.* 2003; 167:603.

60. Comstock GW, Baum C, Snider DE Jr. Isoniazid prophylaxis among Alaskan Eskimos: final report of the Bethel isoniazid studies. *Am Rev Respir Dis.* 1979;119:827.

61. Comstock GW, Hammes LM, Pio A. Isoniazid prophylaxis in Alaskan boarding schools: comparison of two doses. *Am Rev Respir Dis.* 1969;100:773.

62. International Union Against Tuberculosis Committee on Prophylaxis. Efficacy of various durations of isoniazid preventive therapy for tuberculosis: five years of follow-up in the IUAT trial. *Bull WHO.* 1982;60:555.

63. Snider DE Jr, Caras GJ, Kaplan JP. Preventive therapy with isoniazid: cost-effectiveness of different durations of therapy. *JAMA.* 1986;255:1579.

64. Starke JR. Multidrug therapy for tuberculosis in children. *Pediatr Infect Dis J.* 1990;9:785.

65. Abernathy RS, Dutt AK, Stead WW, et al. Short-course chemotherapy for tuberculosis in children. *Pediatrics.* 1983;72:801.

66. Jacobs RF, Abernathy RS. The treatment of tuberculosis in children. *Pediatr Infect Dis.* 1985;4:513.

67. Reis FJ, Bedran MB, Mowra JA, et al. Six-month isoniazid-rifampin treatment for pulmonary tuberculosis in children. *Am Rev Respir Dis.* 1990;142:996.
68. Aquinas SM. Short-course therapy for tuberculosis. *Drugs.* 1982;24:118.
69. Biddulph J. Short-course chemotherapy for childhood tuberculosis. *Pediatr Infect Dis J.* 1990;9:794.
70. Ibanez S, Ross G. Quimioterapia abreviada de 6 meses en tuberculosis pulmonary infantile. *Rev Chil Pediatr.* 1980; 51:249.
71. Kumar L, Dhand R, Singhi PD, et al. A randomized trial of fully intermittent vs. daily followed by intermittent short-course chemotherapy for childhood tuberculosis. *Pediatr Infect Dis J.* 1990;9:802.
72. Tsakalidis D, Pratsidou P, Hitoglou-Makedou A, et al. Intensive short course chemotherapy for treatment of Greek children with tuberculosis. *Pediatr Infect Dis J.* 1992;11:1036–1042.
73. Varudkar BL. Short-course chemotherapy for tuberculosis in children. *Indian J Pediatr.* 1985;52:593.
74. Al-Dossary FS, Ong LT, Correa AG, et al. Treatment of childhood tuberculosis with a six month directly observed regimen of only two weeks of daily therapy. *Pediatr Infect Dis J.* 2002;21:91.
75. Te Water Naude JM, Donald PR, Hussey GO, et al. Twice-weekly vs. daily chemotherapy for childhood tuberculosis. *Pediatr Infect Dis J.* 2000;19:405.
76. Tuberculosis in children: guidelines for diagnosis, prevention and treatment (Statement of the Scientific Committee of the International Union Against Tuberculosis and Lung Disease). *Bull Int Union Tuberc Lung Dis.* 1991;66:61.
77. Jawahar MS, Sivasubramanian S, Vijayan VK, et al. Short course chemotherapy for tuberculous lymphadenitis in children. *Br Med J.* 1990;301:359.
78. Vsiudhiphan P, Chiemchanya S: Tuberculous meningitis in children: treatment with isoniazid and rifampin for twelve months. *J Pediatr.* 1989;114:875.
79. Kendig EL Jr. Tuberculosis among children in the United States. *Pediatrics.* 1978;62:269.
80. Jacobs RF, Sunakorn P, Chotpitayasunonah T, et al. Intensive short course chemotherapy for tuberculous meningitis. *Pediatr Infect Dis J.* 1992;11:194.
81. Centers for Disease Control. Interstate outbreak of drug-resistant tuberculosis involving children: California, Montana, Nevada, Utah *MMWR Morb Mortal Wkly Rep.* 1983;32:516.
82. Riley LW, Arathoon E, Loverde VD. The epidemiologic patterns of drug-resistant *Mycobacterium tuberculosis* infections: A community-based study. *Am Rev Respir Dis.* 1989;139:1282.
83. Steiner P, Rao M, Mitchell M. Primary drug-resistant tuberculosis in children: correlation of drug-susceptibility patterns of matched patient and source-case strains of *Mycobacterium tuberculosis. Am J Dis Child.* 1985;139:780.
84. Schaaf HS, Gie RP, Beyer N, et al. Primary drug-resistant tuberculosis. *Pediatr Infect Dis J.* 2000;19:695.
85. Ridzon R, Kent JH, Valway S, et al. Outbreak of drug-resistant tuberculosis with secondary—generation transmission in a high school in California. *J Pediatr.* 1997;131:863.
86. Steiner P, Rao M. Drug-resistant tuberculosis in children. *Semin Pediatr Infect Dis.* 1993;4:275.
87. Swanson DS, Starke JR. Drug-resistant tuberculosis in pediatrics. *Pediatr Clin North Am.* 1995;42:553.
88. Lobato M, Mohle-Boetani JC, Royce SE. Missed opportunities for preventing tuberculosis among children younger than five years of age. *Pediatrics.* 2000;106:e75.
89. Mohle-Boetani JC, Miller B, Halpern M, et al. School-based screening for tuberculous infection: a cost benefit analysis. *JAMA.* 1995;274:613.
90. Mohle-Boetani, JC, Flood J. Contact investigations and the continued commitment to control tuberculosis. *JAMA.* 2002;287:1040.

30

Pregnancy and the Puerperium

David Fleece
Stephen C. Aronoff

The issue of tuberculosis (TB) during pregnancy and the puerperium is not simply an historical inquiry but rather an increasingly familiar clinical problem facing industrial nations as well as the emerging countries of the world. This chapter focuses on the maternal aspects of tuberculous infection, including transmission to the fetus. For discussion of TB in the newborn, the reader is referred to Chapter 29.

EFFECT OF TUBERCULOSIS ON PREGNANCY

Tuberculosis can affect female reproduction before pregnancy because infection of the genital organs can lead to infertility and abdominal or tubal pregnancy. In the prechemotherapy era, prematurity rates in tuberculous women ranged from 23–44%, with the higher rates in the most severely affected mothers.[1] In a study of 124 women in England with TB complicated by pregnancy during the period 1944–1953, all had healthy babies, although only four of the patients had received chemotherapy.[2] With early recognition and effective chemotherapy, there is no evidence of adverse effect on pregnancy.[3,4] In patients with advanced disease, coinfection with human immunodeficiency virus (HIV), or little to no prenatal care, prematurity, and intrauterine growth retardation (IUGR) occur in approximately 30% of pregnancies.[5,6] Similar results were reported from the Indian subcontinent, where 79 pregnancies complicated by TB had a twofold increase in prematurity and small-for-gestational-age (SGA) status compared with 316 uninfected controls of similar age, parity, and socioeconomic status. Adverse perinatal outcome was associated with late diagnosis, inadequate treatment, and advanced disease.[7]

EFFECTS OF PREGNANCY ON TUBERCULOSIS

Hippocrates believed that pregnancy had a salutary effect on TB. This belief persisted until the middle of the 19th century, when case reports of accelerated progression of disease

during pregnancy surfaced.[8] An often quoted dictum from the 19th century was, "For the virgin no marriage, for the married no pregnancy, for the pregnant no confinement, and for the mother no suckling." Osler[9] recommended that physicians veto the marriage of any girl "whose family history is bad, whose chest expansion is slight, and whose physique is below the standard." There is much truth, indeed, in the remark of Dubois: '*If a woman threatened with phthisis (pulmonary TB) marries, she may bear the first accouchement well; a second, with difficulty; a third, never.*'

A number of reports from the 1950s, however, showed that pregnancy did not predispose to progressive disease. In a report of 250 women with active TB in the pretreatment era, 83.9% remained stable during pregnancy and 9.1% improved. Although only 7% had evidence of progressive disease during pregnancy, an additional 8.2% experienced progression in the year following pregnancy.[10] A study published in the era of chemotherapy had similar results, with a relapse rate of only 3% after completing a course of chemotherapy. As with the earlier study, most of the relapses occurred in the postpartum period.[4]

Pregnancy may mask the symptoms of early TB, such as tachypnea and fatigue, which may, in turn, delay the diagnosis and treatment of the infection. More than half the patients in two studies were asymptomatic and unaware of their disease.[11,12] Failure to recognize and treat the infection in the pregnant woman may lead to congenital infection in the infant. As evidence of this, in some series of congenital TB the mother was evaluated and TB was diagnosed only after the disease was diagnosed in the infant. Pregnancy does not alter the site of disease; most studies report 5–10% of patients with extrapulmonary disease, similar to the rate in nonpregnant patients.[11]

PATHOGENESIS AND CONGENITAL INFECTION

The pathogenesis of TB in the pregnant woman begins as in all other patients. After exposure, usually by inhalation, and local replication, there is dissemination of the organism by lymphatic spread, hematogenous spread, or both. If the organism affects the placenta or genital tract, the child may be congenitally infected. The mycobacterium may be delivered to the infant directly via the umbilical vein or through aspiration of infected amniotic fluid.

Congenital infection, or infection of the fetus, must be distinguished from disease in the newborn acquired postnatally. The original standardized criteria for distinguishing between the two were proposed by Beitzke[13] in 1935 and were as follows:

- Infant has proven tuberculous lesions, and one of the following:
  - Lesions in the first few days of life
  - A primary hepatic complex
  - Exclusion of postnatal transmission by separation at birth of the infant from the mother and other potential sources

Cantwell et al.[14] reviewed congenital TB in 1994, including all published case reports since 1980. They concluded that the original diagnostic criteria had limited use, based, in part, on over-reliance of autopsy or liver biopsy data, as well as the now uncommon practice of isolating the newborn. Therefore, they proposed modified diagnostic criteria, more compatible with modern practice. These consist of the following:

- Infant has proven tuberculous lesions and one of the following:
  - Lesions in the first week of life
  - A primary hepatic complex or caseating hepatic granulomas
  - Tuberculous infection of the placenta or maternal genital tract
  - Exclusion of postnatal transmission by a thorough investigation of contacts and adherence to current infection control guidelines

The authors showed these criteria to have increased diagnostic sensitivity when applied to the cases reported in the literature.

EPIDEMIOLOGY

The epidemiology of TB in pregnancy reflects that of TB at large. Worldwide, the number of cases of TB is slowly increasing, with declining rates in western and central Europe, North and South America and the Middle East more than offset by increases in Sub-Saharan Africa and the former Soviet Union.[15] For the United States, the rising incidence of TB seen during the late 1980s and early 1990s appears to have ended. The case rate (per 100,000 total population) of 10.5 in 1992 declined to 5.2 in 2002. Differing ethnic groups, though, have widely differing rates. The 2002 TB case rates for women of childbearing age from various ethnic groups are found in Table 30-1.[16]

For women of childbearing age, infection with HIV represents a significant risk factor for TB infection. Of 16 pregnant women with TB in New York City reported by Margono and coworkers,[5] 7 of 11 tested were HIV-positive. Also highlighting the increased risk of TB in pregnancy in HIV-infected women was a study of 124 HIV-positive women, of whom 46 were pregnant. Five of the pregnant women (11 %) had a positive tuberculin skin test reaction, and 14 (30%) were anergic.[17]

CLINICAL MANIFESTATIONS

The clinical manifestations of TB in pregnancy are similar to those in nonpregnant women. Good and associates[18] reported that among 27 women with active disease, cough (71%), weight loss (41%), fever (30%), and malaise and fatigue (30%) were the most common symptoms; however, 20% of the women were asymptomatic.

The lungs are the most common site affected and account for approximately 90% of all cases.[11,19] Lymph node, bone, and kidney disease affect most of the remaining patients. HIV infection modifies the type of TB disease to more serious forms. In a study of 16 patients with TB in an area of high HIV prevalence, there were 10 cases of pulmonary disease (5 cavitary), 2 meningeal, 1 mediastinal, 1 renal, 1 gastrointestinal, and 1 pleural.[5]

Table 30-1. Tuberculosis Case Rates Per 100,000 Population for Women of Childbearing Age, United States 2002

Ethnic Group	15–24 Year Olds	25–44 Year Olds
White, non-Hispanic	0.4	1.0
Black, non-Hispanic	7.1	12.1
Hispanic	7.1	8.6
Asian/Pacific Islander	20.8	28.0

Source: CDC. Reported Tuberculosis in the United States, 2002. Atlanta, GA: U.S. Department of Health and Human Services, CDC, September 2003.

DIAGNOSIS

The tuberculin skin test (Mantoux) is the test of choice for diagnosing TB infection in pregnant women. Although pregnant women have suppressed cell-mediated immunity to tuberculin in *in vitro* studies,[20,21] this does not appear to be clinically relevant.[22] Pregnancy does not alter the response to a tuberculin skin test; however, 10–25% of immunocompetent persons with active TB, pregnant or not, will have a negative test result.[23] Because the nonspecific symptoms of TB (increased respiratory rate, fatigue) mimic the physiologic changes in pregnancy and therefore may be missed, TB skin testing should be pursued in high-risk populations. These include minority urban communities, recent immigrants from countries with a high prevalence of TB, intravenous drug users, populations at high risk for HIV infection, and persons already infected with HIV.[24]

HIV-infected persons with active TB have a negative skin test result in 40–60% of cases.[5,24] Skin test negativity is highly correlated with CD4 count and not with pregnancy. A study of pregnant and nonpregnant women infected with HIV showed that the anergy rate to tetanus toxin and mumps was 14 of 46 (30%) in pregnant women and 38 of 78 (49%) in nonpregnant women. Anergy was associated with lower CD4 counts in both groups in this study, and although the nonpregnant women were more likely to be anergic, the CD4 counts were similar in both groups.[17]

A thorough investigation to detect TB should be pursued for all persons with clinical features compatible with TB. Because of the high rate of anergy in HIV-infected patients, all pregnant women at risk for or with known HIV infection should also be evaluated.[24] To rule out active TB, routine chest radiographs with proper shielding of the abdomen after the 12th week of gestation should be performed in women with a positive tuberculin skin test result. Chest radiographs should be performed sooner if symptoms suggest pulmonary TB, even if the skin test result is negative. In addition, examination of specimens for mycobacteria should be performed in all patients with HIV infection and pulmonary disease. A complete review of systems and physical examination should be conducted to exclude extrapulmonary TB.[24,25] In one study, among 16 pregnant women with active TB (7 of whom were known to be HIV-infected), only 6 of 15 had positive skin test results and 6 of 16 had extrapulmonary disease.[5]

TREATMENT

Preventive Therapy

Isoniazid (INH) effectively prevents the progression of latent infection to active disease in individuals infected with susceptible strains. Furthermore, there is no evidence of teratogenic effects on the fetus. The major side effect of INH is hepatitis, which occurs most frequently in persons over 35 years of age. Pregnancy and the postpartum period are also considered independent risk factors for INH toxicity. In a report of 20 deaths due to INH toxicity, 4 were in women who began taking INH in pregnancy and continued after delivery. The incidence of death was estimated to be 1 in 2000 postpartum women taking INH.[26]

The American Thoracic Society states that for most pregnant women, preventive therapy should generally be delayed until after delivery. The exception is for women with recent infection. In this case, preventive therapy should begin when TB is documented but not until after the first trimester. The recommendation to begin therapy after delivery is based on the increased risk of active TB during the postpartum period, notwithstanding the increased toxicity of INH during this period.[27] The Advisory Committee for the Elimination of Tuberculosis Guidelines published in 1990 do not specifically address preventive therapy or treatment of pregnant women.

Because of the high risk of development of active disease in the TB-infected, HIV-positive woman, preventive therapy should be given to all patients who experience purified protein derivative (PPD) conversion and strongly considered for those who have negative test results but are anergic and from high-incidence areas. In all cases, preventive therapy should consist of INH, 300 mg in a single daily dose. Pyridoxine supplementation should be given to all pregnant and breast-feeding women taking INH. In addition, because nursing infants receive approximately 20% of a therapeutic dosage of INH through breast milk, these infants should also receive pyridoxine supplementation because neurotoxicity, including seizures, has been reported in these children.[28,29] Alternatively, breast-feeding mothers may take their medication immediately after breast-feeding and substitute a bottle for the next feeding.

Active Disease

Pregnant women with active TB should begin therapy as soon as the diagnosis is established. The risk of transmission of the organism to the infant outweighs the risks of the drugs to the mother's own health. The preferred initial treatment for pregnant women is INH, rifampin, and ethambutol. Streptomycin should not be used because there is a risk of sensorineural hearing loss in the infant.[30] Pyrazinamide (PZA) is recommended for routine use in pregnant women by the WHO, but has not received such approval in the United States due to a paucity of safety data.[31]

If resistance to the first-line drugs is encountered, the risks and benefits of second-line drugs should be weighed and their use considered. Unfortunately, most second-line medications may have deleterious effects on the fetus. Ethionamide use has been associated with teratogenic effects in animals. Aminoglycosides including kanamycin, capreomycin and amikacin presumably share streptomycin's ototoxic potential. The fluoroquinolones have been shown to damage growing cartilage, and thus should be avoided in pregnancy if at all possible.[31] Treatment duration should be 9 months.

REFERENCES

1. Ratner B, Rostler AE, Salgado PS. Care, feeding and fate of premature and full term infants born of tuberculous mothers. *Am J Dis Child.* 1951;81:471.
2. Pugh DL. The relation of child-bearing and child-rearing to pulmonary tuberculosis. *Br J Tuberc.* 1955;49:206–216.
3. Mehta BR: Pregnancy and tuberculosis. *Dis Chest.* 1961; 39:505–511.
4. Schaefer G, Zervoudakis IA, Fuchs FF, et al. Pregnancy and pulmonary tuberculosis. *Obstet Gynecol.*1975;46:706–715.
5. Margono F. Mroueh J, Garely A, et al. Resurgence of active tuberculosis among pregnant women. *Obstet Gynecol.* 1994;83:911–914.
6. Hamadeh MA, Glassroth J. Tuberculosis and pregnancy. *Chest.* 1992;101:1114–1120.
7. Jana N, Vasishta K, Jindal SK, et al. Perinatal outcome in pregnancies complicated by pulmonary tuberculosis. *Int J Gynaecol Obstet.* 1994;44:119–124.
8. Grisolle A. De l'influence que la grossesse et la phthisie pulmonaire excercent reciproquement l'une sur l'autre. *Arch Gen Med.* 1850;22:41.
9. Osler W. In *The Principles and Practice of Medicine*, 2nd ed. New York, D. Appleton, 1897.
10. Hedvall E. Pregnancy and tuberculosis. *Acta Med Scand.* 1953;147(Suppl 286):1–101.
11. Wilson EA, Thelin TJ, Dilts PV. Tuberculosis complicated by pregnancy. *Am J Obstet Gynecol.* 1972;115:526.
12. Carter EJ, Mates S. Tuberculosis during pregnancy: The Rhode Island experience, 1987 to 1991. *Chest.* 1994;106: 1466–1470.
13. Beitzke H. Ueber die angeborene tuberkuloese infection. *Ergeb Ges Tuberk Forsch.* 1935:7:1–30.
14. Cantwell MF, Shehab ZM, Costello AM et al. Congenital Tuberculosis. *N Engl J Med.* 1994;330:1051–1054.
15. Frieden TR, Sterling TR, Munsiff SS et al. Tuberculosis. *Lancet.* 2003;362(9387):887–899.
16. CDC. Reported Tuberculosis in the United States, 2002. Atlanta, GA: U.S. Department of Health and Human Services, CDC, September 2003.
17. Mofenson L, Rodriguez EM, Hershow R, et al. *Mycobacterium tuberculosis* infection in pregnant and nonpregnant women infected with HIV in the Women and Infants Transmission Study. *Arch Intern Med.* 1995;155:1066–1072.
18. Good JT, Iseman MD, Davidson PT, et al. Tuberculosis in association with pregnancy. *Am J Obstet Gynecol.* 1981;140: 492–498.
19. Hammer GS, Hirshman SZ. Infections in pregnancy. In: Cherry SH, Berkowitz RL, Kase NG, eds. *Medical, Surgical and Gynecologic Complications of Pregnancy*, 3rd ed. Baltimore: Williams & Wilkins; 1985:14–15.
20. Covelli HD, Wilson RT. Immunologic and medical considerations in tuberculin-sensitized pregnant patients. *Am J Obstet Gynecol.* 1978;132:256–259.
21. Tanaka A, Hirota K, Takahashi K, et al. Suppression of cell mediated immunity to cytomegalovirus and tuberculin in pregnancy employing the leukocyte migration inhibition test. *Microbiol Immun.* 1983;27:937–943.
22. Present PA, Comstock GW. Tuberculin sensitivity in pregnancy. *Am Rev Respir Dis.* 1975;112:413–416.
23. Huebner RE, Schein MF, Bass JB. The tuberculin skin test. *Clin Infect Dis.* 1993;17:968–975.
24. Centers for Disease Control. Screening for tuberculosis infection in high risk populations. *MMWR Morb Mortal Wkly Rep.* 1990;39(No. RR-8):1–7.
25. Centers for Disease Control. The use of preventive therapy for tuberculous infection in the United States: Recommendations of the Advisory Committee for Elimination of Tuberculosis. *MMWR Morb Mortal Wkly Rep.* 1990;39(No. RR-8):9–12.
26. Moulding TS, Redeker AG, Kanal GC. Twenty isoniazid-associated deaths in one state. *Am Rev Respir Dis.* 1989;140: 700–705.
27. American Thoracic Society. Treatment of tuberculosis and tuberculosis infection in adults and children. *Am Rev Respir Dis.* 1986;134:355–363.
28. Snider DE, Powell KE. Should mothers taking antituberculous drugs breast feed? *Arch Intern Med.* 1984;144:589–590.
29. McKenzie SA, Macnab AI, Katz G. Neonatal pyridoxine responsive convulsions due to isoniazid therapy. *Arch Dis Child.* 1976;51:567.
30. Snider DE, Layde RM, Johnson MW, et al. Treatment of tuberculosis during pregnancy. *Am Rev Respir Dis.* 1980;122: 65–79.
31. Centers for Disease Control and Prevention. Treatment of Tuberculosis, American Thoracic Society, CDC, and Infectious Diseases Society of America. *MMWR Morb Mortal Wkly Rep.* 2003;52(No. RR-11):62–63.

31

HIV and Tuberculosis

Midori Kato-Maeda
Peter M. Small

INTRODUCTION

Tuberculosis (TB) is an opportunistic infection among patients infected with the human immunodeficiency virus (HIV). In persons infected only with *Mycobacterium tuberculosis* (MTB) the risk of developing TB is approximately 10% during their life time.[1] In contrast, in patients infected with HIV and MTB, the risk of developing TB is 10% per year.[2] This is explained by the synergic interaction of MTB and HIV. HIV induces immunosuppression and therefore is an important risk factor for the progression of MTB infection to disease and for death by TB. Conversely, MTB accelerates the progression of HIV infection. In this chapter, we will review the pathogenesis of the coinfection of HIV and TB, the epidemiology, and the clinical aspects of TB in patients infected with HIV.

PATHOGENESIS OF THE COINFECTION OF MTB-HIV

The principal effect of HIV is immune dysfunction and immune depletion. HIV enters into macrophages facilitated by the attachment of its glycoprotein GP120 to the CD4 receptor and the chemokine receptor CCR5, which is critical in the initial establishment of HIV infection. Eventually HIV infects T-lymphocyte helper cells, facilitated by the CD4 receptor in conjunction with the chemokine receptor CXCR4.[3] It is estimated that a tremendous turnover of viral particles takes place, with some 10 virions produced each day. Another effect of HIV is the induction of mononuclear cell apoptosis.[4] The result is a selective and progressive depletion of CD4+ T lymphocytes and alteration of macrophage function. Eventually, HIV causes profound immunosuppression, at some point manifested as an opportunistic infection, neoplasm, or other life-threatening complication. AIDS is only the last stage of this process.

Because of the dysfunction and depletion of CD4+ T lymphocytes and other components of the cellular immune system, TB is frequently diagnosed in patients with HIV infection. Tuberculosis is observed in all stages of the HIV infection. In early stages, the inflammatory response and the clinical and histopathologic characteristics of TB are similar to those persons who are not infected with HIV, with the presence of granuloma with or without central caseation. Nonetheless, with the progression of the immunosuppression, granulomas are either not well formed or absent. Instead, abundant tubercle bacilli and abscess formation in soft tissues is frequently observed.[5]

Conversely, MTB induces progression of HIV immunosuppression by at least two mechanisms.[6] First, MTB induces the replication of HIV in cells of the monocyte lineage and in acutely infected primary macrophages.[7,8] This phenomena has been attributed to proinflammatory cytokines such as TNFα, which is induced in mononuclear cells by MTB.[7] TNFα accelerates HIV replication through nuclear factor kappa B (NFkB) and p38MAP kinase. It may also be accelerated by the presence of high levels of non-inhibitory β-chemokine (MCP1) and low levels of inhibitory β-chemokines (MIP-1 alpha, MIP-1 beta and RANTES) at the site of MTB infection. This may explain why replication of HIV-1 is more prominent in the sites where MTB is present, independent of systemic HIV activity.[9] Second, MTB activates transcriptionally latent HIV in alveolar macrophages or in monocytes newly recruited to sites of MTB infection.[6] The clinical effect of MTB on HIV replication has been confirmed in a cohort of patients, whose viral load increased on average of 2.5 fold at the time of the diagnosis of TB.[8]

The result of the complex immunologic interaction of HIV and MTB is progressive immunosuppression that increases the risk of TB, both by reactivation of a latent TB infection (LTBI) and by recent infection and rapid evolution to TB. HIV is the strongest risk factor, independent of the number of CD4 cells, to develop reactivation of LTBI. Among intravenous drug users with positive skin tests, 7 of 49 (14%) persons infected with HIV developed active TB within 2 years compared with 0 of 62 not infected with HIV.[2] This rate exceeds the lifetime risk of reactivation in patients without HIV infection.[2] HIV is also a risk factor for having been recently infected.[10] A study performed in New York City demonstrated that 40% of the cases of TB were the result of recent transmission, HIV/AIDS being an independent risk factor. The immunosuppression by HIV accelerates the progression of recently acquired infection to active TB. In Italy, 7 of 18 (35%) patients with HIV exposed to MTB in a nosocomial outbreak developed TB within 60 days.[11] In San Francisco, 37% of the contacts of a smear positive TB patient in a residential facility of patients with AIDS developed active TB by the same strain within 3 months of diagnosis of the first case.[12] Nevertheless, HIV infection does not enhance the infectiousness of individual patients with TB. In fact, the proportion of HIV patients with smear positive pulmonary TB (a known factor for infectiousness) is lower than in HIV negative patients.[13]

EPIDEMIOLOGY

The interaction of HIV/AIDS and MTB has consequences at the individual level, where HIV has changed the clinical course of TB. It also has consequences at the population level; both in the United States as well as in other parts of the world, by increasing the number of cases of TB which has compromised the possibility of controlling this epidemic.[14]

In the United States, by the end of 2002, approximately 500,000 people had died of AIDS.[15] Although the mortality rate decreased 14% from 1998 to 2002, the number of reported new cases of HIV/AIDS was stable, with an estimated 26,464 new cases in 2002. As a result, the number of persons living with AIDS increased to approximately 390,000 persons in 2002 and the number of persons living with HIV is estimated to be between 850,000 and 950,000, one-quarter of whom are unaware of their infection.[16] The epidemic of HIV/AIDS was temporally associated with the resurgence of TB in the United States and other industrialized countries. The increase in TB case rates was more dramatic in the geographic areas and populations such as homeless population[17] that have been most severely affected by AIDS. Although it is clear that the increased susceptibility of HIV-infected people greatly contributed to the increase in TB rates in the United States and worldwide,[18] it must be stressed that this increase was also in part due to waning attention to and decreased funding of control efforts. Indirect evidence for this is the fact that after peaking in 1992, TB rates in the United States began a steady decline despite the increase in the number of cases of HIV/AIDS.[15]

Since 1993, in the United States the rate of TB has been decreasing by an average of 6.8% per year. In 2002, there were 15,072 new cases of TB corresponding to 5.2 cases per 100,000 inhabitants. As the overall rate of TB decreased, the frequency of the coinfection with HIV also decreased. From 1993 to 2001, the percentage of cases of TB with HIV coinfection decreased from 29% to 17% in persons 25–44 years old and from 15% to 9% in all ages.[18] This decrease is attributed to the TB control

measures such as improvements on the completion therapy with Direct Observed Therapy Short-Course (DOTS) and the increase on the detection of cases. It is also attributed to the treatment of HIV infection with antiretrovirals. Early studies showed a reduction of the incidence of TB (RR = 0.6, 95%IC 0.4–1.0),[19,20] which has been more significant with the use of more aggressive antiretroviral treatment such as highly active antiretroviral therapy (HAART) (RR = 0.2, 95%CI 0.1–0.5).[19,20] Although the frequency of the coinfection is decreasing in United States, it is estimated that around 200,000 persons infected with HIV are unaware of their infection[15,21] and 15 million persons have LTBI.[15,21] Because the risk factors for both infections are similar, it is necessary to continue the activities to control these epidemics.

Globally, the potential impact of HIV on TB is staggering. During 2003, the estimated number of new cases of TB was 8.8 million, an increase of incidence of 1.1% per year, and the number of deaths was approximately 2 million.[22] The increase in new cases of TB has been mostly attributed to HIV infection; 9% of all new TB cases in adults were attributed to HIV infection.[23] Of the 35–43 million persons infected with HIV around the world, it is estimated that 14 million are coinfected with TB.[24,25] Most of these cases are occurring in regions with limited resources. In fact, 29.4 million of the HIV patients live in sub-Saharan Africa, representing 8.8% of their population.[24] In this area, it is estimated that 31% of the adult cases of TB are attributable to HIV and the prevalence of HIV among new adult patients with TB is 38%.[23] The epidemic is growing despite the availability of drugs and interventions proven to be efficient to cure TB and control HIV infection.[18] DOTS strategy, which has increased the cure rate of TB is some areas, is not enough in settings where HIV is prevalent.[26] The use of antiretrovirals, which has been shown to have a positive impact in both epidemics,[27] is used by 5% of the patients with HIV in the world, most of them in developed countries.[28] In order to reverse the current trends it is necessary to consider HIV and TB as one entity and design strategies that focus on the management of these infections together.[29,30] The new strategies should be integrated into broader projects to decrease poverty and increase education.[31]

CLINICAL PRESENTATION

HIV does not alter the symptoms classically associated with TB such as fatigue, weight loss, fevers, sweats, cough, and anorexia; however, the symptoms are less

Table 31-1. Clinical Characteristic of TB in Patients Coinfected with HIV

During Early HIV Infection: Typical Features of TB are Frequent.
Usually pulmonary disease with involvement of the upper lobe and presence of cavitation.
Tuberculin skin test positive in >50% of cases.
Good response to therapy.

During Advance HIV Infection:
Any organ can be affected.
Extrapulmonary involvement is common (bone and/or joint, lymphatic, meningeal, pleural, hepatic, renal, splenic, spinal, cutaneous, miliary dissemination) with similar manifestations seen in patients without HIV infection.
Unusual radiographic findings (diffuse infiltration, mid and lower-lung zone infiltrates, intrathoracic adenopathy, pleural effusion, or normal).
PPD test results positive in <40% of cases.
Good response to therapy but early mortality may be high.

specific because other conditions, such as HIV-associated fevers and weight loss, lymphoma, and disseminated histoplasmosis produce symptoms consistent with TB.

Given that much of the pathology of TB results from the host's response to the infection, it is not surprising that the signs of TB vary considerably with the severity of HIV-induced immunosuppression. (Table 31-1) Although TB may develop at any stage in HIV infection, it tends to occur early. With mild immunosuppression, MTB causes disease that closely resembles that in patients without HIV infection. A "classical TB" presentation has been described in prospective studies in which either HIV infected patients were observed for the development of TB or patients with TB were tested for evidence of HIV infection.[32,33] As immunosuppression becomes progressively severe, the clinical presentation of TB becomes more "atypical" with unusual radiographic manifestations and nonreactive tuberculin skin tests, as well as disseminated and extrapulmonary TB.[32,33]

Tuberculosis in patients with HIV can affect any organ. In a prospective study of TB in patients with and without HIV infection (81% with CD4+ T lymphocyte count of 200 cells/mm^3 or lower), the lung was involved similarly in both groups: 74.3% and 78.3%, respectively.[34] The majority of patients with pulmonary involvement had positive cultures for MTB, but the direct sputum examination was positive only in 54.3% of patients with HIV as opposed to nearly 75% in patients without HIV infection. Interestingly, this discrepancy persisted even when only those patients who had either focal infiltrates or cavities apparent on chest radiographs were analyzed. Extrapulmonary TB, either as the sole presentation or concomitant with pulmonary involvement, is more frequent in patients with HIV infection (56.5% vs. 35.7%) and HIV is a strong risk factor for this type of TB (OR 4.93; 95%CI, 1.95–12.46).[35] The most common location among 85 patients in Arkansas was bone and/or joint TB (27%), followed by cervical lymphatic TB (17.7%).[35] Other forms seen were genitourinary, peritoneal, noncervical lymphatic, meningeal, and disseminated disease. Tuberculosis bacteremia, which is extremely rare in patients without HIV, was observed in 20–40% of patients,[36] and tuberculous meningitis in up to 10% of patients with TB and HIV.[2] Other manifestations have been reported such as cutaneous and splenic lesions. The clinical presentation of extrapulmonary TB is similar to immunocompetent patients[35]; however, TB meningitis in patients with HIV infection has more ventricular dilatation and infarcts,[37] and abdominal TB has more visceral lesions and intraabdominal lymphadenopathy (instead of ascites and omental thickening observed in patients without HIV infection).[38] Due to the diversity in the clinical presentation, it is important to consider TB in the differential diagnosis among patients infected with HIV/AIDS with fever.

DIAGNOSIS

Because of the high frequency of coinfection of MTB and HIV, all patients infected with HIV should be screened for LTBI and TB. Also, all patients with TB should be advised to undergo voluntary counseling and testing for HIV infection.[39–41] The methods used to diagnosis LTBI and TB are the same as in patients without HIV infection. However, the interpretation of the tests is complicated by the higher possibility of false negative results (e.g., negative tuberculin skin test, negative smear examination and normal chest x-ray) as well as the lack of specificity of the symptoms.

Diagnosis of LTBI

Skin test with PPD should be performed for screening and when TB is suspected in patients with HIV. Because HIV-induced immunosuppression may blunt the delayed hypersensitivity response, the CDC recommends that any induration greater than 5 mm be classified, as a significant reaction.[42] Anergy is increasingly common with progression of HIV disease. There is no method to evaluate anergy; the use antigens such as mumps or *Candida* are not recommended because of their lack of reliability.

Recently, two new methods to diagnose LTBI have been assessed in clinical studies. One is based on the production of interferon-γ by T-lymphocytes stimulated with MTB. Initial studies demonstrated conflicting results. One study demonstrated that the quantification of interferon-γ was less likely to be false positive over the skin test,[43] whereas other studies did not show any benefits.[44,45] Because this test relies on the ability of the T-lymphocyte immune response, until further evaluation, it is currently not recommended in patients infected with HIV.[46] The second method is also based on the production of interferon-γ in response to ESAT-6 and CFP-10, two highly immunogenic secreted antigens.[16] The results demonstrated less sensitivity but higher specificity compared with tuberculin skin test; however, no studies have been evaluated in patients with HIV infection.

Diagnosis of Tuberculosis

Specimens from any site suspected of being infected with TB should be submitted for mycobacterial smear and culture. The sensitivity of the sputum smear examination is lower, mainly in patients with advanced HIV infection when compared with patients without HIV infection. In one study, the sensitivity was 45% in patients with HIV infection compared with 81% in patients without HIV infection.[47] Currently, it is possible to confirm whether the acid fast bacilli (AFB) observed in a smear is MTB. This method is based on nucleic acid amplification and has a sensitivity of 100% if the sputum smear examination is positive.[48] In contrast, the sensitivity is around 50% if the smear examination is negative and therefore it is recommended in cases with a high clinical suspicion of pulmonary TB.[48,49] A recent study in Kenya demonstrated that the performance was similar in patients with and without HIV infection, when using culture in Lowenstein Jensen media as gold standard. The sensitivity of the

nucleic acid amplification method was 89% in patients with HIV and 95% in patients without HIV infection. In contrast, the sensitivity of the smear examination was 44% and 63%, respectively.[50] Although there is still no definitive data, experts suggests that if two different and adequate sputum samples are negative, the possibility of pulmonary TB is unlikely.[48] If the clinical suspicion of TB is high and the direct smear examination and nucleic acid amplification tests are negative, it is advisable to continue the patient evaluation, including invasive diagnostic procedures to obtain samples for histopathologic and microbiologic studies or to perform a treatment trial. The culture for mycobacterium is considered the gold standard for the diagnosis of TB and is reviewed extensively in this book earlier. The chest radiographs during the early stages of the HIV infection may demonstrate upper-lobe involvement and cavitation. During late stages, it is not rare to find involvement of the mid and lower lung lobes, lymphadenopathy (Fig. 31-1), pleural effusion (Fig. 31-2), and

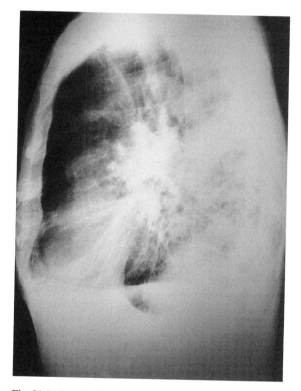

Fig. 31-1. Lateral chest radiograph showing extensive mid and lower lung field involvement and associated lymphadenopathy in a man with AIDS.

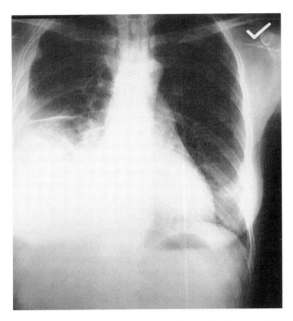

Fig. 31-2. Posteroanterior chest radiograph demonstrating extensive right lower infiltrate associated with pleural effusion.

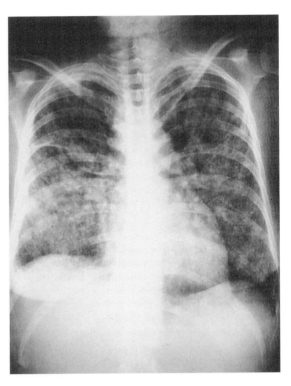

Fig. 31-3. Posteroanterior chest radiograph showing extensive bilateral diffuse infiltrate in a young woman with advanced HIV infection.

diffuse infiltrates (Fig. 31-3). In some cases, the chest radiographs are normal, even when the sputum examination shows acid-fast bacilli.[51]

The diagnosis of extrapulmonary TB is challenging because of the difficulty of obtaining an appropriate sample. Culture and the nucleic acid amplification methods are less sensitive and specific for extrapulmonary TB diagnosis. Sometimes, the diagnosis relies on epidemiologic and clinical manifestations and the response to treatment.[48,52]

TREATMENT OF LTBI

Although the risk for TB has decreased considerably with HAART, it is still twice as high relative to those without HIV infection.[13,20,53] Therefore an attempt should be made to identify and treat all dually infected persons. Treatment should be offered to those with a skin test ≥5 mm who have not received treatment for LTBI. Also, it should be offered to patients infected with HIV who have been in contact with patients with TB, regardless of their skin test and previous history of treatment for TB.[54,55]

The treatment for LTBI is the same as in patients without HIV infection. The treatment should be started after

excluding the presence of active TB with a medical history, physical examination, and chest x-ray. Treatment with isoniazid for six months decreases by 60% (range of 35–76%) the likelihood of patients with HIV and positive skin test to develop TB.[56] The treatment with daily or twice a week dose of isoniazid for 9 months has less drug interactions and secondary effects, but has less compliance because of the length of the treatment. The treatment with daily rifampin for 4 months has a higher drug interaction and should be used cautiously.[57,58] The treatment with rifampin and pyrazinamide should not be used in patients infected with HIV because the high risk of developing liver disease, unless the potential benefits outweigh the risk (high possibility of developing TB and low possibility of complying with the isoniazid treatment).[59,60] If so, patients should be followed clinically, with laboratory monitoring at least every two weeks during the 2 months of treatment. Due to the drug interactions between rifampin and antiretrovirals, the drugs should be adjusted. Although there is no data on treatment for LTBI by multidrug resistant MTB, experts suggest treatment with either pyrazinamide and ethambutol or pyrazinamide and quinolone (e.g., ofloxacin) for 12 months.[58]

TREATMENT OF ACTIVE TUBERCULOSIS

Tuberculosis in HIV-infected patients responds well to therapy. The treatment of TB in patients infected with HIV has been reviewed recently[41,61] and updated frequently on the CDC website.[62] The treatment of pulmonary TB is similar to the treatment for patients without HIV infection, independent of the degree of immunodeficiency.[41] Because of the difficulty distinguishing MTB from *Mycobacterium avium* complex, it is prudent to empirically initiate antituberculosis chemotherapy when sputum samples demonstrate AFB pending microbiologic confirmation. The recommended therapy includes two months (initial phase) with a rifamycin, isoniazid, pyrazinamide, and ethambutol, followed by four months (maintenance phase) with a rifamycin and isoniazid (Table 31-2). Because peripheral neuropathies are common in HIV-infected patients, pyridoxine (25 mg/day) should be prescribed for all patients receiving INH. The recommended rifamycin is rifabutin, which has the same efficacy but fewer drug interactions with antiretrovirals than rifampin.[63–65] Rifampin can be used in settings where rifabutin is not available, with the appropriate adjustment on the antiretroviral

treatment (discussed later). Rifapentine is not recommended because the one week dose was associated with the development of acquired drug resistance.[66] Thiacetazone (a drug used in areas where rifampin is not available) is not recommended due to the risk of severe and sometimes fatal skin reaction in patients with HIV infection.[67] The maintenance phase should be given with three or more doses per week if the CD4+ T lymphocytes counts are less than 100 cells/ul or twice or more per week if the CD4+ T lymphocytes are above 100 cells/ul.[41] Patients with pulmonary TB should be followed with sputum smear examination and culture every month until two consecutive specimens are negative on culture. It is also important to monitor the HIV load to assess the efficacy of the antiretroviral therapy and the evolution of the HIV infection. In general, six months of adequate therapy that includes a rifamycin is recommended, including cases with smear negative pulmonary TB. At the completion of two months of therapy, patients with positive cultures for a fully susceptible MTB should receive maintenance phase (isoniazid and rifamycin) for an additional 3 or 4 months after cultures become negative.[57] If the patient is medically compliant and has pulmonary TB by an antibiotic-susceptible organism, the sputum will be sterilized and the treatment failure and relapse rates will be less than 5%.[68] The risk of death during treatment is higher in patients with HIV infection,

Table 31-2. Recommended Regimen for Tuberculosis Treatment

Drugs/Doses: Intensive Phase	Drugs/Doses: Maintenance Phase	Comments
Isoniazid (300 mg/d) Rifampin (450 mg/d if less than 50 kg, or 600 mg/d if more than 50 k) or Rifabutin 300 mg/d Pyrazinamide (25 mg/kg/d) Ethambutol (25 mg/kg/d) Pyridoxine (25 mg/d)*	Isoniazid (300 mg/d) Rifampin (450 mg/d if less than 50 kg, or 600 mg/d if more than 50 kg) or Rifabutin 300 mg/d 3 times a week if CD4 less than 100 cells/ul or 2 times a week if CD4 more than 100 cells/ul	If sputum remains culture positive after completion of 2 months of treatment, verify susceptibility of the MTB. If susceptible, continue maintenance phase for 3 months more or 4 months after the last positive result.
Isoniazid (300 mg/d) Rifampin (450 mg/d if less than 50 kg, or 600 mg/d if more than 50 kg) or Rifabutin 300 mg/d Pyrazinamide (25 mg/kg/d) Pyridoxine (25 mg/d)*	Isoniazid (300 mg/d) Rifampin (450 mg/d if less than 50 kg, or 600 mg/d if more than 50 kg) or Rifabutin 300 mg/d 3 times a week if CD4 less than 100 cells/ul or 2 times a week if CD4 more than 100 cells/ul	If the frequency of primary drug resistant for isoniazid is less than 4%. Otherwise use ethambutol in the intensive phase.

*To decrease the risk of peripheral neuropathies associated with isoniazid.

but decreases if a rifamycin is used.[69] Directly observed therapy should be the standard of care for all HIV-infected patients because poor compliance is the strongest predictor for failure of TB treatment and because clinicians are poor at predicting compliance.[57]

The treatment of extrapulmonary TB is similar to the treatment recommended in patients without HIV infection. These patients frequently have less than 100/ul CD4+ T lymphocytes and should receive daily or at least three times per week doses during the maintenance phase. Although there is not much evidence, six months of treatment is adequate for most of the cases of extrapulmonary TB, except for TB in the central nervous system disease, which should be treated with regimens containing rifamycin for 9–12 months, and bone and joint infection, which should be treated for 6–9 months.[41] The indications for adjuvant corticosteroids are similar to those in patients without HIV infection, including TB in the central nervous system and pericardium.[39,41]

The management of treatment failure, relapse, multidrug resistant TB and TB in children infected with HIV, is similar to patients without HIV infection and can be reviewed elsewhere in this book.[41] The possibility that patients are infected with organisms that are resistant to multiple antituberculosis agents should be considered in all HIV-infected patients as well as those who have resided in areas that have a high incidence of drug resistance or who have been previously treated for TB. Patients coinfected with HIV and multidrug resistant MTB can improve their survival with two or more effective antituberculosis drugs.[70,71] The treatment of TB in children with HIV should include a minimum of 9 months according to the American Academy of Pediatrics.[41,72]

Timing to Start Antiretrovirals Relative to Tuberculosis Treatment

HAART has improved the prognosis of patients with HIV and TB[20,27]; however, frequently patients with TB have advanced HIV disease and have not started antiretrovirals.[73] In this situation, starting both treatments is not recommended because the risk of drug interactions, side effects, poor compliance, and paradoxical reaction (as discussed later). In contrast, patients already receiving antiretroviral treatment should start antituberculosis drugs as soon as possible, and drugs for both infections should be adjusted based on drug interaction and side effects.[41]

There is no controlled study to define the timing to start antiretrovirals and antituberculosis drugs; however, the general principles are to start the treatment of TB as soon as the diagnosis is made and to hold off on antiretrovirals if possible. The ATS, CDC and IDSA recommend individualizing the decision based on the patient's initial response to antituberculosis treatment, the occurrence of drug side effects and the availability of drugs for both infections.[41] The antiretroviral treatment can be started at any time in patients with CD4+ T >350 cells/ul after the antituberculosis drugs have been started and tolerated. Some authors have recommended to defer HAART until completing the intensive phase in patients with >100 CD4+ T lymphocytes/ul and start the antiretrovirals as soon as possible if the CD4+ T lymphocytes are <100 cells/ul.[74]

Drug Interactions

There are complex interactions between the drugs used to treat TB and HIV infection mainly based on the activity of the cytochrome P450. Summarized information of the drug interactions and dose modifications of antiretrovirals and antituberculosis drugs are shown in Tables 31-3 and 31-4. Because of the constant approval of new antiretrovirals, it is recommended to review updated information on the CDC website.[75] The most important interactions are listed below:

1. Rifamycins induce the activity of the isoenzyme CYP3A4 of the cytochrome P450 system, reducing the serum concentration of protease inhibitors and nonnucleoside reverse transcriptase inhibitors. Rifampin is the most potent inducer, followed by rifapentine (which is not recommended in HIV patients). Rifabutin is the least powerful inducer, and it is recommended in the treatment of TB in HIV patients. Its levels can be monitored to provide better follow up.[76,77]

2. Rifampin decreases the levels of most of the protease inhibitors by 75%. Therefore this combination is not recommended with the exceptions of rifampin with the following protease inhibitors: ritonavir alone, saquinavir combined with ritonavir, and probably lopinavir combined with ritonavir.[76–78](see Table 31-4)

3. If a patient receiving rifampin will be started on protease inhibitors (different to ritonavir alone or in combination) or nonnucleoside reverse transcriptase inhibitors, rifampin should be replaced by rifabutin at least 2 weeks before starting the antiretroviral drugs.[78]

4. Rifampin alters the levels of drugs used commonly in HIV patients like trimethoprim-sulfamethoxazole, dapsone, and azoles.[77]

5. Protease inhibitors decrease the activity of the isoenzyme CYP3A4, increasing the serum concentration

Table 31-3. Effect of Rifampin on the Different Antiretroviral Drugs and Other Drugs Commonly Prescribed in HIV Infected Patients

Effect of Rifampin on:	Resulting Effect
Nucleoside reverse transcriptase inhibitors (NRTIs)	Mild decrease of concentration of zidovudine and possibly abacavir
Protease inhibitor	75% decrease of concentration, except for ritonavir and combinations with ritonavir
Non-nucleoside reverse transcriptase inhibitor (NNRTIs)	Decrease concentration
Enfuvirtide (HIV fusion inhibitor)	None
Trimethoprim-sulfamethoxazole	Decrease concentration
Dapsone	Decrease concentration
Itraconazole, ketoconazole	Decrease concentration

Table 31-4. Dose Adjustment of Rifamycins, Antiretroviral Drugs and Other Commonly Prescribed Drugs

	Rifampin: Normal Dose: 600 mg/Day	Rifabutin: Normal Dose: 300 mg/day
Nucleoside reverse transcriptase inhibitors (NRTIs)	Caution when using zidovudine, lamivudine-abacavir	Normal each
Non-nucleoside reverse transcriptase inhibitors (NNRTIs)		
Efavirenz	Increase efavirenz to 800 mg/d	Increase Rifabutin to 450–600 mg/day
Nevirapine	Use normal dose of each, because therapeutic index of nevirapine is high. Check for hepatotoxicity	Normal each
Delavirdine	Not recommended	Not recommended
Protease Inhibitors		
Amprenavir	Not recommended	Decrease Rifabutin to 150 mg/day
Nelfinavir		
Atazanavir	No data	Decrease Rifabutin to 150 mg/day, three times/wk
Indinavir	Not recommended	Decrease Rifabutin to 150 mg/day Increase indinavir to 1000 mg/8 hours
Saquinavir/ritonavir		Normal of each
Ritonavir	Use full dose ritonavir (400 to 600 mg/12 hours)	Decrease Rifabutin to 150 mg/day, two times/wk
Lopinavir/ritonavir	Increase antiretrovirals to 400/400 mg/12 hours or 800/200 mg/12 hours	Decrease Rifabutin to 150 mg/day, three times/wk
Other drugs		
Trimethoprim-sulfamethoxazole	No data, but probably reasonable to give 160/800 mg/day	

of rifabutin. Therefore the dose of rifabutin should be lowered to 150 mg/day or even 150 mg two or three times a week when combined with protease inhibitors.[41]

6. Efavirenz reduces the concentration of rifabutin by almost 40%; therefore the dose of the antituberculosis drug should be increased to 450–600 mg/day when combined with efavirenz.[79]

Drug Side Effects

The treatment of both TB and HIV infection will require on average 7 drugs. Therefore it is not surprising to observe a high frequency of drug reactions. The frequency of drug side effects varies with the study population. In a study of 188 patients, 45% started antiretroviral treatment while on TB treatment. Adverse reactions occurred in 54% of these patients and one-third changed or interrupted their treatment. The most frequent side effects were peripheral neuropathy (21%), rash (17%), and gastrointestinal upset (10%). Most of the side effects occurred during the first two months.[74] Hepatitis due to antituberculosis drugs is 4-fold more frequent in patients with HIV and 14-fold if infected with HIV and Hepatitis C virus. Therefore it is recommended to screen for hepatitis C in patients with HIV and to do close laboratory monitoring if antituberculosis drugs will be prescribed for these patients.[41,80]

Paradoxical Reaction

Paradoxical reaction is defined as a temporary exacerbation of symptoms, signs or radiographic manifestations of TB after days to weeks of antituberculosis drugs.[81] It can occur in patients with TB lymphadenitis without HIV infection; but it is more frequent in patients infected with HIV and much more frequent if they are receiving antiretroviral agents (2%, 7%, and 36% respectively).[82,83] In patients with HIV infection, this reaction has been observed 2–40 days (median of 15 days) after the initiation of HAART[82] but there is a report of a patient with a paradoxical reaction after 6 weeks of treatment.[84] The reconstitution of the immune response is the most likely explanation of this syndrome, supported by a conversion of the tuberculin skin test from negative to positive and the decrease in the HIV viral load.[82] The clinical presentation ranges from mild manifestations with high fever, lymphadenopathy and worsening of the initial signs and symptoms to life-threatening manifestations such as signs of expansion of central nervous system lesions and increase of pleural effusions or parenchymal infiltrations. The symptoms can be brief or prolonged

with recurrences, but generally are self-limited, lasting 10–40 days.[39] Before considering the diagnosis of paradoxical reaction it is important to rule out treatment failure of TB, drug hypersensitivity, infections and other events such as tumors in the central nervous system. The treatment of mild cases includes the continuation of antiretroviral therapy and in some cases use of nonsteroidal anti-inflammatory drugs. In severe or life-threatening manifestations, it is recommended to temporarily stop the antiretroviral therapy and use a short course of corticosteroids with 1mg/kg of prednisone per day for one to two weeks with a gradual reduction thereafter.[41,78]

INFECTION CONTROL

Infection control measures are an important component of TB prevention in HIV immunosuppressed population. Secondary spread of TB to patients infected with HIV has been documented in residential settings for homeless, hospitals, clinics, among others.[85] Because newly acquired TB infection in HIV-infected patients can progress rapidly to active disease, there should be heightened surveillance for TB in facilities where HIV infected people live. Recommendations for infection control have been established and should be scrupulously followed.[86] In addition, all TB cases should be reported to public health officials so that contacts are investigated appropriately.

FUTURE

It is remarkable how difficult it has been to control the epidemic of TB, a curable disease. Currently, HIV is the most important factor contributing to the increase of cases of TB, complicating its treatment and therefore the control of the epidemic. Nonetheless, in the last 5 years, in the United States and other developed countries, the survival of patients with HIV/AIDS and TB who are diagnosed on time and treated properly has increased dramatically. In contrast, in poor countries, where most of the cases of TB and HIV occur, patients continue to die. Therefore, there is an urgent need to provide antituberculosis treatment and antiretrovirals to these patients. In view of the high rate of HIV and MTB infections, the developing of vaccines and more effective treatments for both infections remains an important future goal.

REFERENCES

1. Vynnycky E, Fine PE. The natural history of tuberculosis: the implications of age-dependent risks of disease and the role of reinfection. *Epidemol Infect.* 1997;119:183–201.

2. Selwyn PA, Hartel D, Lewis VA, et al. A prospective study of the risk of tuberculosis among intravenous drug users with human immunodeficiency virus infection. *N Engl J Med.* 1989;320:545–550.

3. Stebbing J, Gazzard B, Douek DC. Where does HIV live? *N Engl J Med.* 2004;350:1872–1880.

4. Lawn SD, Butera ST, Folks TM. Contribution of immune activation to the pathogenesis and transmission of human immunodeficiency virus type 1 infection. *Clin Microbiol Rev.* 2001;14:753–777.

5. Schluger NW, Rom WN. The host immune response to tuberculosis. *Am J Respir Crit Care Med.* 1998;157:679–691.

6. Toossi Z. Virological and immunological impact of tuberculosis on human immunodeficiency virus type 1 disease. *J Infect Dis.* 2003;188:1146–1155.

7. Goletti D, Weissman D, Jackson RW, et al. Effect of *Mycobacterium tuberculosis* on HIV replication. Role of immune activation. *J Immunol.* 1996;157:1271–1278.

8. Toossi Z, Mayanja-Kizza H, Hirsch CS, et al. Impact of tuberculosis (TB) on HIV-1 activity in dually infected patients. *Clin Exp Immunol.* 2001;123:233–238.

9. Nakata K, Rom WN, Honda Y, et al. *Mycobacterium tuberculosis* enhances human immunodeficiency virus-1 replication in the lung. *Am J Respir Crit Care Med.* 1997;155:996–1003.

10. Alland D, Kalkut GE, Moss AR, et al. Transmission of tuberculosis in New York City. An analysis by DNA fingerprinting and conventional epidemiologic methods. *N Engl J Med.* 1994;330:1710–1716.

11. Di Perri G, Cruciani M, Danzi MC, et al. Nosocomial epidemic of active tuberculosis among HIV-infected patients. *Lancet.* 1989;2:1502–1504.

12. Daley CL, Small PM, Schecter GF, et al. An outbreak of tuberculosis with accelerated progression among persons infected with the human immunodeficiency virus. An analysis using restriction-fragment-length polymorphisms. *N Engl J Med.* 1992;326:231–235.

13. Girardi E, Raviglione MC, Antonucci G, et al. Impact of the HIV epidemic on the spread of other diseases: the case of tuberculosis. *AIDS* (14 Suppl). 2000;3:S47–S56.

14. Steinbrook R. The AIDS Epidemic in 2004. *N Engl J Med.* 2004;351:115–117.

15. National Center for HIV STD and TB Prevention. Table 1. Estimated numbers of diagnoses of HIV/AIDS, by year of diagnosis and selected characteristics of persons, 1999–2002—30 areas with confidential name-based HIV infection reporting, HIV/AIDS Surveillance Report, Vol.14. Atlanta: GA; 2003.

16. Hill PC, Brookes RH, Fox A, et al. Large-scale evaluation of enzyme-linked immunospot assay and skin test for diagnosis of *Mycobacterium tuberculosis* infection against a gradient of exposure in The Gambia. *Clin Infect Dis.* 2004;38:966–973.

17. Moss AR, Hahn JA, Tulsky JP, et al. Tuberculosis in the homeless. A prospective study. *Am J Respir Crit Care Med.* 2000;162:460–464.

18. Iademarco MF, Castro KG. Epidemiology of tuberculosis. *Semin Respir Infect.* 2003;18:225–240.

19. San-Andres FJ, Rubio R, Castilla J, et al. Incidence of acquired immunodeficiency syndrome-associated opportunistic diseases and the effect of treatment on a cohort of 1115 patients infected with human immunodeficiency virus, 1989–1997. *Clin Infect Dis.* 2003;36:1177–1185.

20. Jones JL, Hanson DL, Dworkin MS, et al. HIV-associated tuberculosis in the era of highly active antiretroviral therapy. The Adult/Adolescent Spectrum of HIV Disease Group. *Int J Tuberc Lung Dis.* 2000;4:1026–1031.

21. Tuberculosis elimination revisited. obstacles, opportunities, and a renewed commitment. Advisory Council for the Elimination of Tuberculosis (ACET). *MMWR Morb Mortal Wkly Rep.* 1999;48:1–13.

22. Global Tuberculosis Control -Surveillance, Planning, Financing, WHO Report 2004. WHO/HTM/TB/2004. 331, WHO, 2004.

23. Corbett EL, Watt CJ, Walker N, et al. THE growing burden of tuberculosis: global trends and interactions with the HIV epidemic. *Arch Intern Med.* 2003;163:1009–1021.

24. UNAIDS/WHO. AIDS epidemic update: 2003. Geneva: UNAIDS/WHO; 2003.

25. UNAIDS/WHO. World TB Day, 2004. Geneva: UNAIDS/WHO; 2004.

26. Hill AR, Manikal VM, Riska PF. Effectiveness of directly observed therapy (DOT) for tuberculosis: a review of multinational experience reported in 1990–2000. *Medicine (Baltimore).* 2002;81:179–193.

27. Hung CC, Chen MY, Hsiao CF, et al. Improved outcomes of HIV-1-infected adults with tuberculosis in the era of highly active antiretroviral therapy. *AIDS.* 2003;17:2615–2662.

28. World Health Organization (Europe). HIV/AIDS treatment: antiretroviral therapy, Fact Sheet EURO/06/03: WHO; 2003.

29. Friedland G, Abdool Karim S, Abdool Karim Q, et al. Utility of tuberculosis directly observed therapy programs as sites for access to and provision of antiretroviral therapy in resource-limited countries. *Clin Infect Dis* (38 Suppl). 2004;5:S421–S428.

30. WHO. Two diseases—one patient, HIV and TB—one patient, HIV and TB—one community, one patient. In: WHO, ed. Geneva: WHO; 2003.

31. Godfrey-Faussett P, Ayles H. Can we control tuberculosis in high HIV prevalence settings? *Tuberculosis (Edinb).* 2003;83:68–76.

32. Sunderam G, McDonald RJ, Maniatis T, et al. Tuberculosis as a manifestation of the acquired immunodeficiency syndrome (AIDS). *JAMA.* 1986;256:362–366.

33. Small PM, Schecter GF, Goodman PC, et al. Treatment of tuberculosis in patients with advanced human immunodeficiency virus infection. *N Engl J Med.* 1991;324:289–294.

34. Alpert PL, Munsiff SS, Gourevitch MN, et al. A prospective study of tuberculosis and human immunodeficiency virus infection: clinical manifestations and factors associated with survival. *Clin Infect Dis.* 1997;24:661–668.

35. Yang Z, Kong Y, Wilson F, et al. Identification of risk factors for extrapulmonary tuberculosis. *Clin Infect Dis.* 2004;38:199–205.

36. Barber TW, Craven DE, McCabe WR. Bacteremia due to *Mycobacterium tuberculosis* in patients with human immunodeficiency virus infection. A report of 9 cases and a review of the literature. *Medicine (Baltimore)*. 1990;69:375–383.

37. Schutte CM. Clinical, cerebrospinal fluid and pathological findings and outcomes in HIV-positive and HIV-negative patients with tuberculous meningitis. *Infection*. 2001;29:213–217.

38. Fee MJ, Oo MM, Gabayan AE, et al. Abdominal tuberculosis in patients infected with the human immunodeficiency virus. *Clin Infect Dis*. 1995;20:938–944.

39. Barnes PF, Lakey DL, Burman WJ. Tuberculosis in patients with HIV infection. *Infect Dis Clin North Am*. 2002;16:107–126.

40. Centers for Disease Control and Prevention. Prevention and treatment of tuberculosis among patients infected with human immunodeficiency virus: principles of therapy and revised recommendations. Centers for Disease Control and Prevention. *MMWR Morb Mortal Wkly Rep*.1998;47:1–58.

41. Blumberg HM, Burman WJ, Chaisson RE, et al. American Thoracic Society/Centers for Disease Control and Prevention/Infectious Diseases Society of America: treatment of tuberculosis. *Am J Respir Crit Care Med*. 2003;167:603–662.

42. Targeted tuberculin testing and treatment of latent tuberculosis infection. This official statement of the American Thoracic Society was adopted by the ATS Board of Directors, July 1999. This is a Joint Statement of the American Thoracic Society (ATS) and the Centers for Disease Control and Prevention (CDC). This statement was endorsed by the Council of the Infectious Diseases Society of America. (IDSA), September 1999, and the sections of this statement. *Am J Respir Crit Care Med*. 2000;161: S221–S247.

43. Mazurek GH, LoBue PA, Daley CL, et al. Comparison of a whole-blood interferon gamma assay with tuberculin skin testing for detecting latent *Mycobacterium tuberculosis* infection. *JAMA*. 2001;286:1740–1747.

44. Bellete B, Coberly J, Barnes GL, et al. Evaluation of a whole-blood interferon-gamma release assay for the detection of *Mycobacterium tuberculosis* infection in 2 study populations. *Clin Infect Dis*. 2002;34:1449–1456.

45. Fietta A, Meloni F, Cascina A, et al. Comparison of a whole-blood *interferon-gamma* assay and tuberculin skin testing in patients with active tuberculosis and individuals at high or low risk of Mycobacterium tuberculosis infection. *Am J Infect Control*. 2003;31:347–353.

46. Mazurek GH, Villarino ME. Guidelines for using the QuantiFERON-TB test for diagnosing latent *Mycobacterium tuberculosis* infection. Centers for Disease Control and Prevention. *MMWR Morb Mortal Wkly Rep*. 2003;52:15–18.

47. Klein NC, Duncanson FP, Lenox TH, 3rd, et al. Use of mycobacterial smears in the diagnosis of pulmonary tuberculosis in AIDS/ARC patients. *Chest*. 1989;95:1190–1192.

48. Schluger NW: The diagnosis of tuberculosis. What's old, what's new? *Semin Respir Infect*. 2003;18:241–248.

49. Update. Nucleic acid amplification tests for tuberculosis. *MMWR Morb Mortal Wkly Rep*. 2000;49:593–594.

50. Kivihya-Ndugga L, van Cleeff M, Juma E, et al. Comparison of PCR with the routine procedure for diagnosis of tuberculosis in a population with high prevalences of tuberculosis and human immunodeficiency virus. *J Clin Microbiol*. 2004;42:1012–1015.

51. Perlman DC, el-Sadr WM, Nelson ET, et al. Variation of chest radiographic patterns in pulmonary tuberculosis by degree of human immunodeficiency virus-related immunosuppression. The Terry Beirn Community Programs for Clinical Research on AIDS (CPCRA). The AIDS Clinical Trials Group (ACTG). *Clin Infect Dis*. 1997;25:242–246.

52. Burman WJ, Jones BE. Clinical and radiographic features of HIV-related tuberculosis. *Semin Respir Infect*. 2003;18:263–271.

53. Horsburgh CR, Jr. Priorities for the treatment of latent tuberculosis infection in the United States. *N Engl J Med*. 2004;350:2060–2067.

54. Casado JL, Moreno S, Fortun J, et al. Risk factors for development of tuberculosis after isoniazid chemoprophylaxis in human immunodeficiency virus-infected patients. *Clin Infect Dis*. 2002;34:386–389.

55. Sonnenberg P, Glynn JR, Fielding K, et al. HIV and pulmonary tuberculosis: the impact goes beyond those infected with HIV. *AIDS*. 2004;18:657–662.

56. Bucher HC, Griffith LE, Guyatt GH, et al. Isoniazid prophylaxis for tuberculosis in HIV infection: a meta-analysis of randomized controlled trials. *AIDS*. 1999;13:501–507.

57. Prevention and treatment of tuberculosis among patients infected with human immunodeficiency virus. Principles of therapy and revised recommendations. Centers for Disease Control and Prevention. *MMWR Morb Mortal Wkly Rep*. 1998;47:1–58.

58. Targeted tuberculin testing and treatment of latent tuberculosis infection. American Thoracic Society. *MMWR Morb Mortal Wkly Rep*. 2000;49:1–51.

59. Cohn DL. Treatment of latent tuberculosis infection. *Semin Respir Infect*. 2003;18:249–262.

60. Update. Adverse event data and revised American Thoracic Society/CDC recommendations against the use of rifampin and pyrazinamide for treatment of latent tuberculosis infection—United States, 2003. *MMWR Morb Mortal Wkly Rep*. 2003;52:735–739.

61. de Jong BC, Israelski DM, Corbett EL, et al. Clinical management of tuberculosis in the context of HIV infection. *Ann Rev Med*. 2004;55:283–301.

62. National Center for HIV STD and TB Prevention. TB Guidelines. Available at: http://www.cdc.gov/nchstp/tb/pubs/mmwrhtml/maj_guide.htm. Accessed, April 14, 2005.

63. Gonzalez-Montaner LJ, Natal S, Yongchaiyud P, et al. Rifabutin for the treatment of newly-diagnosed pulmonary tuberculosis: a multinational, randomized, comparative study versus Rifampicin. Rifabutin Study Group. *Tuber Lung Dis*. 1994;75:341–347.

64. McGregor MM, Olliaro P, Wolmarans L, et al. Efficacy and safety of rifabutin in the treatment of patients with newly diagnosed pulmonary tuberculosis. *Am J Respir Crit Care Med*. 1996;154:1462–1467.

65. Schwander S, Rusch-Gerdes S, Mateega A, et al. A pilot study of antituberculosis combinations comparing rifabutin with rifampicin in the treatment of HIV-1 associated tuberculosis. A single-blind randomized evaluation in Ugandan patients with HIV-1 infection and pulmonary tuberculosis. *Tuber Lung Dis.* 1995;76:210–218.

66. Vernon A, Burman W, Benator D, et al. Acquired rifamycin monoresistance in patients with HIV-related tuberculosis treated with once-weekly rifapentine and isoniazid. Tuberculosis Trials Consortium. *Lancet.* 1999;353:1843–1847.

67. Okwera A, Johnson JL, Vjecha MJ, et al. Risk factors for adverse drug reactions during thiacetazone treatment of pulmonary tuberculosis in human immunodeficiency virus infected adults. *Int J Tuberc Lung Dis.* 1997;1:441–445.

68. Kassim S, Sassan-Morokro M, Ackah A, et al. Two-year follow-up of persons with HIV-1- and HIV-2-associated pulmonary tuberculosis treated with short-course chemotherapy in West Africa. *AIDS.* 1995;9:1185–1191.

69. Perriens JH, Colebunders RL, Karahunga C, et al. Increased mortality and tuberculosis treatment failure rate among human immunodeficiency virus (HIV) seropositive compared with HIV seronegative patients with pulmonary tuberculosis treated with "standard" chemotherapy in Kinshasa, Zaire. *Am Rev Respir Dis.* 1991;144:750–755.

70. Park MM, Davis AL, Schluger NW, et al. Outcome of MDR-TB patients, 1983–1993. Prolonged survival with appropriate therapy. *Am J Respir Crit Care Med.* 1996;153: 317–324.

71. Turett GS, Telzak EE, Torian LV, et al. Improved outcomes for patients with multidrug-resistant tuberculosis. *Clin Infect Dis.* 1995;21:1238–1244.

72. American Academy of Pediatrics. Tuberculosis. In: LJ P, ed. *Red Book Report of the Committee on Infectious Disease* (ed 25th). Elk Grove Village, IL: American Academy of Pediatrics; 2000:593–613.

73. Yeni PG, Hammer SM, Carpenter CC, et al. Antiretroviral treatment for adult HIV infection in 2002: updated recommendations of the International AIDS Society-USA Panel. *JAMA.* 2002;288:222–235.

74. Dean GL, Edwards SG, Ives NJ, et al. Treatment of tuberculosis in HIV-infected persons in the era of highly active antiretroviral therapy. *AIDS.* 2002;16:75–83.

75. National Center for HIV STD and TB Prevention. TB/HIV Drug Interactions, Updated Guidelines for the Use of Rifamycins for the Treatment of Tuberculosis Among HIV-Infected Patients Taking Protease Inhibitors or Nonnucleoside Reverse Transcriptase Inhibitors. Available at: http://www. cdc. gov/nchstp/tb/TB_HIV_Drugs/TOC.htm. Accessed April 14, 2005.

76. Updated guidelines for the use of rifabutin or rifampin for the treatment and prevention of tuberculosis among HIV-infected patients taking protease inhibitors or nonnucleoside reverse transcriptase inhibitors. Centers for Disease Control and Prevention. *MMWR Morb Mortal Wkly Rep.* 2000;49:185–189.

77. Niemi M, Backman JT, Fromm MF, et al. Pharmacokinetic interactions with rifampicin: clinical relevance. *Clin Pharmacokinet.* 2003;42:819–850.

78. Burman WJ, Jones BE. Treatment of HIV-related tuberculosis in the era of effective antiretroviral therapy. *Am J Respir Crit Care Med.* 2001;164:7–12.

79. Lopez-Cortes LF, Ruiz-Valderas R, Viciana P, et al. Pharmacokinetic interactions between efavirenz and rifampicin in HIV-infected patients with tuberculosis. *Clin Pharmacokinet.* 2002;41:681–690.

80. Ungo JR, Jones D, Ashkin D, et al. Antituberculosis drug-induced hepatotoxicity. The role of hepatitis C virus and the human immunodeficiency virus. *Am J Respir Crit Care Med.* 1998;157:1871–1876.

81. Cheng VC, Ho PL, Lee RA, et al. Clinical spectrum of paradoxical deterioration during antituberculosis therapy in non-HIV-infected patients. *Eur J Clin Microbiol Infect Dis.* 2002;21:803–809.

82. Narita M, Ashkin D, Hollender ES, et al. Paradoxical worsening of tuberculosis following antiretroviral therapy in patients with AIDS. *Am J Respir Crit Care Med.* 1998;158: 157–161.

83. Kunimoto DY, Chui L, Nobert E, et al. Immune mediated 'HAART' attack during treatment for tuberculosis. Highly active antiretroviral therapy. *Int J Tuberc Lung Dis.* 1999;3: 944–947.

84. Orlovic D, Smego RA, Jr. Paradoxical tuberculous reactions in HIV-infected patients. *Int J Tuberc Lung Dis.* 2001;5: 370–375.

85. Paolo WF, Jr., Nosanchuk JD. Tuberculosis in New York city: recent lessons and a look ahead. *Lancet Infect Dis.* 2004;4:287–293.

86. Sehulster L, Chinn RY. Guidelines for environmental infection control in health-care facilities. Recommendations of CDC and the Healthcare Infection Control Practices Advisory Committee (HICPAC). *MMWR Morb Mortal Wkly Rep.* 2003;52:1–42.

32

Paradoxical Reactions and the Immune Reconstitution Inflammatory Syndrome

Preston Church
Marc A. Judson

INTRODUCTION

The immune response to mycobacterial infection is complex, involving several arms of the immune system. Organs are damaged by mycobacteria directly and also by the necrotic granulomatous immune response of the host to this pathogen. Ideally, mycobacterial infection is met with a balanced immune response that is sufficient to kill organisms but not so severe as to cause excessive tissue injury. Immunosuppression may promote growth of mycobacteria while decreasing tissue injury by the host response to the infection. Conversely, enhancement of the host's immune response may kill more organisms, but may also result in more organ damage.

An example may be seen with highly active antiretroviral therapy (HAART) for HIV-infected individuals with mycobacterial infection. HAART therapy may result in a heightened granulomatous response that helps rid mycobacterial organisms, but the granulomatous inflammation may cause considerable damage. Such paradoxical injurious reactions have been defined as transient worsening or appearance of new signs, symptoms, or radiographic manifestations of tuberculosis (TB) that occur after initiation of treatment, and are not the result of treatment failure or a second process.[1] In HIV-infected individuals, paradoxical reactions are common after the initiation of HAART,[2] and have been called "the immune reconstitution inflammatory syndrome" (IRIS)[3] or "HAART attacks."[4] The following is a review of the basic clinical and immunological aspects of these phenomena.

HOST RESPONSE TO MYCOBACTERIA

Tuberculosis infection is initiated via inhalation of airborne droplet nuclei containing mycobacteria into the terminal airspaces of the lung. The organisms are engulfed by alveolar macrophages with subsequent release proinflammatory cytokines including tumor necrosis factor (TNF), interleukin (IL)-1, and IL-12.[5] This leads to an early inflammatory reaction that includes the recruitment of monocytes from the bloodstream into the infected area of the lung.[5] Eventually, a population of specific T lymphocytes is stimulated to proliferate and participate in a cell-mediated immune reaction.[5] Prior to the development of a specific immune response, the organisms are poorly contained and mycobacteremia occurs with systemic seeding of organisms.[5] The acquired specific immunity to the organism follows: antigen-presenting cells (APC) (alveolar macrophages and dendritic cells), having engulfed mycobacterial proteins, then process them into small peptides so that these peptides can be presented to naïve CD4+ cells via major histocompatibility complex (MHC) Class II molecules.[5] The APC produce cytokines IL-12 and IL-1 that drives a specific immune response. IL-12 biases the immune reaction by causing additional cytokines to be released to cause a T helper 1 (Th1) response.[5] IL-1 stimulates CD4+ lymphocytes to produce IL-2 and upregulate lymphocyte IL-2 surface receptors, resulting in a rapid clonal expansion of specific CD4+ Th1 lymphocytes. These produce interferon-gamma (INF-γ), a cytokine that activates the macrophages that have engulfed mycobacteria to produce a variety of substances, such as reactive oxygen and nitrogen species that are involved in growth inhibition and killing of mycobacteria.[6] The central role of INF-γ secretion by lymphocytes in mycobacterial containment is evidenced by animal models of fatal infections in the absence of this cytokine.[7,8] In addition, disseminated disease has been reported in humans with genetic abnormalities in the INF-γ receptor.[9,10]

Although the intended effect of this immune response is eradication of mycobacteria, viable organisms persist in the lung.[5] Therefore, over the next 7–14 days, an ongoing Th1 response results in further accumulation of macrophages and lymphocytes culminating in granuloma formation.[5,11] The granuloma represent the manifestation of cell-mediated immunity(CMI) to wall off the focus of infection and further limit the spread of TB. Viable bacteria persist within the cells of the granuloma although they fail to progressively replicate, and thereby latent infection is established.[5] These sites of latent infection could become foci of active infection both in the lungs and at distant sites.

TUBERCULOSIS AND THE "PARADOXICAL REACTION"

In the 1950s following the introduction of effective antituberculous chemotherapy, physicians noted that some patients developed a recrudescence of their illness during the first few months of therapy. Initial reports described children who manifested fever and increased pulmonary infiltrates on chest x-ray.[12] Symptoms often occurred during the second or third week of INH and streptomycin and persisted for a week before gradually resolving without modifying or discontinuing therapy.

Subsequent case reports in adults described worsening of pulmonary disease with paradoxical reactions, including new pleural effusions[13] and acute respiratory failure,[14] although substantiation of an enhanced inflammatory response in these cases is clouded by persistent positive cultures for *Mycobacterium tuberculosis*, leaving open the possibility of disease progression. A retrospective review of tuberculous pleural effusions demonstrated paradoxical worsening in 10 of 61 (16%) patients[15] with six of these patients requiring thoracentesis and five requiring corticosteroids.

Paradoxical reactions may occur in up to 25% of patients treated for tuberculous lymphadenitis, characterized by new or enlarging lymphadenopathy, which may be tender or painful.[16–19] Suppuration or cutaneous fistula formation may occur requiring surgical extirpation.[16,17] New or enlarging mass lesions (tuberculomas) are well recognized complications of antituberculous chemotherapy of central nervous system (CNS) TB (both meningitis and tuberculomas)[20–22] and pose significant management problems. The frequency of paradoxical reactions in this setting is unknown but was 50% (4 of 8) in one series.[22] The time to presentation is unpredictable, ranging from 1 week to 27 months after the initiation of antituberculous chemotherapy. Corticosteroids, often used in the first 3 months of CNS TB, may contribute to a delay in the development of this complication.

Although older studies reported paradoxical reactions are common in children (50%)[12] or in lymphadenitis (10–25%),[16–19] recent retrospective[23–25] and prospective[2] series of adults infected with TB found evidence of IRIS in 2–10%. The decline in the reported incidence of IRIS over the last few decades is probably artifactual because initial antituberculous chemotherapy has remained relatively constant over the last 30 years and the studies with a high incidence if IRIS were done in children or in populations predominantly from Africa and southern and southeastern Asia with higher proportions of miliary or extrapulmonary TB.

Distinguishing paradoxical reactions from disease progression, drug fever or secondary complications remains an important issue in TB management. Fever in conjunction with new foci of disease or worsening of pre-existing disease excludes a drug reaction as the cause. In pulmonary and pleural disease, paradoxical reactions follow a typical time course, with a period of definite improvement followed by transient worsening 2–4 weeks later.[12,15] This temporal pattern would not be expected with progressive disease unless concomitant corticosteroids are used, which could also cause transient amelioration. In CNS and lymphatic TB the time to presentation of a paradoxical reaction may occur 2 weeks to 8 months after the initiation of antituberculous therapy, with most episodes presenting by week 12.[18,20–22] Initial improvement may be absent in these patients, necessitating aspiration or biopsy to distinguish paradoxical reaction from treatment failure. Most presentations of paradoxical reaction can be managed "palliatively" with continuation of antituberculous therapy. Corticosteroids are probably indicated for severe pleural and most CNS paradoxical reactions to manage symptoms and CNS edema. The optimum dose and duration has not been established; published recommendations for initial corticosteroid management of pleural and CNS disease are reasonable guidelines.[26]

EFFECT OF HIV AND HAART THERAPY ON THE GRANULOMATOUS RESPONSE

The importance of CD4+ lymphocytes in the control of mycobacteria has been demonstrated in several animal models of where rapidly, progressive, fatal infection has occurred when this class of lymphocytes has been depleted.[27–29]

It is logical to suspect that HIV infection would hamper the granulomatous response to mycobacteria by depleting the number of circulating CD4+ lymphocytes. It has been demonstrated that HIV infected individuals with low CD4+ counts have a decreased secretion of INF-γ and decreased proliferation of peripheral blood mononuclear cells in response to mycobacterial antigens.[30] This most probably explains the impaired granulomatous response to *Mycobacterium tuberculosis* that is seen in HIV infected individuals[31] and also accounts for the high rate of active TB that is seen in this population.[32,33]

HAART has been associated with an increase in the proliferation of peripheral blood mononuclear cells and INF-γ in response to specific mycobacterial antigens.[30] These increases occur over several months and do not reach levels seen in healthy control subjects. Therefore, HAART would be expected to improve immunity to *M. tuberculosis* by increasing the function and number of CD4+ lymphocytes, thereby augmenting the Th1 response to mycobacterial antigens, and improving the granulomatous response to the organism.[11] Although the heightened granulomatous response from HAART would help clear mycobacterial organisms, the granulomatous inflammation itself may cause significant damage, thus resulting in IRIS.

TUBERCULOSIS—IRIS CASE PRESENTATION

A 48-year-old man presented with fever and thrush. His chest radiograph showed an interstitial infiltrate proven to be due to *Pneumocystis carinii* pneumonia and he responded to therapy with trimethoprim-sulfamethoxazole. HIV ELISA and Western blot were positive and his CD4 cell count was 75 cells/microliter. A purified protein derivative (PPD) TB skin test was negative.

One month later, his chest radiograph was normal (Fig. 32-1A). His HIV viral load was 442,000 copies/ml and antiretroviral therapy was initiated with zidovudine, lamivudine and indinavir. After three months on this antiretroviral regimen, his CD4 count had increased to 167 and his viral load had decreased to <400 copies/ml. He then presented with wheezing and cough when lying on his left side. Auscultation of the chest was normal. Radiologic studies demonstrated a mass in the left hilum (Fig. 32-1B,C). Bronchoscopy revealed an endobronchial mass at the orifice of the left upper lobe and biopsy specimens revealed caseating granulomata. Special stains and cultures for acid-fast bacilli (AFB) and fungi were negative. A PPD was now 12 mm. A diagnosis of pulmonary TB was made and the following antituberculous therapy was administered: isoniazid (INH), rifampin and pyrazinamide and subsequently changed to INH, ethambutol and pyrazinamide was for 18 months. His symptoms resolved completely and he remains well seven years later.

COMMENT ON CASE—AN ATYPICAL TUBERCULOSIS IRIS

Two distinct presentations of IRIS are recognized with *M. tuberculosis*. An atypical presentation is similar to the patient presented here in which patients with HIV develop active TB after a successful response to HAART.[34,35] This typically occurs 2–12 weeks following the start of HAART and coincides with a rise in the absolute CD4 count and a decline in HIV viremia.

This type of IRIS occurs more commonly with infection by low virulence organisms such as *Mycobacterium avium* complex.[3] Because of the more virulent nature of *M. tuberculosis* and the greater likelihood of progression to symptomatic disease when CD4 counts are low, the window of

time where infection is subclinical is likely to be small. It is also clear, however, that a substantial number of HIV infected patients with low CD4 counts may harbor latent infection, as shown by tuberculin skin test conversion after restoration of CD4 counts above 200,[36] suggesting that a sizeable HIV infected population is at risk. Since this type of TB-associated IRIS is uncommon, the proper treatment and expected response are not clear. It appears that patients respond to usual antituberculous therapy as expected, although corticosteroids have been used in cases presenting with either miliary disease or severe lung injury.[34]

An important issue in *M. tuberculosis* associated IRIS is the importance of immune reconstitution due to antiretroviral therapy versus the reversal of immune suppressive effects attributable to TB alone (the "paradoxical reaction" described previously). The occurrence of IRIS in the absence of antituberculous therapy suggests that antiretroviral therapy is important in the pathogenesis of IRIS, and that the paradoxical reaction and IRIS are not the same.

TYPICAL TB—ASSOCIATED IRIS

The more common presentation of IRIS occurs after initiating antiretroviral therapy in HIV patients already on treatment for *M. tuberculosis*. This situation commonly arises when patients present with symptomatic TB and are diagnosed with HIV infection as part of the initial evaluation. Four case series compare the incidence of IRIS in HIV infected patients simultaneously or subsequently assigned to HAART the incidence of paradoxical reactions in patients with[2,23,24] or without[24,37] HIV. Incidence rates were 11–36% in the patients receiving HAART and 0–10% in the various control groups. When one patient cohort[2] was reassessed on the basis of radiographic changes alone, the incidence of IRIS was 45%.[38] Three of these studies concluded that the incidence of IRIS in patients receiving HAART was significantly greater than the incidence of paradoxical reactions.[2,24,25] Although the frequency of IRIS was not statistically different in one study,[23] patients receiving HAART required hospitalization because of fever, weight loss and lymphadenitis within 4 weeks of initiating antiretroviral therapy.[23] Some patients subsequently developed mycobacterial psoas abscesses.[23] By contrast, the patients with TB and HIV but not receiving HAART who developed paradoxical worsening had only new or enlarging lymphadenopathy which occurred in the setting of weight gain and resolving pulmonary infiltrates.[23]

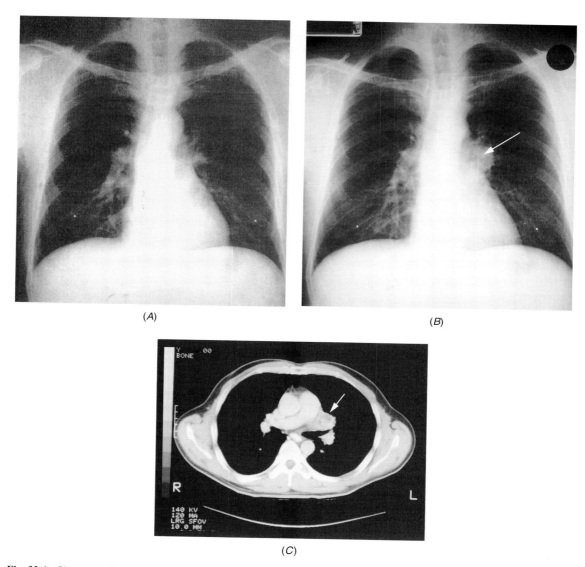

(A)

(B)

(C)

Fig. 32-1. Chest x-ray before (*A*) and 3 months after (*B*) initiation of antiretroviral therapy demonstrating a new left hilar mass (arrow). Chest CT scan (*C*) demonstrates a 2.0 × 2.0 × 2.5 cm heterogeneous mass just anterior to the left upper lobe bronchus. The lung parenchyma is normal and no mediastinal adenopathy is present.

The median time to onset of IRIS is 12 days (range 2–114 days)[2,25,37] after initiation of antiretroviral therapy. Fever is the most common presenting symptom (Table 32-1). Radiographic findings usually include new or worsening lymphadenopathy and worsening localized pulmonary infiltrates.[2,38] Newly recognized foci of infection occur in a significant minority of patients and may include cervical adenopathy,[2,23,25,37] visceral,[37] musculoskeletal[23,37] or subcutaneous abscesses,[2] pleural effusions,[2,25,39] ascites,[2,25,36,39] hepatitis,[39] epididymitis and orchitis,[39] CNS tuberculomas,[25,40] ileitis with intestinal perforation[41] or granulomatous nephritis.[42]

Defining risk factors for developing IRIS have been hindered by the small number of cases. In most reports,

Table 32-1. TB and IRIS

	INCIDENCE		
Ref #	Frequency, HIV+ on HAART	Frequency, HIV+, no HAART	Frequency, HIV−
2	12/33 (36%)	2/28 (7%)	1/55 (2%)
23	3/28 (11%)	3/44 (7%)	
24	6/17 (35%)	0/59	
25	14/50 (28%)		5/50 (10%)
37	16/37 (43%)		
40	6/69 (9%)		

		CLINICAL FEATURES					
Ref #	N	# With Disseminated TB at Initial Diagnosis	Median Time to Onset (Range), Days	Fever	New or Increased Lymphadenopathy	New or Increased Pulmonary Signs/Symptoms	New or Increased CNS Signs Symptoms
2	13		12 (2–40)	9/13	8/13	5/13	0/13
23	3	3/3		3/3	3/3		
24	6			6/6	4/6	2/6	
25	14	9/14	11 (8–18)	4/14	7/14	3/14	2/14
37	16	16/16	12 (2–114)	14/16	11/16	2/16	0/16
40	5		18 (10–59)				5/5

absolute CD4 counts have been lower and viral loads higher at baseline in the group developing IRIS but the values overlap considerably. IRIS is more frequently identified in patients with disseminated infection[23,25,37] and is more likely to occur when antiretroviral therapy is started within 6 weeks of antituberculous therapy.[25] Breton et al.[37] found a trend towards greater elevation in total CD4 count after one month of antiretrovirals in patients who developed IRIS compared with those who did not (+99 cells/microliter vs +35 cells/microliter, p = ns) and a strong correlation with the change in CD4 percentages (median of +11% in patients with IRIS versus 2% in controls, p <0.001, OR 1.34 [1.08–1.56]), suggesting that the quality of and rate of immune response to antiretroviral therapy is a major determinant in the occurrence of IRIS.

None of the studies performed to date can adequately address managing or preventing IRIS. One approach has been to temporarily halt antiretroviral therapy; in some patients resumption of therapy has led to a second episode of IRIS.[2] An alternative approach has been to employ NSAIDs or corticosteroids for more severe symptoms. There is no agreed upon dose but at least one author has suggested an initial dose of 1 mg/kg/day of prednisone with gradual tapering after 1–2 weeks.[43,44]

The use of prednisone in this setting does not appear to be associated with TB treatment failure.[39,43]

Given our current inability to predict which patients will develop IRIS, when should antiretroviral therapy be initiated in the patient on antituberculous chemotherapy? ATS/CDC/IDSA guidelines suggest delaying antiretroviral therapy 4–8 weeks (if possible) in patients with CD4 counts <350 cells/µl.[44] The World Health Organization (WHO) recommends initiating antiretroviral therapy as soon as antituberculous therapy is tolerated in patients with CD4 <50 cells/µl, waiting until 2 months into antituberculous therapy in patients with CD4 counts between 50 and 200 cells/µl, and deferring therapy until the completion of TB treatment in those with counts >200 cells/µl.[45]

MYCOBACTERIUM AVIUM COMPLEX IRIS CASE PRESENTATION

A 40-year-old man with AIDS presented with several months' history of watery diarrhea, weight loss, night sweats and "low grade" fevers. His physical examination revealed oral candidiasis and multiple nontender, mobile, 1-centimeter nodes in the axillae and posterior cervical chains. Cultures of blood and stool, including cultures for mycobacteria, were negative. A chest radiograph was normal; an abdominal CT scan showed 1-centimeter periaortic and retroperitoneal adenopathy. His CD4 count was 42 cells/microliter and viral load >100,000 copies/ml. Antiretroviral therapy with zidovudine, lamivudine, and saquinavir was initiated.

Four weeks later the patient complained of a painful mass in his neck. Examination revealed a warm, tender and fluctuant 3 × 5 centimeter mass in the right posterior neck. His CD4 count was now 200 cells/μl and viral load 2800 copies/ml. Aspiration of the mass yielded 15 ml of pus; gram stain revealed many neutrophils and gram positive rods which were also acid fast. Cultures were ultimately positive for *M. avium* complex. Clarithromycin and ethambutol were initiated and antiretrovirals were continued. His neck pain gradually subsided over the next several weeks and no new lymphadenopathy appeared.

COMMENT ON CASE—*MYCOBACTERIUM AVIUM* COMPLEX IRIS

This case is typical of IRIS associated with *M. avium* complex disease occurring after the initiation of HAART. Patients usually have no prior symptoms of *M. avium* infection and have very low CD4 counts. Several weeks after HAART is initiated symptoms emerge, most commonly lymphadenitis. CD4 counts have usually increased and a prominent inflammatory response with neutrophils is common.

M. AVIUM COMPLEX IRIS

Disseminated *M. avium* complex infections were first recognized in patients with AIDS in 1982.[46] Typical findings of such infections included fever, weight loss, and malaise. In addition, *M. avium* complex was usually recovered from blood or bone marrow culture. A new presentation of *M. avium* complex was first reported in 1989[47] in three patients, started on zidovudine monotherapy. One to three months after initiation of zidovudine all 3 patients developed acute, localized lymphadenitis characterized by swelling, erythema, pain, and tenderness with subsequent isolation of *M. avium* complex from the mass. Systemic illness, including fever, was notably absent and in all cases cultures of blood and bone marrow were negative. French et al.[48] observed localized *M. avium* complex disease developing 1–2 weeks after initiation of zidovudine in 4 patients. In all 4 patients anergy to tuberculin had been documented prior to zidovudine monotherapy with subsequent tuberculin reactivity appearing at the time of symptom onset. Interestingly, all 4 patients lost tuberculin reactivity by

28 weeks of zidovudine and this was associated with the resolution of focal symptoms in all patients and subsequent mycobacteremia in two.

In contrast with *M. tuberculosis*, *M. avium* complex infection is often subclinical in the HIV infected individual due to the low virulence of the organism. In patients with[49,50] or without[47,50,51] evidence of disseminated infection, focal disease, most commonly lymphadenitis, may ensue with the initiation of HAART. Lymphadenitis is characterized by superficial or deep lymph node enlargement, frequently with erythema and tenderness and occasionally by suppuration and formation of draining sinuses.[3,47–51] These findings characteristically present during the first 8 weeks of antiretroviral therapy. Fever may or may not be present but the characteristic wasting seen in disseminated *M. avium* complex is absent at the time of IRIS. Disease onset correlates with rapid rise in CD4 count (median 120 cells/microliter)[50,52] and significant reductions in HIV RNA in the majority of cases. Focal extranodal disease has included granulomatous hepatitis,[52] pneumonitis,[53] pyomyositis with cutaneous abscesses,[54] enteritis,[55] colitis,[52] a paravertebral abscess,[56] and a CNS mass.[57] The majority of extranodal cases also present within the first 8 weeks of antiretroviral therapy. Three reported cases of extranodal IRIS due to *M. avium* occurred 1–2 years after initiation of antiretroviral therapy.[55–57] In each of these cases the patient had been on one or more drugs for the treatment of *M. avium* complex at the time of initiation of HAART, possibly delaying or abrogating onset of IRIS. The frequency of IRIS due to *M. avium* complex is unknown, but in patients with CD4 counts less than 200 cells/microliter at the time HAART is initiated, the overall rate of IRIS may be as high as 25%.

Biopsy of lymph nodes or other involved organs show granulomatous inflammation with caseous necrosis—features not seen in patients with untreated HIV and *M. avium* infection. Acid-fast smears are frequently positive and the organism is usually recovered from cultures of tissue. Blood and bone marrow cultures are usually negative. Management of IRIS due to *M. avium* complex disease should be directed at treating the infection and managing symptoms. The antimicrobial therapy of *M. avium* complex infection is discussed in detail in the chapter 34.[58] For symptom management, a trial of NSAIDs should be considered, but no data exists to document their efficacy in this setting. Thalidomide, a potent TNF-alpha inhibitor, has been suggested as an alternative, based upon efficacy in management of erythema nodosum leprosum, but data to support its effectiveness is lacking. Corticosteroids are effective in reducing fever and local symptoms and are useful for more serious or disabling cases.[59] Although symptoms will resolve with cessation of antiretrovirals, discontinuation of these drugs is discouraged, as relapses frequently occur with the resumption of HAART.[59]

THE GRANULOMATOUS RESPONSE IN SARCOIDOSIS

Our current understanding of sarcoidosis is that its development requires three major events: exposure to antigen, acquired cellular immunity directed against the antigen mediated through APC and antigen-specific T-lymphocytes, and the appearance of immune effector cells that promote a nonspecific inflammatory response.[60] More specifically, alveolar macrophages from patients with pulmonary sarcoidosis show enhanced antigen presenting capacity by the enhanced expression of HLA (MHC)-class II molecules. This is probably induced by interaction with the sarcoidosis antigen(s) and possibly INF-γ.[61] These macrophages recognize, process, and present the putative antigen to CD4+ T-cells of the Th1-type.[61] These activated macrophages produce IL-12 that induces a lymphocyte shift toward a Th1 profile, and causes T-lymphocytes to secrete INF-γ. These activated T-cells release IL-2 and chemotactic factors that recruit monocytes and macrophages to the site of disease activity. IL-2 is also activated and expands various T-cell clones.[62] INF-γ is able to further activate(macrophages and to transform them into giant cells, which are important building blocks of the granuloma.[62,63]

Thus the immunopathogenesis of granuloma formation in sarcoidosis is similar to that seen with pulmonary TB. The major difference is that the antigens responsible for granulomatous inflammation in TB are peptides resulting from digestion and processing of the microorganism, whereas in sarcoidosis the putative antigens are unknown. Like TB, CD4+ cells are essential to granuloma formation.

SARCOIDOSIS IRIS CASE PRESENTATION

A 61-year-old Nigerian woman presented with a five-month history of slowly worsening exertional dyspnea and cough, producing frothy white sputum. She had drenching night sweats and a 20-pound weight loss. She noted enlarged lymph nodes in her neck and left axilla.

Prior history included a diagnosis of sarcoidosis made13 years previously and confirmed by mediastinal lymph node biopsy during a left mastectomy for localized breast cancer. Three years previously she was diagnosed with pulmonary TB and was treated. Fourteen months prior to presentation, she was found to be HIV positive

and started on a three-drug antiretroviral regimen (zidovudine, lamivudine, and nelfinavir).

On physical examination, she had an oral temperature of 101°F, a respiratory rate of 24 and arterial oxygen saturation of 90% on room air by pulse oximetry. Auscultation of the chest was normal. Lymph nodes (about 1 cm) were palpated in the left posterior cervical, left supraclavicular and right axillary locations. Recent CD4 count was 252 cells/microliter with viral load of 782 copies/ml.

A chest radiograph revealed bilateral pulmonary infiltrates (Fig. 32-2). Empiric therapy with trimethoprim-sulfamethoxazole and azithromycin was started. Three smears and cultures for AFB were negative. Bronchoalveolar lavage was negative for pneumocystis, fungi and mycobacteria. INH and rifampin were started for the possible diagnosis of reactivation TB.

One week later the patient underwent open lung biopsy for progressive symptoms. On examination, the lung was noted to have "multiple malignant appearing nodules." Histopathology revealed multiple noncaseating granulomata randomly involving lung parenchyma without a vascular predilection consistent with nodular pulmonary sarcoid. The patient improved on prednisone at an initial dose of 60 mg/day.

COMMENT ON CASE

This patient had reactivation of sarcoidosis following institution of HAART, which is an uncommon presentation. This scenario has occurred more than 15 years after the diagnosis of sarcoidosis in patients who had not previously required treatment.[64] The CD4 count is usually greater than 200 cells/microliter at the time of sarcoidosis reactivation. Patients have responded to 20–30 mg of daily prednisone.[64]

TYPICAL IRIS IN SARCOIDOSIS: CLINICAL ASPECTS

New-onset sarcoidosis is rare in HIV-infected patients.[65] This can probably be explained by the HIV-induced alteration in CMI described above[66,67]; however, several cases of sarcoidosis have been reported after initiation of HAART therapy (Table 32-2).[64,65,67–72] The pathogenesis of this condition is likely to be very similar to the paradoxical reactions seen in HAART-treated HIV-infected patients with TB. It is likely that the antigen(s) that cause sarcoidosis are present in the HIV-infected individual with a low CD4+ count. However, CD4+ lymphocyte number and function is inadequate to mount a significant Th1-induced granulomatous response until HAART

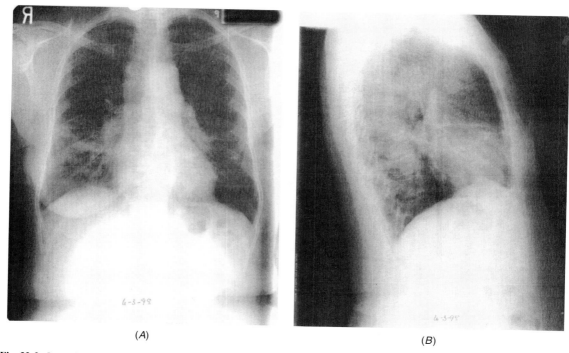

(A)   *(B)*

Fig. 32-2. Lateral and AP chest x-rays demonstrating bilateral interstitial infiltrates, most pronounced in the right middle lobe.

is given. Once HAART induces a granulomatous response, all of the clinical manifestations of sarcoidosis may be seen.

Sarcoidosis has developed in as little as 3 months and as long as $3\frac{1}{2}$ years since starting HAART.[71,72] It has developed with several different antiretroviral regimens.[72] At the time of the diagnosis of sarcoidosis, the CD4+ count has risen in all cases, always exceeded 150 cells/mm^3, and is usually above 200 cells/mm^3.[64,65,71,72]

Sarcoidosis from immune reconstitution mirrors sarcoidosis that is not related to this entity. It most commonly occurs in the lungs, but the liver, spleen, skin, parotid glands, salivary glands, peripheral lymph nodes, and muscle may be involved.[64,65,67–72] The patient may present without symptoms and with only a chest radiographic abnormality,[64,68] or with symptoms of dyspnea, cough, wheezing, or chest pain.[64,71,72] Chest radiographs typically reveal bilateral interstitial infiltrates with or without hilar lymphadenopathy.[64,65,67–72] Spirometry reveals predominantly a restrictive ventilatory defect.[64,68] The serum angiotensin-converting enzyme level is often, although not always, increased.[67,68,71,72] Bronchoalveolar

lavage reveals a lymphocytosis in the bronchoalveolar lavage fluid (BALF). Analysis of lymphocytes in blood and BALF show a movement of CD4+ lymphocytes out of the blood compartment and into the lung compartment, with a low CD4/CD8 ratio in the blood (<1.0) and a high ratio in the BALF (>5.0).[68]

The diagnosis of sarcoidosis in HIV-infected patients must be made with caution, as infectious causes of granulomatous disease must be rigorously excluded. Tuberculin skin testing is not sufficient to exclude TB as it may be negative in up to 25 percent of patients with miliary disease.[73,74] All patients should undergo a diagnostic biopsy, which will show granulomatous inflammation. The specimens need to be examined appropriately for mycobacteria and fungi. The presence of caseating granulomas suggests a diagnosis of TB and not sarcoidosis[75]; however, the finding of noncaseating granulomas does not exclude TB, as this is seen with TB in 20% of cases.[75]

Treatment with prednisone must be undertaken with caution as such therapy may cause significant morbidity (or death) if the granulomatous inflammation is truly the

Table 32-2. Sarcoidosis—Iris Case Reports

SARCOIDOSIS PRIOR TO HIV-HAART

Ref #	N	Time from Sarcoidosis DX to Sarcoidosis Exacerbation	1st Documented CD4 (Cells/μl)	CD4 (cells/μl) at Sarcoidosis Exacerbation	Organs Involved	CXR Findings
34	2	15–30 + years	178/unknown	250/371	Lung, Liver	Bilateral infiltrates
35	1	3 years	194	341	Lung, ear	Focal nodules

SARCOIDOSIS AFTER HIV-HAART

Ref #	N	Time to Development After HAART	1st Documented CD4 (Cells/μl)	CD4 (cells/μl) at Sarcoidosis Exacerbation	Organs Involved	CXR Findings
35	2	4 years	26/11	199/126	Lung	Hilar adenopathy, cavitary nodules
38	2	3/15 months	19/275	219/318	Lung, salivary gland	
40	1	16 months		550	Lung	Bilateral infiltrates
37	1	Unknown	200	503	Lung	Hilar adenopathy
42	8	29+ 16 months	<300 in all	418 + 234 (increased in all)	Lung (all), salivary glands, liver, spleen	Scadding stages: I-2, II-2, III-4
41	1	20 months	130	510	Lung, skin	II
39	1	14 months	5	235	Lung	I

result of infection. On occasion, the disease the sarcoidosis-IRIS will remit on its own without therapy,[67,72] and this should be considered if the patient is asymptomatic. Corticosteroids in doses of 20– 50 mg/day have been successful in inducing a clinical response.[64,71,72]

effectively clear TB antigens and the unknown antigens of sarcoidosis, this inflammatory response may be directly injurious to the host. In these cases, the clinician faces the difficult clinical dilemma of balancing the benefits of an improved host response while trying to avoid its potential injurious consequences.

SUMMARY

The immune reconstitution inflammatory syndrome (IRIS) represents an augmentation of the patient's ability to mount a granulomatous response to specific antigens. For the patient with HIV, this occurs via a HAART-induced increase in the number and function of CD4+ cells. Such cells are a key element in the granulomatous response. Although the heightened granulomatous response may

REFERENCES

1. Burman WJ, Jones BE. Treatment of HIV-related tuberculosis in the era of effective antiretroviral therapy. *Am J Respir Crit Care Med.* 2000;m164:7–12.
2. Narita M, Ashkin D, Hollender DS, et al. Paradoxical worsening of tuberculosis following antiretroviral therapy in patients with AIDS. *Am J Respir Crit Care Med.* 1998;158: 157–161.

3. Shelburne SA, Hamill RJ. The immune reconstitution inflammatory syndrome. *AIDS Rev.* 2003;5:67–79.

4. Kumimoto DY, Chui L, Norbert E, et al. Immune mediated "HAART" attack during treatment for tuberculosis. *Br J Tuberc Lung Dis.* 1999;3:944–947.

5. Mason CM, Ali J. Immunity against mycobacteria. *Semin Respir Crit Care Med.* 2004;25:53–61.

6. Schluger NW, Rom WN. The host immune response to tuberculosis. *Am Rev respire Crit Care Med.* 1998;157:679–691.

7. Cooper A, Dalton D, Stewart T, et al. Disseminated tuberculosis in interferon γ gene-depleted mice. *J Exp Med.* 1993;178:2243–2247.

8. Flynn J, Chan J, Triebold K, et al. An essential role for interferon γ in resistance to *Mycobacterium tuberculosis* infection. *J Exp Med.* 1993;178:2249–2254.

9. Jouanguy E, Altare F, Lamhamedi S, et al. interferon-γ-receptor deficiency in an infant with fatal bacilli Calmette-Guerin infection. *N Engl J Med.* 1996;335:1956–1961.

10. Ottenhoff T, Kumararame D, Casanova J. Novel human immunodeficiencies reveal the essential role of type-1 cytokines in immunity ro intracellular bacteria. *Immunol Today.* 1998;19:491–494.

11. Judson MA. Highly active antiretroviral therapy for HIV with tuberculosis: pardon the granuloma. *Chest.* 2002;122:399–400.

12. Choremis CD, Padiatellis C, Zoumboulakis D et al. Transitory exacerbation of fever and roentgenographic findings during treatment of tuberculosis in children. *Am Rev Tuberc.* 1955;72:527–536.

13. Matthy RA, Neff TA, Iseman MD. Tuberculous pleural effusions developing during chemotherapy for pulmonary tuberculosis. *Am Rev Resp Dis.* 1974;109:469–472.

14. Onwubalili JK, Scott GM, Smith H. Acute respiratory distress related to chemotherapy of advanced pulmonary tuberculosis: a study of 2 cases and review of the literature. *Q J Med.* 1986;59:599–610.

15. Al-Majed SA. Study of paradoxical response to chemotherapy in tuberculous pleural effusion. *Respir Med.* 1996;90:211–214.

16. Byrd RB, Bopp RK, Gracey DR, Puritz EM. The role of surgery in tuberculosis lymphadenitis is adults. *Am Rev Resp Dis.* 1971;103:816–820.

17. Campbell IA, Dyson AJ. Lymph node tuberculosis: a comparison of various methods of treatment. *Tubercle.* 1977;58:171–179.

18. British Thoracic society research committee. Short course chemotherapy for tuberculosis of lymph nodes: a controlled trial. *BMJ.* 1985;290:1106–1108.

19. Chin Y-M, Lee P-Y, Su W-J, Perug R-P. Lymph node tuberculosis: 7 year experience in Veterans General Hospital, Taipei, Taiwan. *Tuberc Lung Dis.* 1992;73:368–371.

20. Teoh R, Humphries MJ, O'Mahoney G. Symptomatic intracranial tuberculoma developing during treatment of tuberculosis: a report of 10 patients and review of the literature. *Q J Med.* 1987;241:449–460.

21. Afghani B, Lieberman JM. Paradoxical enlargement or development of intracranial tuberculomas during therapy: case report and review. *Clin Infect Dis.* 1994;19:1092–1099.

22. Labhard N, Nicod L, Zellweger JP. Cerebral tuberculosis in the immunocompetent host: 8 cases observed in Switzerland. *Tuber Lung Dis.* 1994;75:454–459.

23. Wendel KA, Alwood KS, Gachuhi R, et al. Paradoxical worsening of tuberculosis in HIV-infected persons. *Chest.* 2001;120:193–197.

24. Navas E, Martin-Dávila P, Moreno L, et al. Paradoxical reactions of tuberculosis in patients with the acquired immunodeficiency syndrome who are treated with highly active antiretroviral therapy. *Arch Intern Med.* 2002;162:97–99.

25. Breen RAM, Smith CJ, Bettinson H, et al. Paradoxical reactions during tuberculosis treatment in patients with and without HIV co-infection. *Thorax.* 2004;59:704–707.

26. Dooley DP, Carpenter JL, Rademacher S. Adjunctive corticosteroid therapy for tuberculosis: a critical reappraisal of the literature. *Clin Infect Dis.* 1997;25:872–887.

27. Muller I, Cobbold S, Waldmann H, et al. Impaired resistance to *Mycobacterium tuberculosis* infection after selective in vivo depletion of L3T4+ and Lyt-2+ T cells. *Infect Immunol.* 1987;55:2037–2041.

28. Scanga C, Mohan V, Yu K, et al. Depletion of CD4+ T cells causes reactivation of interferon γ and nitric oxide synthase 2. *J Exp Med.* 2000;192:347–358.

29. Saunders B, Frank A, Orme I, et al. CD4 is required for the development of a protective granulomatous response to pulmonary tuberculosis. *Cell Immunol.* 2002;216:65–72.

30. Schluger NW, Perez D, Liu YM. Reconstitution of immune response to tuberculosis in patients with HIV infection who receive antiretroviral therapy. *Chest.* 2002;122:597–602.

31. Lawn SD, Butera ST, Shinnick TM. Tuberculosis unleashed: the impact of human immunodeficiency virus infection on the host granulomatous response to Mycobacterium tuberculosis. *Microbes Infect.* 2002;4:635–646.

32. Barnes P, Bloch A, Davidson P, et al. Tuberculosis in patients with human immunodeficiency virus infection. *N Engl J Med.* 1991;324:1644–1650.

33. Graham N, Chaisson R. Tuberculosis and HIV infection: epidemiology, pathogenesis, and clinical aspects. *Ann Allergy.* 1993;71:421–428.

34. Goldsack NR, Allen S, Lipman MCI. Adult respiratory distress syndrome as a severe immune reconstitution disease following the commencement of highly active antiretroviral therapy. *Sex Transm Infect.* 2003;79:337–338.

35. Crump JA, Tyrer MJ, Lloyd-Owen SJ, et al. Miliary tuberculosis with paradoxical expansion of intracranial tuberculomas complicating human immunodeficiency virus infection in a patient receiving highly active antiretroviral therapy. *Clin Infect Dis.* 1998;26:1008–1009.

36. Girardi E, Palmieri F, Zaccarelli M, et al. High incidence of tuberculin skin test conversion among HIV-infected persons who have a favorable immunologic response to HAART

[abstract]. 9th Conference on Retroviruses and Opportunistic Infections, Seattle, WA: 2002:282. Abstract 624.

37. Breton G, Duval X, Estellat C, et al. Factors associated with immune reconstitution inflammatory syndrome during tuberculosis in HIV-1 infected patients [Abstract]. 11th Conference on Retroviruses and Opportunistic Infections, San Fransisco, CA: 2004:348. Abstract 757.

38. Fishman JE, Saraf-Lavi E, Narita M, et al. Pulmonary tuberculosis in AIDS patients: transient chest radiographic worsening after initiation of antiretroviral therapy. *AJR Am J Roentgenol.* 2000;174:43–49.

39. Furrer H, Malinverni R. Systemic inflammatory reaction after starting highly active antiretroviral therapy in AIDS patients treated for extrapulmonary tuberculosis. *Am J Med.* 1999;106:371–372.

40. Hollender E, Narita M, Ashkin D, et al. CNS manifestations of paradoxical reaction in HIV+ TB patients on HAART [Abstract] 7th Conference on Retroviruses and Opportunistic Infections. San Fransisco, CA: 2000. Abstract 258.

41. Geux AC, Bucher HC, Demartines N, et al. Inflammatory bowel perforation during immune restoration after one year of antiretroviral and antituberculosis therapy in an HIV-1 infected patient. *Dis Colon Rectum.* 2002;45: 977–978.

42. Jehle AW, Khanna N, Sigle JP, et al. Acute renal failure on immune reconstitution in an HIV-positive patient with miliary tuberculosis. *Clin Infect Dis.* 2004;38:e32–e35.

43. de Jong BC, Israelski DM, Corbett EL, Small PM. Clinical management of tuberculosis in the context of HIV infection. *Ann Rev Med.* 2004;55:283–301.

44. Treatment of tuberculosis: American Thoracic Society, CDC and IDSA. *MMWR Morb Mortal Wkly Rep.* 2003;52 (RR-11):1–77.

45. Pedral-Sampaio DB, Netto EM, Brites C. Treating tuberculosis in AIDS patients: when to start and how long to keep giving drugs? *AIDS.* 2002;16:75–83.

46. Zakowski P, Fligiel S, Berlin GW et al. Disseminated *Mycobacterium avium-intracellulare* infection in homosexual men dying of acquired immunodeficiency. *JAMA.* 1982;248: 2980–2982.

47. Barbaro DJ, Orcutt VL, Coldiron BM. *Mycobacterium avium-Mycobacterium intracellulare* infection limited to the skin and lymph nodes in patients with AIDS. *Rev Infect Dis.* 1989;11:625–628.

48. French MAH, Mallal SA, Dawkins RL. Zidovudine-induced restoration of cell-mediated immunity to mycobacteria in immunodeficient HIV-infected patients. *AIDS.* 1992;6: 1293–1297.

49. Race EM, Adelson-Mitty J, Kriegel GR et al. Focal mycobacterial lymphadenitis following initiation of protease-inhibitor therapy in patients with adbanced HIV-1 disease. *Lancet.* 1998;351:252–255.

50. Phillips P, Kwiatkowski MB, Copland M et al. Mycobacterial lymphadenitis associated with the initiation of combination antiretroviral therapy. *J Acquir Immun Defic Syndr Hum Retrovirol.* 1999;20:122–128.

51. Cabié A, Abel S, Brebion A et al. Mycobacterial lymphadenitis after initiation of highly active antiretroviral therapy. *Eur J Clin Microbiol Infect Dis.* 1998;17: 812–813.

52. Shelburne SA, Hamill RA, Rodriguez-Barradas MC et al. Immune reconstitution inflammatory syndrome: emergence of a uniquye syndrome during highly active antiretroviral therapy. *Medicine.* 2002;81:213–227.

53. Salama C, Policart M, Venkataraman M. Isolated pulmonary *Mycobacterium avium* comples infection in patients with human immunodeficiency virus infection: case reports and literature review. *Clin Infect Dis.* 2003;37:e35–e40.

54. Lawn SD, Bicanic TA, Macallan DC. Pyomyositis and cutaneous abscesses due to *Mycobacterium avium*: an immune reconstitution manifestation in a patient with AIDS. *Clin Infect Dis.* 2004;38:461–463.

55. Cinti SK, Kaul DR, Sax PE et al. Recurrence of *Mycobacterium avium* infection in patients receiving highly active antiretroviral therapy and antimycobacterial agents. *Clin Infect Dis.* 2000;30:511–514.

56. Currier JS, Williams PI, Koletar SL et al. Discontinuation of *Mycobacterium avioum* complex prophylaxis in patients with antiretroviral-induced increases in CD4+ cell count. *Ann Intern Med.* 2000;133:493–503.

57. Murray R, Mallal S, Heath C et al. Cerebral *Mycobacterium avium* infection in an HIV-infected patient following immune reconstitution and cessation of therapy for disseminated *Mycobacterium avium* complex infection. *Eur J Clin Microbiol Infect Dis.* 2001;20:199–201.

58. Karakousis PG, Moore RD, Chaisson RE. *Mycobacterium avium* complex in patients with HIV infection in the era of highly active antiretroviral therapy. *Lancet Infect Dis.* 2004;4:557–565.

59. Desimone JA, Babinchak TJ, Kaulback KR et al. Treatment of *Mycobacterium avium* complex immune reconstitution disease in HIV-1 infected individuals. *AIDS Patient Care and STDs.* 2003;17:617–622.

60. Newman LS, Rose CS, Maier LA. Sarcoidosis. *N Engl J Med.* 1997;336:1224–1234.

61. Costabel U. Sarcoidosis: clinical update. *Eur Respir J.* 2001;18:Suppl 32, 56s–68s.

62. Konishi K, Moller D, Saltini C, et al. Spontaneous expression of the interleukin 2 receptor gene and presence of functional interleukin 2 receptors on T lymphocytes in the blood of individuals with active pulmonary sarcoidosis. *J Clin Invest.* 1988;82:775–781.

63. Steffen M, Petersen J, Oldigs M, et al. Increased secretion of tumor necrosis factor-alpha, interleukin-1-beta, and interleukin-6 by alveolar macrophages from patients with sarcoidosis. *J Allergy Clin Immunol.* 1993;91:939–949.

64. Lenner R, Bregman Z, Teirstein AS. Recurrent pulmonary sarcoidosis in HIV-infected patients receiving highly active antiretroviral therapy. *Chest.* 2001;119:978–981.

65. Haramati LB, Lee G, Singh, et al. Newly diagnosed pulmonary sarcoidosis in HIV-infected patients. *Radiology.* 2001;218:242–246.

66. Granieri J, Wisnieski JJ, Graham BC, et al. Sarcoid myelopathy in a patient with human immunodeficiency virus infection. *South Med J.* 1995;88:591–595.

67. Mirmirani P, Maurer TA, Herndier B, et al. Sarcoidosis in a patient with AIDS: a manifestation of immune restoration syndrome. *J Am Acad Dermatol.* 1999;41:285–286.

68. Naccache J, Antoine M, Wislez M, et al. Sarcoid-like pulmonary disorder in human immunodeficiency virus-infected patients receiving antiretroviral therapy. *Am J Respir Crit Care Med.* 1999;159:2009–2013.

69. Gomez V, Smith PR, Burack J, et al. Sarcoidosis after anti-retroviral therapy in a patient with acquired immunodeficiency syndrome. *Clin Infect Dis.* 2000;31:1278–1280.

70. Wittram C, Fogg J, Farber H. Immune restoration syndrome manifested by pulmonary sarcoidosis. *AJR.* 2001:1427.

71. Trevenzoli M, Cattelan AM, Marina F, et al. Sarcoidosis and HIV infection: a case report and a report a review of the literature. *Postgrad Med J.* 2003;79:535–538.

72. Foulon G, Wislez M, Naccache JM, et al. Sarcoidosis in HIV-infected patients in the era of Highly active antiviral therapy. *Clin Infect Dis.* 2004;38:418–425.

73. Munt PW. Miliary tuberculosis in the chemotherapy era: with a clinical review in 69 American adults. *Medicine.* 1972;51:139–155.

74. Geppert EF, Leff A. The pathogenesis of pulmonary and military tuberculosis. *Arch Intern Med.* 1979;139:1381–1383.

75. Brice EAW, Friedlander W, Bateman ED, et al. Serum angiotensin-converting enzyme activity, concentration, and specific activity in granulomatous interstitial lung disease, tuberculosis, and COPD. *Chest.* 1995;107:706–710.

33

Nontuberculous Mycobacteria—Introduction

Henry Yeager, Jr.
Karl E. Farah

INTRODUCTION

Microorganisms related to the bacteria that cause tuberculosis (TB) and leprosy are abundant in our environment, and have been known at least ever since shortly after the discovery of the tubercle bacillus in the late 1800s. It was not until the development of effective antibiotics for TB, however, in the 1940s and 1950s, that wide-spread culturing of mycobacteria was done, and the diseases associated with nontuberculous mycobacteria (NTM) began to be appreciated.[1] The one exception to the above statement is that the leprosy bacillus still has not been satisfactorily cultured *in vitro*.[2] The third most common mycobacterial disease in Africa, and presumably other parts of the world, is said to be Buruli or Barnesdale ulcer, caused by *Mycobacterium ulcerans*.[3]

NTM have been variously described by the adjectives as "atypical", "anonymous", "mycobacteria other than TB (MOTT)", "environmental", "environmental opportunistic", and, seemingly most commonly in the medical literature, "nontuberculous" or "NTM". They are present in soils, natural waters and water systems, amebae, fish, various birds, and animals. Falkinham and his associates and other investigators have isolated them from aerosols and dust, especially peat-rich dust.[4]

MICROBIOLOGY

In the 1950s, NTM were classified by Timpe and Runyon according to their rate of growth and colony pigment formation.[5] Types I, II, and III, took more than 7 days to grow in culture, and were further distinguished by their colony pigment formation. If the pigments were produced on exposure to light only, then they are called photochromogens (Type I); or even if produced when grown in the dark, then they are called scotochromogens (Type II). And if they were not strongly pigmented, then they are called nonphotochromogens (Type III). The "rapid growers" (Type IV) grow out in less than 7 days time, but still more slowly than many bacteria (Fig. 33-1). This classification is not used very frequently now, and at present it is urged that species identification be done when possible, since this influences the choice of appropriate treatment. There are over 100 species recognized now, and a significant portion of all NTM isolates are not presently speciated.[6]

On microscopy, NTM have a generally indistinguishable appearance from *Mycobacterium tuberculosis*. Cultures should be inoculated unto one or more solid media (Löwenstein-Jensen or Middlebrook 7H10/7H11) and into a liquid medium as well, such as the BACTEC system. Skin and/or soft tissue samples should be incubated at 95°F (35°C) and at 82.4–89.6°F (28–32°C) because many pathogens which infect these tissues, such as *M. marinum* and *M. haemophilum*, may grow only at the lower temperatures.

Established biochemical techniques may need to be used in species identification in situations where access to molecular identification techniques is not possible. The American Society of Microbiology series of technical publications, such as the "Clinical Microbiology Procedures Handbook, 2nd Edition", are available on CD-ROM and on line (http://www.asmpress.org). Newer analytical tools, if available, may play a key role in species identification—for an excellent review see Ref. 6.

EPIDEMIOLOGY

The prevalence of NTM can only be estimated since they are not "reportable" to health authorities in many parts of the world. Though, there is increasing evidence that NTM infection rates and actual disease are increasing, well summarized in a review in 2002.[7] Many factors may have contributed to this rise, for instance, an increase in the specimens submitted for AFB analysis, better recognition of NTM disease, and finally, improved laboratory

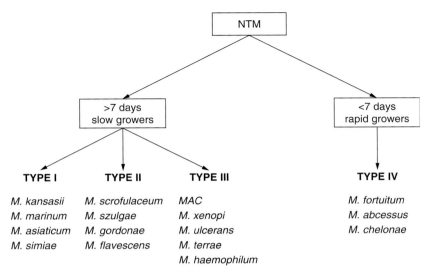

Fig. 33-1. Classification according to Timpe and Runyon.

techniques, which have made the identification and isolation of NTM more accurate and rapid.

As summarized by Marras and Daley,[7] North American and European rates of NTM infection and disease range from 1–15/10^5, and 0.1–2/10^5, respectively. Most common organisms are the *Mycobacterium avium* complex (MAC), made up of *M. avium* and *Mycobacterium intracellulare*, followed by "rapid growers" and *Mycobacterium kansasii*. In the U.S., the southeastern regions seem to have the most infection and disease with MAC. *M. kansasii* is more common in parts of the Midwest and in the Texas-Louisiana-Oklahoma areas. Other pathogens occasionally causing pulmonary disease include *Mycobacterium fortuitum, Mycobacterium szulgai, Mycobacterium simiae, Mycobacterium xenopi, Mycobacterium malmoense, Mycobacterium celatum, Mycobacterium asiaticum,* and *Mycobacterium shimoidei. Mycobacterium xenopi* is second to MAC as cause of lung disease in areas of Canada, the United Kingdom and some other areas of Europe, whereas *Mycobacterium malmoense* is second to MAC in Scandinavia and areas of Northern Europe (Table 33-1).[8]

In general, there has been a consensus that the reported rates of NTM infection and disease are probably underestimated, given that people without significant symptoms are not likely to have intensive investigation to detect infection. Furthermore, it has been speculated that infection with TB and Bacille Calmette-Guérin (BCG) vaccination may provide cross-immunity protection against NTM infection; in fact, many investigations have observed decreasing rates of TB, concomitant with the increase of NTM. Consistent with this idea, studies from Sweden and the Czech Republic since the end of compulsory BCG vaccination in infants have shown a marked rise in NTM cervical lymphadenitis.

PATHOGENESIS

In the early decades of our learning about NTM lung infections, they seemed to occur only in persons who had previous lung disease and in persons with COPD, TB, histoplasmosis, other causes of bronchiectasis, or previously altered systemic immunity, mostly type 4 cell-mediated immunity. A clear-cut increase in disseminated NTM infections occurred in AIDS patients with a CD-4 count less than 50. At first disseminated NTM disease was noted to occur in persons either with hematological malignancies (i.e., MAC in hairy-cell leukemia), or in immunosuppresed persons with organ transplants. In the 1980s with the HIV/AIDS era, the occurrence of widespread abdominal and hematogenous MAC, *M. kansasii* and other infections with NTM greatly increased the medical community's awareness of these pathogens. In recent years, the presence of one or two genes for cystic fibrosis[9] and what has been called a Marfan-like body type, (lean and lanky, with pectus excavatum, and/or scoliosis, and other deformities of the thoracic cage, and mitral valve

Table 33-1. Features of the Common Species

Clinical Disease	Common Etiologies	Geography	Morphologic Features
Pulmonary disease	*M. avium* complex	Worldwide	Usually not pigmented; slow growth (>7 days)
	M. kansasii	USA, coal mining regions, Europe	Pigmented; often large and beaded on acid fast stain
	M. abcessus	Worldwide but mostly USA	Rapid growth (<7 d); not pigmented
Lymphadenitis	*M. xenopi*	Europe, Canada	Slow growth; pigmented
	M. malmoense	UK, northern Europe	Slow growth; not pigmented
	M. avium complex	Worldwide	Usually not pigmented
	M. scrofulaceum	Worldwide	Pigmented
	M. malmoense	UK, northern Europe (especially Scandinavia)	Slow growth
Cutaneous disease	*M. marinum*	Worldwide	Photochromogen; requires low temperatures (28–30°C) for isolation
	M. fortuitum *M. chelonae* *M. abcessus*	Worldwide, mostly USA	Rapid growth; not pigmented
	M. ulcerans	Australia, tropics, Africa, SE Asia	Grows slowly; pigmented
Disseminated disease	*M. avium* complex	Worldwide	
	M. kansasii	USA	
	M. chelonae	USA	
	M. haemophilum	USA, Australia	Requires iron to culture

prolapse) have been shown to be additional risk factors for NTM pulmonary infection.[10,11]

Lowell Young, Luis Bermudez and colleagues have outlined the likely cellular pathogenesis of the most common NTM infections in a series of elegant research studies.[12] NTM strains can get into the body either through the gastrointestinal or respiratory mucosal membranes, or, less commonly, by inoculation. In HIV-infected patients, there seems to be preferential entry through the gastrointestinal tract. MAC can withstand normal gastric acidity, and tend to be taken up by the lining cells of the small intestine, especially the enterocytes of the terminal ileum. Fibronectin-attachment protein lets MAC use fibronectin to "bridge" or "join" bacteria to integrin receptors on mucosal cells. The receptor(s) by which MAC get into the intestinal cell is unknown. There is a change in MAC phenotype inside the epithelial cell, whereby, after it exits these cells, it is better able to withstand the antimicrobial properties of the macrophage. In AIDS patients, MAC presumably go to intestinal lymph nodes, only to disseminate later if host defenses deteriorate.

In the respiratory tract, NTM are inhaled, from water (such as in persons taking shower baths), from dirt, dust, or other aerosols, and most of the time are handled by innate host defenses, mainly mucociliary clearance and cough, and do not cause disease. Presumably in tracheobronchial passages that have excess secretions and do not clear properly, there is an opportunity for biofilm to be laid down, a characteristic for which NTM are known.[12] Once the alveolar spaces are reached, NTM are postulated to colonize Type 2 alveolar cells and alveolar macrophages. Once inside cells, NTM are able to survive, at least in part by interfering with fusion of phagosomes and lysosomes, and by as yet other means. In immunocompetent hosts, CD4 lymphocytes and NK cells can interact with infected mononuclear cells and kill the bacteria. The role of neutrophils is controversial, and may not be very substantial; antibodies do not seem to play any significant role.[12]

PULMONARY DISEASE

Pulmonary disease is the most common clinical manifestation of NTM infection in the U.S. Signs and symptoms of NTM pulmonary disease are not specific, and the evaluation tends to be complicated by the symptoms caused by coexistent disease. There are several fairly distinct types: (1) the longest recognized, infection in previously damaged lung, such as may occur in COPD, pneumoconiosis, bronchiectasis, previous mycobacterial diseases, cystic fibrosis; chronic aspiration syndromes, and so forth; (2) primary lung disease in the middle aged and elderly, with presumed subtle deficiencies in host defense; (3) lung infiltrates, masses and/or nodules simulating lung malignancies or other infections, seen usually in patients with HIV or other immunedeficiencies; and, (4) hypersensitivity pneumonitis.[13]

In the first type, symptoms usually include chronic cough, sputum production and fatigue. Less commonly, malaise, dyspnea, fever, hemoptysis, and weight loss occur, usually with advanced disease. In general, the radiographic appearance cannot be used to distinguish between classic post-primary TB and cavitary upper lobe disease caused by nontuberculous mycobacteria (at least MAC).

In the second type, Primary "Lady Windermere's syndrome" occurs in middle aged or elderly women, overwhelmingly white or Asian, without any preceding lung disease. However, these often have thoracic cage and other connective tissue abnormalities, pectus abnormalities, scoliosis, mitral valve prolapse, etc. They usually develop a chronic cough, with or without production of sputum, eventually along with systemic symptoms of fatigue, weight loss, etc. The radiologic picture is that of nodular bronchiectasis, involving the middle lobe and lingula predominantly.[14]

In the third type, there may symptoms and radiographic changes typical of a pneumonitis or a single or multiple lung parenchymal nodules, often with mediastinal lymphadenopathy, in the case of an HIV-coinfected patient.[15] In the older nonimmunocompromised patient, MAC, or rarely other NTM, may present as a mass or nodule in a subject who usually will have been a smoker and is at risk for lung cancer.[16]

In the fourth type, typical hypersensitivity pneumonitis caused by NTM has been seen in persons in two different types of activities, one occupational (metal working in automobile manufacturing) and one leisure-related (being exposed in indoor swimming pool). Exposure to mycobacterial aerosols has been a common feature of the outbreaks.[17]

LYMPHATIC INFECTION

Lymphadenitis is the most common manifestation of NTM disease in children. Involvement of the submandibular, submaxillary, cervical, or preauricular lymph nodes in children between 1–5 years old is the typical presentation. NTM rarely affect immuno-competent adults, in whom *M. tuberculosis* is a more common cause of agent of mycobacterial lymphadenitis. The disease occurs generally without systemic symptoms; the child is afebrile, and the involved nodes are generally unilateral and nontender. It follows an insidious course, and the lymph node(s) may be swollen for weeks or even months. The causative organism is most commonly MAC; *M. scrofulaceum* was the predominant etiology before the 1970s. Other NTM are uncommon causes of lymphadenitis. *M. tuberculosis* accounts for only 10–20 % of all the mycobacterial lymphadenitis in this age group in the U.S.[17] The differential diagnosis includes bacterial abscess, cat-scratch disease, TB and malignancy. Distinguishing tuberculous from NTM lymphadenitis is important, due to the different course of action required for each. The diagnosis may be difficult to confirm, as positive cultures occur in 50–85% of cases, but it is based on the appearance of caseating granuloma in histopathology, with or without AFB, and a negative or weakly reactive PPD skin test. Simple diagnostic biopsy or incision and drainage are to be avoided because they may be complicated by fistula formation with chronic drainage. Fine needle aspiration is controversial. Excisional biopsy is both diagnostic and probably the best treatment option currently. For other types of NTM head and neck infection, see Ref. 18. In past years skin tests have shown promise on a research basis with antigens prepared from NTM.[19] It is likely that, in the future, blood tests depending on the release of gamma-interferon from T lymphocytes in the presence of suitable NTM antigens may prove to be useful in diagnosis. Such are already proving to be useful in the diagnosis of latent TB.[20]

SKIN AND SOFT TISSUE INFECTION

NTM skin and soft tissue infections are most commonly caused by *M. fortuitum*, *M. abcessus*, *M. marinum*, and in developing nations, *M. ulcerans*. The first three are probably the result of direct exposure to contaminated water sources through inoculation after trauma, surgery, or injections. Nosocomial infections have been associated with cardiac bypass surgery and augmentation mammoplasty and long-term use of intravenous or peritoneal catheters. Most often, these infections occur 4–6 weeks after a localized trauma like stepping on a nail. Infection after trauma to the skin by *M. marinum* is called "swimming pool granuloma." A small papule or nodule begins 2–3 weeks after inoculation. There may be spontaneous resolution or the formation of an abscess.

First discovered in Buruli, Uganda during the 1950s, Buruli ulcer (BU) disease is now an emerging disease that is evidently on the increase in tropical wetlands areas of Africa, Australia, and elsewhere. BU is caused by *M. ulcerans*, a NTM classified as type III in the Timpe/ Runyon classification. Little is known about the epidemiology and pathogenesis of BU disease. It is believed that infection is related to specific trauma to the skin, and that aquatic insects may have a role in its transmission to humans. Clinically, the mode of presentation may be variable: nodules, plaques, and ulcers may occur. Bone involvement may be seen. The distribution of active lesions involves the lower (62 %) and upper limbs (31%) mainly, and other parts of the body rarely. The clinical diagnosis can be confirmed by one of the following: direct smear examination for acid-fast bacilli (AFB), culture, IS2404 polymerase chain reaction (PCR) and histopathologic examination. This infection is the only one caused by a pathogenic mycobacterium in which the predominant cellular response is neutrophilic. Due to the minimal resources and capacities in endemic areas, diagnosis is unfortunately often only clinical. While some health workers suggest that clinical features are sufficient to diagnose BU, many think that the disease is often misdiagnosed, due to absence of concrete proof of disease. Currently, surgery is the only proven effective treatment in *M. ulcerans* disease. In less severe cases antimycobacterial antibiotics may be effective, however.[21]

INFECTION OF BONES AND JOINTS

Bursae, joints, tendon sheaths, and bone infections due to nontuberculous mycobacteria have been described following accidental trauma and orthopedic procedures. They usually present as painful swelling of an extremity, or part of an extremity, associated with movement limitation. Sometimes synovial thickening and crepitus may be present. Physical examination and x-ray imaging are neither specific nor reliable. Diagnosis is based on the culture of the organism, although a positive AFB smear and/or a characteristic histopathology may be highly predictive. *M. marinum* and MAC have been associated with tenosynovitis of the hand. In the past, *M. abcessus* or *M. fortuitum* were related to osteomyelitis of the sternum after open-heart surgery.

Immune-suppressed recipients of solid organ transplants are at high risk of infections such as cutaneous lesions, tenosynovitis, or arthritis late in the post transplant period. Surgery and antimicrobial therapy are usually curative.[22]

DISSEMINATED DISEASE

Disseminated disease from NTM was occasionally seen in the pre-HIV-AIDS era. The total number seen greatly increased, however, after the advent of HIV, in the 1980s, before the advent of highly active retroviral therapy and antibiotic chemoprophylaxis.

The large number of bloodstream infections in HIV-AIDS patients usually occurred when patients had CD4 counts of less than 50/ml. MAC was by far the most frequent etiologic agent; other NTM such as *M. kansasii, M. gordonae, M. malmoense,* and *M. haemophilum* were also occasionally implicated. Aside from blood, bone marrow, liver, spleen, lymph nodes, and sometimes other organs were affected. Common symptoms included fever, weight loss, diarrhea, and abdominal pain. Anemia and elevated alkaline phosphatase were strongly associated with positive cultures for NTM. A recent paper found that at Hopkins, the rate of disseminated MAC in HIV has fallen from 16% to 1%, with risk factors of younger age, no use of HAART, and enrollment before 1996.[15] Diagnosis is done by culturing the organism from any normally sterile site such as blood, bone marrow, liver, or lymph nodes.

The non-HIV patients with NTM disseminated disease include patients with impaired immunity due to genetic defects affecting their immune defenses, such as: severe combined immunodeficiency (SCID), abnormalities of gamma-interferon or interleukin-12, their receptors and so forth, persons suffering from blood/lymphatic malignancies, those with immunodeficiencies acquired from large doses of immunosuppressives given for organ transplants, or various inflammatory disorders. A common problem has been intravenous catheter infections in patients who have had hematopoietic stem cell transplants. Common etiologic agents have been MAC, *M. haemophilum, M. fortuitum, M. chelonae,* and *M. abscessus.* Patients present generally with fever, weight loss, bone pain, and a variety of skin lesions. Diagnosis is confirmed by culturing the organism from blood, bone marrow, or skin lesion.[23]

DIAGNOSIS OF DISEASE

A series of statements has been offered by the American Thoracic Society for the diagnosis of pulmonary disease caused by NTM. The last of these was published in 1997,[24] and a revision is underway at the time of writing of this chapter. For pulmonary disease, it has been difficult to tell whether a positive culture represents laboratory contamination, in some cases, colonization, or true disease. A combination of clinical, radiologic, and bacteriologic features has been suggested for diagnosis of pulmonary NTM infections. For extra-pulmonary disease, a combination of clinical and bacteriologic criteria (such as isolation of organisms from normally sterile sites), sometimes helped by pathologic confirmation, is used.[6]

REFERENCES

1. Chapman JS. The Atypical Mycobacteria and Human Mycobacterioses. New York: Plenum Publishing Co; 1977.

2. Hagge DA, Ray NA, Krahenbuhl JL, et al. An *in vitro* model for the lepromatous leprosy granuloma: fate of *M. leprae* from target macrophages after interaction with normal and activated effector macrophages. *J Immunol.* 2004;172:7771–7779.

3. WHO. Buruli ulcer—*Mycobacterium ulcerans* infection. Asiedu K, Scherpbier R, Raviglione M, ed. Geneva: WHO; 2000.

4. Primm TP, Lucero CA, Falkinham JO III. Health impacts of environmental mycobacteria. *Clin Micro Rev.* 2004;17:98.

5. Timpe A, Runyon EH. The relationship of atypical acid-fast bacteria to human disease: a preliminary report. *J Lab Clin Med.* 1954;44:202–209.

6. Brown-Elliott BA, Griffith DE, Wallace RJ Jr. Diagnosis of nontuberculous mycobacterial infection. *Clin Lab Med.* 2002;22:911–925.

7. Marras TK, Daley CL. Epidemiology of human pulmonary infection with nontuberculous mycobacteria. *Clin Chest Med.* 2002;23:553–567.

8. Falkinham JO III. Mycobacterial aerosols and respiratory disease. *Emerging Infect Dis.* 2003;9:763–767.

9. Griffith DE. Emergence of nontuberculous mycobacteria as pathogens in cystic fibrosis. *Am J Respir Crit Care Med.* 2003;167:810–812.

10. Iseman MD, Buschman DL, Ackerson LM. Pectus excavatum and scoliosis. Thoracic anomalies associated with pulmonary disease caused by *Mycobacterium avium* complex. *Am Rev Resp Dis.* 1991;144:914–916.

11. Guide SV, Holland SM. Host susceptibility factors in mycobacterial infection. Genetics and body morphotype. *Infect Dis Clin N Amer.* 2002;16:163–186.

12. McGarvey JM, Bermudez LE. Pathogenesis of nontuberculous mycobacterial infections. *Clin Chest Med.* 2002;23:2002.

13. Wittram C, Weisbrod GL. *Mycobacterium avium* complex lung disease in immunocompetent patients: radiography-CT correlation. *Brit J Radiol.* 2002;75;340–344.

14. Chalermskulrat W, Gilbey JG, Donohue JF. Nontuberculous mycobacteria in women, young and old. *Clin Chest Med.* 2002;23:675–686.

15. Karakousis PC, Moore RD, Chaisson RE. *Mycobacterium avium* complex in patients with HIV infection in the era of highly active antiretroviral therapy. *Lancet Infect Dis.* 2004;4:557–565.

16. Kobashi Y, Yoshida K, Miyashita N, et al. Pulmonary *Mycobacterium avium* disease with a solitary pulmonary nodule requiring differentiation form recurrence of pulmonary adenocarcinoma. *Intern Med.* 2004;43:855–860.

17. Falkinham JO iii, Mycobacterial aerosols and respiratory disease. *Emerg Inf Dis.* 2003;9:763–767.

18. Albright JT, Pransky SM. Nontuberculous mycobacterial infections of the head and neck. *Pediatr Clin North Am.* 2003;50:503–514.

19. Hersh AL, Tosteson AN, von Reyn CF. Dual skin testing for latent tuberculosis infection: a decision analysis. *Am J Prev Med.* 2003;24:254–259.

20. Mori T, Sakatani M, Yamagishi F, et al. Specific detection of tuberculosis infection: an interferon-γ–based assay using new antigens. *Am J Respir Crit Care Med.* 2004;170:59–64.

21. Noeske J, Kuaban C, Rondini S et al. Buruli ulcer disease in Cameroon rediscovered. *Am J Trop Med Hyg.* 2004;70: 520–526.

22. Meier JL, Beekman SE. Mycobacterial and fungal infections of bone and joints. *Curr Opin Rheumatol.* 1995;7:329–336.

23. Doucette K, Fishman JA. Nontuberculous mycobacterial infection in hematopoietic stem cell and solid organ transplant recipients. *Clin Infect Dis.* 2004;38:1428–1439.

24. Wallace RJ Jr, Cook JL, Glassroth J et al. American Thoracic Society Statement: diagnosis and treatment of disease caused by nontuberculous mycobacteria. *Am J Resp Crit Care Med.* 1997;156:S1–S25.

34

Mycobacterium Avium Complex Disease

Jason E. Stout

Carol Dukes Hamilton

ECOLOGY AND EPIDEMIOLOGY OF MAC

Ecology and Transmission

Robert Koch announced the studies that proved the tubercle bacillus caused tuberculosis (TB) in 1882. Investigators identified other mycobacteria species in the ensuing years by examining environmental as well as human and animal materials. It was not until the TB epidemic began to wane in the U.S. and Europe, however, that the pathogenic nature of some of these nontuberculous mycobacteria (NTM) began to be recognized and characterized. In 1979, Emanuel Wolinsky published a summary of the early recognition of NTMs and the extensive ecologic and epidemiologic studies performed after 1950.[1] As is true today, *Mycobacterium kansasii* and *Mycobacterium avium-intracellulare-scrofulaceum* complex were the organisms most commonly associated with diseases in humans. U.S.-based studies have found significant geographic variability in the frequency with which *M. avium-intracellulare* (MAC) and other NTMs are isolated in the environment, and there remains little to no evidence that the NTM are transmitted person-to-person.

A survey of U.S. state public health laboratories in 1979 showed that the highest MAC isolation rates (>4.8 per 100,000 population) were in Florida, North Carolina, Maryland, Connecticut, Kansas and Arizona. All the Gulf States had rates between 3.3 and 4.8 per 100,000 population (Figs. 34-1 and 34-2).[2] *M. tuberculosis* case rates at the same time were 9.7 per 100,000 population.[2] Further evidence of environmental exposure to NTM was demonstrated when U.S. Navy recruits were studied for skin test reactivity to antigens prepared from *M. intracellulare* (PPD-B) and *M. scrofulaceum* (PPD-G). There was a pronounced clustering of reactors in the southeastern U.S.[3] More recently, Von Reyn and colleagues used dual skin testing with *M. avium* sensitin (MAS) and *M. tuberculosis* purified protein derivative (PPD) to test asymptomatic health care workers and medical students from northern and southern U.S. sites. They found that MAS-dominant reactions, indicating

exposure to MAC, and possibly other nontuberculous mycobacteria, were significantly more common among subjects in the south than in subjects in the north (46% vs. 33%, p < 0.001).[4]

Organisms belonging to the *M. avium* complex are commonly isolated from water,[5–7] house dust,[8] and soil.[9,10] They are relatively resistant to chemical disinfection by chlorine, chloramine, and ozone[11,12]; as a result the organisms can often be found in water distribution systems.[13] The two major species in the complex, *M. avium* and *M. intracellulare*, may occupy slightly different environmental niches. In one study, *M. avium* was frequently isolated from drinking water samples, while *M. intracellulare* was primarily isolated from biofilms inside the water distribution system.[13]

HIV-infected Populations

There are laboratory and clinical data suggesting that *M. avium*, which is by far the most common species to infect patients with HIV, is probably acquired via the gastrointestinal tract.[14] MAC strains isolated from hospital water have been described as very similar to strains isolated from AIDS patients with MAC disease treated in those hospitals.[15–18] In the laboratory, a MAC strain found in drinking water provided to simian immunodeficiency virus-infected macaques matched the strain that was isolated from the macaques' bloodstream.[19] In a separate study, gastrointestinal inoculation of *M. avium* into immunosuppressed rodents resulted in bacteremic dissemination of the organism to the spleen and bone marrow, analogous to human disease.[20–22] The predominance of *M. avium* in disseminated disease may be partially explained by the fact that *M. avium* is somewhat more resistant to gastric acid than *M. intracellulare*, and *M. avium* invades intestinal cells in both cell culture and a mouse model significantly more efficiently than *M. intracellulare*.[23] In addition, gastrointestinal colonization with strains that demonstrate greater invasion of gastrointestinal cells and macrophages *in vitro* is associated with disseminated MAC disease.[24] While it is often assumed that disease occurs as a result of relatively recent exposure, a recent study in rhesus macaques suggested that latent infection might occur with subsequent reactivation causing disseminated MAC disease.[25]

General Populations

In contrast to HIV-associated disseminated MAC disease, it is thought that immunocompetent patients with pulmonary MAC are usually infected with *M. intracellulare*

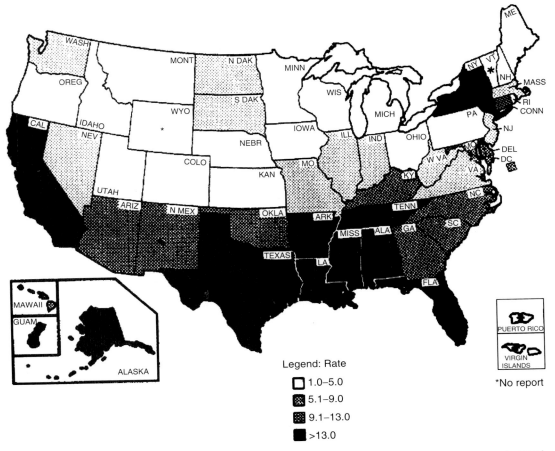

Fig. 34-1. Isolation rates (per 100,000 population) for *Mycobacterium tuberculosis* in the United States, by state, in 1980.[2]

(as opposed to *M. avium*),[26–28] and most likely acquire their infection by the respiratory route. Nonetheless, person-to-person transmission of MAC does not seem to occur. *M. intracellulare* is preferentially isolated from environmental aerosols,[5,29] and one study associated contaminated hospital water with MAC respiratory colonization among hospitalized patients with chronic lung disease.[30] The predilection for MAC pulmonary disease to involve the right middle lobe and lingula,[31,32] which are common anatomic sites of aspiration, implies that aspiration may also be an important mechanism for infection. Although the organisms have been recovered from cigarettes[33] before and after smoking, no cases of MAC disease have been associated with shared cigarettes.

When clusters of patients infected with similar isolates are found, the link is usually a common water source.[15,34–36]

Inhalation of infectious aerosols is most clearly responsible for disease among persons with a particular syndrome of diffuse pulmonary infiltrates and granulomatous inflammation, termed "hot tub lung." The syndrome has been associated with exposure to poorly cleaned and maintained hot tubs,[37] or after introduction into the hot tub by contaminated soil on the skin of persons who did not shower prior to using the hot tub.[38,39] In several reported series, multiple family members have developed disease from the same hot tub.[39] In these clusters, MAC is usually isolated from both the hot tub water and from the patients' lungs,[38–41] and molecular strain typing has confirmed that the strains from the hot tub and patients' lungs are identical.[39]

Humans appear to acquire MAC infection at an early age. Studies in the U.S. and Europe have shown that humoral and cell-mediated immune recognition of MAC

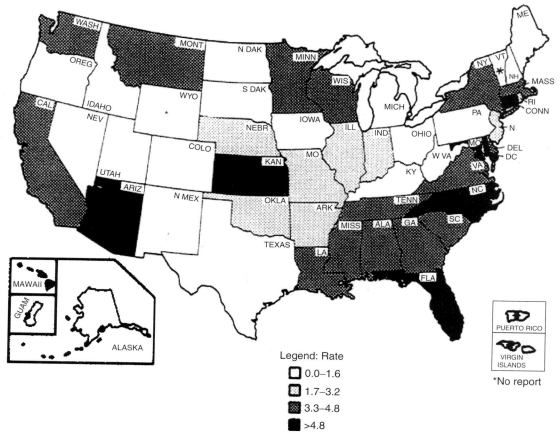

Fig. 34-2. Isolation rates (per 100,000 population) for *Mycobacterium avium complex* in the United States, by state, in 1980.[2]

antigens increases with age, and there are striking differences between those <6 years of age and the older age groups.[42,43]

While respiratory and even gastrointestinal exposure to MAC appears to be common, especially in the southeastern U.S., subsequent infection rarely translates to frank disease. When disease occurs, the clinical manifestations differ dramatically depending on the age, gender and medical comorbidities of the host (Fig. 34-3). The incidence and epidemiology of the different groups will be discussed separately.

Epidemiology

HIV-infected Populations

In 1984, NIH investigators reported findings from 30 men with a clinical diagnosis of AIDS, 16 of who were

investigated because of unremitting fevers and weight loss. They found 8 patients with disseminated MAC (DMAC), and found that over time they remained persistently bacteremic.[44] This and other early studies of AIDS defined DMAC as an important AIDS-associated opportunistic infection (OI).[45] It became evident that DMAC occurred at the extreme of CD4 lymphopenia, and was highly associated with mortality within the following year.[46–50] The Swiss HIV Cohort Study specifically looked at DMAC in a prospectively followed cohort of 6290 HIV-infected subjects between 1987 and 1995. They found 2-year probabilities of developing DMAC to be 22% among those whose first CD4 count was <50 cells/mm^3 and 11% if their CD4 count was 50–99 cells/mm^3.[51] Furthermore, they found that the cumulative probability of MAC disease after 2 years of follow up increased from 9.8% (95% CI 4.4–15.2%) to 29.8% (95% CI 20.8–38.8%)

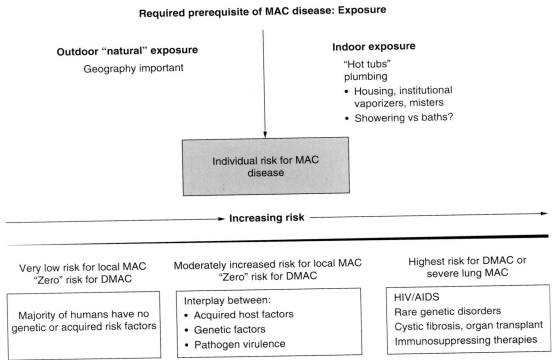

Fig. 34-3. Interplay between environmental exposure, host susceptibility and pathogen virulence.

among those entering the cohort in later years (1993–1995 compared to 1987–1989). There was no improvement in survival over the same time period, median survival following diagnosis of DMAC being 7.9 months. As AIDS reports accumulated in the 1980s, the percentage of AIDS cases with DMAC reported to the Centers for Disease Control (CDC) increased from 4.7% in 1987[52] to 7.6% by the end of 1990.[50]

There has clearly been a change in the epidemiology of DMAC over the life of the AIDS epidemic in the U.S. and Europe.[53] Potent combination ("highly active") anti-retroviral therapy (HAART) came into widespread use between 1995 and 1997, and overall HIV-associated mortality rates began declining by 1996.[54–56] Data from a multicenter study, the HIV Outpatient Study Cohort, noted a dramatic increase in the use of protease-inhibitor containing regimens, from 2% of patients taking HIV therapy in mid-1995 to 82% by mid-1997.[56] Though the rates of prophylaxis for DMAC remained the same over the time period of the study, the incidence of DMAC declined from as high as 20 per 100 person-years, to

<5 per 10 person-years between 1994–1997. DMAC in Atlanta, Georgia, decreased from a peak of 198 cases in 1995, to only 66 cases in 2000. Rates in Sao Paulo, Brazil decreased from >20% in 1995–96 to <7% by 1998, and correlated with increased availability to HAART.[57]

Today, those who develop DMAC in resource-rich countries are usually not on either HAART or primary MAC prophylaxis, either out of personal choice or due to a variety of barriers to health care. Once a person is diagnosed with DMAC, the greatest correlation with subsequent survival is initiation of HAART; treatment with a macrolide-containing DMAC treatment regimen is also associated with improved survival.[58–60]

In developing countries, the highly virulent pathogen, *M. tuberculosis*, is a common cause of death in HIV/AIDS that occurs relatively early in a person's experience with HIV. In these resource poor settings, it is assumed that an HIV-infected person's likelihood of living long enough to "experience" DMAC and other OI common in the U.S. and Europe is low, resulting in few reports of DMAC in Sub-Saharan Africa, for example.

General Populations

The epidemiology of pulmonary MAC in HIV-seronegative persons has not been as extensively studied as the epidemiology of DMAC because in most areas, pulmonary MAC (unlike HIV/AIDS) is not a disease required to be reported to public health authorities. From the 1950s through the 1970s, MAC-related pulmonary disease was reported most commonly in older men[61,62] with preceding lung injury including silicosis and other pneumoconiosis, previous or coexisting tuberculosis or fungal lung diseases, tobacco-associated chronic bronchitis or obstructive pulmonary disease (COPD), or bronchiectasis.[61,63,64] A nationwide U.S. survey performed between 1981–1983 obtained an estimated prevalence of 0.8 cases of MAC pulmonary disease per 100,000 population.[61] Patients were primarily male (56%), over 45 years of age (88%), and of those with clinical information provided, 40% had underlying COPD. A study in Japan between 1971–1984 reported an annual incidence of 1.29 cases of MAC pulmonary disease per 100,000 population, with no secular trend. Similar to patients in the United States, patients were primarily male (64%) and elderly (mean age 63 years for men, 66 years for women).[62] A more recent study of pulmonary MAC in Northern Territory, Australia between 1989–1997 reported an annual incidence of 2.1 cases per 100,000 population, with an increase in the number of cases over time.[63] Again, patients were predominantly male and over 50 years of age. No recent large, epidemiologic studies have been performed in the United States, but the rate of isolation of MAC from respiratory specimens has been rising, and is greater than the rate of *M. tuberculosis* isolation in parts of the U.S.[65,66] The demographics of patients with MAC pulmonary disease in recent case series have also shifted from primarily elderly males with tobacco-related lung disease to elderly females, many of whom have no underlying pulmonary disease.[67–70] The magnitude and significance of this demographic shift are unclear, but it may partially reflect greater awareness of the different clinical manifestations of MAC pulmonary disease in women.

MAC is one of several NTM to cause extrapulmonary disease in HIV-uninfected hosts. Lymphadenitis is the most common manifestation of MAC in immunocompetent hosts, occurring most commonly in young children. Interestingly, prior to 1970, *M. scrofulaceum* was the most common NTM causing lymphadenitis, but the epidemiology has changed and MAC causes 60–85% of these cases in the U.S.[61,71] MAC can also infect other organ systems, causing diverse syndromes including osteomyelitis, septic arthritis, skin and soft tissues

infections and middle ear disease (see clinical section below).

HOST AND PATHOGEN FACTORS ASSOCIATED WITH MAC DISEASE

Once they gain entry into the host, MAC organisms may produce a range of clinical manifestations from asymptomatic colonization to severe, disseminated disease. Any clinical manifestations resulting from MAC infection depend significantly on the interaction between the particular organism and the host. Both parameters will be explored.

Host Factors

MAC and other NTM are common in the environment, yet few people develop clinical disease. Thus, susceptibility to MAC is the exception rather than the rule. The first-line of defense is clearly the lung macrophage, which must be activated to effectively phagocytose and destroy the organism. The complex networks of activating and modulating influences within the immune system determine the effectiveness of these effector cells. HIV-associated acquired immunodeficiency helped demonstrate the critical role that CD4-positive T-helper lymphocytes (CD4 cells) have in maintaining host resistance to MAC, among other opportunistic infections. Disseminated MAC occurs exclusively among patients with profound depletion of CD4 + T-lymphocytes; almost all patients with disseminated MAC have CD4 + T-lymphocyte counts of <100 cells/mm^3, with the median T-cell count in many studies in the 20–40 range.[72–74] HIV infected patients with disseminated MAC disease have higher HIV RNA levels than similar patients without disseminated MAC.[75] This observation can be partially explained by a reciprocal interaction between HIV and MAC in human monocytes. *In vitro*, MAC infection enhances replication of HIV in human monocytes through NF-κB-dependent mechanisms that are independent of cytokine induction.[76] Conversely, HIV infection of human macrophages increases intracellular growth of MAC organisms inside these macrophages.[77]

CD4 cell decline is also associated with a cascade of dysfunction within the cell-mediated immune, or TH1, pathway, including alterations in cytokine levels and responsiveness. Mouse models have been used to investigate disseminated BCG, *M. tuberculosis* and MAC, and these studies have shown the importance of CD4 and CD8 T-cells and their associated cytokines in controlling infection, again because of their pro-activating effect on macrophages and monocytes. Studies of

Toll-like receptors (TLR) show they are important players in innate host defense, and some may have pathogen-specific importance for mycobacteria.[78–80] IL-12,[81] IFN-γ, and TNF-α are important in macrophage activation and regulation, and nitric oxide is an important mediator of lethality for the intracellular pathogen.[82,83]

In addition to acquired host vulnerability to MAC, there are likely genetically determined differences in humans. Certain inbred mice are particularly vulnerable to mycobacteria, and this vulnerability has been mapped to a gene called the *bcg* locus.[84] The human correlate, previously termed *NRAMP1*, now called "the solute carrier family 11" (SLC11A1), has been examined for association with *M. tuberculosis* disease in large populations. The results have been mixed, depending on the population studied, leading most to believe that susceptibility/resistance to TB to be a complex interplay between multiple genes, and modulated by other host and pathogen factors.[85] The same is likely true for host susceptibility to other mycobacteria.

Experiments of nature have contributed to our understanding of genetic determinants of immunity to mycobacteria. There are a series of Mendelian immune disorders that predispose humans to mycobacterial infections due to either absence or dysfunction of T cells, altered NF-κB signaling, or disorders of the IL-12/interferon-γ (IFN-γ) axis. "Mendelian susceptibility to mycobacterial disease" (MSMD) comprises several disorders related to IFN-γ production deficits, or poor responsiveness to IFN-γ due to receptor abnormalities or deficiencies.[84,86] While informative, these Mendelian disorders account for a very small number of cases of MAC. As an example, one group analyzed 8 women with MAC who had no recognized underlying immunodeficiency, looking for alleles in the *NRAMP1* and *IFN-γR1* coding regions to account for their predisposition to MAC disease. They found no evidence for a genetic defect in either gene.[87] As follow-up, other Japanese investigators evaluated both the organism and host among siblings found to both have pulmonary MAC. They evaluated strain similarity between MAC isolates from each sibling pair, and, using restriction fragment polymorphisms (RFLP), looked for polymorphisms in the *NRAMP1* region of each sibling's cDNA. They found no evidence of particularly virulent MAC strains nor unusual alleles in the *NRAMP1* gene to explain the phenomenon.[88] On the other hand, investigators in Japan have found two HLA antigens associated with having MAC disease compared to control Japanese populations. They found HLA-DR6 in 50.8% of cases versus 20.2% of controls, and HLA-A33 in 28.8% of cases versus

12.5% of controls.[89] In a different analysis among Japanese patients with pulmonary MAC, HLA-A26 antigen was associated with pulmonary deterioration.[90]

In summary, the critical effector cell for controlling MAC is the lung macrophage, which ingests the mycobacteria.[91] Once engulfed by the macrophage, the bacteria's fate—destruction, persistence, or replication—is determined by the cell's state of immune activation, which is determined by interactions between cells in the TH1 pathway and their associated cytokines (Figure 34-3), particularly the IL-12/interferon-γ (IFN-γ) axis. Numerous other cytokines (e.g., IL-18, IL-23, IL-29), receptors (e.g., vitamin D receptor) and unidentified cofactors,[92] may also be important. Perturbations in cytokine production, protein conformation or receptors, increase the likelihood that the bacteria will replicate and cause disease. A number of excellent reviews are available that focus on host immunity to MAC and other mycobacteria, to which the reader is referred.[93]

Pathogen Factors

Different subgroups of organisms within the *Mycobacterium avium* complex are associated with different manifestations of disease; whether these clinical differences represent differential pathogenicity of the organisms, differences in environmental niches, or differences in host susceptibilities is unclear. It is becoming increasingly clear that species and subspecies differences within MAC have clinical importance.

The *M. avium* complex consists of two defined species, *M. avium* and *M. intracellulare*, and a third group of "X" organisms that are not assigned to either species. The two species within the MAC group are morphologically and biochemically indistinguishable.[94] Differentiating between the two MAC species was traditionally performed by serotyping.[95] Twenty eight serovars have been described, with serovars 1–6, 8–11, and 21 assigned to *M. avium*, serovars 7, 12–20, and 25 assigned to *M. intracellulare*, and other serovars not assigned to either species.[96] Unfortunately, the results of serotyping were not consistent between different laboratories,[97] and serotyping is not possible for all MAC organisms.[98] Fortunately, newer molecular methods have overcome these limitations. Two commercially available DNA probes (Gen-Probe, San Diego, CA) are available to specifically identify *M. avium* and *M. intracellulare*.[96] Other methods employed to differentiate MAC strains include phage typing,[99] multilocus enzyme electrophoresis analysis,[100,101] restriction fragment length polymorphism (RFLP) analysis of insertion elements such as IS1245[102] and others,[103,104] and nucleotide sequencing of regions of the 65-kilodalton heat shock protein (*hsp65*),[105] and the internal transcribed spacer located between the genes encoding 16S and 23S rRNAs (16S-23S ITS).[106]

Agreement between these various methods has not always been consistent. In studies examining human and animal MAC isolates from Australia,[101] and the U.S.[100] there was no clear correspondence between the results of serotyping and multienzyme electrophoresis. Nevertheless, subgroups obtained by sequencing *hsp65* and the 16S-23S ITS have correlated reasonably well.[105] Both of these methods have divided MAC into over 20 subgroups[107–109] and their nomenclature is described in Table 34-1.[109]

Substrain speciation of MAC isolates is important for exploring pathogenetic mechanisms underlying different forms of disease. Disseminated MAC disease is predominantly (80–95%) caused by *M. avium*, while isolates from patients with pulmonary disease are more evenly divided between *M. avium* and *M. intracellulare*.[26,109–113] In particular, the most common *M. avium* strain isolated from AIDS patients with disseminated MAC is Mav-B (79–90%), followed by Mav-A (5–16%) and Mav-E (0–5%).[109,114–116] These three strains were also the most common isolates found in HIV-uninfected children with MAC lymphadenitis in two studies,[109,114–116] although in another study, the majority of isolates (69%) belonged to the species *M. intracellulare*.[117]

M. avium, particularly the Mav-A/Mav-B strains, may be more likely to cause disseminated disease in AIDS patients because of specific virulence factors. Two putative virulence factors have been identified in *M. avium*: *mig*[118] and hemolysin.[119] Expression of the *mig*, or macrophage-induced gene, occurs only when the organisms are replicating within macrophages.[120] Secretion of the 30 kilodalton Mig protein is induced by the acid environment present inside the macrophage. While the exact function of the protein is unknown, variation in the *mig* gene correlates with the ability of *M. avium* to replicate in human macrophages,[121] and survival of *mig*-transfected *M. smegmatis* inside macrophages[118] is enhanced compared to wild-type *M. smegmatis* strains. In at least one study, the *mig* gene was present in *M. avium* strains but absent from *M. intracellulare* strains,[110] which correlates with the proclivity of these two species to cause disseminated disease. Hemolysin is a magnesium-dependent, cell wall-associated protein that may be important for intracellular survival. Expression of hemolysin has been strongly associated with *M. avium* strains responsible for disseminated disease in both AIDS and other immunosuppressed patients;[119] *M. avium* and *M. intracellulare* strains associated with pulmonary disease generally did not express hemolysin. More recent data has demonstrated that human isolates of Mav-A and Mav-B obtained from patients with both disseminated and pulmonary disease are strong producers of hemolysin, while animal isolates in the Mav-A and Mav-C groups were significantly less hemolytic.[122]

A key component of the virulence of MAC organisms may be the ability of the organisms to invade human epithelial cells.[123] This invasion likely occurs by MAC proteins that adhere to fibronectin and other extracellular matrix proteins.[124] Colonial morphology on solid media has been traditionally correlated with relative invasiveness of MAC organisms. MAC strains with smooth, flat, and transparent colonial morphology seem to be more virulent than strains with domed and opaque morphology in some studies.[125–127] Colonial morphology appears to be determined by the glycopeptidolipid content of the mycobacterial wall, and differences in glycopeptidolipid seem to be associated with differential inhibition of intracellular killing of *M. avium*.[128] The less virulent *M. avium* strains, as identified by colony morphology, appear to induce more IL-18 expression by the infected monocyte, resulting in more IFN-γ production and greater inhibition of mycobacterial growth, than more virulent strains.[129]

Table 34-1. Nomenclature for MAC Substrains based on Molecular Typing Methodology

	16S-23S ITS Classification	*hsp65* **Classification**
M. avium	Mav-A through Mav-E	*hsp65.1, hsp65.2, hsp65.20, hsp65.21, hsp65.34*
M. intracellulare	Min-A through Min-D	*hsp65.3–hsp65.7, hsp65.18, hsp65.22, hsp65.32*
Nonavium/ nonintracellulare	MAC-A through MAC-H	*hsp65.8, hsp65.10, hsp65.13, hsp65.28, hsp65.29*

The resulting milieu, rich in IFN-γ, also may explain why these less virulent strains appear to be phagocytized by human monocytes more readily than more virulent strains.[127]

CLINICAL SYNDROMES ASSOCIATED WITH MAC

MAC in the Setting of HIV/AIDS

Pulmonary: Colonization versus Disease

Pulmonary parenchymal disease caused by MAC is uncommon among patients with AIDS[130]; however, prospective studies have examined whether pulmonary or GI colonization with MAC might predict subsequent DMAC. One study showed that in patients with CD4 counts <50, 67% of those who had MAC in sputum or stool developed DMAC within 1 year, though few developed pulmonary disease per se. However, of those who developed DMAC, only about a third had preceding positive stool or sputum cultures. Tuberculosis, not MAC, should be the greatest concern for the clinician who receives a report showing acid-fast bacilli on the sputum smear from a patient with HIV/AIDS. While the finding of MAC in sputum might cause concern for future dissemination, TB is an imminent threat to the patient, and to those in his or her home, clinic, hospital, or work environment. In settings where HAART is available, the cost effectiveness of checking for MAC in sputum or stool is dwarfed by the benefits of starting HAART to prevent the emergence of DMAC. If HAART is ineffective, due to HIV multidrug resistance, for example, or CD4 lymphocyte improvement is delayed in a particular individual, MAC prophylaxis is still an important adjunct to care, and is cost-effective.[131]

Disseminated MAC

Initially, there was confusion about whether MAC was causative of symptoms and eventual death among those suffering from AIDS. MAC was easily cultured from lymph nodes, bone marrow, sputum, and other organ systems when looked for in patients with late stage AIDS.[132] Still, the frequent finding of concurrent pathogens, such as cytomegalovirus, and the paucity of typical granulomatous inflammatory response, made its role in symptomatology and clinical deterioration unclear. When investigators used newer broth culture techniques to look for the organism in the blood, they found that the patients were almost uniformly mycobacteremic, illustrating the overwhelming nature of their infection.[44]

It became clear that DMAC was one of the entities that could cause the end-of-life event known as "wasting syndrome". In an attempt to tease out the impact of DMAC itself from the generalized immune deterioration in advanced AIDS, one group performed a case control study of patients with one episode of *Pneumocystis carinii* pneumonia (PCP) as well as respiratory and sterile body cultures for mycobacteria. Survival of cases (with DMAC) and controls was indexed to their first episode of PCP. Median survival was shorter in those with DMAC (107 days; 95% confidence interval [CI] 55–179) compared to those with negative MAC cultures (275 days; 95% CI 230–319, $P < 0.01$).[49] Other studies confirmed this finding, and also found that poor survival was associated with lack of antiretroviral therapy, the level of anemia, and lack of antimycobacterial chemotherapy.[48] A prospective observational study examined the impact of treatment of DMAC on survival among patients with AIDS in the pre-HAART era and confirmed earlier findings that patients with AIDS who developed DMAC were more likely to die, but that those receiving antimycobacterial therapy had improved survival (median 263 compared to 139 days, $p < 0.001$).[133] Unfortunately, 23% of those with DMAC died within 29 days of diagnosis, and most of these persons had not yet had time to initiate DMAC therapy.

Clinically, patients who have DMAC in the setting of AIDS have persistent, high-grade fevers, profound night sweats, weight loss, anorexia, fatigue, and diarrhea often associated with cramping abdominal pain.[48] Laboratory abnormalities classically have reflected the disseminated nature of the disease with profound anemia out of proportion to neutropenia or thrombocytopenia, and elevated transaminases and alkaline phosphatase. Either because of improved diagnosis or concurrent antiretroviral therapy, these laboratory abnormalities may be less common among patients with DMAC diagnosed in the present day than among those diagnosed earlier in the HIV/AIDS epidemic. For example, a recent study found that over the period 1991–1997, patients presenting with DMAC were significantly less likely to have anemia or an elevated alkaline phosphatase.[58] Radiographic findings frequently demonstrate diffuse adenopathy on chest or abdominal CT scans. Bone marrow biopsy may show granulomas, though these may be poorly formed, and acid-fast stain of the bone marrow often shows evidence of unchecked mycobacterial replication, easily confirmed by microbiologic culture. Culture of blood is the easiest diagnostic method, and reflects the high level bacteremia, with a projected sensitivity of 90% with a single blood culture.[134] Autopsy results in one series of 44 patients with documented MAC bacteremia showed that 31 (70%) also had histologic findings of MAC in other organs, and this was associated with elevated hepatocellular enzymes to a statistically significant degree.[135] The organism can be cultured from essentially every body site at autopsy in those with DMAC at death.[136]

Profound anemia frequently accompanies patients with HIV/AIDS and DMAC, while the other cell lines remain relatively intact. Investigators found that bone marrow cellularity and appearance, as well as erythropoietin levels, were indistinguishable between patients with AIDS with and without DMAC. However, bone marrow mononuclear cells were able to generate fewer erythroid progenitor colonies, and sera from patients with DMAC was markedly inhibitory to the erythroid progenitors as compared to sera from patients with AIDS but without DMAC.[137] One study seeking a model to predict DMAC in patients with AIDS found in a multivariate analysis that among those whose CD4 count was <50 cells/mm^3, there were 3 independent predictors of DMAC: fever on >30 days in the preceding 3 months, hematocrit of <30%, and a serum albumin concentration of <3.0 g/dl.[73]

MAC in General Populations

Pulmonary: Colonization versus Disease

In persons without HIV/AIDS, the most common site of MAC infection is the respiratory tract. MAC pulmonary infection has a wide spectrum of clinical manifestations, ranging from asymptomatic colonization to progressive, symptomatic disease (Table 34-2). Understanding of this spectrum has increased significantly during the past 50 years. Seminal work by Dr. Ernest Runyon and others published in the 1940s and 50s described both asymptomatic colonization and a chronic pulmonary disease with clinical manifestations similar to tuberculosis.[137] This chronic pulmonary disease, now often called "classic" MAC pulmonary disease, primarily affected white males over the age of 50 with underlying pulmonary diseases such as silicosis, prior pneumonia, or a history of pulmonary tuberculosis (Fig. 34-4). The clinical syndrome was often insidious in onset; prominent manifestations included chronic cough, hemoptysis, weight loss, and low grade fever.[138–140] The disease was generally slowly progressive, frequently did

Table 34-2. Spectrum of Pulmonary Disease Caused by MAC

Type of Disease	Host Characteristics	Demographics	Radiographic Features
"Classic"	Underlying lung disease, especially chronic obstructive pulmonary disease	Males over 50	Cavitation, often upper lobes involved, fibronodular infiltrates
"New"	No underlying lung disease, possibly associated with thoracic deformities	Elderly females	Multiple nodules associated with areas of bronchiectasis; predilection for right middle lobe/lingula
Pediatric	Healthy children	Usually under 5 years of age, no gender/racial proclivity	Intrathoracic lymphadenopathy, focal atelectasis
Pulmonary/disseminated	Late-stage HIV infection, bone marrow transplants, other immunodeficiency (severe combined immunodeficiency, interleukin-12 or γ-interferon deficiency)	No age/gender/racial proclivity	Multiple nodules, diffuse interstitial infiltrate, cavitation in setting of disseminated MAC
Hot tub lung	Generally immunocompetent	No age/gender/racial proclivity	Bilateral interstitial +/– alveolar infiltrates, ground glass appearance on CT scan

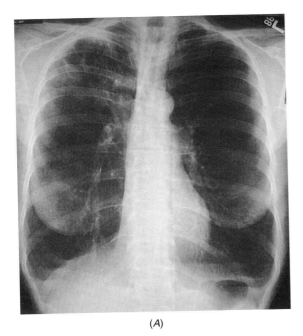

(A)

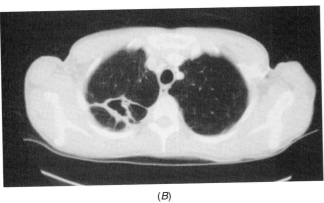

(B)

Fig. 34-4. Chest radiograph (*A*) and CT scan (*B*) from a patient with "classic" type pulmonary MAC. The chest radiograph demonstrates fibronodular upper lobe opacities, and cavitation is evident on the CT scan.

not respond well to available antituberculous agents,[64,138,139,141,142] and was frequently treated with adjunctive surgical resection. Most of these patients had positive tuberculin skin tests, but when concurrent testing with PPD-B antigen (derived from the "Battey bacillus" aka *M. intracellulare*) was performed, the reaction to PPD-B was generally larger than to the PPD-S tuberculin reagent.[138,141] No distinctive physical examination findings were reported. Cavitation was present on chest radiographs in most cases; calcification and pleural effusions were also occasionally observed.[138,140,142,143]

The disease generally ran an indolent course despite ineffective therapy, and patients usually died from other underlying illnesses. In one series of 100 patients evaluated between 1968–1972 with 10 years longitudinal follow up, 26 patients demonstrated improvement, 55 were clinically stable, and 19 had progressive symptoms and radiographic findings. Twenty-nine of the 100 patients died during follow up, but only 4 persons were felt to have died directly because of MAC pulmonary disease.[64,144] Dyspnea on initial presentation and presence of coexisting lung disease have been associated with increased mortality among patients with MAC pulmonary disease.[145]

During the late 1970s and 1980s, understanding of the range of reported clinical manifestations of MAC in the lung significantly increased. In one series of 20 patients with solitary, granulomatous pulmonary nodules, 12 (60%) grew MAC, whereas only 1 grew *M. tuberculosis*.[146] Most of these patients were asymptomatic. Nontuberculous mycobacteria grew from open lung biopsies obtained from 40 patients at the same medical center during the same time period (1969–1980); 24 grew MAC, and 16 of these 24 patients biopsy specimens were solitary pulmonary nodules. Thirteen of these 16 patients had no other medical problems, and only one of the 16 had a prior history of any predisposing lung disease.[147] A report by Prince, et al.[67] in 1989 described a series of 21 patients with pulmonary MAC disease who had no predisposing medical conditions. Unlike previous series, these patients were overwhelmingly (86%) female. They presented with an indolent cough that had been present for a long period (average 25.6 weeks) prior to diagnosis. Most of the patients had no other symptoms. The radiographic pattern of disease was also different than what had previously been described. Most of the patients had multiple pulmonary nodules, and only 24% had cavities on chest radiographs (Fig. 34-5). In most patients the disease was very slowly progressive, and often 2–3 years passed before radiographic progression was noted. Four of the 21 patients died directly of MAC pulmonary disease.

Subsequent reports from the past 2 decades have confirmed that elderly, primarily Caucasian females constitute a majority of patients with MAC pulmonary disease.[148,149] These female patients often have no known underlying pulmonary disease, and often are non-smokers.[67,149–151] One study noted higher rates of pectus excavatum and scoliosis in the MAC patients than in either a comparison group with tuberculosis or in the general population.[152] However, the MAC patients in this study were seen at a major referral center for mycobacterial diseases, so referral bias may be responsible for this association. Some of these patients had isolated involvement of the right middle lobe and lingula, often with associated bronchiectasis (Fig. 34-6). This pattern has been named the Lady Windermere's Syndrome, after a fastidious character in the play *Lady Windermere's Fan* by Oscar Wilde.[32] The presumption is that patients with this syndrome voluntarily suppress the cough reflex, resulting in aspiration and damage to the right middle lobe and/or lingula. Despite anecdotal connections between cough suppression and this syndrome,[153] the pathogenesis of MAC pulmonary disease in these patients is unclear.

As awareness of MAC as a respiratory pathogen has increased among clinicians, more affected populations with unique disease manifestations have been identified. Patients with cystic fibrosis are one such population. These patients almost always have bronchiectasis, and frequently have nodular infiltrates on chest CT presumed to be due to mucus impaction. Because of the overwhelming respiratory manifestations of cystic fibrosis and associated superinfections, it is very difficult to tease out what part of the clinical picture might be attributable to MAC infection. Recent data have demonstrated that a significant proportion of these patients' lungs are at least colonized with MAC. In a large, multicenter, cross-sectional study of patients with cystic

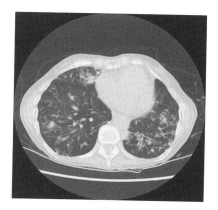

Fig. 34-5. Chest CT scan from a patient with "new" type pulmonary MAC, demonstrating multiple pulmonary nodules throughout both lungs.

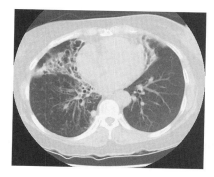

Fig. 34-6. "Lady Windermere" pattern of MAC pulmonary disease, with prominent bronchiectasis affecting the right middle lobe and lingula.

fibrosis, 13% had pulmonary colonization with at least one nontuberculous mycobacterium, and 72% of these mycobacteria were MAC.[154] Interestingly, in this study MAC colonization was associated with older age, higher FEV1, higher rates of colonization by *Staphylococcus aureus*, lower rates of colonization by *Pseudomonas aeruginosa*, and an overall better prognosis. In a nested-cohort study, the same authors found that cystic fibrosis patients with positive sputum cultures for nontuberculous mycobacteria (primarily MAC) had the same rate of decline in FEV1 as cystic fibrosis patients without positive sputum cultures for nontuberculous mycobacteria. However, cystic fibrosis patients who met the American Thoracic Society for nontuberculous mycobacterial pulmonary disease were significantly more likely to have progressive high-resolution chest CT changes over time, consistent with progression of nontuberculous mycobacterial pulmonary disease.[155] Further research is needed in this area to better understand the role of MAC and other nontuberculous mycobacteria in deterioration of lung function and symptomatology among patients with cystic fibrosis.

Until recently, MAC was not reported to be a significant cause of pulmonary disease among immunocompetent, healthy children; however, an increasing number of case reports describe a syndrome of subacute respiratory symptoms associated with mediastinal adenopathy and/or endobronchial lesions with frequent partial lung collapse. Two percent of children in a two-year prospective surveillance study in the Netherlands with nontuberculous mycobacterial infection had mediastinal lymphadenopathy, and 3% had pulmonary abnormalities.[156] A recent review of the literature found 43 published cases of intrathoracic disease caused by nontuberculous mycobacteria among otherwise healthy children between 1930 and 2003.[157] Of these, 29 patients were infected by MAC organisms. Interestingly, over half the cases were published after 1990, suggesting either an increasing prevalence of MAC pulmonary disease in children or increased awareness of this clinical entity. Most children with intrathoracic MAC disease are under 5 years of age, but children up to 14 years old have been affected. Children with intrathoracic MAC disease generally present with cough, wheezing (due to bronchial obstruction), and respiratory distress (sometimes). Approximately half these children will have constitutional symptoms including fever, night sweats, anorexia, and weight loss. Radiographs frequently demonstrate hilar lymphadenopathy, air trapping, or focal infiltrates. Bronchoscopy or surgical biopsy is often required to make the diagnosis, although gastric lavage has been useful in some cases.

Finally, an entirely different form of MAC pulmonary disease has been described since the late 1990s.[38,158] This disease, usually termed "hot tub lung," occupies a gray area between infection and a hypersensitivity reaction to the organism. Patients with hot tub lung are usually immunocompetent persons who have repeated exposures to indoor hot tubs. They develop progressive dyspnea, often accompanied by nonproductive cough, fever, and chills.[38,39,159] Chest radiography demonstrates diffuse infiltrates with a ground-glass appearance; multiple small nodules may be seen as well. Lung biopsy reveals granulomatous inflammation with or without acid-fast bacilli. Sputum or lung biopsy cultures usually are positive for MAC; in a minority of cases other nontuberculous mycobacteria such as *M. fortuitum* may be responsible.[39,159] Outbreaks of hot tub lung affecting multiple family members and/or close associates have been reported,[38,39] so detection of one case should prompt evaluation of other persons who have had consistent exposure to the same hot tub. Whether the hot tub lung syndrome actually represents infection, hypersensitivity pneumonitis, or both is a subject of active debate,[37] as many patients recover spontaneously once exposure to the hot tub ceases.

Extrapulmonary Disease

In addition to pulmonary disease, MAC has been reported to cause symptomatic disease at a number of other sites. The lymph nodes are by far the most common extrapulmonary site of disease. MAC lymphadenitis primarily afflicts healthy children with normal immune systems. A recent 2-year prospective surveillance study of nontuberculous mycobacterial disease among children in the Netherlands reported an incidence of 0.77 cases of disease per 100,000 children.[156] Eighty percent of the affected children were under 5 years of age, and in 92% the site of infection was the cervical lymph nodes. Females were affected more often than males (61% vs. 39%). Among children with a diagnosis of nontuberculous mycobacterial infection and a positive mycobacterial culture, 67% grew MAC. In general, MAC lymphadenitis affects the anterior cervical lymph nodes, is unilateral, affects primarily children between the ages of 1 and 4, and has a tendency to occur more often in the winter and spring than in other seasons.[71,160,161] Most affected children have positive tuberculin skin tests, which makes the syndrome difficult to differentiate from tuberculosis.[71,156,162] The majority of children in this and other series[161–163] have presented with an enlarging neck mass with no systemic symptoms and no evidence of MAC infection elsewhere in the body. Without treatment, the lymph nodes often spontaneously regress, but on occasion they will suppurate and erode through the overlying skin, creating chronic fistulas and scarring.[1,71,160,164]

Focal extrapulmonary MAC disease outside the lymph nodes is relatively rare; however, MAC has been reported to cause a wide variety of manifestations. Among these uncommon manifestations, musculoskeletal and cutaneous infections are the most frequently reported. In particular, MAC can cause a chronic tenosynovitis, usually of the hand or arm. Patients with this syndrome usually present with stiffness, swelling, and pain of the affected extremity. A history of prior trauma to the affected extremity can sometimes be elicited, but often the source of the infection is unclear. Systemic symptoms are uncommon, and laboratory studies are frequently unrevealing. Patients often experience significant diagnostic delays, and frequently receive multiple empiric corticosteroid injections, which may exacerbate the underlying infection. Mycobacterial culture of synovial biopsies is essential for diagnosis, as pathology frequently demonstrates granulomatous inflammation but no acid-fast bacilli.[165–167] In addition to tenosynovitis, MAC may cause septic arthritis[168] and osteomyelitis[169]; these manifestations are quite rare and usually occur in immunocompromised hosts or in patients who have had prior trauma to the affected area.[170] MAC can also cause primary cutaneous disease without evidence of systemic dissemination in both immunocompetent and immunocompromised hosts. The clinical manifestations have included papulonodular lesions on the trunk and thighs,[171] erythematous patches with pustules on the abdomen, legs, and buttocks,[172] and plaques on the face resembling lupus vulgaris.[173] An outbreak of cutaneous MAC disease has been reported in 3 immunocompetent family members, associated with common exposure to a circulating, constantly heated bath water system.[174] Cutaneous MAC disease is chronic and very slowly progressive in all cases, with onset ranging from 4 months to 10 years prior to diagnosis. Biopsies usually demonstrate granulomatous inflammation, but acid-fast bacilli are usually not seen, and culture is required for diagnosis.

DIAGNOSTIC CONSIDERATIONS

Microbiologic

The diagnosis of MAC pulmonary disease can be difficult because the signs and symptoms are frequently subtle and nonspecific. A combination of clinical, radiographic, and microbiologic data is necessary to make the diagnosis with confidence. The American Thoracic Society published criteria for diagnosis of MAC pulmonary disease in 1997 (Box 34-1).[134] Their criteria emphasize the importance of establishing the chronicity of symptoms associated with microbiologic or radiographic evidence of parenchymal damage. Unfortunately, these criteria are based on expert opinion, and most experts would agree that clinical studies are needed to assess their validity and long-term patient outcomes.

Box 34-1. The 1997 American Thoracic Society Diagnostic Criteria for Nontuberculous Mycobacterial Lung Disease[134]

Symptomatic Patient
Infiltrate, nodular, or cavitary disease on chest radiograph, or high-resolution computed tomography scan that shows multifocal bronchiectasis and/or multiple small nodules

Microbiologic Criteria:
If three sputum/bronchial wash results are available from the previous 12 months:
  Three positive cultures with negative acid-fast smear results or
  Two positive cultures and one positive acid-fast smear
If only one bronchial wash is available:
  Positive culture with 2+, 3+, or 4+ acid-fast smear or 2+, 3+, or 4+ growth on solid media
If sputum/bronchial wash evaluations are nondiagnostic or another disease cannot be excluded:
  Transbronchial or lung biopsy yielding a nontuberculous mycobacteria
  Biopsy showing mycobacterial histopathologic features (granulomatous inflammation and/or acid-fast bacilli) and one or more sputums or bronchial washings are positive for a nontuberculous mycobacterium even in low numbers

Radiographic

High-resolution chest CT is vital to diagnosis and management of MAC pulmonary disease, particularly in patients with nodular/bronchiectatic disease. In one study of 26 consecutive patients with chest CT scans demonstrating clusters of small nodules in the lung periphery associated with bronchiectasis, 13 (50%) were eventually diagnosed with MAC pulmonary disease.[31] Furthermore, 8 of these patients had cavities noted on CT that were not readily apparent on plain radiographs. Notably, only 6 of these patients had MAC grow from sputum; bronchoscopy and/or open lung biopsy was necessary to make the diagnosis in the others. Cavitation on CT has been associated with positive sputum cultures; patients without cavities may require more invasive procedures to obtain microbiologic confirmation of MAC pulmonary disease.[175] Another study of 100 unselected patients with bronchiectasis on chest CT reported that this constellation of radiographic findings—bronchiectasis plus peripheral parenchymal nodules—was 80% sensitive and 87% specific for the diagnosis of MAC pulmonary disease.[150] In recent years, this constellation has been the most common radiographic presentation of MAC pulmonary disease; for example, in two series published in the early 1990s, bronchiectasis and nodules were seen in 70–94% of patients, while cavities were seen in 0–28%.[176,177]

In light of the difficulties in obtaining a clear-cut diagnosis of MAC pulmonary disease, particularly given the propensity for this disease to afflict relatively elderly and frail patients, less invasive diagnostic methods are needed. Immunologic testing of blood specimens, either examining cellular or humoral responses, may offer one such method. A group of Japanese investigators have studied an enzyme immunoassay system that detects antibody responses to glycopeptidolipid antigens specific for MAC. In an early study of this technique among a mixed group of healthy patients and patients with mycobacterial infections, this test had a sensitivity of 92% and a specificity of 97% for diagnosis of MAC pulmonary disease. Furthermore, the level of these antibodies declined significantly among patients with MAC who converted sputum cultures from positive to negative.[178] Confirmation of this work and exploration of similar techniques offers the promise of significant advances in diagnosis and management of MAC pulmonary disease.

THERAPY FOR MAC DISEASE

Basic Principles

MAC organisms are resistant to many antibiotic agents, and treatment is complicated by the need for long-term therapy in frequently frail patients who are often taking multiple other medications concurrently. Agents with proven or potential clinical utility for MAC treatment are listed in Table 34-3. In general, it is advisable to administer a second-generation macrolide (clarithromycin or azithromycin) in combination with one or more other agents to reduce the likelihood that drug-resistant MAC strains will emerge on therapy. Monitoring for side effects and long-term toxicity related to antimicrobial agents is essential. Many of the drugs used for MAC therapy have potentially significant drug interactions with other commonly used medications; some of the most common of these interactions are noted in Table 34-4.

Drug Susceptibility Testing

The use of susceptibility testing to guide treatment of MAC disease is controversial. Correlation between *in vitro* drug susceptibility and clinical outcomes has only been clearly demonstrated for macrolides.[70,199] Furthermore, treatment of clarithromycin-resistant MAC with clarithromycin does result in reduced levels of mycobacteremia, at least in mice.[200] Studies attempting to correlate results of antimicrobial susceptibility testing of MAC to other drugs with clinical outcomes have described mixed results.[201,202] The latest recommendation from the National Committee for Clinical Laboratory Standards advises that antimicrobial susceptibility testing for MAC should be performed only for the macrolides, and only in the following circumstances[203]:

1. The patient has received prior macrolide therapy
2. The patient developed MAC bacteremia while receiving macrolide prophylaxis
3. The patient developed a relapse of MAC disease while receiving macrolide therapy
4. The MAC isolate is an initial, clinically significant isolate used to determine baseline drug resistance

Drug susceptibility testing of MAC isolates should be performed at a laboratory with significant experience in these techniques, as the reproducibility of these results is lower at inexperienced laboratories.[204]

Treatment in the Setting of HIV/AIDS

Treatment of Disseminated MAC

The most important component of treatment of disseminated MAC infection in persons with advanced HIV disease is control of the underlying HIV disease. Median survival among patients in one study who received

Table 34-3. Antimicrobial Agents Useful for Treatment of MAC Infection

Drug	Common Side Effects
Likely Useful	
Macrolides	
Azithromycin	Diarrhea, nausea, abdominal pain, rash, elevated hepatic transaminases, tinnitus, hearing loss
Clarithromycin	Diarrhea, nausea, abnormal taste, dyspepsia, abdominal pain, headache, rash, hearing loss, elevated hepatic transaminases, QT prolongation
Ethambutol	Decreased visual acuity (optic neuritis), rash
Rifamycins	
Rifampin	Abdominal pain, nausea, rash, elevated hepatic transaminases, hyperbilirubinemia, "flu-like syndrome," leukopenia, thrombocytopenia, interstitial nephritis, orange secretions
Rifabutin	Abdominal pain, nausea, rash, abnormal taste, arthralgias, uveitis, leukopenia, thrombocytopenia, "flu-like syndrome," elevated hepatic transaminases, orange secretions
Aminoglycosides	
Amikacin	Both drugs: Vestibulotoxicity (particularly streptomycin), cochlear toxicity (hearing loss), nephrotoxicity (less so with streptomycin than amikacin), rash, fever, muscle weakness (neuromuscular blockade)
Streptomycin	
Fluoroquinolones	
Ciprofloxacin	Nausea, vomiting, abdominal pain, rash, abnormal liver transaminases, central nervous system effects (delirium, dizziness, insomnia), tendonitis/tendon rupture, QT prolongation
Gatifloxacin	
Levofloxacin	
Moxifloxacin	
Potentially Useful	
Clofazimine	Abdominal pain, diarrhea, nausea, vomiting, skin discoloration, rash, dry skin, conjunctival and corneal pigmentation, eye irritation
Interferon-γ	Fever, myalgias, elevated hepatic transaminases, neutropenia, thrombocytopenia, delirium, gait disturbances
Linezolid	Diarrhea, nausea, headache, myelosuppression, lactic acidosis, optic neuropathy, peripheral neuropathy
Mefloquine	Dizziness, myalgia, nausea, vomiting, headache, rash, hair loss, sleep disorders, psychosis, cardiac conduction abnormalities, elevated hepatic transaminases
Telithromycin	Diarrhea, nausea, dizziness, visual disturbances, QT prolongation, elevated hepatic transaminases, exacerbation of myasthenia gravis

Source: Data from references 179–195.

macrolide-based antimycobacterial therapy for MAC in the pre-HAART era was 8.6 months.[205] Mortality rates in other studies of disseminated MAC with low rates of concurrent HAART use were also very high.[206,207] Since the introduction of HAART, survival after diagnosis of disseminated MAC has improved significantly.[59] This improvement in survival has been independently associated with prescription of HAART.[58]

Initial therapy for disseminated MAC should include at least a macrolide (clarithromycin or azithromycin) plus ethambutol (Table 34-5). Macrolide-based therapy has been associated with significant improvements in survival after diagnosis of disseminated MAC.[205] Clarithromycin monotherapy has been associated with emergence of clarithromycin-resistant organisms,[199] and the addition of ethambutol at a dose of 15 mg/kg daily significantly reduces relapses and emergence of clarithromycin resistance.[208] Clarithromycin should be used at a dose of 500 mg twice daily (or 1000 mg of the extended-release formulation once daily), as higher doses have been associated with increased mortality.[206] Azithromycin, at a dose of 600 mg daily, may also be used,[207] although this agent may be less effective at sterilizing blood cultures than clarithromycin.[209] The primary

Table 34-4. Common Drug Interactions for Drugs Used to Treat MAC Infection

Primary Drug	Second Drug	Interaction
Clarithromycin (Inhibits cytochrome P450 3A4 enzyme)	Rifabutin	↑ Rifabutin AUC, higher risk for uveitis ↓ Clarithromycin AUC
	Rifampin	↓ Clarithromycin AUC
	Fluoroquinolones	Both classes cause QT prolongation; use with caution
	Protease inhibitors	↑ Clarithromycin AUC
	Efavirenz	↑ Clarithromycin AUC, ↑ risk of rash
	Nevirapine	↓ Clarithromycin AUC
Rifabutin	Protease inhibitors	↑ Rifabutin AUC; decrease in AUC of some protease inhibitors (indinavir, saquinavir)
	Efavirenz	↓ Rifabutin AUC (rifabutin dose increase to 450–600 mg daily recommended)
	Clarithromycin	See above
Rifampin	Protease inhibitors	↓ Protease inhibitor AUC; coadministration generally not recommended
	Efavirenz	↓ Efavirenz AUC, but can be coadministered
	Nevirapine	↓ Nevirapine AUC
	Clarithromycin	See above
	Mefloquine	↓ Mefloquine AUC
	Telithromycin	↓ Telithromycin AUC
Linezolid	Antidepressants, particularly serotonin reuptake inhibitors	Possible serotonin syndrome due to monoamine oxidase inhibition by linezolid

AUC = Area under the curve.
Source: Data from references 179–182, 184–188,190–198.

consideration for which macrolide to use will be driven by tolerability and possible drug-drug interactions.

Many clinicians use a third drug in addition to a macrolide and ethambutol for treatment of disseminated MAC. Rifabutin has been most commonly used as this third drug. In one randomized, placebo-controlled trial, bacteriologic response and survival were no different between patients treated with or without rifabutin (300 mg daily) added to a regimen of clarithromycin 500 mg twice daily and ethambutol 1200 mg once daily.[210] Nevertheless, a more recent three-arm, randomized, controlled trial reported that survival among patients assigned to a 3-drug regimen consisting of clarithromycin, ethambutol, and rifabutin was better than among patients assigned either to clarithromycin plus ethambutol or clarithromycin plus rifabutin.[211] Still, microbiologic and clinical responses to therapy were not statistically different among the 3 arms. Drug interactions between rifabutin and other components of therapy are a

significant consideration (Table 34-4). In particular, a high rate of rifabutin-associated uveitis has been reported when clarithromycin and high-dose rifabutin (600 mg daily) were coadministered.[205] Uveitis was noted at a much lower rate when the rifabutin dose was lowered to 300 mg daily.[210,212] A fluoroquinolone is also a reasonable choice as a third agent, and one retrospective study suggested a survival advantage when ciprofloxacin was added to clarithromycin and ethambutol for treatment of disseminated MAC.[213] The newer fluoroquinolones, moxifloxacin and gatifloxacin, have demonstrated *in vitro* activity against MAC that is superior to ciprofloxacin or levofloxacin,[214–217] but published clinical experience with these compounds is lacking. Amikacin, at a dose of 15 mg/kg daily, may also be useful as part of a multidrug regimen to treat disseminated MAC,[218–220] but no large studies have been performed to validate its utility. Addition of clofazimine to clarithromycin and ethambutol has been associated an increase in mortality

Table 34-5. Recommendations for Medical Treatment of MAC Disease

Type of Disease	Recommended Therapy
Prophylaxis for disseminated MAC	Azithromycin 1200 mg po once weekly **OR** Clarithromycin 500 mg po qd or bid

Disseminated MAC	Clarithromycin 500 mg po bid* **OR** azithromycin 500–600 mg po qd
	     PLUS
	 Ethambutol 15 mg/kg po qd +/–
	 Rifabutin 300–450 mg po qd **OR** fluoroquinolone (ciprofloxacin 750 mg
	     po bid, levofloxacin 750 mg po qd, moxifloxacin 400 mg po qd,
	     gatifloxacin 400 mg po qd)
	 PLUS ANTIRETROVIRAL THERAPY FOR PATIENTS
	     WITH HIV

Pulmonary MAC	*Intermittent dosing*
	 Clarithromycin 500 mg po bid* **OR** azithromycin
	     250–500 mg po thrice weekly **PLUS**
	 Ethambutol 15–25 mg po thrice weekly **PLUS**
	 Rifabutin 300–600 mg po thrice weekly **PLUS OR MINUS**
	 Aminoglycoside (streptomycin 500–1000 mg or amikacin 15 mg/kg
	     2–3 times weekly) for the first 2 months
	 Daily dosing
	 Clarithromycin 500 mg po bid* **OR** azithromycin 250–500 mg po
	     QD **PLUS**
	 Ethambutol 25 mg/kg po QD × 2 months, then 15 mg/kg po QD **PLUS**
	 Rifabutin 150–300 mg po QD **PLUS OR MINUS**
	 Aminoglycoside (streptomycin 500–1000 mg or amikacin 15 mg/kg
	     2–3 times weekly) for the first 2 months

*Clarithromycin may be administered as 1000 mg of the XL formulation instead of 500 mg twice daily of the usual formulation.

compared with no clofazimine, so clofazimine should generally not be used for treatment of disseminated MAC.[221] Other compounds have *in vitro* activity against MAC, but clinical experience with these has been very limited. IFN-γ as adjunctive therapy was tried in 2 HIV-infected patients with disseminated MAC, but produced only transient clinical improvement.[222] Both linezolid and mefloquine have *in vitro* activity against MAC,[216,223] and addition of these 2 drugs to clarithromycin, moxifloxacin, granulocyte-macrophage colony stimulating factor, and ethambutol resulted in successful treatment of a patient with chronic lymphocytic leukemia and disseminated MAC.[224]

Other adjunctive therapies that have been used in very limited numbers of patients include granulocyte-macrophage colony stimulating factor (GM-CSF) and corticosteroids. GM-CSF augments MAC phagocytosis and intracellular killing of MAC by macrophages *in vitro* and *in vivo*, and was associated with delayed time to blood culture positivity in one HIV-infected patient.[225] A study of GM-CSF added to azithromycin in a group of 8 patients with advanced HIV demonstrated enhanced mycobacterial killing by these patients' macrophages, but nonsignificant decreases in mycobacteremia.[226] Corticosteroids have been studied in small, uncontrolled series; one study of 5 patients with advanced HIV and refractory MAC demonstrated clinical improvement when 2 mg of dexamethasone was given daily in addition to antimycobacterial therapy.[227]

Disseminated MAC is a relatively rare disease in persons without HIV, and there are no large studies to direct therapy in HIV-seronegative persons. It is reasonable to apply the same general principles of therapy to HIV-seronegative patients with disseminated MAC.

IFN-γ may have a particular role in treatment of disseminated MAC among patients with certain types of congenital and acquired immunodeficiencies. In a study of 7 patients with refractory, disseminated nontuberculous mycobacterial infection, the addition of IFN-γ produced significant clinical benefit.[228] Among patients who have disseminated MAC in the setting of bone marrow or solid organ transplantation, reduction of the level of immunosuppression may also be helpful.[229,230] In this patient population, the use of rifamycins is often problematic due to multiple drug interactions with immunosuppresive medications, and a fluoroquinolone may be preferable as a third agent.

Treatment of patients with refractory disease or relapse is difficult, and the elements of management will differ depending on the underlying disease. In the setting of advanced HIV infection, aggressive HIV treatment is the most important element, and improving HIV control alone may suffice to control disseminated MAC. Susceptibility testing of the MAC isolate can be helpful, keeping the above caveats in mind. In the setting of failure or relapse, therapeutic drug monitoring to ensure adequate absorption of orally administered antimicrobial agents may be helpful.[231] Addition of 2 new agents with activity against MAC, if possible, is a reasonable approach to these patients, but data to support this approach is lacking.

For patients with advanced HIV who have a good response to antiretroviral therapy, treatment of disseminated MAC disease may be discontinued in some cases. Cure of disseminated MAC infection has been reported with concurrent effective antiretroviral therapy.[232,233] Patients who have a sustained increase in the CD4 count to over 100 cells/mm^3 for at least 6 months, and who have completed at least 12 months of antimycobacterial therapy, may be considered for discontinuation of MAC therapy.[232,234] The patient should be asymptomatic, with documentation of a negative mycobacterial blood culture, prior to discontinuation of therapy. Caution should be used when considering discontinuation of therapy in patients whose immune reconstitution has not been robust, as relapses in this setting have been reported.[235] These patients should be closely monitored for relapse, particularly if the CD4 count falls below 100 cells/mm^3.

Management of Immune Reconstitution Inflammatory Syndromes

Clinicians are increasingly recognizing that HIV-infected patients may develop new focal manifestations or clinical deterioration of MAC disease associated with immune reconstitution. These clinical manifestations have been termed immune reconstitution inflammatory syndromes (IRIS), and have been described in association with multiple pathogens including tuberculosis,[236,237] cytomegalovirus,[238] *Pneumocystis jirovecii*, aspergillus, hepatitis B, and hepatitis C, among others.[239] The incidence of IRIS associated with disseminated MAC is unknown, but MAC accounts for a significant proportion of IRIS cases among HIV-infected persons.[239] The manifestations of MAC-associated IRIS are diverse; many patients experience new onset of fever and malaise, but focal manifestations vary widely. Common manifestations include lymphadenopathy in the abdomen or mediastinum, new focal lung infiltrates, or nodules.[240] Other reports have described focal cervical lymphadenitis with spontaneous drainage,[241] pyomyositis with cutaneous abscesses,[242] and brain abscess.[243] The syndrome usually occurs within the first 3 months after the initiation of effective antiretroviral therapy, and usually is associated with significant increases in the CD4 count after initiation of antiretrovirals.[239] There is no firm data to guide management of the syndrome. Case reports have described good outcomes with focal drainage of localized abscesses,[241,242] surgical excision of a focal brain lesion,[243] and systemic corticosteroids;[239] in all cases concurrent MAC therapy was prescribed. In our experience and that of others,[244] symptomatic therapy with nonsteroidal inflammatory agents, corticosteroids, and drainage of focal collections in addition to antimycobacterial therapy is sufficient for most patients. In a few cases with severe symptoms, temporary discontinuation of antiretroviral therapy while attempting to reduce the MAC burden with antimycobacterial agents may be necessary, but there is no data to demonstrate the efficacy or safety of this approach.

Prophylaxis for Disseminated MAC in Patients with Advanced HIV Disease

Persons with advanced HIV are at significant risk to develop disseminated MAC. The incidence of disseminated MAC among HIV-infected patients with CD4 counts of less than 100/mm^3 is approximately 20% per year without antiretroviral therapy or prophylactic antibiotics.[245] Azithromycin, clarithromycin, and rifabutin have all been clearly effective in reducing the risk of disseminated MAC in patients with such low CD4 counts. Two randomized, double-blind, placebo-controlled trials of rifabutin 300 mg daily vs. placebo demonstrated an approximately 50% reduction of the risk of development of disseminated MAC.[246] There was a nonsignificant trend toward improved survival in the rifabutin arms of these studies. A randomized, double-blind, study comparing clarithromycin 500 mg twice daily to placebo demonstrated a 69% reduction in the incidence of disseminated MAC disease and a significant 25% reduction in mortality.[247] Clarithromycin both at this dosing schedule and at a dose of 500 mg once daily was superior to rifabutin, and adding rifabutin to clarithromycin was no more effective than using clarithromycin alone.[248,249] Azithromycin at a dose of 1200 mg once weekly was also more effective than rifabutin,[250] and although no direct comparisons have been performed it appears to be approximately as effective as clarithromycin in prevention of disseminated MAC. When once-weekly azithromycin was compared to placebo, patients in the azithromycin arm had a 66% reduction in the incidence of disseminated MAC.[251] Adding rifabutin 300 mg daily to azithromycin 1200 mg weekly further reduced the incidence of disseminated MAC over either drug alone, but was associated with an increase in drug-associated toxicity.[250] The current USPHS/IDSA guidelines recommend either azithromycin 1200 mg once weekly or clarithromycin 500 mg twice daily as first-line therapy for disseminated MAC prophylaxis among HIV-infected patients with CD4 counts of less than 50/mm^3 (Table 34-5).[234] Clarithromycin 500 mg once daily or rifabutin 300 mg once daily are reasonable second-line alternatives. Prophylaxis may be discontinued safely in patients whose CD4 counts rise to consistently over 100 cells/mm^3 for at least 3 months.[234,252]

Treatment in General Populations

Treatment of Pulmonary MAC

The data for treatment of pulmonary MAC in HIV-seronegative patients is limited by the paucity of randomized, controlled trials. Older, noncomparative studies in which patients were treated with combinations of conventional antituberculous agents reported highly variable outcomes. Patients in these studies did not necessarily have uniform definitions of disease, radiographic response, or cure. In most cases, conversion of sputum cultures to negative was the primary outcome. Sputum conversion rates using standard antituberculous agents, primarily in populations with classic MAC pulmonary disease, ranged from 38–91% across studies published between 1967 and 1988.[141,142,253–256] A more recent randomized, controlled trial compared 2 years of isoniazid, rifampin, and ethambutol to 2 years of rifampin plus

ethambutol in 75 patients from the United Kingdom and Scandinavia.[257,258] Study patients primarily had classic MAC pulmonary disease; 61% had preexisting lung disease and 61% had cavitary disease. Cure was defined as having negative sputum cultures in the last 3 months of treatment, with persistently negative sputum cultures during 3 years of follow-up. At the end of 5 years, 10/37 (27%) patients in the rifampin/ethambutol arm were cured, compared with 13/38 (34%) in the isoniazid/rifampin/ethambutol arm (p = 0.67). Of note, 27 (36%) patients had died at the end of 5-year follow up, and 21 (28%) were considered treatment failures or relapses. Only 3 of the deaths were directly attributed to MAC disease. *In vitro* susceptibility testing of the MAC organisms to multiple antituberculous agents was performed using the modal resistance method, but had no significant correlation with treatment outcome.

The study comparing isoniazid, rifampin, and ethambutol to rifampin plus ethambutol represents the only published randomized, controlled trial of different medical regimens to treat MAC pulmonary disease in HIV-seronegative patients. After that trial was started, it was discovered that the new macrolides (azithromycin and clarithromycin) possess significant activity against MAC. Furthermore, in the United States, rifabutin is often used as a component of pulmonary MAC treatment instead of rifampin because of better *in vitro* activity and somewhat less induction of cytochrome P450 metabolism.[259] An early study of 30 patients with MAC pulmonary disease reported that 58% of patients who completed a 4-month course of clarithromycin monotherapy 500 mg twice daily converted sputum cultures to negative, and another 21% had a significant reduction in the number of MAC colonies grown in sputum culture.[260] A majority of these patients had classic MAC pulmonary disease: 60% were male, and 65% had fibrocavitary disease on chest radiographs. Of note, only 20 of the initial 30 patients completed the study and were assessed for sputum conversion. Isolates obtained after relapse or end of therapy from 3 (16%) of these 20 patients had developed high-level clarithromycin resistance. A similar study examined azithromycin monotherapy, 600 mg once daily for 4 months. Twenty-nine patients entered the study, of whom 23 (79%) completed the full course of treatment. Among these 23 patients, 38% converted sputum cultures to negative, and another 38% had a significant reduction in the number of MAC colonies in their sputum.[261] Again, the majority of patients in this study were male (52%), 48% had fibrocavitary disease on chest radiographs, and 65% were former or current smokers. Acquired macrolide resistance was not noted in this study. In both of these studies, gastrointestinal side effects were common, and changes in hearing were not infrequent.

These two studies strongly suggest that clarithromycin and azithromycin have clinical utility for treatment of pulmonary MAC. An open-label study of high-dose clarithromycin (30 mg/kg daily) with or without other medications in 45 French patients reported a 71% sputum culture conversion rate, but treatment regimens were heterogeneous and 49% of patients had received other antimycobacterial treatment.[69] Richard Wallace and colleagues published the results of the first 50 patients they treated with a clarithromycin-based regimen consisting of clarithromycin 500 mg twice daily, rifampin or rifabutin, ethambutol, and initial streptomycin in 1996.[262] Eleven (22%) of these patients dropped out of the study in the first 3 months, but of the remaining 39, 36 (92%) converted sputum cultures to negative. Relapse occurred in 4 of these patients, and isolates from 6 of the 39 (15%) patients became clarithromycin resistant. Of note, one or more drugs were discontinued in 16 of 39 (41%) patients because of side effects. A second study performed in Japan enrolled sequential HIV-seronegative patients with pulmonary MAC disease between 1992–97.[70] Patients were treated with clarithromycin 10 mg/kg, ethambutol 15 mg/kg, and rifampin 10 mg/kg daily. For the first 2–6 months, kanamycin 20 mg/kg was administered intramuscularly 3 times weekly, followed by either ofloxacin 10 mg/kg daily or levofloxacin 5 mg/kg daily thereafter. Patients were treated for 24 months total, and if patients had difficulty with the planned treatment regimen, other antituberculous agents including enviomycin (a polypeptide similar to capreomycin), isoniazid, or ethionamide could be used in place of one or more of the drugs in the standard regimen. Forty-six patients participated in the study, of whom 32 (70%) were female, 22 (48%) had underlying pulmonary conditions, and only 18 (39%) had cavitary disease. Only 29 of the 46 patients were actually begun on the planned treatment regimen; the remainder used a modified regimen because of preexisting conditions or refusal to take the standard regimen. Thirty-nine (85%) patients completed at least 6 months of treatment, and only 21 (54%) completed a full 24 months. Twenty two (48%) of the original 46 patients converted their sputum cultures to negative and remained culture negative at the end of the study. Both of these studies enrolled patients whose pretreatment MAC isolates demonstrated *in vitro* resistance to clarithromycin, and patients in both studies infected with clarithromycin-resistant MAC had significantly lower culture conversion rates than patients infected with clarithromycin-susceptible MAC.

Daily administration of multiple-drug regimens for pulmonary MAC is both expensive and often poorly tolerated. To circumvent these issues, David Griffith and colleagues studied both clarithromycin- and azithromycin-based intermittent regimens for treatment of pulmonary MAC disease. They first examined 21 patients prescribed a regimen of azithromycin 600 mg three times weekly, plus rifabutin 300 mg and ethambutol 25 mg/kg daily for two months, followed by ethambutol 15 mg/kg thereafter. Patients also received streptomycin 500–1000 mg intramuscularly 2–3 times weekly during the first two months. One (5%) patient had adjunctive surgical resection. After 6 months of therapy, 14 (67%) patients had converted sputum cultures to negative, and no patient had developed macrolide resistance. A second group of 47 patients were prescribed azithromycin 600 mg, rifabutin 300–600 mg, ethambutol 25 mg/kg all three times weekly, with streptomycin 500–1000 mg intramuscularly two to three times weekly for the first two months. Three (6%) had surgical resection. At the end of 6 months, 24 (51%) patients had converted sputum cultures to negative, and no emergence of macrolide resistance was noted. Long-term follow up of patients in these two groups, plus another group prescribed daily azithromycin with the same companion drugs (N = 32) suggested that daily and thrice-weekly azithromycin-based regimens were roughly comparable. Fifty-nine percent of patients who took daily azithromycin-based therapy attained treatment success, defined as 12 consecutive months of negative sputum cultures while the patient was on therapy. Fifty-five percent of patients who took thrice-weekly azithromycin with daily companion drugs and 65% of patients who took all drugs thrice weekly met criteria for treatment success. The differences in rates of treatment success among these 3 groups were not statistically significant. Furthermore, drug toxicity was significantly less with intermittent administration of azithromycin.[68]

Based on these encouraging results, the same authors studied an intermittent clarithromycin-containing regimen for HIV-seronegative patients with MAC pulmonary disease.[263] Patients were prescribed clarithromycin 1000 mg, rifabutin 300–600 mg, and ethambutol 25 mg/kg three times weekly. Fifty-nine patients were enrolled, of whom 41 (69%) completed at least 6 months of therapy. After 6 months of therapy, 32 (54%) patients converted sputum cultures to negative. Notably, 13 (22%) patients discontinued either clarithromycin or rifabutin because of drug-related adverse events, and 22 (37%) required a decrease in the dosage of either clarithromycin or rifabutin because of drug-related adverse events. No emergence of clarithromycin resistance was noted.

Despite these seminal contributions to understanding of the medical management of MAC pulmonary disease, much remains to be learned. No randomized, controlled trials of macrolide-based therapy have been performed. Radiographic and clinical outcomes in all of the preceding studies of macrolides were not standardized, and loss to follow-up was a significant problem. Many patients with MAC pulmonary disease only receive microbiologic confirmation by use of bronchoscopy or other invasive procedures because they do not effectively produce sputum,[31,70] so sputum conversion is not an outcome that can be effectively used to assess treatment efficacy. As noted above, drug intolerance in the generally frail, elderly group of patients with pulmonary MAC is a major barrier to effective therapy. Interactions between other medications that patients are taking and antimycobacterial agents, particularly clarithromycin and rifabutin, also present significant challenges to medical therapy (Table 34-4). Despite these caveats, recommendations for first-line therapy of pulmonary MAC are presented in Table 34-5.

Lung resection surgery has been used as an adjunct to medical treatment. Surgery may be useful in the setting of patients with localized pulmonary disease who are refractory to medical therapy, or who do not tolerate medical therapy. In one recent series of 28 patients who had pulmonary resection for MAC, perioperative complications occurred in 9 (32%).[264] Complications included persistent air leak requiring repeat operation (5 patients), bronchopleural fistula (1 patient), atelectasis (1 patient), and postoperative death (2 patients). Eight patients had pneumonectomies, and 20 had single lobectomies. Of 26 surviving patients, 24 (92%) had persistently negative postoperative sputum cultures. In a second series of 21 patients, postoperative complications occurred in 6 (29%), but no perioperative deaths were reported. Eighty-seven percent of patients were considered disease-free at 3 years of follow-up.[265] Patients described in these series are carefully selected, and surgery was performed at referral centers with extensive experience in treatment of pulmonary MAC.

Several other classes of drugs have promise for treatment of pulmonary MAC, but clinical evidence for their use is limited. Perhaps the most promising class of drugs is the fluoroquinolones, particularly the new agents moxifloxacin and gatifloxacin. Fluoroquinolones have good *in vitro* activity against MAC,[214,215,217,266,267] and a retrospective study of treatment of patients with disseminated MAC suggested that the addition of ciprofloxacin to clarithromycin and ethambutol was associated with improved survival.[142] Yet, no comparative studies exist to assess the efficacy of fluoroquinolones in treatment of pulmonary MAC. In our clinical experience, the fluoroquinolones represent a reasonable alternative as third drug (in addition to a macrolide and ethambutol) for patients who have intolerance or unacceptable drug interactions with rifabutin. Aminoglycosides, particularly amikacin, are also frequently used as part of multidrug regimens, but no studies exist to document the benefit of using these agents. Other drugs with good *in vitro* activity against MAC, but limited published data to support their use in treatment of pulmonary MAC disease, include linezolid,[216,224] mefloquine,[223,224] and telithromycin.[268] Inhaled antibiotics represent an interesting approach to treatment of pulmonary MAC, with potential for high drug concentrations at the site of disease but low systemic toxicity. Inhaled amikacin has been used by some experts in addition to oral medications,[269] but no published data exist to clearly support its safety and efficacy. Inhaled IFN-γ has produced transient improvement in a few patients,[270] but a recent randomized, placebo-controlled phase II trial of aerosolized interferon-γ-1b three times weekly in addition to standard antimycobacterial therapy was stopped early due to lack of efficacy (Larry Davis, Pharm.D., Intermune, personal communication).

We generally use a multifaceted treatment strategy for our patients with MAC pulmonary disease. Many of these patients are elderly, frail, and are intolerant of multiple medications. In our experience, many patients tolerate rifabutin poorly, and have underlying diseases that make parenteral aminoglycosides unattractive. We frequently use a three-drug regimen for initial therapy that includes a macrolide, ethambutol, and moxifloxacin. Many of our patients tolerate thrice-weekly therapy better than daily therapy, both because of side effects and high medication costs. Adjunctive therapy with bronchodilators, mucus clearance devices, and pulmonary rehabilitation is helpful for many patients, particularly patients with bronchiectasis and chronic, productive cough. Baseline vision and hearing testing is important to monitor potential toxicity from long-term use of the macrolides and ethambutol, respectively. For patients with significant comorbidities, poor drug tolerance, and limited projected lifespan, suppressive therapy with two drugs (macrolide + ethambutol) or close observation with symptomatic therapy is reasonable.

Treatment of Extrapulmonary MAC

Extrapulmonary MAC infection is relatively uncommon, and no large trials exist to guide treatment of most forms. Children with lymphadenitis usually do well with surgical excision alone, so excisional biopsy is the first-line treatment for cervical lymphadenitis due to MAC.[71,160,163,271] For other sites of disease, the same general principles of therapy used to treat disseminated MAC are reasonable. First-line therapy should include at least a macrolide plus ethambutol, with a third drug (rifabutin, fluoroquinolone) added for extensive disease. An aminoglycoside, particularly amikacin or streptomycin, also may be helpful in the initial stages of therapy. Patients with tenosynovitis often require extensive debridement in addition to medical therapy for cure of their disease.[165,167] Patients with extrapulmonary MAC disease have often been treated with 12–24 months of multi-drug therapy, depending on the site of disease, underlying immunosuppression, and clinical response.

CONCLUSION

MAC organisms are commonly found in the environment, but cause disease in relatively few of those who are infected. *M. avium*, the most common species to infect patients with HIV/AIDS, is probably acquired via the gastrointestinal tract, while *M. intracellulare* is likely acquired by the respiratory tract. DMAC is almost exclusively seen in patients with late stage AIDS, and can be treated with either clarithromycin or azithromycin in combination with ethambutol, with or without rifabutin or a fluoroquinolone. The most important intervention in this setting, however, is to gain HIV viral control with the use of potent antiretroviral therapy. Pulmonary MAC is seen most often in elderly patients, and the epidemiology has shifted from primarily older men to a demographic that includes women with underlying bronchiectasis. Differentiating colonization from MAC pulmonary disease can be challenging, and successful treatment requires a multi-pronged approach that includes antibiotics, aggressive pulmonary hygiene and sometimes resection of the diseased lung. Further studies, including randomized trials, are needed to better define the most important characteristics that predict the patient's likely pace of progression or stability, and to optimize treatment.

REFERENCES

1. Wolinsky E. Nontuberculous mycobacteria and associated diseases. *Am Rev Respir Dis.* 1979;119:107–159.
2. Good RC and Snider DE, Jr. Isolation of nontuberculous mycobacteria in the United States, 1980. *J Infect Dis.* 1982;146:829–833
3. Edwards LB, Acquaviva FA, Livesay VT, et al. An atlas of sensitivity to tuberculin, PPD-B, and histoplasmin in the United States. *Am Rev Respir Dis.* 1969;99: S1–S132.
4. Von Reyn CF, Horsburgh CR, Olivier KN, et al. Skin test reactions to *Mycobacterium tuberculosis* purified protein derivative and *Mycobacterium avium* sensitin among health care workers and medical students in the United States. *Int J Tuberc Lung Dis.* 2001;5:1122–1128.
5. Parker BC, Ford MA, Gruft H, et al. Epidemiology of infection by nontuberculous mycobacteria. IV. Preferential aerosolization of *Mycobacterium intracellulare* from natural waters. *Am Rev Respir Dis.* 1983;128:652–656.
6. Von Reyn CF, Waddell RD, Eaton T, et al. Isolation of *Mycobacterium avium* complex from water in the United States, Finland, Zaire, and Kenya. *J Clin Microbiol.* 1993;31: 3227–3230.
7. Katila ML, Iivanainen E, Torkko P, et al. Isolation of potentially pathogenic mycobacteria in the Finnish environment. *Scand J Infect Dis-Supplementum.* 1995;98: 9–11.
8. Ichiyama S, Shimokata K, and Tsukamura M. The isolation of *Mycobacterium avium* complex from soil, water, and dusts. *Microbiol Immunol.* 1988;32:733–739.
9. Brooks RW, Parker BC, Gruft H, et al. Epidemiology of infection by nontuberculous mycobacteria. V. Numbers in eastern United States soils and correlation with soil characteristics. *Am Rev Respir Dis.* 1984;130:630–633.
10. Kirschner RA, Jr., Parker BC, and Falkinham JO, III. Epidemiology of infection by nontuberculous mycobacteria. *Mycobacterium avium*, *Mycobacterium intracellulare*, and *Mycobacterium scrofulaceum* in acid, brown-water swamps of the southeastern United States and their association with environmental variables. *Am Rev Respir Dis.* 1992;145: 271–275.
11. Taylor RH, Falkinham JO, III, Norton CD, et al. Chlorine, chloramine, chlorine dioxide, and ozone susceptibility of *Mycobacterium avium*. *Appl Environ Microbiol.* 2000;66: 1702–1705.
12. Falkinham JO, III. Factors influencing the chlorine susceptibility of *Mycobacterium avium*, *Mycobacterium intracellulare*, and *Mycobacterium scrofulaceum*. *Appl Environ Microbiol.* 2003;69:5685–5689.
13. Falkinham JO, III, Norton CD, and LeChevallier MW. Factors influencing numbers of *Mycobacterium avium*, *Mycobacterium intracellulare*, and other Mycobacteria in drinking water distribution systems. *Appl Environ Microbiol.* 2001;67:1225–1231.
14. Damsker B and Bottone EJ. *Mycobacterium avium-Mycobacterium intracellulare* from the intestinal tracts of patients with the acquired immunodeficiency syndrome: concepts regarding acquisition and pathogenesis. *J Infect Dis.* 1985;151:179–181.
15. Von Reyn CF, Maslow JN, Barber TW, et al. Persistent colonisation of potable water as a source of *Mycobacterium avium* infection in AIDS. *Lancet.* 1994;343: 1137–1141.

16. Aronson T, Holtzman A, Glover N, et al. Comparison of large restriction fragments of *Mycobacterium avium* isolates recovered from AIDS and non-AIDS patients with those of isolates from potable water. *J Clin Microbiol.* 1999;37:1008–1012.

17. du Moulin GC, Stottmeier KD, Pelletier PA, et al. Concentration of *Mycobacterium avium* by hospital hot water systems. *JAMA.* 1988;260:1599–1601.

18. Tobin-D'Angelo MJ, Blass MA, del Rio C, et al. Hospital water as a source of *Mycobacterium avium* complex isolates in respiratory specimens. *J Infect Dis.* 2004;189:98–104.

19. Mansfield KG and Lackner AA. Simian immunodeficiency virus-inoculated macaques acquire *Mycobacterium avium* from potable water during AIDS. *J Infect Dis.* 1997;175:184–187.

20. Orme IM, Furney SK, and Roberts AD. Dissemination of enteric *Mycobacterium avium* infections in mice rendered immunodeficient by thymectomy and CD4 depletion or by prior infection with murine AIDS retroviruses. *Infect Immun.* 1992;60:4747–4753.

21. Bermudez LE, Petrofsky M, Kolonoski P, et al. An animal model of *Mycobacterium avium* complex disseminated infection after colonization of the intestinal tract. *J Infect Dis.* 1992;165:75–79.

22. Brown ST, Edwards FF, Bernard EM, et al. Progressive disseminated infection with *Mycobacterium avium* complex after intravenous and oral challenge in cyclosporine-treated rats. *J Infect Dis.* 1991;164:922–927.

23. McGarvey JA and Bermudez LE. Phenotypic and genomic analyses of the *Mycobacterium avium* complex reveal differences in gastrointestinal invasion and genomic composition. *Infect Immun.* 2001;69(12):7242–7249.

24. Ohkusu K, Bermudez LE, Nash KA, et al. Differential Virulence of *Mycobacterium avium* Strains Isolated from HIV-Infected Patients with Disseminated M. avium Complex Disease. *J Infect Dis.* 2004;190:1347–1354.

25. Maslow JN, Brar I, Smith G, et al. Latent infection as a source of disseminated disease caused by organisms of the *Mycobacterium avium* complex in simian immunodeficiency virus-infected rhesus macaques. *J Infect Dis.* 2003;187:1748–1755.

26. Guthertz LS, Damsker B, Bottone EJ, et al. Mycobacterium avium and Mycobacterium intracellulare infections in patients with and without AIDS. *J Infect Dis.* 1989;160:1037–1041.

27. Wallace Jr RJ, Zhang Y, Brown-Elliott BA, et al. Repeat positive cultures in Mycobacterium intracellulare lung disease after macrolide therapy represent new infections in patients with nodular bronchiectasis. *J Infect Dis.* 2002;186:266–273.

28. Wallace RJ, Jr., Zhang Y, Brown BA, et al. Polyclonal *Mycobacterium avium* complex infections in patients with nodular bronchiectasis. *Am J Respir Crit Care Med.* 1998;158:1235–1244.

29. Wendt SL, George KL, Parker BC, et al. Epidemiology of infection by nontuberculous Mycobacteria. III. Isolation of potentially pathogenic mycobacteria from aerosols. *Am Rev Respir Dis.* 1980;122:259–263.

30. Lavy A, Rusu R, and Shaheen S. *Mycobacterium avium-intracellulare* in clinical specimens: etiological factor or contaminant? *Isr J Med Sci.* 1990;26:374–378.

31. Tanaka E, Amitani R, Niimi A, et al. Yield of computed tomography and bronchoscopy for the diagnosis of *Mycobacterium avium* complex pulmonary disease. *Am J Respir Crit Care Med.* 1997;155:2041–2046.

32. Reich JM and Johnson RE. *Mycobacterium avium* complex pulmonary disease presenting as an isolated lingular or middle lobe pattern. The Lady Windermere's syndrome. *Chest.* 1992;101:1605–1609.

33. Eaton T, Falkinham JO, III, and Von Reyn CF. Recovery of *Mycobacterium avium* from cigarettes. *J Clin Microbiol.* 1995;33:2757–2758.

34. Telles MA, Yates MD, Curcio M, et al. Molecular epidemiology of *Mycobacterium avium* complex isolated from patients with and without AIDS in Brazil and England. *Epidemiol Infect.* 1999;122:435–440.

35. Kunimoto DY, Peppler MS, Talbot J, et al. Analysis of *Mycobacterium avium* complex isolates from blood samples of AIDS patients by pulsed-field gel electrophoresis. *J Clin Microbiol.* 2003;41:498–499.

36. Legrand E, Sola C, Verdol B, et al. Genetic diversity of *Mycobacterium avium* recovered from AIDS patients in the Caribbean as studied by a consensus IS1245-RFLP method and pulsed-field gel electrophoresis. *Res Microbiol.* 2000;151:271–283.

37. Aksamit TR. Hot tub lung: infection, inflammation, or both? *Semin Respir Infect.* 2003;18:33–39.

38. Embil J, Warren P, Yakrus M, et al. Pulmonary illness associated with exposure to Mycobacterium-avium complex in hot tub water. Hypersensitivity pneumonitis or infection? *Chest.* 1997;111:813–816.

39. Mangione EJ, Huitt G, Lenaway D, et al. Nontuberculous mycobacterial disease following hot tub exposure. *Emerg Infect Dis.* 2001;7:1039–1042.

40. Rickman OB, Ryu JH, Fidler ME, et al. Hypersensitivity pneumonitis associated with *Mycobacterium avium* complex and hot tub use. *Mayo Clin Proc.* 2002;77:1233–1237.

41. Case records of the Massachusetts General Hospital. Weekly clinicopathological exercises. Case 27-2000. A 61-year-old with rapidly progressive dyspnea. *N Engl J Med.* 2000;343:642–649.

42. Fairchok MP, Rouse JH, and Morris SL. Age-dependent humoral responses of children to mycobacterial antigens. *Clin Diagn Lab Immunol.* 1995;2:443–447.

43. Larsson LO, Skoogh BE, Bentzon MW, et al. Sensitivity to sensitins and tuberculin in Swedish children. II. A study of preschool children. *Tubercle.* 1991;72:37–42.

44. Macher AM, Kovacs JA, Gill V, et al. Bacteremia due to *Mycobacterium avium-intracellulare* in the acquired immunodeficiency syndrome. *Ann Intern Med.* 1983;99:782–785.

45. Fauci AS, Macher AM, Longo DL, et al. NIH conference. Acquired immunodeficiency syndrome: epidemiologic, clinical, immunologic, and therapeutic considerations. *Ann Intern Med.* 1984;100:92–106.

46. Chaisson RE, Moore RD, Richman DD, et al. Incidence and natural history of *Mycobacterium avium*-complex infections in patients with advanced human immunodeficiency virus disease treated with zidovudine. The Zidovudine Epidemiology Study Group. *Am Rev Respir Dis.* 1992;146:285–289.

47. Chin DP, Hopewell PC, Yajko DM, et al. *Mycobacterium avium* complex in the respiratory or gastrointestinal tract and the risk of M. avium complex bacteremia in patients with human immunodeficiency virus infection. *J Infect Dis.* 1994;169:289–295.

48. Horsburgh CR, Jr., Metchock B, Gordon SM, et al. Predictors of survival in patients with AIDS and disseminated *Mycobacterium avium* complex disease. *J Infect Dis.* 1994;170:573–577.

49. Jacobson MA, Hopewell PC, Yajko DM, et al. Natural history of disseminated *Mycobacterium avium* complex infection in AIDS. *J Infect Dis.* 1991;164:994–998.

50. Horsburgh CR, Jr. *Mycobacterium avium* complex infection in the acquired immunodeficiency syndrome. *N Engl J Med.* 1991;324:1332–1338.

51. Low N, Pfluger D, Egger M, et al. Disseminated *Mycobacterium avium* complex disease in the Swiss HIV cohort study: Increasing incidence, unchanged prognosis. *AIDS.* 1997;11:1165–1171.

52. Selik RM, Starcher ET, Curran JW. Opportunistic diseases reported in AIDS patients: frequencies, associations, and trends. *AIDS.* 1987;1:175–182.

53. McNaghten AD, Hanson DL, Jones JL, et al. Effects of antiretroviral therapy and opportunistic illness primary chemoprophylaxis on survival after AIDS diagnosis. Adult/Adolescent Spectrum of Disease Group. *AIDS.* 1999;13:1687–1695.

54. Forrest DM, Seminari E, Hogg RS, et al. The inicidence and spectrum of AIDS-defining illnesses in persons treated with antiretroviral drugs. *Clin Infect Dis.* 1998;27: 1379–1385.

55. Ives NJ, Gazzard BG, and Easterbrook PJ. The changing pattern of AIDS-defining illnesses with the introduction of highly active antiretroviral therapy (HAART) in a London clinic. *J Infect.* 2001;42:134–139.

56. Palella FJJ, DeLaney KM, Moorman AC, et al. Declining morbidity and mortality among patients with advanced human immunodeficiency virus infection. *N Engl J Med.* 1998;338:853–860.

57. Hadad DJ, Palaci M, Pignatari AC, et al. Mycobacteraemia among HIV-1-infected patients in Sao Paulo, Brazil: 1995 to 1998. *Epidemiol Infect.* 2004;132:151–155.

58. Horsburgh CR, Jr., Gettings J, Alexander LN, et al. Disseminated *Mycobacterium avium* complex disease among patients infected with human immunodeficiency virus, 1985–2000. *Clin Infect Dis.* 2001;33:1938–1943.

59. Karakousis PC, Moore RD, and Chaisson RE. *Mycobacterium avium* complex in patients with HIV infection in the era of highly active antiretroviral therapy. *Lancet Infect Dis.* 2004;4:557–565.

60. Kaplan JE, Hanson D, Dworkin MS, et al. Epidemiology of human immunodeficiency virus-associated opportunistic infections in the United States in the era of highly active antiretroviral therapy. *Clin Infect Dis.* 30 Suppl 1: S5–S14, 2000.

61. O'Brien RJ, Geiter LJ, and Snider DE, Jr. The epidemiology of nontuberculous mycobacterial diseases in the United States. Results from a national survey. *Am Rev Respir Dis.* 1987;135:1007–1014.

62. Tsukamura M, Kita N, Shimoide H, et al. Studies on the epidemiology of nontuberculous mycobacteriosis in Japan. *Am Rev Respir Dis.* 1988;137:1280–1284.

63. O'Brien DP, Currie BJ, and Krause VL. Nontuberculous mycobacterial disease in northern Australia: a case series and review of the literature. *Clin Infect Dis.* 2000;31: 958–967.

64. Rosenzweig DY. Pulmonary mycobacterial infections due to Mycobacterium intracellulare- avium complex. Clinical features and course in 100 consecutive cases. *Chest.* 1979;75:115–119.

65. du Moulin GC, Sherman IH, Hoaglin DC, et al. *Mycobacterium avium* complex, an emerging pathogen in Massachusetts. *J Clin Microbiol.* 1985;22:9–12.

66. Cox JN, Brenner ER, and Bryan CS. Changing patterns of mycobacterial disease at a teaching community hospital. *Infect Control Hosp Epidemiol.* 1994;15:513–515.

67. Prince DS, Peterson DD, Steiner RM, et al. Infection with *Mycobacterium avium* complex in patients without predisposing conditions. *N Engl J Med.* 1989;321:863–868.

68. Griffith DE, Brown BA, Girard WM, et al. Azithromycin-containing regimens for treatment of *Mycobacterium avium* complex lung disease. *Clin Infect Dis.* 2001;32: 1547–1553.

69. Dautzenberg B, Piperno D, Diot P, et al. Clarithromycin in the treatment of *Mycobacterium avium* lung infections in patients without AIDS. Clarithromycin Study Group of France. *Chest.* 1995;107:1035–1040.

70. Tanaka E, Kimoto T, Tsuyuguchi K, et al. Effect of clarithromycin regimen for *Mycobacterium avium* complex pulmonary disease. *Am J Respir Crit Care Med.* 1999;160: 866–872.

71. Wolinsky E: Mycobacterial lymphadenitis in children: a prospective study of 105 nontuberculous cases with long-term follow-up. *Clin Infect Dis.* 1995;20:954–963.

72. Tumbarello M, Tacconelli E, de Donati KG, et al. Changes in incidence and risk factors of *Mycobacterium avium* complex infections in patients with AIDS in the era of new antiretroviral therapies. *European J Clin Microbiol & Infectious Diseases.* 1920;498–501.

73. Chin DP, Reingold AL, Horsburgh CR, Jr. et al. Predicting *Mycobacterium avium* complex bacteremia in patients infected with human immunodeficiency virus: a

prospectively validated model. *Clin Infect Dis.* 1994;19: 668–674.

74. Gordin FM, Cohn DL, Sullam PM, et al. Early manifestations of disseminated *Mycobacterium avium* complex disease: a prospective evaluation. *J Infect Dis.* 1997;176: 126–132.

75. Tsukaguchi K, Yoneda T, Okamura H, et al. Defective T cell function for inhibition of growth of *Mycobacterium avium*-intracellulare complex (MAC) in patients with MAC disease: restoration by cytokines. *J Infect Dis.* 2000;182:1664–1671.

76. Ghassemi M, Asadi FK, Andersen BR, et al. Mycobacterium avium induces HIV upregulation through mechanisms independent of cytokine induction. *AIDS Res Hum Retroviruses.* 2000;16:435–440.

77. Kallenius G, Koivula T, Rydgard KJ, et al. Human immunodeficiency virus type 1 enhances intracellular growth of *Mycobacterium avium* in human macrophages. *Infect Immun.* 1992;60:2453–2458.

78. Gomes MS, Florido M, Cordeiro JV, et al. Limited role of the Toll-like receptor-2 in resistance to *Mycobacterium avium.* *Immunology.* 2004;111:179–185.

79. Janssens S and Beyaert R: Role of Toll-like receptors in pathogen recognition. *Clin Microbiol Rev.* 2003;16: 637–646.

80. Sabroe I, Read RC, Whyte MK, et al. Toll-like receptors in health and disease: complex questions remain. *J Immunol.* 2003;171:1630–1635.

81. Silva RA, Florido M, and Appelberg R. Interleukin-12 primes CD4+ T cells for interferon-gamma production and protective immunity during *Mycobacterium avium* infection. *Immunology.* 2001;103:368–374.

82. Bhattacharyya A, Pathak S, Kundu M, et al. Mitogen-activated protein kinases regulate *Mycobacterium avium*-induced tumor necrosis factor-alpha release from macrophages. *FEMS Immunol Med Microbiol.* 2002;34: 73–80.

83. Ehlers S, Benini J, Kutsch S, et al. Fatal granuloma necrosis without exacerbated mycobacterial growth in tumor necrosis factor receptor p55 gene-deficient mice intravenously infected with *Mycobacterium avium.* *Infect Immun.* 1999;67:3571–3579.

84. Skamene E, Schurr E, and Gros P. Infection genomics: Nramp1 as a major determinant of natural resistance to intracellular infections. *Annu Rev Med.* 1998;49:275–287.

85. Fitness J, Floyd S, Warndorff DK, et al. Large-scale candidate gene study of tuberculosis susceptibility in the Karonga district of northern Malawi. *Am J Trop Med Hyg.* 2004;71:341–349.

86. Casanova JL and Abel L. Genetic dissection of immunity to mycobacteria: The human model. *Ann Rev Immunol.* 2002;20:581–620.

87. Huang JH, Oefner PJ, Adi V, et al. Analyses of the NRAMP1 and INF-gammaR1 genes in women with *Mycobacterium avium-intracellulare* pulmonary disease. *Am J Respir Crit Care Med.* 1998;157:377–381.

88. Tanaka E, Kimoto T, Matsumoto H, et al. Familial pulmonary *Mycobacterium avium* complex disease. *Am J Respir Crit Care Med.* 2000;161:1643–1647.

89. Takahashi M, Ishizaka A, Nakamura H, et al. Specific HLA in pulmonary MAC infection in a Japanese population. *Am J Respir Crit Care Med.* 2000;162(1):316–318.

90. Kubo K, Yamazaki Y, Hanaoka M, et al. Analysis of HLA antigens in *Mycobacterium avium-intracellulare* pulmonary infection. *Am J Respir Crit Care Med.* 2000;161: 1368–1371.

91. Rook GAW. Macrophages and *Mycobacterium tuberculosis*: The key to pathogenesis. *Immunol Ser.* 1994;60: 249–261.

92. Florido M, Goncalves AS, Silva RA, et al. Resistance of virulent *Mycobacterium avium* to gamma interferon-mediated antimicrobial activity suggests additional signals for induction of mycobacteriostasis. *Infect Immun.* 1999;67:3610–3618.

93. Ottenhoff THM, Verreck FAW, Lichtenauer-Kaligis EGR, et al. Genetics, cytokines and human infectious disease: lessons from weakly pathogenic mycobacteria and salmonellae. *Nat Genet.* 2002;32:97–104.

94. Inderlied CB, Kemper CA, and Bermudez LE. The *Mycobacterium avium* complex. *Clin Microbiol Rev.* 1993;6:266–310.

95. Schaefer WB. Serologic identification and classification of the atypical mycobacteria by their agglutination. *Am Rev Respir Dis.* 1965;92:85–93.

96. Saito H, Tomioka H, Sato K, et al. Identification of various serovar strains of *Mycobacterium avium* complex by using DNA probes specific for *Mycobacterium avium* and Mycobacterium intracellulare. *J Clin Microbiol.* 1990;28: 1694–1697.

97. Wayne LG, Good RC, Tsang A, et al. Serovar determination and molecular taxonomic correlation in *Mycobacterium avium*, Mycobacterium intracellulare, and Mycobacterium scrofulaceum: a cooperative study of the International Working Group on Mycobacterial Taxonomy. *Int J Syst Bacteriol.* 1993;43:482–489.

98. Yakrus MA and Good RC. Geographic distribution, frequency, and specimen source of *Mycobacterium avium* complex serotypes isolated from patients with acquired immunodeficiency syndrome. *J Clin Microbiol.* 1990;28: 926–929.

99. Crawford JT and Bates JH. Phage typing of the *Mycobacterium avium-intracellulare-scrofulaceum complex.* A study of strains of diverse geographic and host origin. *Am Rev Respir Dis.* 1985;132:386–389.

100. Wasem CF, McCarthy CM, and Murray LW. Multilocus enzyme electrophoresis analysis of the *Mycobacterium avium* complex and other mycobacteria. *J Clin Microbiol.* 1991;29:264–271.

101. Feizabadi MM, Robertson ID, Cousins DV, et al. Genetic characterization of *Mycobacterium avium* isolates recovered from humans and animals in Australia. *Epidemiol Infect.* 1996;116:41–49.

102. Guerrero C, Bernasconi C, Burki D, et al. A novel insertion element from *Mycobacterium avium*, IS1245, is a specific target for analysis of strain relatedness. *J Clin Microbiol.* 1995;33:304–307.

103. Pavlik I, Svastova P, Bartl J, et al. Relationship between IS901 in the *Mycobacterium avium* complex strains isolated from birds, animals, humans, and the environment and virulence for poultry. *Clin Diagn Lab Immunol.* 2000;7:212–217.

104. Roiz MP, Palenque E, Guerrero C, et al. Use of restriction fragment length polymorphism as a genetic marker for typing *Mycobacterium avium* strains. *J Clin Microbiol.* 1995;33:1389–1391.

105. Swanson DS, Kapur V, Stockbauer K, et al. Subspecific differentiation of *Mycobacterium avium* complex strains by automated sequencing of a region of the gene (hsp65) encoding a 65-kilodalton heat shock protein. *Int J Syst Bacteriol.* 1997;47:414–419.

106. Frothingham R and Wilson KH. Sequence-based differentiation of strains in the *Mycobacterium avium* complex. *J Bacteriol.* 1993;175:2818–2825.

107. Kapur V, Li LL, Hamrick MR, et al. Rapid Mycobacterium species assignment and unambiguous identification of mutations associated with antimicrobial resistance in *Mycobacterium tuberculosis* by automated DNA sequencing. *Arch Pathol Lab Med.* 1995;119:131–138.

108. Pai S, Esen N, Pan X, et al. Routine rapid Mycobacterium species assignment based on species-specific allelic variation in the 65-kilodalton heat shock protein gene (hsp65). *Arch Pathol Lab Med.* 1997;121:859–864.

109. De Smet KA, Brown IN, Yates M, et al. Ribosomal internal transcribed spacer sequences are identical among *Mycobacterium avium-intracellulare* complex isolates from AIDS patients, but vary among isolates from elderly pulmonary disease patients. *Microbiology.* 1995;141(Pt 10): 2739–2747.

110. Beggs ML, Stevanova R, and Eisenach KD. Species identification of *Mycobacterium avium* complex isolates by a variety of molecular techniques. *J Clin Microbiol.* 2000;38: 508–512.

111. Torrelles JB, Chatterjee D, Lonca JG, et al. Serovars of *Mycobacterium avium* complex isolated from AIDS and non-AIDS patients in Spain. *J Appl Microbiol.* 2000;88: 266–279.

112. Cangelosi GA, Freeman RJ, Lewis KN, et al. Evaluation of a high-throughput repetitive-sequence-based PCR system for DNA fingerprinting of *Mycobacterium tuberculosis* and *Mycobacterium avium* complex strains. *J Clin Microbiol.* 2004;42:2685–2693.

113. Raszka WV, Jr., Skillman LP, McEvoy PL, et al. Isolation of nontuberculous, non-avium mycobacteria from patients infected with human immunodeficiency virus. *Clin Infect Dis.* 1995;20:73–76.

114. Frothingham R and Wilson KH. Molecular phylogeny of the *Mycobacterium avium* complex demonstrates clinically meaningful divisions. *J Infect Dis.* 1994;169:305–312.

115. Frothingham R, Meeker-O'Connell WA, Cobb AJ, et al. Association of *Mycobacterium avium* sequevars Mav-B and Mav-E with disseminated disease in immunodeficient hosts. *38th annual meeting of the Infectious Diseases Society of America,* 2000. Abstract 558.

116. Hazra R, Lee SH, Maslow JN, et al. Related strains of *Mycobacterium avium* cause disease in children with AIDS and in children with lymphadenitis. *J Infect Dis.* 2000;181:1298–1303.

117. Swanson DS, Pan X, Kline MW, et al. Genetic diversity among *Mycobacterium avium* complex strains recovered from children with and without human immunodeficiency virus infection. *J Infect Dis.* 1998;178:776–782.

118. Plum G, Brenden M, Clark-Curtiss JE, et al. Cloning, sequencing, and expression of the mig gene of Mycobacterium avium, which codes for a secreted macrophage-induced protein. *Infect Immun.* 1997;65:4548–4557.

119. Maslow JN, Dawson D, Carlin EA, et al. Hemolysin as a virulence factor for systemic infection with isolates of *Mycobacterium avium* complex. *J Clin Microbiol.* 1999; 37:445–446.

120. Plum G and Clark-Curtiss JE. Induction of *Mycobacterium avium* gene expression following phagocytosis by human macrophages. *Infect Immun.* 1994;62:476–483.

121. Meyer M, von Grunberg PW, Knoop T, et al. The macrophage-induced gene *mig* as a marker for clinical pathogenicity and in vitro virulence of *Mycobacterium avium* complex strains. *Infect Immun.* 1998;66: 4549–4552.

122. Rindi L, Bonanni D, Lari N, et al. Most human isolates of *Mycobacterium avium* Mav-A and Mav-B are strong producers of hemolysin, a putative virulence factor. *J Clin Microbiol.* 2003;41:5738–5740.

123. Bermudez LE, Shelton K, and Young LS. Comparison of the ability of *Mycobacterium avium*, M. smegmatis and M. tuberculosis to invade and replicate within HEp-2 epithelial cells. *Tuber Lung Dis.* 1995;76:240–247.

124. Ratliff TL, McCarthy R, Telle WB, et al. Purification of a mycobacterial adhesin for fibronectin. *Infect Immun.* 1993;61:1889–1894.

125. Crowle AJ, Tsang AY, Vatter AE, et al. Comparison of 15 laboratory and patient-derived strains of *Mycobacterium avium* for ability to infect and multiply in cultured human macrophages. *J Clin Microbiol.* 1986;24:812–821.

126. Schaefer WB, Davis CL, and Cohn ML. Pathogenicity of transparent, opaque, and rough variants of *Mycobacterium avium* in chickens and mice. *Am Rev Respir Dis.* 1970;102: 499–506.

127. Shiratsuchi H, Johnson JL, Toba H, et al. Strain- and donor-related differences in the interaction of *Mycobacterium avium* with human monocytes and its modulation by interferon-gamma. *J Infect Dis.* 1990;162:932–938.

128. Tassell SK, Pourshafie M, Wright EL, et al. Modified lymphocyte response to mitogens induced by the lipopeptide fragment derived from *Mycobacterium avium* serovar-specific glycopeptidolipids. *Infect Immun.* 1992;60:706–711.

129. Shiratsuchi H and Ellner JJ. Expression of IL-18 by *Mycobacterium avium*-infected human monocytes; association with M. avium virulence. *Clin Exp Immunol.* 2001;123:203–209.

130. Hocqueloux L, Lesprit P, Herrmann JL, et al. Pulmonary *Mycobacterium avium* complex disease without dissemination in HIV-infected patients. *Chest.* 1998;113:542–548.

131. Yazdanpanah Y, Goldie SJ, Paltiel AD, et al. Prevention of human immunodeficiency virus-related opportunistic infections in France: a cost-effectiveness analysis. *Clin Infect Dis.* 2003;36:86–96.

132. Greene JB, Sidhu GS, Lewin S, et al. *Mycobacterium avium-intracellulare*: a cause of disseminated life-threatening infection in homosexuals and drug abusers. *Ann Intern Med.* 1982;97:539–546.

133. Chin DP, Reingold AL, Stone EN, et al. The impact of *Mycobacterium avium* complex bacteremia and its treatment on survival of AIDS patients—a prospective study. *J Infect Dis.* 1994;170:578–584.

134. American Thoracic Society. Diagnosis and treatment of disease caused by nontuberculous mycobacteria. *Am J Respir Crit Care Med.* 1997;156:S1–S25.

135. Torriani FJ, McCutchan JA, Bozzette SA , et al. Autopsy findings in AIDS patients with *Mycobacterium avium* complex bacteremia. *J Infect Dis.* 1994;170:1601–1605.

136. Hawkins CC, Gold JW, Whimbey E, et al. *Mycobacterium avium* complex infections in patients with the acquired immunodeficiency syndrome. *Ann Intern Med.* 1986;105:184–188.

137. Gascon P, Sathe SS, and Rameshwar P. Impaired erythropoiesis in the acquired immunodeficiency syndrome with disseminated *Mycobacterium avium* complex. *Am J Med.* 1993;94:41–48.

143. Runyon EH. Anonymous mycobacteria in pulmonary disease. *Medical Clinics of North America.* 1959;43:273–290.

138. Lewis AGJr, Lasche EM, Armstrong AL, et al. A clinical study of the chronic lung disease due to nonphotochromogenic acid-fast bacilli. *Ann Intern Med.* 1960;53:273–285.

139. Bates JH. A study of pulmonary disease associated with mycobacteria other than *Mycobacterium tuberculosis*: Clinical characteristics. *Am Rev Respir Dis.* 1967;96:1151–1157.

140. Kim TC, Arora NS, Aldrich TK, et al. Atypical mycobacterial infections: a clinical study of 92 patients. *South Med J.* 1981;74:1304–1308.

141. Fischer DA, Lester W, and Schaefer WB. Infections with atypical mycobacteria. Five years' experience at the National Jewish Hospital. *Am Rev Respir Dis.* 1968;98:29–34.

142. Tsukamura M and Ichiyama S. Comparison of antituberculosis drug regimens for lung disease caused by *Mycobacterium avium* complex. *Chest.* 1988;93:821–823.

144. Rosenzweig DY and Schlueter DP. Spectrum of clinical disease in pulmonary infection with *Mycobacterium avium-intracellulare*. *Rev Infect Dis.* 1981;3:1046–1051.

145. Engbaek HC, Vergmann B, and Bentzon MW. Lung disease caused by *Mycobacterium avium/Mycobacterium intracellulare*. An analysis of Danish patients during the period 1962-1976. *Eur J Respir Dis.* 1981;62:72–83.

146. Gribetz AR, Damsker B, Bottone EJ, et al. Solitary pulmonary nodules due to nontuberculous mycobacterial infection. *Am J Med.* 1981;70:39–43.

147. Marchevsky A, Damsker B, Gribetz A, et al. The spectrum of pathology of nontuberculous mycobacterial infections in open-lung biopsy specimens. *Am J Clin Pathol.* 1982;78:695–700.

148. Reich JM and Johnson RE. *Mycobacterium avium* complex pulmonary disease. Incidence, presentation, and response to therapy in a community setting. *Am Rev Respir Dis.* 1991;143:1381–1385.

149. Huang JH, Kao PN, Adi V, et al. *Mycobacterium avium-intracellulare* pulmonary infection in HIV-negative patients without preexisting lung disease: diagnostic and management limitations. *Chest.* 1999;115:1033–1040.

150. Swensen SJ, Hartman TE, and Williams DE. Computed tomographic diagnosis of *Mycobacterium avium-intracellulare* complex in patients with bronchiectasis. *Chest.* 1994;105:49–52.

151. Watanabe K, Fujimura M, Kasahara K, et al. Characteristics of pulmonary *Mycobacterium avium-intracellulare* complex (MAC) infection in comparison with those of tuberculosis. *Respiratory Medicine.* 2003;97:654–659.

152. Iseman MD, Buschman DL, and Ackerson LM. Pectus excavatum and scoliosis. Thoracic anomalies associated with pulmonary disease caused by *Mycobacterium avium* complex. *Am Rev Respir Dis.* 1991;144:914–916.

153. Dhillon SS and Watanakunakorn C. Lady Windermere's syndrome: middle lobe bronchiectasis and *Mycobacterium avium* complex infection due to voluntary cough suppression. *Clin Infect Dis.* 2000;30:572–575.

154. Olivier KN, Weber DJ, Wallace RJ, Jr. et al. Nontuberculous mycobacteria. I: Multicenter prevalence study in cystic fibrosis. *Am J Respir Crit Care Med.* 2003;167:828–834.

155. Olivier KN, Weber DJ, Lee JH, et al. Nontuberculous mycobacteria. II: nested-cohort study of impact on cystic fibrosis lung disease. *Am J Respir Crit Care Med.* 2003;167:835–840.

156. Haverkamp MH, Arend SM, Lindeboom JA, et al. Nontuberculous mycobacterial infection in children: a 2-year prospective surveillance study in the Netherlands. *Clin Infect Dis.* 2004;39:450–456.

157. Nolt D, Michaels MG, and Wald ER. Intrathoracic disease from nontuberculous mycobacteria in children: two cases and a review of the literature. *Pediatrics.* 112:e434–2003.

158. Kahana LM, Kay JM, Yakrus MA, et al. *Mycobacterium avium* complex infection in an immunocompetent young adult related to hot tub exposure. *Chest.* 1997;111:242–245.

159. Khoor A, Leslie KO, Tazelaar HD, et al. Diffuse pulmonary disease caused by nontuberculous mycobacteria in

immunocompetent people (hot tub lung). *Am J Clin Pathol.* 2001;115:755–762.

160. Schaad UB, Votteler TP, McCracken GH, Jr. et al. Management of atypical mycobacterial lymphadenitis in childhood: a review based on 380 cases. *J Pediatr* 1979;95:356–360.

161. Panesar J, Higgins K, Daya H, et al. Nontuberculous mycobacterial cervical adenitis: a ten-year retrospective review. *Laryngoscope.* 2003;113:149–154.

162. Rahal A, Abela A, Arcand PH, et al. Nontuberculous mycobacterial adenitis of the head and neck in children: experience from a tertiary care pediatric center. *Laryngoscope.* 2001;111:1791–1796.

163. Flint D, Mahadevan M, Barber C, et al. Cervical lymphadenitis due to nontuberculous mycobacteria: surgical treatment and review. *Int J Pediatr Otorhinol.* 2000;53: 187–194.

164. Taha AM, Davidson PT, and Bailey WC. Surgical treatment of atypical mycobacterial lymphadenitis in children. *Pediatr Infect Dis.* 1985;4:664–667.

165. Anim-Appiah D, Bono B, Fleegler E , et al. *Mycobacterium avium* complex tenosynovitis of the wrist and hand. *Arthritis Rheum.* 2004;51:140–142.

166. Hellinger WC, Smilack JD, Greider JL, Jr., et al. Localized soft-tissue infections with *Mycobacterium avium/Mycobacterium intracellulare* complex in immunocompetent patients: granulomatous tenosynovitis of the hand or wrist. *Clin Infect Dis.* 1995;21:65–69.

167. Lefevre P, Gilot P, Godiscal H, et al. Mycobacterium intracellulare as a cause of a recurrent granulomatous tenosynovitis of the hand. *Diagn Microbiol Infect Dis.* 2000;38:127–129.

168. Bridges MJ and McGarry F.Two cases of *Mycobacterium avium* septic arthritis. *Ann Rheum Dis.* 2002;61:186–187.

169. Mehta JB, Emery MW, Girish M, et al. Atypical Pott's disease: localized infection of the thoracic spine due to *Mycobacterium avium-intracellulare* in a patient without human immunodeficiency virus infection. *South Med J.* 2003;96:685–688.

170. Chan ED, Kong PM, Fennelly K, et al. Vertebral osteomyelitis due to infection with nontuberculous Mycobacterium species after blunt trauma to the back: 3 examples of the principle of locus minoris resistentiae. *Clin Infect Dis.* 2001;32:1506–1510.

171. Komatsu H, Terunuma A, Tabata N, et al. *Mycobacterium avium* infection of the skin associated with lichen scrofulosorum: report of three cases. *Br J Dermatol.* 1999;141: 554–557.

172. Satta R, Retanda G, and Cottoni F. *Mycobacterium avium* complex: cutaneous infection in an immunocompetent host. *Acta Derm Venereol.* 1999;79:249–250.

173. Kullavanijaya P, Sirimachan S, and Surarak S. Primary cutaneous infection with *Mycobacterium avium intracellulare* complex resembling lupus vulgaris. *Br J Dermatol.* 1997;136:264–266.

174. Sugita Y, Ishii N, Katsuno M, et al. Familial cluster of cutaneous *Mycobacterium avium* infection resulting from use of a circulating, constantly heated bath water system. *Br J Dermatol.* 2000;142:789–793.

175. Corbett EL, Blumberg L, Churchyard GJ, et al. Nontuberculous mycobacteria: defining disease in a prospective cohort of South African miners. *Am J Respir Crit Care Med.* 1999;160:15–21.

176. Hartman TE, Swensen SJ, and Williams DE. Mycobacterium avium-intracellulare complex: evaluation with CT. *Radiology.* 1993;187:23–26.

177. Primack SL, Logan PM, Hartman TE, et al. Pulmonary tuberculosis and *Mycobacterium avium-intracellulare*: a comparison of CT findings. *Radiology.* 1995;194:413–417.

178. Kitada S, Maekura R, Toyoshima N, et al. Serodiagnosis of pulmonary disease due to *Mycobacterium avium* complex with an enzyme immunoassay that uses a mixture of glycopeptidolipid antigens. *Clin Infect Dis.* 2002;35: 1328–1335.

179. Biaxin package insert. Available at: http://www.fda.gov/cder/foi/label/2000/50662S29lbl.pdf, Last update 10-12-2000. Accessed November 14, 2004.

180. Zithromax package insert. Available at: http://www.fda.gov/cder/foi/label/2004/50710slr017,021,50711slr015,017_zithromax_lbl.pdf, Last update 1-15-2004. Accessed November 11, 2004.

181. Rifampin package insert. Available at: http://www.fda.gov/cder/foi/label/2000/50662S29lbl.pdf, Last update 1999. Accessed November 14, 2004.255.

182. Myambutol package insert. Available at: http://www.fda.gov/cder/foi/label/2004/16320slr060_myambutol_lbl.pdf, Last update 3-24-2004. Accessed November 14, 2004.

183. Mycobutin package insert. Available at: http://www.pfizer.com/download/uspi_mycobutin.pdf, Last update 2004, Accessed November 11, 2004.

184. PDR Drug information for streptomycin. Available at: http://www.drugs.com/PDR/Streptomycin_Sulfate_Injection.html, Last update 1998, Accessed November 14, 2004.

185. Cipro package insert. Available at: http://www.fda.gov/cder/foi/label/2004/19537s053,054,20780s017,018lbl.pdf, Last update 7-14-2004, Accessed November 11, 2004.

186. Levaquin package insert. Available at: http://www.fda.gov/cder/foi/label/2004/20634s035,20635s035,21721s003lbl.pdf, Last update 11-24-2004, Accessed November 14, 2004.

187. Avelox package insert. Available at: http://www.fda.gov/cder/foi/label/2004/21277s019,21085s024lbl.pdf , Last update 7-28-2004, Accessed November 14, 2004.

188. Tequin package insert. Available at: http://www.fda.gov/cder/foi/label/2004/21061s023,024,21062s026,037lbl.pdf, Last update 9-14-2004, Accessed November 14, 2004.

189. Lamprene package insert. Available at: http://www.fda.gov/cder/foi/label/2003/19500slr010_lamprene_lbl.pdf, Last update 2002, Accessed November 14, 2004.

190. Actimmune package insert. Available at: http://www. actimmune.com/pdf/pi.pdf, Last update 2004, Accessed November 14, 2004.

191. Zyvox package insert. Available at: http://www.pfizer. com/download/uspi_zyvox.pdf, Last update 2004, Accessed November 14, 2004.

192. Lariam package insert. Available at: http://www.fda.gov/ cder/foi/label/2003/19591slr022_lariam_lbl.pdf, Last update 8-15-2003, Accessed November 14, 2004.

193. Ketek package insert. Available at: http://www.fda.gov/ cder/foi/label/2004/21144_ketek_lbl.pdf, Last update 4-1-2004, Accessed November 15, 2004.

194. Frothingham R. Rates of torsades de pointes associated with ciprofloxacin, ofloxacin, levofloxacin, gatifloxacin, and moxifloxacin. *Pharmacotherapy.* 2001;21:1468–1472.

195. Brown BA, Griffith DE, Girard W, et al. Relationship of adverse events to serum drug levels in patients receiving high-dose azithromycin for mycobacterial lung disease. *Clin Infect Dis.* 1997;24:958–964.

196. Mycobutin package insert. Available at: http://www.fda. gov/cder/foi/label/2001/50689s11s13lbl.pdf, Last update 11-9-2001. Accessed November 11, 2004.

197. Lamprene package insert. Available at: http://www.fda. gov/cder/foi/label/2003/19500slr010_lamprene_lbl.pdf, Last update 2002. Accessed November 14, 2004.

198. Wallace RJ, Jr., Brown BA, Griffith DE, et al. Reduced serum levels of clarithromycin in patients treated with multidrug regimens including rifampin or rifabutin for Mycobacterium avium-M. intracellulare infection. *J Infect Dis.* 1995;171:747–750.

199. Chaisson RE, Benson CA, Dube MP, et al. Clarithromycin therapy for bacteremic *Mycobacterium avium* complex disease. A randomized, double-blind, dose-ranging study in patients with AIDS. AIDS Clinical Trials Group Protocol 157 Study Team. *Ann Intern Med.* 1994;121:905–911.

200. Bermudez LE, Nash K, Petrofsky M, et al. Clarithromycin-resistant *Mycobacterium avium* is still susceptible to treatment with clarithromycin and is virulent in mice. *Antimicrobial Agents Chemother.* 2000;44:2619–2622.

201. Sison JP, Yao Y, Kemper CA, et al. Treatment of *Mycobacterium avium* complex infection: do the results of in vitro susceptibility tests predict therapeutic outcome in humans? *J Infect Dis.* 1996;173:677–683.

202. Horsburgh CR, Jr., Mason UG, III, Heifets LB, et al. Response to therapy of pulmonary *Mycobacterium avium-intracellulare* infection correlates with results of in vitro susceptibility testing. *Am Rev Respir Dis.* 135:418–421.

203. Woods GL. Susceptibility testing for mycobacteria. *Clin Infect Dis.* 2000;31:1209–1215.

204. Woods GL, Williams-Bouyer N, Wallace RJ Jr. et al. Multisite reproducibility of results obtained by two broth dilution methods for susceptibility testing of *Mycobacterium avium* complex. *J Clin Microbiol.* 2003;41(2):627–631.

205. Shafran SD, Singer J, Zarowny DP, et al. A comparison of two regimens for the treatment of *Mycobacterium avium* complex bacteremia in AIDS: rifabutin, ethambutol, and clarithromycin versus rifampin, ethambutol, clofazimine, and ciprofloxacin. Canadian HIV Trials Network Protocol 010 Study Group. *N Engl J Med.* 1996;335:377–383.

206. Cohn DL, Fisher EJ, Peng GT, et al. A prospective randomized trial of four three-drug regimens in the treatment of disseminated *Mycobacterium avium* complex disease in AIDS patients: excess mortality associated with high-dose clarithromycin. Terry Beirn Community Programs for Clinical Research on AIDS. *Clin Infect Dis.* 1999;29: 125–133.

207. Dunne M, Fessel J, Kumar P, et al. A randomized, double-blind trial comparing azithromycin and clarithromycin in the treatment of disseminated *Mycobacterium avium* infection in patients with human immunodeficiency virus. *Clin Infect Dis.* 2000;31:1245–1252.

208. Dube MP, Sattler FR, Torriani FJ, et al. A randomized evaluation of ethambutol for prevention of relapse and drug resistance during treatment of *Mycobacterium avium* complex bacteremia with clarithromycin-based combination therapy. California Collaborative Treatment Group. *J Infect Dis.* 1997;176:1225–1232.

209. Ward TT, Rimland D, Kauffman C, et al. Randomized, open-label trial of azithromycin plus ethambutol vs. clarithromycin plus ethambutol as therapy for *Mycobacterium avium* complex bacteremia in patients with human immunodeficiency virus infection. Veterans Affairs HIV Research Consortium. *Clin Infect Dis.* 1998;27:1278–1285.

210. Gordin FM, Sullam PM, Shafran SD, et al. A randomized, placebo-controlled study of rifabutin added to a regimen of clarithromycin and ethambutol for treatment of disseminated infection with *Mycobacterium avium* complex. *Clin Infect Dis.* 1999;28:1080–1085.

211. Benson CA, Williams PL, Currier JS, et al. A prospective, randomized trial examining the efficacy and safety of clarithromycin in combination with ethambutol, rifabutin, or both for the treatment of disseminated *Mycobacterium avium* complex disease in persons with acquired immunodeficiency syndrome. *Clin Infect Dis.* 2003;37:1234–1243.

212. Shafran SD, Singer J, Zarowny DP, et al. Determinants of rifabutin-associated uveitis in patients treated with rifabutin, clarithromycin, and ethambutol for *Mycobacterium avium* complex bacteremia: a multivariate analysis. Canadian HIV Trials Network Protocol 010 Study Group. *J Infect Dis.* 1998;177:252–255.

213. Keiser P, Nassar N, Skiest D, et al. A retrospective study of the addition of ciprofloxacin to clarithromycin and ethambutol in the treatment of disseminated *Mycobacterium avium* complex infection. *Int J STD AIDS.* 1999;10: 791–794.

214. Tomioka H, Sano C, Sato K, et al. Antimicrobial activities of clarithromycin, gatifloxacin and sitafloxacin, in combination with various antimycobacterial drugs against extracellular and intramacrophage *Mycobacterium avium* complex. *Int J Antimicrob Agents.* 1919:139–145.

215. Tomioka H, Sato K, Kajitani H, et al. Comparative antimicrobial activities of the newly synthesized quinolone WQ-3034, levofloxacin, sparfloxacin, and ciprofloxacin against *Mycobacterium tuberculosis* and *Mycobacterium avium* complex. *Antimicrobial Agents Chemother.* 2000;44:283–286.

216. Rodriguez Diaz JC, Lopez M, Ruiz M, et al. In vitro activity of new fluoroquinolones and linezolid against nontuberculous mycobacteria. *Int J Antimicrob Agents.* 2003;21:585–588.

217. Bermudez LE, Inderlied CB, Kolonoski P, et al. Activity of moxifloxacin by itself and in combination with ethambutol, rifabutin, and azithromycin in vitro and in vivo against *Mycobacterium avium. Antimicrobial Agents Chemother.* 2001;45:217–222.

218. Roger PM, Carles M, Agussol-Foin I, et al. Efficacy and safety of an intravenous induction therapy for treatment of disseminated *Mycobacterium avium* complex infection in AIDS patients: a pilot study. *J Antimicrob Chemother.* 1999;44:129–131.

219. Parenti DM, Williams PL, Hafner R, et al. A phase II/III trial of antimicrobial therapy with or without amikacin in the treatment of disseminated *Mycobacterium avium* infection in HIV-infected individuals. AIDS Clinical Trials Group Protocol 135 Study Team. *AIDS.* 1998;12:2439–2446.

220. Chiu J, Nussbaum J, Bozzette S, et al. Treatment of disseminated *Mycobacterium avium* complex infection in AIDS with amikacin, ethambutol, rifampin, and ciprofloxacin. California Collaborative Treatment Group. *Ann Intern Med.* 1990;113:358–361.

221. Chaisson RE, Keiser P, Pierce M, et al. Clarithromycin and ethambutol with or without clofazimine for the treatment of bacteremic *Mycobacterium avium* complex disease in patients with HIV infection. *AIDS.* 1997;11:311–317.

222. Lauw FN, Der Meer JT, de Metz J, et al. No beneficial effect of interferon-gamma treatment in 2 human immunodeficiency virus-infected patients with *Mycobacterium avium* complex infection. *Clin Infect Dis.* 2001;32:e81–e82.

223. Bermudez LE, Kolonoski P, Wu M, et al. Mefloquine is active in vitro and in vivo against *Mycobacterium avium* complex. *Antimicrobial Agents Chemother.* 1999;43(8):1870–1874, 43:1870–1874.

224. Nannini EC, Keating M, Binstock P, et al. Successful treatment of refractory disseminated *Mycobacterium avium* complex infection with the addition of linezolid and mefloquine. *J Infect.* 2002;44:201–203.

225. Kedzierska K, Mak J, Mijch A, et al. Granulocyte-macrophage colony-stimulating factor augments phagocytosis of *Mycobacterium avium* complex by human immunodeficiency virus type 1-infected monocytes/macrophages in vitro and in vivo. *J Infect Dis.* 2000;181:390–394.

226. Kemper CA, Bermudez LE, and Deresinski SC. Immunomodulatory treatment of *Mycobacterium avium* complex bacteremia in patients with AIDS by use of recombinant granulocyte-macrophage colony-stimulating factor. *J Infect Dis.* 1998;177:914–920.

227. Wormser GP, Horowitz H, and Dworkin B. Low-dose dexamethasone as adjunctive therapy for disseminated *Mycobacterium avium* complex infections in AIDS patients. *Antimicrobial Agents Chemother.* 1994;38:2215–2217.

228. Holland SM, Eisenstein EM, Kuhns DB, et al. Treatment of refractory disseminated nontuberculous mycobacterial infection with interferon gamma. A preliminary report. *N Engl J Med.* 1994;330:1348–1355.

229. Doucette K and Fishman JA. Nontuberculous mycobacterial infection in hematopoietic stem cell and solid organ transplant recipients. *Clin Infect Dis.* 2004;38:1428–1439.

230. Munoz RM, Alonso-Pulpon L, Yebra M, et al. Intestinal involvement by nontuberculous mycobacteria after heart transplantation. *Clin Infect Dis.* 2000;30:603–605.

231. Peloquin CA. *Mycobacterium avium* complex infection. Pharmacokinetic and pharmacodynamic considerations that may improve clinical outcomes. *Clin Pharmacokinet.* 1997;32:132–144.

232. Aberg JA, Yajko DM, and Jacobson MA. Eradication of AIDS-related disseminated *Mycobacterium avium* complex infection after 12 months of antimycobacterial therapy combined with highly active antiretroviral therapy. *J Infect Dis.* 1998;178:1446–1449.

233. Hadad DJ, Lewi DS, Pignatari AC, et al. Resolution of *Mycobacterium avium* complex bacteremia following highly active antiretroviral therapy. *Clin Infect Dis.* 1998;26:758–759.

234. U.S. Public Health Service (USPHS) and Infectious Diseases Society of America (IDSA). . Guidelines for the Prevention of Opportunistic Infections in Persons Infected with Human Immunodeficiency Virus. Available at: http://aidsinfo.nih.gov/guidelines/op_infections/OI_1128 01.html#disseminated_infection, Last update 11-28-2001. Accessed November 18, 2004.

235. Cinti SK, Kaul DR, Sax PE, et al. Recurrence of *Mycobacterium avium* infection in patients receiving highly active antiretroviral therapy and antimycobacterial agents. *Clin Infect Dis.* 2000;30:511–514.

236. Furrer H and Malinverni R. Systemic inflammatory reaction after starting highly active antiretroviral therapy in AIDS patients treated for extrapulmonary tuberculosis. *Am J Med.* 1999;106:371–372.

237. Narita M, Ashkin D, Hollender ES, et al. Paradoxical worsening of tuberculosis following antiretroviral therapy in patients with AIDS. *Am J Respir Crit Care Med.* 1998;158:157–161.

238. Karavellas MP, Lowder CY, Macdonald C, et al. Immune recovery vitritis associated with inactive cytomegalovirus retinitis: a new syndrome. *Arch Ophthalmol.* 1998;116:169–175.

239. Cheng VC, Yuen KY, Chan WM, et al. Immune reconstitution disease involving the innate and adaptive response. *Clin Infect Dis.* 2000;30:882–892.

240. Foudraine NA, Hovenkamp E, Notermans DW, et al. Immunopathology as a result of highly active antiretroviral therapy in HIV-1-infected patients. *AIDS*. 1999;13: 177–184.

241. Price LM and O'Mahony C. Focal adenitis developing after immune reconstitution with HAART. *Int J STD AIDS*. 2000;11:685–686.

242. Lawn SD, Bicanic TA, and Macallan DC. Pyomyositis and cutaneous abscesses due to *Mycobacterium avium*: an immune reconstitution manifestation in a patient with AIDS. *Clin Infect Dis*. 2004;38:461–463.

243. Berger P, Lepidi H, Drogoul-Vey MP, et al. *Mycobacterium avium* brain abscess at the initiation of highly active anti-retroviral therapy. *Eur J Clin Microbiol Infect Dis*. 2004;23: 142–144.

244. Desimone JA, Jr., Babinchak TJ, Kaulback KR, et al. Treatment of *Mycobacterium avium* complex immune reconstitution disease in HIV-1-infected individuals. *AIDS Patient Care STDS*. 2003;17:617–622.

245. Nightingale SD, Byrd LT, Southern PM, et al. Incidence of *Mycobacterium avium-intracellulare* complex bacteremia in human immunodeficiency virus-positive patients. *J Infect Dis*. 1992;165:1082–1085.

246. Nightingale SD, Cameron DW, Gordin FM , et al. Two controlled trials of rifabutin prophylaxis against *Mycobacterium avium* complex infection in AIDS. *N Engl J Med*. 1993;329: 828–833.

247. Pierce M, Crampton S, Henry D, et al. A randomized trial of clarithromycin as prophylaxis against disseminated *Mycobacterium avium* complex infection in patients with advanced acquired immunodeficiency syndrome. *N Engl J Med*. 1996;335:384–391.

248. Benson CA, Williams PL, Cohn DL, et al. Clarithromycin or rifabutin alone or in combination for primary prophylaxis of *Mycobacterium avium* complex disease in patients with AIDS: A randomized, double-blind, placebo-controlled trial. The AIDS Clinical Trials Group 196/Terry Beirn Community Programs for Clinical Research on AIDS 009 Protocol Team. *J Infect Dis*. 2000;181:1289–1297.

249. Hewitt RG, Papandonatos GD, Shelton MJ, et al. Prevention of disseminated *Mycobacterium avium* complex infection with reduced dose clarithromycin in patients with advanced HIV disease. *AIDS*. 1999;13:1367–1372.

250. Havlir DV, Dube MP, Sattler FR, et al. Prophylaxis against disseminated *Mycobacterium avium* complex with weekly azithromycin, daily rifabutin, or both. California Collaborative Treatment Group. *N Engl J Med*. 1996;335:392–398.

251. Oldfield EC, III, Fessel WJ, Dunne MW, et al. Once weekly azithromycin therapy for prevention of *Mycobacterium avium* complex infection in patients with AIDS: a randomized, double-blind, placebo-controlled multicenter trial. *Clin Infect Dis*. 1998;26:611–619.

252. El Sadr WM, Burman WJ, Grant LB, et al. Discontinuation of prophylaxis for *Mycobacterium avium* complex disease in HIV-infected patients who have a response to antiretroviral therapy. Terry Beirn Community Programs for Clinical Research on AIDS. *N Engl J Med*. 2000;342:1085–1092.

253. Dutt AK and Stead WW. Long-term results of medical treatment in Mycobacterium intracellulare infection. *Am J Med*. 1979;67:449–453.

254. Davidson PT, Khanijo V, Goble M, et al. Treatment of disease due to Mycobacterium intracellulare. *Rev Infect Dis*. 1981;3:1052–1059.

255. Ahn CH, Ahn SS, Anderson RA, et al. A four-drug regimen for initial treatment of cavitary disease caused by *Mycobacterium avium* complex. *Am Rev Respir Dis*. 1986;134:438–441.

256. Etzkorn ET, Aldarondo S, McAllister CK, et al. Medical therapy of *Mycobacterium avium-intracellulare* pulmonary disease. *Am Rev Respir Dis*. 1986;134:442–445.

257. Pulmonary disease caused by *Mycobacterium avium-intracellulare* in HIV-negative patients. five-year follow-up of patients receiving standardised treatment. *Int J Tuberc Lung Dis*. 2002;6:628–634.

258. First randomised trial of treatments for pulmonary disease caused by *M. avium* intracellulare, *M. malmoense*, and *M. xenopi* in HIV negative patients. rifampicin, ethambutol and isoniazid versus rifampicin and ethambutol. *Thorax*. 2001;56:167–172.

259. Woodley CL and Kilburn JO. In vitro susceptibility of *Mycobacterium avium* complex and *Mycobacterium tuberculosis* strains to a spiro-piperidyl rifamycin. *Am Rev Respir Dis*. 1982;126:586–587.

260. Wallace RJ, Jr., Brown BA, Griffith DE, et al. Initial clarithromycin monotherapy for *Mycobacterium avium-intracellulare* complex lung disease. *Am J Respir Crit Care Med*. 1994;149:1335–1341.

261. Griffith DE, Brown BA, Girard WM, et al. Azithromycin activity against *Mycobacterium avium* complex lung disease in patients who were not infected with human immunodeficiency virus. *Clin Infect Dis*. 1996;23:983–989.

262. Wallace RJ, Jr., Brown BA, Griffith DE, et al. Clarithromycin regimens for pulmonary *Mycobacterium avium* complex. The first 50 patients. *Am J Respir Crit Care Med*. 1996;153:1766–1772.

263. Griffith DE, Brown BA, Cegielski P, et al. Early results (at 6 months) with intermittent clarithromycin-including regimens for lung disease due to *Mycobacterium avium* complex. *Clin Infect Dis*. 2000;30:288–292.

264. Nelson KG, Griffith DE, Brown BA, et al. Results of operation in *Mycobacterium avium-intracellulare* lung disease. *Ann Thorac Surg*. 1998;66:325–330.

265. Shiraishi Y, Nakajima Y, Takasuna K, et al. Surgery for *Mycobacterium avium* complex lung disease in the clarithromycin era. *Eur J Cardiothorac Surg*. 2002;21: 314–318.

266. Sato K, Tomioka H, Akaki T, et al. Antimicrobial activities of levofloxacin, clarithromycin, and KRM-1648 against *Mycobacterium tuberculosis* and *Mycobacterium avium* complex replicating within Mono Mac 6 human macrophage

and A-549 type II alveolar cell lines. *Int J Antimicrob Agents.* 2000;16:25–29.

267. Kaur D and Khuller GK. In vitro, ex-vivo and in vivo activities of ethambutol and sparfloxacin alone and in combination against mycobacteria. *Int J Antimicrob Agents.* 2001;17:51–55.

268. Bermudez LE, Inderlied CB, Kolonoski P, et al. Telithromycin is active against *Mycobacterium avium* in mice despite lacking significant activity in standard in vitro and macrophage assays and is associated with low frequency of resistance during treatment. *Antimicrobial Agents Chemother.* 2001;45:2210–2214.

269. Iseman MD. Medical management of pulmonary disease caused by *Mycobacterium avium* complex. *Clin Chest Med.* 2002;23:633–641.

270. Chatte G, Panteix G, Perrin-Fayolle M, et al. Aerosolized interferon gamma for *Mycobacterium avium*-complex lung disease. *Am J Respir Crit Care Med.* 1995;152:1094–1096.

271. Starke JR. Management of nontuberculous mycobacterial cervical adenitis. *Pediatr Infect Dis J.* 1919;674–675.

35

Rapidly Growing Mycobacteria

Barbara A. Brown-Elliott
Richard J. Wallace Jr.

TAXONOMY

Historical Background

The history of the major pathogenic species of rapidly growing mycobacteria (RGM) can be traced back to the early 20th century[1] when Friedmann recovered *Mycobacterium chelonae* from the lungs of two sea turtles (hence, the name *chelonae* from the Latin "of a turtle"). Fifty years later, the closely related *M. abscessus* was first reported as a cause of human skin and soft tissue infection in a patient with multiple soft tissue abscesses of a lower extremity.[2]

Mycobacterium fortuitum was originally recovered from frogs in 1905 and named *M. ranae*; however, in 1938 da Costa Cruz gave the name *M. fortuitum* to what he thought was a new mycobacterial species isolated from a patient with a skin abscess following local vitamin injections.[3] Subsequently the two organisms were proven to be the same with the illegitimate name *M. fortuitum* retained as the species name on the request of Dr. Ernest Runyon.[4]

Early taxonomic studies that utilized phenotypic analysis concluded that the two species *M. fortuitum* and *M. chelonae* were composed of several "subspecies" (i.e., *M. chelonae* subspecies *chelonae*, *M. chelonae* subspecies *abscessus*) or "biovariants" (*M. fortuitum* biovariant *fortuitum*, *M. fortuitum* biovariant *peregrinum*, and *M. fortuitum* third biovariant complex).[5]

More recent taxonomic studies that utilized molecular analysis with DNA-DNA hybridization and 16S ribosomal sequencing have shown that these "biovars" and "subspecies" are in fact separate species, and most have been renamed without the subgroup designation.[6]

Current Classification

Currently, the RGM are grouped into the *M. fortuitum* group, the *M. chelonae/abscessus* group, the *Mycobacterium smegmatis* group, and pigmented RGM. There are now more than 50 recognized species, representing approximately 50% of all recognized mycobacterial species. The three most important clinical pathogenic species that represent more than 80% of clinical isolates of RGM are *M. fortuitum*, *M. chelonae*, and *M. abscessus*.[7,8] As of 2004, there are another 11 less frequent, but definite human pathogenic species that have been associated with more than five cases of human disease. These include *M. peregrinum* (formerly pipemidic acid susceptible Type 1), *M. porcinum*, *M. houstonense*, *M. senegalense*, *M. immunogenum*, *M. goodii*, *M. wolinskyi*, *M. boenickei*, *M. smegmatis*, *M. mageritense*, and *M. mucogenicum* (see Table 35-1).[6,9–18] These 14 species of RGM are nonpigmented (with the exception of some isolates of *M. goodii and M. smegmatis* which form a very late pigment).[9,14] Approximately 36 other species of RGM including pigmented (chromogenic) species have been recognized (especially with the introduction of molecular technology) but these have rarely been a cause of clinical disease (see Table 35-1).[19,20]

EPIDEMIOLOGY

Community Acquired Disease

The RGM are ubiquitous.[20,21] Human infections have been reported from most developed areas of the world, and RGM have been isolated from 30–78% of soil samples from various geographical regions in the United States.[22,23] Most reported cases of disease have been from the United States, with most clustered outbreaks and studies of selected diseases, having shown a strong disease localization in the southern United States.[24–26] Community acquired localized skin, soft tissue, and/or bone disease often follows a traumatic injury with potential soil contamination (e.g., stepping on a nail, motor vehicle accident with an open fracture, etc.). The reservoir for RGM pulmonary disease is unknown.[27]

Recently RGM lower extremity skin infections involving *M. fortuitum*, *M. mageritense*, and a newly described species, *M. cosmeticum* associated with the use of contaminated, nail salon, whirlpool, footbaths has also been described.[28,29,29a]

Nosocomial/Health Care Associated Disease

Exposure to tap water appears to be the major risk factor for nosocomial (health care associated) disease.[22,30,31] Most outbreaks of healthcare associated infections or pseudo-infections have been epidemiologically associated with various water sources, including water-based solutions,

Table 35-1. Currently Recognized Species of Rapidly Growing Mycobacteria

Nonpigmented Species	Pigmented Species	
1. Common Pathogens	None	
M. chelonae		
M. abscessus		
M. fortuitum		
2. Infrequent But Proven Pathogens		
M. fortuitum third biovariant complex		
M. mageritense (formerly sorbitol +)		
M. houstonense (formerly sorbitol +)		
M. porcinum (formerly sorbitol −)		
M. boenickei (formerly sorbitol −)		
M. immunogenum		
M. mucogenicum		
M. peregrinum		
M. senegalense (formerly M. peregrinum Type II)		
M. smegmatis group		
M. wolinskyi	*M. smegmatis**	
	*M. goodii**	
3. Rare† or Unproven Pathogens†		
M. brumae‡	*M. agri*	*M. holsaticum*
M. chitae‡	*M. aichiense*	*M. komossense*
M. confluentis‡	*M. aurum*	*M. madagascariense*
M. fallax‡	*M. austroafricanum*	*M. murale*
M. moriokaense‡	*M. chlorophenicolicum*	*M. neoaurum*
M. septicum†	*M. chubuense*	*M. novocastrense*
M. neworleansense†	*M. cosmeticum*	*M. obuense*
M. brisbanense†	*M. diernhoferi*	*M. parafortuitum*
	M. duvalii	*M. phlei*
	M. elephantis	*M. psychrotolerans*
	M. flavescens	*M. rhodesiae*
	M. fredericksbergense	*M. sphagni*
	M. gadium	*M. thermoresistible*
	M. gilvum	*M. tokaiense*
	M. hassiacum	*M. vaccae*
	M. hodleri	*M. vanbaalenii*

*Late pigmentation.
†Associated with human disease, but fewer than five cases.
‡Unassociated with human disease.
+Positive.
−Negative.

distilled water, tap water, ice, and ice water.[22,32–34] DNA fingerprinting for some of these outbreaks has confirmed molecular identity between water and human isolates. Water or water-based solutions may also be responsible for sporadic health care associated infections due to *M. fortuitum*, *M. chelonae*, and *M. abscessus*. These include catheter-related infections, sternal wound infections following cardiac bypass surgery, and infected augmentation mammaplasty sites.[24–26]

One study of hemodialysis centers in the United States showed that 55% of incoming city water contained mycobacteria, of which rapidly growing species were the most common.[35] Biofilms, which are the slimy layers that occur at water-solid interfaces, appear to be present in most pipes and tubings and up to 90% of these from community piped water systems contain mycobacteria.[36] The utilization of pulsed field gel electrophoresis and randomly amplified polymorphic DNA PCR methods for analyzing genomic DNA large restriction fragment patterns has made possible the identification of specific strains of RGM and thus improved the investigation of nosocomial outbreaks.[37–39]

Outbreaks involving RGM have been described for more than 30 years, and continue to be problematic.[34,38–40,39a] These include pseudo-outbreaks of *M. abscessus* or *M. immunogenum* related to contaminated automated bronchoscopes disinfection machines, contaminated gastric endoscopes, and laboratory contamination.[15,31,32,40] Large outbreaks of post-injection abscesses involving *M. abscessus* have also been reported by Villanueva and colleagues from Colombia,[41] Zhibang et al. in China,[42] Galil et al.[43] and Tiwari et al.[34] from the United States.

Infections with RGM species including *M. chelonae* and *M. fortuitum* appear to have a special association with cosmetic surgery procedures, especially liposuction and breast augmentation. In December 1998, the CDC reported nine patients in eight hospitals in Venezuela had acquired postliposuction and liposculpture infections caused by RGM including *M. fortuitum*, *M. abscessus*, and *M. chelonae*.[44] Meyers and colleagues noted 34 out of 82 (41%) patients who underwent liposuction by a single practitioner in a 6 month period in California developed cutaneous abscesses due to *M. chelonae*.[45] A recent outbreak following breast augmentation procedures and liposuction has been reported from the Dominican Republic.[39a] Outbreaks involving infection with RGM following acupuncture treatment have also been detailed by Woo et al., and Tang et al.[46,47] Case reports and outbreaks of lower extremity furunculosis involving *M. fortuitum*, *M. abscessus*, and less common species such as *M. mageritense* have also been recently

reported associated with contaminated water baths at nail salons.[29,39a]

LABORATORY IDENTIFICATION

Phenotypic Methods, High Performance Liquid Chromatography (HPLC)

Laboratory identification of RGM as belonging to the *M. fortuitum* complex (includes the three major pathogenic species of *M. fortuitum*, *M. chelonae*, and *M. abscessus*) has been relatively simple, and is based on growth in <7 days, typical gram stain and colony morphology, acid-fastness, the absence of pigmentation and a positive aryl-sulfatase at three days.[10,11,48,49] The *M. smegmatis* group shares the same properties except for a negative 3 day arylsulfatase.[9,14] Table 35-2 shows a scheme for differentiation for the common RGM species. Unfortunately identification to the species level in the clinical laboratory has been given little priority and is only performed by a few reference laboratories. Because of species differences in the types of clinical disease they produce (e.g., *M. chelonae* typically produces disseminated cutaneous disease in the setting of chronic corticosteroid therapy, *M. fortuitum* does not) and, most importantly, predictable species differences in drug susceptibilities (e.g., ciprofloxacin is highly active against all isolates of *M. fortuitum* but not *M. chelonae* or *M. abscessus*),[10,50,51] it is no longer good clinical practice to send out a report of an isolate with a final identification as "*M. fortuitum* complex" or "*M. chelonae*" (referring to either *M. chelonae* or *M. abscessus*) as if no distinction between the two species exists. Identification to the species level is needed for most clinical isolates.[7,52,53]

This reluctance in part reflects the absence of simple accurate methods to recognize the common species. No commercial DNA probes are available, and high performance liquid chromatography cannot identify most REM to species. Biochemical tests including nitrate reduction, iron uptake, and carbohydrate utilization (mannitol, inositol, sorbitol, rhamnose, and citrate) as well as antimicrobial susceptibilities are currently a minimum for phenotypic identification of these species.[10,48]

Molecular Methods

Restriction fragment length polymorphism (RFLP) analysis of selected gene targets such as *hsp65* and the *rpoB* gene and sequencing of variable regions of the 16S rRNA gene as well as other secondary gene targets such as the *hsp65* gene are being used increasingly by many larger reference laboratories.[19,54] Studies using PCR

Table 35-2. Laboratory Features of the Most Commonly Encountered Species of RGM

Species or Complex	Prior Designation	Pigment	3-Day Arylsulfatase	Nitrate Reduction	Iron Uptake	Sole Carbon Sources			Citrate	5% NaCl	Unique hsp65 RFLP PCR Pattern
						Mannitol	Inositol	Sorbitol			
M. abscessus	*M. chelonae* subsp. *abscessus*	–	+	–	–	–	–	–	–	+/–	+
M. chelonae	*M. chelonae* subsp. *chelonae*, *M. chelonei*	–	+	–	–	–	–	–	+	–	+
M. immunogenum	*M. immunogenum*	–	+	–	–	–	–	–	–	–	+
M. fortuitum	*M. fortuitum* biovar *fortuitum*	–	+	+	+	–	–	–	–	+	+
M. peregrinum	*M. fortuitum* biovar *peregrinum* (Type I, pipemidic acid susceptible)	–	+	+	+	+	–	–	–	+	*
M. senegalense	*M. fortuitum* biovar *peregrinum* (Type II, pipemidic acid resistant)	–	+	+	+	+	–	–	–	+	+
M. mageritense	(sorbitol + group)	–	+	+	+	+	+	+	–	+	+
M. houstonense	(sorbitol + group)	–	+	+	+	+	+	+	–	+	+
M. porcinum	(sorbitol – group)	–	+	+	+	+	+	–	–	+	+
M. boenickei	(sorbitol – group)	–	+	+	+†	+	+	–	–	+	+
M. mucogenicum	*M. chelonae*-like organism, MCLO	–	+	±	+†	+	–	–	+	–	+
M. smegmatis	*M. smegmatis* sensu stricto, Type I	+/–	–	+	+	+	+	+	+/–	+	+
M. wolinskyi	*M. smegmatis*, (Type III)	–	–	+	+	+	+	+	+/–	+	+
M. goodii	*M. smegmatis*, (Type II)	+	–	+	+	+	+	+	+/–	+	+

M. peregrinum (formerly Type I) has the same PRA pattern as *M. boenickei* whereas *M. senegalense* (formerly *M. peregrinum* Type II) has the same PRA pattern as *M. houstonense*, and *M. farcinogenes* (a slowly growing NTM).

†Tan appearance.

+ = Positive.

– = Negative.

amplification and restriction endonuclease analysis (PRA) of a 441 bp portion of the 65-Kilodalton heat shock protein (*hsp65*) gene sequence showed single unique restriction fragment length polymorphism (RFLP) patterns for all common species of RGM.[52,53] Using other restriction endonuclease patterns, additional species of RGM may also be identified. Although some modifications or improvements may be necessary to implement this PRA technology for species identification of the RGM into a clinical laboratory, it is readily adaptable to a reference laboratory. PRA seems particularly adaptable to the clinical laboratory for identifying isolates, which yield equivocal results when other identification techniques are used.[53]

Partial gene sequencing is being used increasingly because of the speed of the procedure and the analytical nature of the results. This procedure works well for established species, but there are many species yet to be identified. 16S r-RNA gene sequencing and *hsp65* gene sequence analysis is often necessary to identify or differentiate many of the newly described species.[19]

ANTIMICROBIAL SUSCEPTIBILITY

Current antimicrobial regimens for treatment of disease caused by the RGM are based upon their unique *in vitro* susceptibility patterns.[11,49–51,55–57] Isolates of RGM are not susceptible to the first line antituberculous drugs and require susceptibility testing in specialized mycobacterial laboratories. Laboratory guidelines for susceptibility testing of the RGM have recently been published, including definitions of susceptible and resistant MICs for the recommended drugs.[57] The eight current drugs which should be tested for susceptibility include amikacin, cefoxitin, imipenem, a sulfonamide alone or trimethoprim/sulfamethoxazole, clarithromycin, ciprofloxacin, doxycycline and tobramycin (the latter only for isolates of

M. chelonae). Optional agents include gatifloxacin, moxifloxacin, and linezolid.[55]

Isolates of *M. fortuitum, M. smegmatis,* and *M. mucogenicum* are generally the most susceptible of the more common species of RGM.[9–11,49–51] They are susceptible to amikacin, cefoxitin, imipenem, ciprofloxacin, sulfonamides, and the new 8-methoxyfluoro-quinolones (gatifloxacin and moxifloxacin) with about 50% of the *M. fortuitum* isolates susceptible to doxycycline. Both minocycline and doxycycline are preferred over tetracycline because of greater *in vitro* activity. Clarithromycin inhibits all isolates of *M. chelonae, M. abscessus,* and *M. fortuitum* at a concentration of 4 µg/ml except for approximately 20% of isolates of *M. fortuitum.*[55] Isolates of the *M. smegmatis* group, *M. houstonense,* and *M. mageritense* are resistant.[6,14,16] Clarithromycin is much more active *in vitro* and clinically than the parent macrolide erythromycin, and has replaced it.[55] Recent studies have shown that RGM species that are intrinsically resistant to clarithromycin (e.g., *M. smegmatis*) contain an inducible erythromycin methylase (*erm*) gene that methylates the 23S rRNA macrolide binding site.[58] Interestingly, all isolates of *M. fortuitum* have this gene,[58] which raises questions about its effectiveness for therapy with this species despite MICs often (80%) at "susceptible" drug concentration.

In contrast, isolates of *M. abscessus* and *M. chelonae* are very drug resistant and generally susceptible or intermediate only to amikacin, imipenem, and clarithromycin.[50,51] Isolates of *M. abscessus* are moderately susceptible to cefoxitin (MIC <64 µg/ml) whereas isolates of *M. chelonae* are highly resistant (MIC >256 µg/ml). Additionally, isolates of *M. chelonae* have lower MICs to tobramycin than amikacin, and it is the only species of RGM for which amikacin is not the preferred aminoglycoside. Approximately 20% of the strains of *M. chelonae* are also susceptible to achievable serum levels of ciprofloxacin and/or doxycycline[49–51] (see Tables 35-3 and 35-4).

Table 35-3. Antimicrobials Used for Treatment of Commonly Encountered Species of RGM

Species	Drugs (untreated strains are 100% susceptible unless otherwise noted)
M. fortuitum	Amikacin, ciprofloxacin, imipenem, sulfonamide or trimethoprim/sulfamethoxazole, tigecycline, cefoxitin,† gatifloxacin, clarithromycin (80%), doxycycline (50%), linezolid (86%)
M. abscessus	Amikacin, clarithromycin, tigecycline,* cefoxitin (99%), imipenem (60%), doxycycline (<5%), ciprofloxacin (<5%), gatifloxacin (13%), linezolid (23%)
M. chelonae	Tobramycin, tigecycline clarithromycin, amikacin (70%), imipenem (60%), doxycycline (25%), ciprofloxacin (25%), gatifloxacin (78%), linezolid (54%)

*Investigational (non-FDA approved).
†Includes both susceptide and intermediate strains.

Table 35-4. General Principles of Therapy of RGM Disease

Clinical Setting	Drug Treatment
Pulmonary Disease	
(a) *M. fortuitum*	(a) short term IV treatment (3–6 weeks), then multiple PO medicines for minimum 6 months of negative cultures.
(b) *M. abscessus*	(b) Incurable with drugs. Clinical improvement with clarithromycin or short-term low-dose amikacin and cefoxitin.
Localized Skin/Soft Tissue/Bone Disease	
(a) *M. fortuitum,* *M. chelonae, M. abscessus*	(a) IV treatment for extensive disease (3–6 weeks), followed by PO medicines; PO medicines only for minor disease. Remove catheter or foreign body. Treat 6 months total for significant disease, including all cases with osteomyelitis.
	(b) Linezolid oral or IV treatment has also been successful for *M. chelonae.*
Disseminated (cutaneous) Disease	
(a) *M. chelonae*	(a) Once daily low-dose tobramycin or intermittent imipenem plus clarithromycin for first 3–6 weeks, then clarithromycin only complete 6 mo. Linezolid oral or IV, a potential alternative second agent.
(b) *M. abscessus*	(b) Same as *M. chelonae* except use amikacin in place of tobramycin, and cefoxitin may replace imipenem.

Recently other antimicrobials have been studied which may provide additional therapeutic benefit for treatment of infections due to RGM. These include gatifloxacin, which appears to have better overall activity against the RGM when compared to ciprofloxacin, although most isolates of *M. abscessus* are still resistant.[59]

Additionally, a new oxazolidinone, linezolid, has been shown to have *in vitro* activity against the *M. fortuitum* group (modal MIC was 4 μg/ml) and *M. chelonae* (modal MIC was 8 μg/ml).[60] Linezolid has been used subsequently in the treatment of infections due to RGM including disseminated *M. chelonae* with acquired mutational resistance to clarithromycin.[61]

Finally, a new glycycycline compound which is a derivative of minocycline, tigecycline (formerly GAR 936),

has shown excellent *in vitro* activity with all MICS <1μg/mL against all species of RGM tested including *M. chelonae, M. abscessus*, and tetracycline susceptible and resistant *M. fortuitum* group.[62] It is currently undergoing human clinical trials.

CLINICAL DISEASE

Localized Post-Traumatic Wound Infections

The best known clinical disease syndrome due to RGM is a localized wound infection following accidental trauma.[60,63–65] Table 35-5 shows a list of the types of injury responsible for infections due to RGM. All involve some form of penetrating trauma such as open fracture

Table 35-5. Species or Taxonomic Group and their Common Clinical Diseases

Group	M. fortuitum	M. chelonae	M. abscessus
	Localized post traumatic infections	Disseminated skin infections	Chronic lung infections
	Catheter infections	Localized post traumatic wound infections	Localized post traumatic wound infections
	Surgical wound infections: cardiac surgery, augmentation mammaplasty	Catheter infections	Catheter infections
		Corneal infections	Disseminated skin infections

and stepping on a nail, often followed by osteomyelitis.[65] After an incubation period of 3–6 weeks, local redness and swelling with spontaneous drainage usually occurs. Systemic symptoms such as fever, chills, malaise, and fatigue are usually absent. The drainage is usually thin and watery but occasionally may be thick and purulent. Sinus tract formations with intermittent drainage is common.

The most common pathogens are *M. fortuitum* and members of the *M. fortuitum* third biovariant complex (*M. porcinum, M. houstonense*) in patients with infected open fractures.[6,10,18] These latter infections frequently are polymicrobial, reflecting the heavy nature of the environmental contamination. Essentially all species of RGM including *M. smegmatis*, and the pigmented rapid growers, however, have been associated with this type of infection.[9,11,14,64,66]

Surgical Wound Infections

Surgical wound infections present in a similar fashion to accidental trauma. After an incubation period of 2–8 weeks, the healing wound will develop serous drainage and redness. Localized nodular areas adjacent to the incision may develop which are often painful, and may require incision and drainage. Low-grade fever of 99°–101°F may develop if the wound is extensive. Breast surgery and cardiac surgery are the most common types of surgery to be followed by this complication. Most isolates are *M. fortuitum*, but occasionally other species are involved. Essentially any type of surgery has been followed by RGM infections, including cataract excision, corneal graft,[67] laser surgery,[68] extremity amputations, dacryocystorhinostomy, plastic surgery of the face,[69] prosthetic hip or knee insertions, coronary artery bypass;[25,70] excision of basal cell carcinoma,[71] and as previously mentioned, cosmetic surgeries including liposuction and liposculpture.[26,44,45]

Catheter-Related Infections

The most common healthcare-associated disease since the 1990s has been central venous catheter infections. These may manifest as occult bacteremia, granulomatous hepatitis, septic lung infiltrates, tunnel infections, or exit site infections.[72] The timing of these infections has not been established, but most have been in place at least several months. The usual etiologic agent is *M. fortuitum*.[73] Other long term catheters have been associated with RGM infections, including chronic peritoneal dialysis catheters, hemodialysis catheters, nasolacrimal duct catheters, and ventriculoperitoneal shunts.[6,74,75]

Disseminated Cutaneous Infections

Rapidly growing mycobacteria produce a clinical syndrome that is rarely seen with other nontuberculous mycobacteria. This is the presence of multiple noncontiguous nodular draining skin lesions on one or more extremities. Two basic types of disease are seen. In patients with chronic nonfatal diseases that require chronic steroid therapy, multiple skin lesions develop and tend to be a nuisance rather than life threatening. These almost always involve the lower extremity, and are most often due to *M. chelonae*.[50] Steroid doses may be as low as 5–10 mg prednisone daily. The most common underlying disease is rheumatoid arthritis, but may also include organ transplants, and chronic autoimmune disorders.[50] The patients are often asymptomatic except for the local discomfort of the lesions. Disseminated skin lesions are also seen in patients with rapidly fatal disorders, especially poorly controlled leukemias and lymphoma.[72,74] Their disseminated infection tends to be systemic, with positive cultures of blood and bone marrow. A portal of entry for the organism is rarely identified, but may be a central catheter. This second type of disease is usually caused by *M. abscessus*, and combined with the underlying disease was often fatal in the era before good drugs for therapy were available. Interestingly, *M. fortuitum* is rarely associated with either type of disseminated disease.[72,76]

Chronic Pulmonary Infections

Perhaps because of the frequency of performing mycobacterial cultures with chronic lung infiltrates, this is one of the best known syndromes due to RGM.[27,75] The typical patient is an elderly nonsmoking female who presents with chronic cough and fatigue. By high-resolution computerized tomography (HRCT) of the chest, most patients have patchy cylindrical bronchiectasis and small nodules of <5 mm involving the right middle lobe and lingula. This radiographic pattern is referred to as nodular bronchiectasis, and was first recognized in patients with *M. avium* complex. However, an identical radiographic picture is seen with *M. abscessus*. More than 80% of RGM cases are due to *M. abscessus*.[77] Interestingly, up to 20% of patients will also have *M. avium* complex simultaneously or at different times. The disease tends to be very slowly progressive, with minimal morbidity. Hemoptysis may be present, and fever may occur with more advanced disease.

Several other pulmonary syndromes are recognized. One is a post-tuberculous disease where infection involves the portion of the lung previously damaged by another mycobacteria, especially tuberculosis (TB). Patients with achalasia and chronic vomiting manifest a relatively acute respiratory syndrome associated with high fevers, striking leucocytosis of 20,000 to 40,000 WBC/cu mm, and alveolar infiltrates. Histopathologically lipoid pneumonia is usually present and may be the major risk factor.

The final syndrome is that of positive respiratory cultures in patients with cystic fibrosis.[78–80] Some patients have unremitting fever, some increased hemoptysis or shortness of breath, while others show no apparent change in their clinical symptoms. Much is to be learned about this latter syndrome. Over the past 15 years, documentation of patients with *M. abscessus* lung disease and underlying cystic fibrosis (CF) has been increasing.[81] Although some patients appear to have transient carriage, other patients remain culture positive,[80] with significant symptoms.[82]

Cullen and coworkers reported an unusual case of indolent carriage of *M. abscessus* that only appeared to become clinically active after 13 years.[78] A recent survey of patients with CF revealed that pulmonary infections with RGM, most often *M. abscessus*, are increasingly reported. In assessing 21 U.S. centers for CF, the study showed 16% of the patients had cultures positive for *M. abscessus*. This group of patients, when compared to those with CF but without NTM, tended to be older (26 vs 22 years), had a higher FEV1 (60 vs 54%), a higher frequency of *Staphylococcus aureus* and a lower frequency of *Pseudomonas aeruginosa*.[83] Fauroux et al., also indicated that these characteristics are also frequently associated with worsening clinical status.[79] See Table 35-6 for a list of pulmonary syndromes and their findings.

Central Nervous System Infections

Only a small number of cases of CNS infection due to the RGM have been documented.[84,85] These cases include those associated with infection with a foreign body following a motor vehicle accident, lumbar dissectomy, chronic otitis media, brain abscess, chronic mastoiditis, deep wound infection, and infection of a ventriculoatrial shunt. The majority of these cases are related to infections with *M. fortuitum*.[85]

DRUG THERAPY/DRUG RESISTANCE

Therapy for RGM infections has not been established by clinical trials except for clarithromycin monotherapy for infections due to *M. chelonae*.[86] Current recommendations are based on uncontrolled case series and individual experience. Mutational drug resistance which develops on therapy is a concern for ribosomal active drugs such as clarithromycin and amikacin for *M. chelonae* and *M. abscessus* which have only one

Table 35-6. Pulmonary Syndromes Associated with Positive Respiratory Cultures for RGM

Finding	Interpretation
1. single AFB smear negative culture (+) specimen with low organism colony counts	1. ?transient colonization or contamination
2. multiple culture (+) specimens	
(a) elderly nonsmoking patients no risk factors bilateral streaky infiltrates on chest radiograph	2. (a) probable nodular bronchiectasis (confirm by HRCT)*
(b) prior TB, now with increased infiltrate in same area	(b) post-tuberculous infection
(c) achalasia with chronic vomiting and bilateral interstitial/alveolar infiltrates or known lipoid pneumonia	(c) chronic pneumonitis
(d) cystic fibrosis	(d) ?focal pneumonitis ?colonization (HRCT may be helpful in determination)

*HRCT = high resolution computerized tomography.

chromosomal copy of the ribosome (all other RGM have two copies.)[87] Mutational resistance is also a concern for the quinolones. Hence, therapy with these agents should include combination therapy when possible for extensive disease with presumed large numbers of organisms. Acquired mutational resistance with the tetracyclines and sulfonamide monotherapy has not been described.

The general recommendation for serious wound infections is combination therapy with initial parenteral therapy for *M. chelonae* and *M. abscessus* until clinically improved to be followed by oral therapy. The usual duration of therapy is six months. Abscess drainage and surgical débridement is important. *M. abscessus* lung disease is currently incurable with drugs; therefore intermittent therapy to produce disease suppression is generally attempted. See Tables 35-3 and 35-4 for a summary of drugs and therapeutic approaches.

REFERENCES

1. Cobbett L. An acid-fast bacillus obtained from a pustular eruption. *Br Med J.* 1918;2:158.
2. Moore M, Frerichs JB. An unusual acid fast infection of the knee with subcutaneous, abscess-like lesions of the gluteal region: report of a case study with a study of the organism, *Mycobacterium abscessus. J Invest Dermatol.* 1953;20:133.
3. da Costa Cruz J. *Mycobacterium fortuitum*: new acid fast bacillus pathogenic for man. *Acta Med Rio de Jaeniro.* 1938;1:297.
4. Runyon H. Conservation of the specific epithet *fortuitum* in the name of the organism known as *Mycobacterium fortuitum* da Costa Cruz. *Int J Sys Bacteriol.* 1972;22:50.
5. Kusunoki S, Ezaki T. Proposal of the *Mycobacterium peregrinum* sp. nov., nom, rev., and elevation of *Mycobacterium chelonae* subsp. *abscessus* (Kubica et al.) to species status: *Mycobacterium abscessus* comb. nov. *Int J Syst Bacteriol.* 1992;42:240.
6. Schinsky MF, Morey RE, Steigerwalt AG, et al. Taxonomic variation in the *Mycobacterium fortuitum* third-biovariant complex: Description of *Mycobacterium boenickei* sp. nov., *Mycobacterium houstonense* sp. nov., *Mycobacterium neworleansense* sp. nov., *Mycobacterium brisbanense* sp. nov., and recognition of *Mycobacterium porcinum* from human clinical isolates. *Int. J. Syst. Evol. Microbiol.* 2004;54:1653.
7. Wallace RJ Jr. Recent changes in taxonomy and disease manifestations of the rapidly growing mycobacteria. *Eur J Clin Microbiol Infect Dis.* 1994;13:953.
8. Brown-Elliott BA, Wallace RJ Jr. Clinical and taxonomic status of pathogenic nonpigmented or late-pigmenting rapidly growing mycobacteria. *Clin. Microbiol. Rev.* 2002;15:716.
9. Wallace RJ Jr, Nash DR, Tsukamura M, Blacklock ZM, Silcox VA: Human disease due to *Mycobacterium smegmatis. J Infect Dis.* 1988;158:52.
10. Wallace RJ Jr, Brown BA, Silcox VA, et al. Clinical disease, drug susceptibility, and biochemical pattens of the unnamed third biovariant complex of *Mycobacterium fortuitum. J Infect Dis.* 1991;163:598.
11. Wallace RJ Jr., Silcox VA, Tsukamura M, et al. Clinical significance, biochemical features, and susceptibility patterns of sporadic isolates of the *Mycobacterium chelonae*-like organism. *J. Clin. Microbiol.* 1993;31:3231.
12. Springer B, Böttger EC, Kirschner P, et al. Phylogeny of the *Mycobacterium chelonae*-like organism based on partial sequencing of the 16S rRNA gene and proposal of *Mycobacterium mucogenicum* sp. nov. *Intern J Syst Bacteriol.* 1995;45:262.
13. Domenech P, Jimenez MS, Menendez MC, et al. *Mycobacterium mageritense* sp. nov. *Int J Syst Bacteriol.* 1997;47:535.
14. Brown BA, Springer B, Steingrube VA, et al. *Mycobacterium wolinskyi* sp. nov. and *Mycobacterium goodii* sp. nov., two new rapidly growing species related to *Mycobacterium smegmatis* and associated with human wound infections: a cooperative study from the International Working Group on Mycobacterial Taxonomy. *Int. J. Syst. Bacteriol.* 1999;49:1493.
15. Wilson RW, Steingrube VA, Böttger EC, et al. *Mycobacterium immunogenum* sp. nov. a novel species related to *Mycobacterium abscessus* and associated with clinical disease, pseudo-outbreaks, and contaminated metalworking fluids: an international cooperative study on mycobacterial taxonomy. *Int. J. Syst. Evol. Microbiol.* 2001;51:1751.
16. Wallace RJ Jr., Brown-Elliott BA, Hall L, et al. Clinical and laboratory features of *Mycobacterium mageritense. J Clin Microbiol.* 2002;40:2930.
17. Wallace RJ Jr., Brown-Elliott BA, Hall L, et al. Polyphasic characterization of *Mycobacterium peregrinum* type II: Demonstration as a human pathogen and recognition as human isolates of *Mycobacterium senegalense*. 2004;(in preparation).
18. Wallace RJ Jr, Brown-Elliott BA, Wilson RW, et al. Clinical and laboratory features of *Mycobacterium porcinum. J Clin Microbiol.* 2004;(in press).
19. Tortoli E. Impact of genotypic studies on mycobacterial taxonomy: the new mycobacteria of the 1990s. *Clin Microbiol Rev.* 2003;16:319.
20. Trujillo ME, Velázquez E, Kroppenstedt RM, et al. *Mycobacterium psychrotolerans* sp. nov., isolated from a pond near a uranium mine. *Int J Syst Epidimiol Microbiol.* 2004;(in press).
21. Wallace RJ Jr. Nontuberculous mycobacteria and water: a love affair with increasing clinical importance. *Infect Dis Clin.* 1987;1:677.
22. Wolinsky E. State of the art: nontuberculous mycobacterial and associated disease. *Am Rev Respir Dis.* 1979;119:107.
23. Falkinham JO. Epidemiology of infection by nontuberculous mycobacteria. *Clin Microbiol Rev.* 1996;9:177.
24. Wallace RJ Jr, Steele LC, Labidi A, et al. Heterogeneity among isolates of rapidly growing mycobacteria responsible

for infections following augmentation mammaplasty despite case clustering in Texas and other southern coastal states. *J Infect Dis.* 1989;160:281.

25. Wallace RJ Jr, Musser JM, Hull SI, et al. Diversity and sources of rapidly growing mycobacteria associated with infections following cardiac surgery. *J Infect Dis.* 1989;159:708.

26. Wallace RJ Jr, Koppaka VR. Nontuberculous mycobacteria. In: *Hospital Epidemiology and Infection Control*, 3rd ed., C.G. Mayhall, ed. Lippincott Williams & Wilkins, Philadelphia, PA. 2004;38:667–683.

27. Griffith DE, Wallace RJ Jr. Diagnosis and treatment of rapidly growing mycobacterial lung disease. *Pulm Crit Care Update.* 1993;8(21).

28. Winthrop KL, Albridge K, South D, et al. The clinical management and outcome of nail salon-acquired *Mycobacterium fortuitum* skin infection. *Clin Infect Dis.* 2004;38:38.

29. Cooksey RC, de Waard JH, Yakrus MA, et al. *Mycobacterium cosmeticum* sp. nov., a novel rapidly growing species isolated from a cosmetic infection and from a nail salon (in press).

29a. Gira AK, Reisenauer AH, Hammock L, et al. Furunculosis due to *Mycobacterium mageritense* associated with footbaths at a nail salon. *J Clin Microbiol.* 2004;42:1813.

30. Covert TC, Rodgers MR, Reyes AL, et al. Occurrence of nontuberculous mycobacteria in environmental samples. *Appl Environ Microbiol.* 1999;65:2492.

31. Phillips MS, von Reyn CF. Nosocomial infections due to nontuberculous mycobacteria. *Clin Infect Dis.* 2001;33:1363.

32. Fraser VJ, Jones M, Murray PR, et al. Contamination of flexible fiberoptic bronchoscopes with *Mycobacterium chelonae* linked to an automated bronchoscope disinfection machine. *Am Rev Respir Dis.* 1992;145:853.

33. Gubler JGH, Salfinger M, von Graevenitz A. Pseudoepidemic of nontuberculous mycobacteria due to a contaminated bronchoscope cleaning machine: report of an outbreak and review of the literature. *Chest.* 1992;101:1245.

34. Tiwari TSP, Ray B, Jost KC Jr, et al. Forty years of disinfectant failure: Outbreak of postinjection *Mycobacterium abscessus* infection caused by contamination of benzalkonium chloride. *Clin Infect Dis.* 2003;36:954–962.

35. Carson LA, Bland LA, Cusick LB, et al. Prevalence of nontuberculous mycobacteria in water supplies of hemodialysis centers. *App Environ Microbiol.* 1988;54:3122.

36. Schulze-Röbbecke R, Janning B, Fischeder R. Occurrence of mycobacteria in biofilm samples. *Tuberc Lung Dis.* 1992;73:141.

37. Hector JSR, Pang Y, Mazurek GH, et al. Large restriction fragment patterns of genomic *Mycobacterium fortuitum* DNA as strain-specific markers and their use in epidemiologic investigation of four nosocomial outbreaks. *J Clin Microbiol.* 1992;30:1250.

38. Wallace RJ Jr., Zhang Y, Brown BA, et al. DNA large restriction fragment patterns of sporadic and epidemic nosocomial strains of *Mycobacterium chelonae* and *Mycobacterium abscessus*. *J Clin Microbiol.* 1993;31:2697.

39. Zhang Y, Rajagopalan M, Brown BA, et al. Randomly amplified polymorphic DNA PCR for comparison of

Mycobacterium abscessus strains from nosocomial outbreaks. *J Clin Microbiol.* 1997;35:3132.

39a. Centers for Disease Control and Prevention. Nontuberculous mycobacterial infections after cosmetic surgery-Santo Domingo, Dominican Republic, 2003–2004. *MMWR Morb Mortal Wkly Rep.* 2004;53:509.

40. Lai KK, Brown BA, Westerling JA, et al. Long-term laboratory contamination by *Mycobacterium abscessus* resulting in two pseudo-outbreaks: recognition with use of random amplified polymorphic DNA (RAPD) polymerase chain reaction. *Clin Infect Dis.* 1998;27:169.

41. Villaneuva A, Calderon RV, Vargas BA, et al. Report on an outbreak of post-injection abscesses due to *Mycobacterium abscessus*, including management with surgery and clarithromycin therapy and comparison of strains by random amplified polymorphic DNA polymerase chain reaction. *Clin Infect Dis.* 1997;24:1147.

42. Zhibang Y, BiXia Z, Qishan L, et al. Large-scale outbreak of infection with *Mycobacterium chelonae* subsp. *abscessus* after penicillin injection. *J Clin Microbiol.* 2002;40:2626.

43. Galil K, Miller LA, Yakrus MA, et al. Abscesses due to *Mycobacterium abscessus* linked to injection of unapproved alternative medication. *Emerg Infect Dis.* 1999;5:681.

44. Centers for Disease Control and Prevention. Rapidly growing mycobacterial infection following liposuction and liposculpture—Caracas, Venezuela, 1996–1998. *MMWR Morb Mortal Wkly Rep.* 1998;47:1065.

45. Meyers H, Brown-Elliott BA, Moore D, et al. An outbreak of *Mycobacterium chelonae* infection following liposuction. *Clin Infect Dis.* 2002;34:1500.

46. Woo PCY, Leung K-W, Wong SSY, et al. Relatively alcohol-resistant mycobacteria are emerging pathogens in patients receiving acupuncture treatment. *J Clin Microbiol.* 2002;40:1219.

47. Tang P, Murray C, Alterman C, et al. An outbreak of acupuncture-associated cutaneous *Mycobacterium abscessus*. *ICAAC*, Chicago, 2003:K–1423.

48. Silcox VA, Good RC, Floyd MM: Identification of clinically significant *Mycobacterium fortuitum* complex isolates. *J Clin Microbiol.* 1981;14:686.

49. Wallace RJ Jr, Brown BA, Onyi GO. Susceptibilities of *Mycobacterium fortuitum* biovar. *fortuitum* and the two subgroups of *Mycobacterium chelonae* to imipenem, cefmetazole, cefoxitin, and amoxicillin-clavulanic acid. *Antimicrob Agents Chemother.* 1991;35:773.

50. Wallace RJ Jr, Brown BA, Onyi GO. Skin, soft tissue, and bone infections due to *Mycobacterium chelonae chelonae*: importance of prior corticosteroid therapy, frequency of disseminated infections, and resistance to oral antimicrobials other than clarithromycin. *J Infect Dis.* 1992;166:405.

51. Swenson JM, Wallace RJ Jr, Silcox VA, et al. Antimicrobial susceptibility of five subgroups of *Mycobacterium fortuitum* and *Mycobacterium chelonae*. *Antimicrob Agents Chemother.* 1985;28:807.

52. Telenti A, Marchesi F, Balz M, et al. Rapid identification of mycobacteria to the species level by polymerase chain

reaction and restriction enzyme analysis. *J Clin Microbiol.* 1993;31:175.

53. Steingrube VA, Gibson JL, Brown BA, et al. PCR amplification and restriction endonuclease analysis of a 65-Kilodalton heat shock protein gene sequence for taxonomic separation of rapidly growing mycobacteria. *J Clin Microbiol.* 1995;33:149.

54. Ringuet H, Akoua-Koffi C, Honore S, et al. *hsp65* sequencing for identification of rapidly growing mycobacteria. *J Clin Microbiol.* 1999;37:852.

55. Brown BA, Wallace RJ Jr, Onyi G, et al. Activities of four macrolides, including clarithromycin, against *Mycobacterium fortuitum, Mycobacterium chelonae,* and *M. chelonae*-like organisms. *Antimicrob Agents Chemother.* 1992;36:180.

56. Wallace RJ Jr, Cook JL , Glassroth J, et al. American Thoracic Society Statement: Diagnosis and treatment of disease caused by nontuberculous mycobacteria. *Am Respir Crit Care Med.* 1997;156:S1.

57. NCCLS. Susceptibility testing of mycobacteria, nocardiae, and other aerobic actinomycetes. Approved Standard. NCCLS document M24-A, 2003.

58. Nash KA, Zhang Y, Brown-Elliott BA, et al. Molecular basis of intrinsic macrolide resistance in clinical isolates of *Mycobacterium fortuitum. J Antimicrob Chemother.* 2005; 55:170.

59. Brown-Elliott BA, Wallace RJ Jr, Crist CJ, et al. Comparison of in vitro activities of gatifloxacin and ciprofloxacin against four taxa of rapidly growing mycobacteria. *Antimicrob Agents Chemother.* 2002;46:3283.

60. Wallace RJ Jr, Brown-Elliott BA, Ward SC, et al. Activities of linezolid against rapidly growing mycobacteria. *Antimicrob Agents Chemother.* 2001;45:764.

61. Brown-Elliott BA, Wallace RJ Jr, Blinkhorn R, et al. Successful treatment of disseminated *Mycobacterium chelonae* infection with linezolid. *Clin Infect Dis.* 2001;33:1433.

62. Wallace RJ Jr, Brown-Elliott BA, Crist CJ, et al.Comparison of the in vitro activity of the glycylcycline tigecycline (formerly GAR-936) with those of tetracycline, minocycline, and doxycycline against isolates of nontuberculous mycobacteria. *Antimicrob Agents Chemother.* 2002;46:3164.

63. Turenne CY, Suchak AA, Wolfe JN, et al. Soft tissue infection caused by a novel pigmented, rapidly growing *Mycobacterium* species. *J Clin Microbiol.* 2003;41:2779–2782.

64. Burns JL, Malhotra U, Lingappa J, et al. Unusual presentations of nontuberculous mycobacterial infections in children. *Pediatr Infect Dis J.* 1997;16:802.

65. Miron D, Lev El A, Zuker M, Lumelsky D, et al. *Mycobacterium fortuitum* osteomyelitis of the cuboid after nail puncture wound. *Ped Infect Dis J.* 2000;19:483.

66. Friedman ND, Sexton DJ. Bursitis due to *Mycobacterium goodii*, a recently described, rapidly growing mycobacterium. *J Clin Microbiol.* 2001;39:404.

67. Sudesh S, Cohen EJ, Schwartz LW, et al. *Mycobacterium chelonae* infection in a corneal graft. *Arch Ophthalmol.* 2000;118:294.

68. Reviglio V, Rodriguez ML, Picotti GS, et al. *Mycobacterium chelonae* keratitis following laser in situ keratomileusis. *J Refrac Surg.* 1998;14:357.

69. Pennekamp A, Pfyffer GE, Wüest J, et al. *Mycobacterium smegmatis* infection in a healthy woman following a facelift: case report and review of the literature. *Ann Plast Surg.* 1997;39:80.

70. Cutay AM, Horowitz HW, Pooley RW, et al. Infection of epicardial pacemaker wires due to *Mycobacterium abscessus. Clin Infect Dis.* 1998;26:520.

71. Saluja A, Peters NT, Lowe L, et al. A surgical wound infection due to *Mycobacterium chelonae* successfully treated with clarithromycin. *Dermatol Surg.* 1997;23:539.

72. Choueiry MA, Scurto PL, Flynn PM, et al. Disseminated infection due to *Mycobacterium fortuitum* in a patient with desmoid tumor. *Clin Infect Dis.* 1998;26:237.

73. Raad II, Vartivarian S, Khan A, et al. Catheter-related infections caused by the *Mycobacterium fortuitum* complex: 15 cases and review. *Rev Infect Dis.* 1991;13:1120.

74. Levendoglu-Tugal O, Munoz J, Brudnicki A, et al. Infections due to nontuberculous mycobacteria in children with leukemia. *Clin Infect Dis.* 1998;27:1227.

75. Al Shaalan M, Law BJ, Israels SJ, et al. *Mycobacterium fortuitum* interstitial pneumonia with vasculitis in a child with Wilms' tumor. *Pediatr Infect Dis J.* 1997;16:996.

76. Chetchotisakd P, Mootsikapun P, Anunnatsiri S, et al. Disseminated infection due to rapidly growing mycobacteria in immunocompetent hosts presenting with chronic lymphadenopathy: A previously unrecognized clinical entity. *Clin Infect Dis.* 2000;30:29.

77. Griffith DE, Girard WM, Wallace, RJ Jr. Clinical features of pulmonary disease caused by rapidly growing mycobacteria: An analysis of 154 patients. *Am Rev Respir Dis.* 1993;147: 1271.

78. Cullen AR, Cannon CL, Mark EJ, et al. *Mycobacterium abscessus* infection in cystic fibrosis. *Am J Respir Crit Care Med.* 2000;161:641.

79. Fauroux B, Delaisi B, Clément A, et al. Mycobacterial lung disease in cystic fibrosis: A prospective study. *Pediatr Infect Dis J.* 1997;16:354.

80. Saiman L, Siegel J. Infection control in cystic fibrosis. *Clin Microbiol Rev.* 2004;17:57.

81. Bange F-C, Brown BA, Smaczny C, et al. Lack of transmission of *Mycobacterium abscessus* among patients with cystic fibrosis attending a single clinic. *Clin Infect Dis.* 2001;32:1648.

82. Sanguinetti M, Ardito F, Fiscarelli E, et al. Fatal pulmonary infection due to multidrug-resistant *Mycobacterium abscessus* in a patient with cystic fibrosis. *J Clin Microbiol.* 2001;39:816.

83. Olivier KN, Weber DJ, Wallace RJ Jr, et al. Nontuberculous mycobacteria: 1. Multicenter prevalence study in cystic fibrosis. *Am J Resp Crit Care Med.* 2003;167:828.

84. Flor A, Capdevila JA, Martin N, Gavaldà J, Pahissa A: Nontuberculous mycobacterial meningitis: Report of two cases and review. *Clin Infect Dis.* 1996;23:1266.

85. Cegielski JP, Wallace RJ Jr. Infections due to nontuberculous mycobacteria. In: *Infections of the Central Nervous System*, 2nd ed., WM Scheld, RJ Whitley, DT Durack, eds. Lippincott-Raven Publishers, Philadephia, 1997;24:445.

86. Wallace RJ, Tanner D, Brennan PJ, et al. Clinical trial of clarithromycin for cutaneous (disseminated) infection due to *Mycobacterium chelonae. Ann Int Med.* 1993; 119:482.

87. Wallace RJ Jr, Meier A, Brown BA, et al. Genetic basis for clarithromycin resistance among isolates of *Mycobacterium chelonae* and *Mycobacterium abscessus. Antimicrob Agents Chemother.* 1996;40:1676.

36

Mycobacterium kansasii

Ian A. Campbell
Eleri Davies

INTRODUCTION

Mycobacterium kansasii is an environmental organism which can be isolated from a wide variety of sources including tap water.[1,2] It is not surprising therefore that it can be readily isolated from clinical specimens where it is present as a casual contaminant; however in some patients particularly those with preexisting lung damage, it can cause serious pulmonary disease and in a small number of patients, it has affected lymph nodes, tendon sheaths and skin.

The fact that *M. kansasii* can be present as a casual contaminant causes problems in determining the significance of its isolation from clinical specimens. Broadly speaking, a single isolate from a series of specimens is highly unlikely to be clinically significant whereas multiple isolates obtained from a sequence of specimens are highly significant.

The species was first described by Handuroy[3] and its clear cut relationship to disease was established by the work of Timpe and Runyon in 1954 and Runyon in 1959.[4,5] In the latter paper Runyon divided the "atypical" mycobacteria isolated from clinical specimens into four groups, the first of which (Group 1) contained the photochromogens and thus, by definition, *M. kansasii*. Following Runyon's work it rapidly became evident that in some parts of the world *M. kansasii* was the opportunist mycobacterium which most frequently caused disease. In 1975 a study by the British Thoracic and Tuberculosis Association (BTTA)[6] reported that of 70 males infected with opportunist mycobacteria in England and Wales, *M. kansasii* was the causative organism in 53. Marks showed that there was a significant association between infection with *M. kansasii* and certain types of dusty work.[7] In the BTTA study, current, rather than past, dust exposure was associated with *M. kansasii* infection and was more frequent than in tuberculosis (TB).[6]

The infectivity of *M. kansasii* is low. Depending upon where we live, many of us come in contact with the organism every day and no doubt inhale it in droplet nuclei from taps and showers; however, the incidence of disease remains low. In addition, despite the fact that some patients produce sputum, which is positive on direct smear, only one instance of patient-to-patient transmission has been reported.[8]

In the laboratory, *M. kansasii* is readily identified by its photochromogenicity. There are other mycobacteria, such as *Mycobacterium marinum*, that produce their pigment only on exposure to light. In an experienced laboratory there should be little chance that these two species will be confused.

LABORATORY DIAGNOSIS

Microscopy and Culture

Specimens are examined by the same techniques that are used for the detection and isolation of *Mycobacterium tuberculosis*.[9]

For direct microscopy, sputum smears are stained with the Ziehl-Neelsen or auramine stains in the usual way. On a positive smear the morphology of the bacilli is usually indistinguishable from that of *M. tuberculosis* and the specimen is reported as acid-fast bacilli (AFB) present. Occasionally, the bacilli are long and beaded and, with experience, a more definitive report can be given. In other specimens, such as tissue or pus, this distinctive morphology is rarely if ever visible.

Specimens for culture are pretreated with acid or alkali to remove contaminating bacteria that would otherwise rapidly overgrow the cultures. They are then inoculated into a solid egg medium, such as Löwenstein-Jensen, or onto Middlebrook 7H agar. Alternatively one of the automated methods may be used, such as the BACTEC 460 radiometric system, the BACTEC MGIT (Mycobacteria Growth Indicator Tube) or the MB/BacT (Biomerieux).

Cultures are incubated for at least six weeks at 37°C, after which a report of a negative results can be issued. If colonies are noted during the weekly examination of the slopes or a positive growth index is obtained in an automated system, then further tests are required to confirm the identity of the organism. As the slopes will normally have been incubated in the dark the characteristic yellow pigment will not have been produced, nor is it seen in liquid culture. Hence the appearance of the colonies of *M. kansasii* is not sufficiently distinctive for a positive identification to be made without further tests.

Identification

A ZN stained smear of the growth reveals long beaded bacilli that to the trained eye immediately suggest *M. kansasii*. To confirm the identity it is sufficient to show that the strain grows well at 37°C and not so well at 25°C, that it is sensitive to thiacetazone and that it produces a bright yellow pigment on exposure to light. No other mycobacterium met in clinical practice will have these characteristics.[10] Developments in molecular biology have resulted in specific nucleic acid (NA) probes being used to rapidly identify *M. kansasii* directly from cultures of viable organisms.[11] Recent developments in DNA strip technology, which is based on the reverse hybridization of PCR products to their complementary probes located on strips, have allowed rapid identification directly from cultures of many of the clinically significant mycobacterial species, including *M. kansasii*.[12,13] This method is more sensitive than the NA probes but takes a little longer and is technically more demanding One of the currently available DNA strip systems (INNO-LiPA Mycobacteria, Innogenetics, Ghent, Belgium) is able to split *M. kansasii* into its five subtypes. This has the potential of providing further helpful information to guide patient management.[14,15] Other identification methods include examination of the strain's superficial lipids using thin layer chromatography[16] or 16s rRNA sequencing. RFLP typing could be useful in determining if a patient has relapsed disease or has acquired new infection.

Sensitivity Tests

The relationship between the sensitivity of most opportunist mycobacteria tested to single drugs *in vitro* and their *in vivo* response is complicated. Fortunately, in this respect *M. kansasii* is more like *M. tuberculosis* than other opportunist mycobacteria in that *in vitro* sensitivity is mirrored by *in vivo* response. The techniques used to determine the sensitivity of *M. tuberculosis* strains to the normally available drugs are therefore applicable to *M. kansasii*. Thus the modal resistance method of Marks[17] or the BACTEC 460 automated system may be used.[18] Strains from untreated patients are usually sensitive to rifampicin, ethambutol, ethionamide (prothionamide), cycloserine, capreomycin, and to the newer macrolides.[19] There is a low level of resistance to streptomycin and they are fully resistant to isoniazid and pyrazinamide.

EPIDEMIOLOGY

As with other opportunist mycobacteria, the true incidence of infection with *M. kansasii* is difficult, if not impossible, to determine. Systems for notification vary from country to country, but in none of them is *M. kansasii* infection a statutorily notifiable disease, unlike infections due to *M. tuberculosis*. Prior to the human immunodeficiency virus (HIV) epidemic, *M. kansasii* was the commonest of the opportunist mycobacterial species encountered in Western Europe, Texas and the upper central states of the United States of America (USA), whereas *Mycobacterium avium intracellulare scrofulaceum* (MAIS) predominated in south-eastern USA, Western Australia and Japan.[20–23] In England and Wales as a whole *M. kansasii* was the commonest species, but in London and the south-east of England *Mycobacterium xenopi* was isolated more frequently than *M. kansasii* or the MAIS complex.[24,25] In England and Wales a laboratory-based reporting system for the opportunist mycobacteria has been in existence since 1981. This shows that, on average, there are 54 new cases of pulmonary disease caused by *M. kansasii* every year. This figure has remained steady, in contrast with the figures for the MAIS complex, which have increased markedly as a result of patients with acquired immunodeficiency syndrome (AIDS). It is not understood why AIDS patients are more likely to be infected with the MAIS complex rather than other opportunist mycobacteria such as *M. kansasii*, to which they are equally exposed.

CLINICAL FEATURES

Patients usually present with a subacute or chronic pattern of symptoms which may include one or more of cough, phlegm, hemoptysis, breathlessness, night sweats, malaise, fatigue and weight loss, but between 10–40% may be asymptomatic.[26–28] The majority have coexisting lung disease such as chronic bronchitis and emphysema, bronchiectasis, or pneumoconiosis.[6,26,29–33] The disease is at least three times commoner in men than in women[20–27] and is found more in middle to old age.[28,32–35] Peptic ulcer, previous gastroduodenal surgery, and conditions associated with reduction in immune response are said to predispose to *M. kansasii* infection but it is not certain whether these are true associations. Fever is not uncommon but usually the physical signs, if present at all, are those of chronic bronchitis and emphysema.

Symptoms and signs are not sufficiently different to allow differentiation between infection with *M. kansasii* and infection with *M. tuberculosis*. Hemoptysis occurs in around 30%, more frequently than in pulmonary TB whereas diabetes mellitus and alcohol in excess of 14 units per week are seen more in patients with tuberculous infection.[26–28] Evans and Colville found no significant differences between the two infections in drug history (including immunosuppressives), past or present smoking, social class, marital status, occupational exposures, history of chest disease, or coexisting lung disease.[28]

Sputum was positive on direct smear in 60% of the 173 patients in the British Thoracic Society's study,[32] in 48% of the Czech patients,[33] and in 63% of the Nottingham patients, much the same as for *M. tuberculosis.*[28]

RADIOLOGICAL FEATURES

In the large study by the British Thoracic Society (BTS) cavitation was seen in 88% of the pre-treatment chest radiographs and in half of these one or more of the cavities were >2 cm. in diameter. In 48% of the patients disease was bilateral and 3 or more lung zones were affected in 46%. Shadowing was limited to one or both upper zones in 28%. Other pulmonary, pleural and/or cardiac diseases were evident in 61%.[32] Pleural effusion was extremely rare, as reported in an earlier series[36] and described again more recently.[37] Christensen et al. also noted that hilar and/or mediastinal lymphadenopathy was rare.[38] In those studies comparing the radiological appearances of *M. tuberculosis, M. kansasii* and other opportunist mycobacteria, pleural effusion and lower lobe involvement were noted more frequently in patients with *M. tuberculosis* but all agreed that in an individual patient the radiological appearances do not allow physicians to distinguish one infection from another.[36–39]

TREATMENT AND OUTCOME

Despite earlier skepticism about whether the disease warranted treatment and about whether chemotherapy or surgery was better, it was accepted by the 1970s that *M. kansasii* infection generally responded well to antimycobacterial therapy,[40] in contrast to disease caused by other opportunist mycobacteria.[41–43] The report by Banks et al. emphasized the importance of rifampicin and ethambutol: among 30 patients treated for periods ranging from 3–24 months there was 100% cure and none relapsed during follow-up for a mean of 5 years.[26]

In 1994 the BTS reported the results of a prospective study in 173 patients of 9 months treatment with rifampicin and ethambutol: there was only one failure of treatment, a man who admitted noncompliance with chemotherapy. The sputum conversion rates during treatment are shown in Table 36-1. By the end of treatment the patients had gained an average of 2.2 kg. Two-thirds consistently showed satisfactory clinical progress during and after treatment. Of the remainder in only 20% was there a period of unsatisfactory clinical

Table 36-1. Sputum Smear and Culture Results During Treatment

	Months of Treatment			
	3	**7**	**8**	**9**
Culture-positive %	11	2	0.6	0
Culture-negative %	53	67	55	68
No sputum coming up or none sent %	36	31	44	32
Positive smear with negative culture %	2	0.6	0	0.6

progress attributed to *M. kansasii*. Radiological healing occurred within three years of completing treatment in 80%. Of 154 patients entering the posttreatment follow-up period, 15 developed positive cultures in the 51 months after the end of chemotherapy (Table 36-2). Eight of these relapses were thought to have been influenced by factors such as lack of compliance with treatment, malnourishment, corticosteroid therapy, severe bronchiectasis and the development of laryngeal carcinoma, which was then treated with radiotherapy. In a further three patients, the radiological features at the time of the new positive cultures suggested reinfection rather than relapse. Thus in only 4 patients (2.3%) was there no reasonable explanation for relapse. Relapse rates were no different between those patients who had initially received isoniazid as a third drug (before the diagnosis had been confirmed as *M. kansasii*) and those who had received only rifampicin and ethambutol. All of the relapses/reinfections responded to further treatment with rifampicin and ethambutol.[32]

Another prospective study, in which a 12-month regimen of ethambutol, rifampicin, and isoniazid was used, reported that 2.5% of the patients relapsed in follow-up periods that varied between 3 and 5 years.[29] The retrospective study in Czechoslovakia reported an 8% relapse rate among 471 patients treated with various antimycobacterial regimens and followed up for periods of between 1–7 years.[33] In Australia no relapses were found among 32 patients treated for up to two years with various regimens, most of which contained rifampicin and ethambutol, and followed up for a mean of five years (range 6 months to 16 years): reinfection was thought to have occurred in one patient who had been free of disease for 12 years.[31] In Barcelona, 28 patients, treated for 6–18 months with regimens incorporating ethambutol, rifampicin, and isoniazid, and followed up for 12–30 months after the end of chemotherapy, there was

Table 36-2. *M. kansasii*: Relapse Rates in Seven Studies

No. Patients	Retrospective (R)		Prospective (P)	
	Duration Rx	**Regimens**	**Follow-up**	**Relapse**
28 (R)	12–18 months	EHR	12–30 months	4%
30 (R)	3–24 months	90% ER	Up to 10 year	0
32 (R)	Up to 24 months	Various	6 months to 16 year	0
39 (R)	Up to 22 months	ER +/– H +/– Z initially	6 months to 9 year	0
471 (R)	9–12 months	Various	Up to 5 hr	8%
40 (P)	12 months	HER	50% for 3 year	2.5%
			30% for 5 year	
173 (P)	9 months	ER +/– H +/– Z +/– S initially	5 year	9%

only one relapse (3.5%).[27] No relapses were noted in a study by Evans et al. of 39 patients treated with rifampicin and ethambutol for an average of about 10 months, most also receiving isoniazid for the majority of the period. Follow-up after chemotherapy averaged around 18 months (Table 36-2).[28]

In the current state of knowledge it would seem that a regimen of 9 months of ethambutol and rifampicin should be sufficient for the majority of patients, but for those with overtly compromised defenses, therapy should probably be continued for 15–24 months or until the sputum has been negative on culture for 12 months. If patients fail to respond to ethambutol and rifampicin then prothionamide and/or streptomycin can be added. Patients suspected of noncompliance with treatment should be followed up indefinitely and any relapse should be retreated with 15–24 months of ethambutol and rifampicin. Macrolides have been shown to be active *in vivo* against *M. kansasii* but their place in treatment remains to be determined by clinical trial.

During the five years of the BTS study 23% of 173 patients died, but in none was *M. kansasii* implicated as the cause of death. High death rates from causes other than *M. kansasii* infection were found by Banks et al. (37%)[21] and by Pang (30%).[31] In the large survey by Kaustova et al., 53 of 471 (11%) died during the period covered by the survey, a period which ranged from 2–7 years and in 4 (0.8%) the deaths were attributed to *M. kansasii*.[33] In the comparative study from Nottingham, Evans et al. noted that 21% of the patients with *M. kansasii* died during a period of observation ranging from 6–108 months (mean observation period = 37 months), compared with 23% in those with *M. tuberculosis* (mean observation period = 26 months,

range 2–104). In two of the four patients with *M. kansasii* who died before treatment was started, the infection was thought to have contributed to death: one of these patients had Hodgkin's lymphoma and the other thyrotoxicosis. In another patient who died three weeks into treatment, *M. kansasii* infection was given as the cause of death. So, between 2% and 6% died because of *M. kansasii* infection, compared with 9% (8 of 87) dying because of *M. tuberculosis*.[28] In a BTS study, death rates in patients with disease caused by other species of opportunist mycobacteria ranged between 34% and 69%; as for *M. kansasii*, the deaths directly attributed to those other species (4–7%) were considerably less than the overall deaths.[41–43] Pulmonary disease caused by *M. kansasii* thus carries a better prognosis than that caused by the other opportunist mycobacteria.

EXTRA-PULMONARY DISEASE

The diagnosis of superficial lymph node, skin/wound, bone/joint or genitourinary infection with *M. kansasii* depends, as for pulmonary disease, on the isolation and identification of the organism from a specimen of the affected tissue. In the large Czech study, extrapulmonary disease was noted in only 0.6% of the patients,[33] but in England and Wales between 1982 and 1994, 9% of 759 *M. kansasii* infections were extrapulmonary.[44]

Lymph node infection with opportunist mycobacteria, predominantly a disease of young children, is usually caused by the MAIS complex and only rarely caused by *M. kansasii*. The enlarged nodes are usually painless and unaccompanied by systemic upset. The condition is treated by excision of the affected nodes in preference to chemotherapy.[45–47] If disease recurs, there should be further excision of the nodes followed by chemotherapy with rifampicin and ethambutol for 9–24 months. Aspiration of the node, or excision and drainage, should be avoided because such procedures may leave a persistently discharging sinus and sometimes leave scarring.

Infection at sites other than the superficial lymph nodes should be treated with rifampicin and ethambutol. There are insufficient data to give good guidance about duration of chemotherapy: it would seem reasonable to treat for 9 months in the first instance. Discussion about the inclusion of isoniazid and/or a macrolide is as yet informed only by anecdote and/or by *in vitro* work.

M. KANSASII AND HIV INFECTION

M. kansasii is infrequently encountered in the HIV positive/AIDs populations in whom, of the opportunist mycobacteria, the MAIS complex is the predominant pathogen.[44] As for MAIS, infection may be localized to the lung but it is more likely to be disseminated and accompanied by bacteremia. There is no good *in vivo* evidence to suggest that any other regimen is better than rifampicin and ethambutol.[48] It is not known whether such therapy will affect life expectancy in these patients, but it is usually given on the basis of reducing symptoms. If immunocompetence can be restored by highly active antiretroviral therapy (HAART) theoretically it should be possible to discontinue antimycobacterial therapy once cultures have been negative for 12 months or more. Otherwise it would seem reasonable to continue treatment indefinitely.

REFERENCES

1. Joynson D. Water: the natural habitat of *Mycobacterium kansasii*. *Tubercle*. 1979;60–77.
2. McSwiggan DA, Collins CH. The isolation of *M. kansasii* and *M. xenopi* from water systems. *Tubercle*. 1974;55:291.
3. Handuroy P. Derniers *Aspects du Mond des Mycobacteries*. Paris: Masson; 1955.
4. Timpe A, Runyon EH. The relationship of "atypical" acid-fast bacteria to human disease: A preliminary report. *J Lab Clin Med*. 1954;44:202.
5. Runyon EH. Anonymous mycobacteria in pulmonary disease. *Med Clin North Am*. 1959;43:273.
6. British Thoracic and Tuberculosis Association. Opportunist mycobacterial pulmonary infection and occupational dust exposure: An investigation in England and Wales. *Tubercle*. 1975;56:295.
7. Marks J. Occupation and *M. kansasii* infection in Cardiff residents. *Tubercle*. 1975;56:311.
8. Penny ME, Cole RB, Gray J. Two cases of *Mycobaterium kansasii* infection occurring in the same household. *Tubercle*. 1982;63:129.
9. Jenkins PA. The microbiology of tuberculosis. In: Davies PDO, ed. *Clinical Tuberculosis*. London: Chapman and Hall; 1994:34.
10. Marks J. Classification of mycobacteria in relation to clinical significance. *Tubercle*. 1972;53:259.
11. Reisner BS, Gatson AM, Woods GL. Use of Gen-Probe AccuProbes to identify Mycobacterium avium complex, *Mycobacterium tuberculosis* complex, *Mycobacterium kansasii*, and Mycobacterium gordonae directly from BACTEC TB broth cultures. *J Clin Microbiol*. 1994; 32:2995.
12. Makinen J, Sarkola A, Marjamaki M, et al. Evaluation of GenoType and LiPA Mycobacteria assays for identification of Finnish Mycobacterial isolates. *J Clin Microbiol*. 2002;40:3478.
13. Padilla E, Gonzalez V, Manterola JM, et al. Comparative evaluation of the new version of the INNO-LiPA Mycobacteria and GenoType Mycobacterium assays for identification of Mycobacterium species from MB/BacT liquid cultures artificially inoculated with Mycobacterial strains. *J Clin Microbiol*. 2004;42:3083.
14. Alcaide F, Richter I, Bernasconi C, et al. Heterogeneity and clonality among isolates of *Mycobacterium kansasii*: implications for epidemiological and pathogenicity studies. *J Clin Microbiol*. 1997;35:1959–1964.
15. Picardeau M, Prod'Hom G, Raskine L, et al. Genotypic characterisation of five subspecies of *Mycobacterium kansasii*. *J Clin Microbiol*. 1997;35:25–32.
16. Szulga T, Jenkins PA, Marks J. Thin layer chromatography of mycobacterial lipids as an aid to classification: *M. kansasii* and M. marinum (balnei). *Tubercle*. 1966;47:130.
17. Marks J. The design of sensitivity tests on tubercle bacilli. *Tubercle*. 1961;42:314.
18. Lazlo A, Gill P, Handzel V, et al. Conventional and radiometric drug susceptibility testing of *Mycobacterium tuberculosis* complex. *J Clin Microbiol*. 1983;18:1335.
19. Yew WW, Piddock LJV, Li MSK et al. *In vitro* activity of quinolones and macrolides against mycobacteria. *J Antimicrob Chemother*. 1994;34:343.
20. Jenkins PA. Non-tuberculous mycobacteria and disease. *Eur J Respir Dis*. 1981;62:69.
21. Selkon JB. Atypical mycobacteria: A review. *Tubercle*. 1969;50(Suppl):70.
22. Edwards FGB. Disease caused by "atypical" (opportunist) mycobacteria: A whole population review. *Tubercle*. 1970;51:285.
23. Tsukamura M, Kita N, Skimoide H, et al. Studies on the epidemiology of nontuberculous mycobacteriosis in Japan. *Am Rev Respir Dis*. 1988;137:1280.
24. Marks J, Schwabacher HB. Infection due to *M. xenopi*. *Br Med J*. 1965;1:32.
25. Grange JM, Yates MD. Infections caused by opportunist mycobacteria: A review. *J Soc Med*. 1986;79:226.

26. Banks J, Hunter AM, Campbell IA, et al. Pulmonary infection with *Mycobacterium kansasii* in Wales, 1970-9: Review of treatment and response. *Thorax.* 1983;38:271.

27. Sauret J, Hernandez-Flix S, Castro E, et al. Treatment of pulmonary disease caused by *Mycobacterium kansasii*: Results of 18 vs. 12 months chemotherapy. *Tuberc Lung Dis.* 1995;76:104.

28. Evans SA, Colville A, Evans AJ, et al. Pulmonary *Mycobacterium kansasii* infection: Comparison of the clinical features, treatment and outcome with pulmonary tuberculosis. *Thorax.* 1996;51:1248.

29. Ahn CH, Lowell JR, Ahn SS, et al. Short-course chemotherapy for pulmonary disease caused by *Mycobacterium kansasii*. *Am Rev Respir Dis.* 1983;128:1048.

30. Schraufanagel DE, Leech JA, Pollak B. *Mycobacterium kansasii*: Colonisation and disease. *Br J Dis Chest.* 1986; 80:131.

31. Pang SC. *Mycobacterium kansasii* infections in Western Australia (1982–1987). *Respir Med.* 1991;85:213.

32. Research Committee, British Thoracic Society. Mycobacterium kansasii pulmonary infection: A prospective study of the result of 9 months' treatment with rifampicin and ethambutol. *Thorax.* 1994;49:442.

33. Kaustova J, Chmelik M, Ettlova D, et al. Disease due to *Mycobacterium kansasii* in Czech Republic 1984–1989. *Tuberc Lung Dis.* 1995;76:205.

34. Bates JH. A study of pulmonary disease associated with mycobacteria other than *Mycobacterium tuberculosis*: Clinical characteristics. *Am Rev Respir Dis.* 1967;96:1151.

35. Waldermar G, Johanson JR, Nicholson DP. Pulmonary disease due to *Mycobacterium kansasii*: An analysis of some factors affecting prognosis. *Am Rev Respir Dis.* 1969;99:73.

36. Christensen EE, Dietz GW, Ahn CH, et al. Initial roentgenographic manifestations of pulmonary *Mycobacterium tuberculosis*, *M. kansasii* and *M. intracellularis*. *Chest.* 1971;80:132.

37. Evans AJ, Crisp AJ, Hubbard RB, et al. Pulmonary *Mycobacterium kansasii* infection: Comparison of radiological appearances with pulmonary tuberculosis. *Thorax.* 1996;51:1243.

38. Christensen EE, Dietz GW, Ahn CH, et al. Radiographic manifestations of pulmonary *Mycobacterium kansasii* infections. *Am J Roentgenol.* 1978;131:985.

39. Zvetina JR, Demos PC, Maliwan N. Pulmonary cavitations in *Mycobacterium kansasii*: Distinction from *M. tuberculosis*. *AJR Am J Roentgenol.* 1984;143:127.

40. Wolinsky E. Non-tuberculous mycobacteria and associated diseases. *Am Rev Respir Dis.* 1979;119:107.

41. The Research Committee of the British Thoracic Society. Pulmonary disease caused by *Mycobacterium avium-intracellulare* in HIV-negative patients: five-year follow-up of patients receiving standardized treatment. *Int J Tuberc Lung Dis.* 2002;6(7):628.

42. The Research Committee of the British Thoracic Society. Pulmonary disease caused by *M. malmoense* in HIV-negative patients: 5-yr follow-up of patients receiving standardized treatment. *Eur Respir J.* 2003;21:478.

43. Jenkins PA, Campbell IA and Research Committee of the British Thoracic Society. Pulmonary disease caused by Mycobacterium xenopi in HIV-negative patients: five year follow-up of patients receiving standardized treatment. *Respir Med.* 2003;97:439.

44. Lamden K, Watson JM, Knerer G, et al. Opportunist mycobacteria in England and Wales: 1982–1994. CDR Review. 1996;6:147.

45. Prissick FH, Masson AM. Cervical lymphadenitis in children caused by chromogenic mycobacteria. *Can Med Assoc J.* 1956;75:798.

46. McKellar A. Diagnosis in management of atypical mycobacterial lymphadenitis in children. *J Pediatr Surg.* 1976;11:85.

47. White NP, Bangash H, Goel KM, et al. Non-tuberculous mycobacterial lymphadenitis. *Arch Dis Child.* 1986;61:368.

48. Sub-committee of the Joint Tuberculosis Committee of the British Thoracic Society: Management of opportunist mycobacterial infections: Joint Tuberculosis Committee guidelines 1999. *Thorax.* 2000;55(3):210.

37

Mycobacterium marinum

Emmanuelle Cambau
Alexandra Aubry
Vincent Jarlier

INTRODUCTION AND HISTORY

The first report of a mycobacterium isolated in fish, supposed to be *Mycobacterium marinum*, has been attributed to Bataillon et al. (1897) who isolated acid-fast bacilli named *Mycobacterium piscium* from a tuberculous lesion in a common carp (*Cyprinus carpio*).[1] *Mycobacterium marinum* was originally isolated and identified from marine at the Philadelphia Aquarium.[2] Initially *M. marinum* was thought to infect marine fish only, and was named accordingly, but it is now known to be a ubiquitous species. The original freshwater isolate of *M. piscium* was, possibly, a *M. marinum* variant. In the early literature, various other *Mycobacterium* species may be encountered, such as *Mycobacterium platypoecilus*, *Mycobacterium anabanti*, and *Mycobacterium balnei*. Comparative sugar fermentative reaction together with published morphological, cultural, and pathogenesis data suggested that they were all synonymous of *M. marinum*[3,4] even if *M. piscium* has not been recognized as a valid species, since its type culture was no longer available.

Human infection due to *M. marinum* was reported as a tuberculoid infection in people using public swimming pools in Sweden (1939) and in the US (1951).[5] Linell and Norden identified the causative organism in 1954 after 80 persons had showed the same granulomatous skin lesions.[6] These early findings led to the disease's once-common name of "swimming pool granuloma." Today, however, due to sanitary chlorination practices, these kinds of outbreaks are seen very rarely. The names "fish tank granuloma" and "fish handler's disease" are now used because of the association with home aquariums and water-related activities such as swimming, fishing and boating.[7]

Scientific interest in *M. marinum* is mainly due to its genetic relation with *M. tuberculosis* and because experimental infection of *M. marinum* in goldfish (*Carassius auratus*) mimics tuberculosis (TB).[8]

FUNDAMENTAL BIOLOGY OF *M. MARINUM*

Taxonomy

M. marinum is one of the 90–100 species of the genus *Mycobacterium*,[9] the only genus of the *Mycobacteriaceae* family. *M. marinum* is an atypical mycobacteria or non tuberculous mycobacteria (NTM) or mycobacteria other than *M. tuberculosis* (MOTT). According to the Runyon's classification, it belongs to the group I composed of photochromogenic species. Although it can grow in less than 7 days, its characteristics are far different from the so-called rapidly growing species of mycobacteria, such as *Mycobacterium chelonae* or *Mycobacterium fortuitum*. Since it carries a single rRNA operon[10] and its 16S rRNA sequence contains the molecular signature of slow growing mycobacteria,[11] it definitely belongs to the slow growing group of mycobacteria. *M. marinum* is a pathogenic mycobacteria, which makes it, along with its related species *Mycobacterium ulcerans*, apart from the other NTM that are opportunistic pathogens.[12]

From phylogenetic analysis based on the 16SrRNA, *M. marinum* lies on a branch of the genus that is close to the branch containing members of the *M. tuberculosis* complex. DNA-DNA hybridization and mycolic acids studies confirm that *M. marinum* is one of the two species (still along with *M. ulcerans*) most closely related to the *M. tuberculosis* complex.[13–15]

Genetics

The study of the *M. marinum* genome has been undertaken at Sanger Institute and is currently complete although not published yet (www.sanger.ac.uk/Projects/M_marinum). The length of *M. marinum* genome is 6.5 Mbs, which is larger than that of *M. tuberculosis* (4.4 Mbs), that of *M. leprae* (3.3 Mbs) and that of *M. ulcerans* (5.8 Mbs),[16,17] (Burulist web server at Pasteur Institute http://genopole.pasteur.fr/). Like *M. tuberculosis* and other slow-growing mycobacteria, *M. marinum* has a single rRNA operon[10] located downstream from the *murA* gene as in the *M. tuberculosis* genome. Overall, *M. marinum* genetics are very close to those of *M. ulcerans* with a high similarity (more than 99% similarity in 16SrRNA) for all housekeeping and structural genes such as those coding for the ribosomal operon, RNA polymerase (*rpoB*), DNA gyrase (*gyrA* and *gyrB*) and the heat shock protein 65 kDa (*hsp*). The minor nucleotide differences in some of these genes that are observed have been related to strain variation and cannot differentiate *M. marinum* from *M. ulcerans*.[14,17–19] The conclusion is, that *M. marinum* seems to be *M. ulceran's* ancestor.[17] Divergence would have occurred along with the gain by *M. ulcerans* of genes such as the "polyketide synthase" encoding the virulence factor mycolactone,[20] and of the insertion sequences IS 2404 and 2606 that do not exist in *M. marinum*.[17,18] The presence in *M. marinum* of insertion sequences homologous to IS 1245 and IS 1311[21] needs to be confirmed by the genome analysis.

Molecular biology of *M. marinum* has been developed because it is less pathogenic and grows faster than *M. tuberculosis* and thus is a suitable model for TB pathogenesis.[27] Genetic manipulations such as transformation and transposition have been successful.[23,24] About 30 virulence genes have been brought up by gene expression either in cultured macrophages or in granuloma.[22,25,26] Mutations in the virulence genes are often complemented by the corresponding gene of *M. tuberculosis* that demonstrates the high relatedness of the genome of the two species.

Pathogenesis

The availability of fish models (Goldfish, Zebrafish) mimicking a natural mycobacterial infection[27–29] enables the study of the pathogen-host interaction. A new model of infection has been described in *Drosophila melanogaster*, where *M. marinum* infection is lethal at a low dose.[30]

Both *M. tuberculosis* and *M. marinum* are intracellular pathogens that proliferate within macrophages in a non-acid (pH 6.1-6.5) phagosome that does not fuse with the lysosome.[22,31,32] Taking into account that both species are also genetically related, it is probable that analogous molecular mechanisms are involved in the survival of these organisms in a hostile cell environment. *M. marinum* is therefore a very useful model system for studying intracellular survival of mycobacteria and possible other host–pathogen interactions associated with TB.[29,33] The organism is able to survive, replicate in macrophages and even escape from the phagosomes into the cytoplasm where it can induce actin polymerization leading to direct cell spread.[34,35] Ultra-structure studies have showed that *M. marinum* stays within activated macrophages in granulomas.

Some of the genes that seem to be important in the capacity to replicate in macrophages and to explain the persistence in granulomas are homologous to the PE-PGRS family of genes discovered in *M. tuberculosis* genome.[25] Recently, *pimF*, a mannosyltranferase and *kasB*, a keto-acyl carrier protein synthase, showed to be essential for the initial cell entry step and cell wall impermeability to host defense molecules.[33,36]

Biochemical Features

The cell wall of *M. marinum* is mainly composed of keto-mycolates and methoxy-mycolates that differentiate from those of *M. tuberculosis* and of other mycobacteria except *M. ulcerans*.[14,37]

The study of extracellular products of *M. marinum* showed a mucinase activity while lipase and RNase activities were detected for *Mycobacterium chelonae* and *Mycobacterium fortuitum*.[38]

Photochromogenicity is due to the active production of beta-carotene mediated by the gene *crtB*, and can be inhibited by chloramphenicol.[9]

MICROBIOLOGICAL CHARACTERS OF *M. MARINUM*

Characters Common to Mycobacteria

Under the microscope, *M. marinum* cannot be distinguished from *M. tuberculosis*. It is a pleomorphic rod (1.0–4.0 µm × 0.2–0.6 µm), not motile, true branching, difficult to stain by usual methods but appears as an acid-fast bacillus after staining by the reference carbol fuchsin or Ziehl-Neelsen method.[39] Like other mycobacteria, *M. marinum* is a strict aerobe. Its preferred carbon sources are glycerol, pyruvate and glucose but ethanol can be also used by *M. marinum*.

Specific Characters of M. marinum

Culture

M. marinum has an optimal growth temperature at 30°C, whereas small colonies or no growth are observed at 37°C.

In primary culture, the growth rate might be slow and positive culture may be obtained only after several weeks' incubation. In subculture, growth rate is between 1 and 2 weeks but can reach 4–5 days because of its rapid ability to adapt to laboratory conditions.

M. marinum grows in all the media used for mycobacterial growth (egg-based, broth, agar-based) without any additives, and also on blood containing agar. After subcultures, some of the strains may even grow on ordinary culture media.

Although like other mycobacteria its growth is dependent on oxygen, 2–5% carbon dioxide in the gas phase above the medium improves the growth of *M. marinum*.

Phenotypic Characters

Colonies of *M. marinum* are typically smooth or intermediate, white or beige when the media is kept at the obscurity and yellow to orange after exposure to light (photochromogen).[39,40] This places it in the group I of Runyon's classification along with *M. kansasii*. Differentiation between these two pathogenic NTM is then done on the basis of biochemical characteristics. The absence of production of nitrate reductase, and growth on medium containing thiacetazone is in favor of *M. marinum*.

Molecular Identification

Molecular biology techniques have been only fairly recently been applied to *M. marinum*. Molecular methods are an alternative for speciation offering the advantages of being rapid and accurate. Today, nucleic acid probes, such as AccuProbe used for *M. tuberculosis* complex identification, are not available for *M. marinum*. PCR-based methods have been developed. Their disadvantages are false-positivity related to the PCR technique itself, and relative high cost compared to classic tools. One of these methods has been commercially developed as INNOLiPA Mycobacteria (Innogenetics). It is based on the amplification of the 16S-23S rRNA spacer, and reverse hybridization to 23 different sequences specific of different mycobacterial species.[41] Indeed, it cannot differentiate *M. marinum* from *M. ulcerans* since the rRNA sequences are similar (see genetics).

Genotyping

Although infection due to *M. marinum* is not contagious between humans, strain genotyping has been undertaken for three reasons: first, to relate environmental strains to strains isolated in infected humans; second, to differentiate strains in aquaculture isolated among fish or water living animals[19] and; third, to demonstrate relapse or reinfection.[42] The technique used was pulse field gel electrophoresis. PCR based methods have been tested but showed low discriminative properties.[21]

M. MARINUM INFECTION

Manifestations of *M. marinum* Disease

Fish Disease

M. marinum disease in fish may occur in either an acute or a chronic form. The acute fulminating disease is rare and is characterized by rapid morbidity and mortality with few clinical signs. *M. marinum* infection is more often chronic progressive disease that may take years to develop into a noticeable illness. Affected fish show behavioral changes such as separating from other fish, and refusing food. They may have skin ulcerations or pigment alterations, and develop spinal curvature. Unilateral or bilateral exophthalmia is also a typical feature.

In fish, *M. marinum* infection is a systemic disease that can affect virtually any organ system, but especially the spleen, kidney and liver.[38]

Human Disease

Due to the optimal growth at 30°C and poor growth at 37°C, human infections with *M. marinum* are localized primarily to the skin. Systemic dissemination is exceptional and has been reported to occur only in immunocompromised patients.[6,43] Infection in HIV positive patients is usually not different from infection in HIV negative patients.

M. marinum infection has different clinical presentations (Table 37-1). Most commonly (about 60% of the cases),[44] *M. marinum* is a cutaneous disease as a solitary papulonodule on a finger or hand. In 25% of the cases, *M. marinum* disease takes on a "sporotrichoid" form[44,45] (Fig. 37-1). This occurs when the infection spreads along the lymphatic vessels to the regional lymph node producing multiple nodules resembling sporotrichosis. Occasionally skin lesions appear as pustular, noduloulcerative, granulomatous, or verrucous plaques.

Deep infections such as tenosynovitis (the most frequent), osteomyelitis, arthritis, and bursitis occur in 20–40% of the cases[44–47] (Fig. 37-2). They result from the extension of a cutaneous infection or direct inoculation of the organism. Infection does not disseminate by a hematogenous route and general symptoms are lacking. Localized adenopathy is rare (15% of the cases).[44]

There is often a several month delay between the onset of the lesions and the patient's seeking medical care[48] because the lesions are subacute or chronic and usually painless. Moreover, the lesions can be self-limited and may heal spontaneously, though healing can take months to several years. Initial misdiagnosis of osteo-articular form of *M. marinum* infection can led to intralesional injection of corticosteroid that favors local dissemination.[46] These forms are often associated with poor prognosis.[49]

Extremities of the upper limbs, such as finger or hand, are the most common sites of infection in relation to fish or water animal exposure. The patients that have skin

Table 37-1. Published Studies of *M. marinum* Infections that Include More than 10 Patients[50]

Reference	No. of Patients (no. with deep infection)	% Fish Exposure	% Cured	Duration (mean)	Antibiotic treatment			
					Monotherapy		Combination Therapy (no)	Surgery (% cured)
					No.	Antibiotic, No. of Patients (% cured)		
Aubry 2002	63 (18)	84%	87%	3.5 months	23	M = 19(100%) C = 4(100%)	40	30 (16%)
Casal 2001	39	90%	99%	2–4 months	20	M = 12 (nd), R = 4 (nd)	7	nd
Edelstein 1994	31 (0)	NA	81%	4 months	19	M = 14(71%), D = 3(67%) T = 1(100%, Co = 1(100%)	8	nd
Bonafe 1992	27 (1)	93%	>74%	3.8 months	NA		NA	NA
Chow 1987	24 (24)	87.5%	83%	9 months	0		24	10 (70%)
Kozin 1994 (100%)	12 (6)	100%	100%	6 months	6–7	D = 5 (100%), Co = 2 (100%), R = 1 (100%)	5–6	12
Even-paz 1976*	10 (0)	0%	44%	NA	0		0	0
Ang 2000†	38 (NA)	45%	81%	3.5 months	22	Co = 19 (93), M = 3 (100%)	12	1 (100%)

NA = nonavailable, M = minocycline, C = clarithromycin, R = rifampin, D = doxycycline, T = tetracycline, Co = cotrimoxazole.

*100% swimming pool exposure.

†Only one culture-confirmed case.

Source: Arend SM, van Meijgaarden KE, de Boer K, et al. Tuberculin skin testing and *in vitro* T cell responses to ESAT-6 and culture filterate protein 10 after infection with *Mycobacterium marinum* or *M. kansasii. J Infect Dis.* 2002;186(12): 1797–1807.

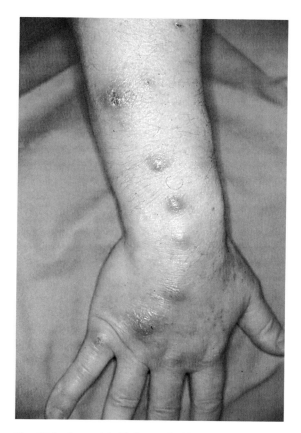

Fig. 37-1. Sporotrichoid form of skin lesions typical of *M. marinum* infection. (Courtesy: Hervé Darie, Noisy le Grand).

lesions on the lower limb are swimming pool cases or indirect cases. *M. marinum* is assumed to be introduced in the skin accidentally through preexisting wounds or abrasion. History of preceding minor trauma is common and an occupation or hobby that resulted in a likely environmental water exposure is the rule: however, since the incubation period is very long, on the average 3 weeks up to 9 months[44,51] minor abrasions or wounds that preceded the contact are usually not recalled at the time of the diagnosis.

Immunity

Tuberculin skin testing is usually positive because of cross-reaction with *M. tuberculosis*.[50] It may suggest a mycobacterial infection, but will not distinguish *M. marinum* from TB or other mycobacterial infections and is therefore of little utility in the workup.

Immunological responses to antigens more specific of TB, such as ESAT-6 and CFP-10 than can differentiate between TB and BCG vaccination, are also positive for *M. marinum* infected patients.[52]

Diagnosis

The diagnosis can be difficult for the clinician[47] because the presentation is often insidious and non specific. If key historical information, such as fish exposure, is not obtained, the diagnosis is commonly delayed.[51] Diagnosing an infection due to *M. marinum* requires a high index of suspicion, a properly obtained exposure history, and knowledge of the laboratory growth characteristics of the organism (Fig. 37-3).

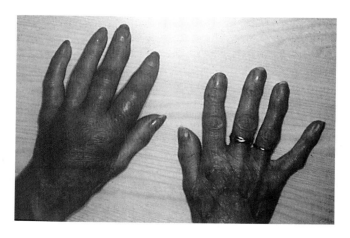

Fig. 37-2. Typical skin lesion of the finger that occurred 8–30 days after fish tank exposure and that disseminated to the subcutaneous and intraarticular tissues. (Courtesy: Eric Caumes, Paris).

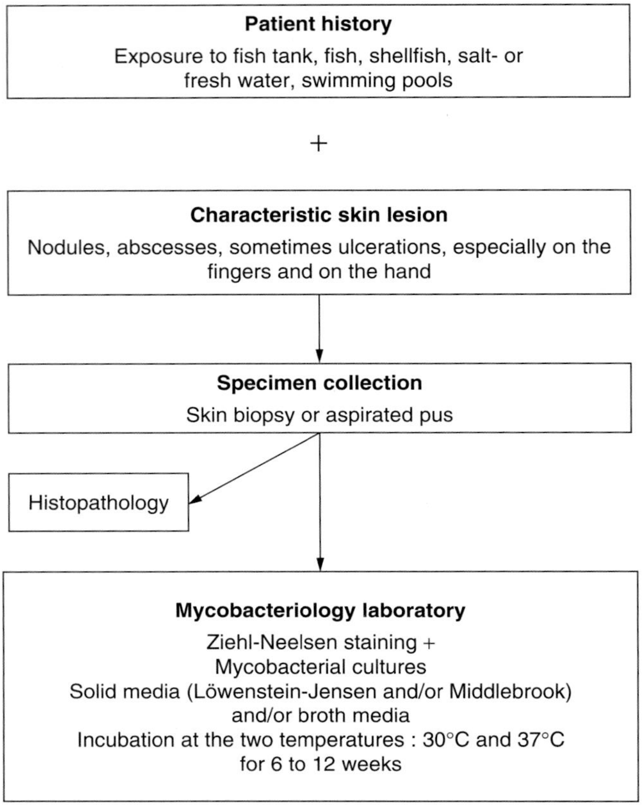

```
┌─────────────────────────────────────────────────┐
│                Patient history                   │
│   Exposure to fish tank, fish, shellfish, salt- or│
│        fresh water, swimming pools               │
└─────────────────────────────────────────────────┘
                        +
┌─────────────────────────────────────────────────┐
│            Characteristic skin lesion            │
│ Nodules, abscesses, sometimes ulcerations, especially on the │
│             fingers and on the hand              │
└─────────────────────────────────────────────────┘
                        │
                        ▼
┌─────────────────────────────────────────────────┐
│               Specimen collection               │
│           Skin biopsy or aspirated pus           │
└─────────────────────────────────────────────────┘
        │
┌──────────────────┐
│  Histopathology  │
└──────────────────┘
                        │
                        ▼
┌─────────────────────────────────────────────────┐
│          Mycobacteriology laboratory            │
│            Ziehl-Neelsen staining +              │
│             Mycobacterial cultures               │
│  Solid media (Löwenstein-Jensen and/or Middlebrook)│
│               and/or broth media                 │
│  Incubation at the two temperatures : 30°C and 37°C│
│               for 6 to 12 weeks                  │
└─────────────────────────────────────────────────┘
```

Fig. 37-3. Microbiological diagnosis of human infection due to *M. marinum*.

Differential diagnosis includes infection due to other atypical mycobacteria known to cause cutaneous infection such as *M. chelonae*, *M. ulcerans*, *M. haemophilum*, *M. fortuitum*, and *M. tuberculosis*; and other infectious and non-infectious diseases such as sporotrichosis, sarcoidosis, skin tumors, and foreign body reactions.

Though the diagnosis can be suspected clinically, especially when exposure is established, the diagnosis relies on isolation of a mycobacterium subsequently identified as *M. marinum*.

Clinical Significance

Isolation of *M. marinum* has a clinical significance whatever the number of colonies or the smear positivity of the specimen since it usually does not grow from the laboratory environment or from the uninfected human body. This important point differentiates *M. marinum* infection from infections due to other NTM such as *M. fortuitum* or *M. chelonae*.[53] Thus correct identification is required.[39,40]

Bacteriological Findings

Microscopic examination of the specimen after Ziehl-Neelsen staining is positive in only 30% of the cases. Even when positive, smear microscopy cannot distinguish *M. marinum* from other mycobacteria including species of the *M. tuberculosis* complex.

A definite diagnosis is obtained by a positive culture. Cultures are reported as positive in 70–80% of the cases, but this number could be increased with attention to the specimen collection and proper incubation temperature. The microbiologist should be aware of suspicion of *M. marinum* infection to perform appropriate cultures at 30°C.

Collection of Specimens

The majority of specimens containing *M. marinum* are from the skin, either skin biopsy or aspirates of pus. Swabs should be avoided for many reasons.[45] Other specimens are articular fluids or subcutaneous tissues and exudates often obtained per surgery. Specimens must be collected before chemotherapy begins. The container should be sterile and should not contain any fixative or preservative. The collected specimen should be kept at 4°C if delivery is delayed to the laboratory. Since *M. marinum* infection is not a multibacillary infection, it is necessary to collect the largest possible volume, especially in the case of skin biopsy or surgery.

Isolation Procedures

Laboratory processing for *M. marinum* disease diagnosis is not an emergency. Level 2 laboratory might be sufficient for isolation although level 3 might be required for identification.[39]

Safety measures are required for handling specimens and cultures: wearing gloves, disinfection of the material and benches, and avoiding use of needles, so that accidental inoculation does not occur.

Skin biopsy or wound fluids might be contaminated with skin flora, such as staphylococci, and consequently require a decontamination procedure (standard NALC-2% NaOH procedure or 4% HCl decontamination) prior to culture. Specimen from sterile deep structures (i.e. articular fluid) might be inoculated directly without decontamination.[39,54]

Since *M. marinum* grows poorly at 37°C, cultures may be negative because incubators are usually set at 37°C. The aspirate or biopsy should be cultured at 30–32°C and incubation should stand 6-12 weeks. Because of other possible mycobacterial diagnosis, specimens should also be incubated at 37°C.

After successful isolation of a photochromogenic mycobacteria, further differentiation between *M. marinum* and other organisms in Runyon group I is required (see above).

Methods based on molecular biology are limited by the high homology between *M. marinum* and *M. ulcerans*. It should associate analysis of 16S rRNA or another conserved genes analysis (*hsp65, gyrA, rpoB,* INNOLiPA) to PCR detection of IS2404,[18,55,56] especially in the absence of photochromogen colonies, and with broth culture.

Histological Findings

Tissue biopsy for histopathology is important but suggests mycobacteriosis in only half the cases since histologic changes depend on the age of the lesion.

Granulomas suggest the diagnosis but are not pathognomonic and are also present in other mycobacterial infections. They are often absent or poorly formed. During the first months, there is a nonspecific inflammatory infiltrate. Later, granulomata with multinucleated giant cell are common findings (Fig. 37-4). Fibrinoid necrosis, but not true caseation, can be observed. Langhans giant cells are seen only occasionally. Hyperkeratosis with focal parakeratosis, hyperplasia, and liquefaction degeneration of the basal layer can be observed.[57]

Although acid fast bacilli are seldom seen in the histological sections,[38] staining should be attempted.

ANTIMICROBIAL SUSCEPTIBILITIES AND TREATMENT
Mode of Action and Resistance Mechanisms in *M. marinum*

The permeability of the *M. marinum* cell wall has not been investigated but was demonstrated to vary at least 10-fold between mycobacterial species, *M. tuberculosis* being 10-fold more permeable than *M. chelonae*.[58] Considering the natural multidrug resistance of *M. marinum* (discussed later), permeability of its cell wall could be close to that of *M. chelonae*. This low permeability probably allows survival in an unfavorable environments.

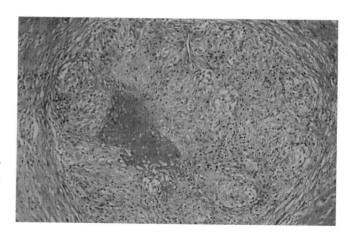

Fig. 37-4. Active disease histopathologic section of tissue from a patient with a *Mycobacterium marinum* infection. The lesion shows granulomatous infiltrate with epithelioid and giant cells. (Courtesy: Bernard Cribier, Strasbourg.)

Enzymes known to hydrolyze antibiotics such as B-lactams, aminoglycosides or macrolides, have not been described in *M. marinum*, but might exist as in other atypical mycobacteria. Annotation of the genome will demonstrate if genes homologous to those encoding theses enzymes are present in *M. marinum*.

The affinity of specific targets for antibiotics, such as ribosomes for macrolides and tetracyclines, RNA polymerase for rifampin and DNA gyrase for quinolones has not been measured.

In vitro Susceptibility to Antibiotics (Table 37-2)

From the studies dealing with a large number of strains and applying a standard method of testing, *M. marinum* has a natural multidrug resistance pattern.[59,60] Indeed, *M. marinum* is resistant to the antituberculous drugs isoniazid, ethambutol and pyrazinamide in most studies. Rifampin and rifabutin are the most active drugs in term of MICs. MICs of minocycline, doxycycline, clarithromycin, linezolid, sparfloxacin, moxifloxacin, imipenem, sulfamethoxazole, and amikacin are close to the susceptibility breakpoints and thus these drugs may have moderate activity.

MICs of trimethoprim, azithromycin, telithromycin, quinupristin-dalfopristin, ciprofloxacin, gemifloxacin, ofloxacin, and levofloxacin are above the concentrations usually obtained *in vivo*, and consequently *M. marinum* may be considered as resistant to them.[61–63]

All the strains have a similar susceptibility pattern since for each drug, the MIC_{50}, geometric mean MIC and modal MIC are very close.[59,62] This constitutes the natural or intrinsic susceptibility pattern of *M. marinum* (Table 37-2).

Acquired resistance has not been described in *M. marinum* so far for any of those antibiotics, even in relapsed cases. Slight differences with the above pattern of natural antibiotic susceptibility that might be observed are usually due to differences in the method or the technique of susceptibility testing.

Susceptibility Testing

Etest has been demonstrated to be an accurate and precise method of MIC determination for bacteria other than mycobacteria,[64] for rapidly growing mycobacterial species and even for some of the slowly growing mycobacterial species.[65–69] Different authors questioned the reliability of the Etest for *M. marinum* and also for

Table 37-2. Minimal Inhibitory Concentrations (μg/ml) of 17 Antibiotics against 54 Strains of *Mycobacterium marinum* determined by the Agar Dilution Method

Antibiotic	MIC_{50}	MIC_{90}	Modal MIC	Geometric mean ± SD	Range
Rifampin	0.25	0.5	0.25	0.24 ± 1.7	0.125–4
Rifabutin	0.06	0.06	0.06	0.06 ± 1.8	0.015–1
Isoniazid	4	8	4	5.6 ± 1.5	4–16
Ethambutol	2	4	2	1.7 ± 1.6	1–4
Amikacin	2	4	4	1 ± 1.7	1–8
Doxycycline	8	16	8	5.7 ± 2	0.5–16
Minocycline	2	4	2	2.9 ± 1.7	0.5–8
Clarithromycin	1	4	2	1.2 ± 2.3	0.5–4
Azithromycin	32	128	32	NA	8–>128
Ofloxacin	4	16	4	6.1 ± 1.7	2–32
Ciprofloxacin	4	8	4	3.8 ± 1.8	1–16
Levofloxacin	4	8	4	4.5 ± 1.7	2–32
Sparfloxacin	1	2	1	1 ± 1.8	0.5–4
Moxifloxacin	0.5	1	0.5	0.6 ± 1.7	0.25–4
Sulfamethoxazole	8	128	8	NA	4–>128
Trimethoprim	64	128	128	67.4 ± 2.3	16–512
Imipenem	2	8	2	2.6 ± 2.6	0.5–16

NA = not applicable. (upper MICs above the highest concentration tested)
Source: Aubry A, Chosidow O, Caumes E, et al. Sixty-three Cases of *Mycobacterium marinum* Infection: Clinical Features, Treatment, and Antibiotic Susceptibility of Causative Isolates. Arch Intern Med. 2002;162(15):1746–52.

other mycobacteria claiming it may cause reports of false resistance.[59,62] Agreement between MICs, yielded by either the Etest method or the agar dilution method used as reference, depends on the antibiotic and was 83% for minocycline, 59% for rifampin, 43% for clarithromycin, and 24% for sparfloxacin.[59,70] Moreover, reproducibility with the Etest was low, in contrast to that with the agar dilution method. In conclusion, Etest is not recommended for *M. marinum* antibiotic susceptibility testing and agar dilution method remains the method recommended.

Since no primary (acquired) resistance has been described so far, routine susceptibility testing seems unnecessary except for relapsed cases as recommended for other atypical mycobacteria.[53,71]

Antimicrobial Therapy of *M. marinum* Infections

Patients infected with *M. marinum* are usually treated with antibiotics (Table 37-1). Different antibiotic regimens have been reported.[46] The choice of the regimen appeared to be based more on personal experience and preference of individual authors than on the demonstrated efficacy.[46] Antibiotic efficacy is unknown since (a) cases are reported separately in the literature, (b) no therapeutic trial has been carried out and (c) *M. marinum* infection may be cured spontaneously.[72–74]

A variety of antibiotics have been used, including tetracyclines, cotrimoxazole, rifampin plus ethambutol and more rarely clarithromycin, levofloxacin, and amikacin.[46,71,75,76] Cure as well as failure has been described with all of these drugs.[46,75,77] Overall, most of the patients are cured after therapy that included tetracyclines or clarithromycin and rifampin, but failures have been also observed. Failure was rarely observed with tetracyclines, but most of the patients treated by tetracyclines, and especially by tetracyclines alone, had mild infection limited to skin and soft tissue. On the other hand, rifampin and rifabutin, which are the only antibiotics with low MICs that are close to those found for *M. tuberculosis*, were usually given in complicated cases with extension of the infection to deeper structures, such as tenosynovitis and osteoarthritis, and did not cure all cases. In our study, failure was related to deep infections (72% only were cured) and to ulcerative lesions.[44]

The *in vivo* activity of the new fluoroquinolones, moxifloxacin, and gatifloxacin, whose MICs are lower than classical fluoroquinolones and which are very potent antituberculous drugs, has still to be demonstrated. The efficacy of linezolid, which shows low MICs, needs to be tested *in vivo*.

Until there are *in vivo* experiments in the animal model or therapeutical trials in humans are available, it is reasonable to recommend tetracyclines for *M. marinum* infection limited to the skin, and the combination of rifampin and clarithromycin for infection involving deeper structures.

No failures have been related to acquired resistance to any antibiotic. Since acquired resistance in mycobacteria is usually described for drugs with potent activity, such as streptomycin resistance for *M. tuberculosis*,[78] or clarithromycin resistance for *M. avium*,[79] the absence of acquired resistance in *M. marinum* might indicate that none of the antibiotics used so far has potent activity *in vivo*.

In the literature, the duration of antimicrobial therapy in *M. marinum* infection from 2 weeks to 18 months, depending on several factors such as the extension and severity of infection, the presence of underlying disorders and the clinical response.[46,47] In many patients with mild disease, infection resolves spontaneously, although complete resolution may take up to several years.[45,46] In our study,[44] the duration of therapy ranged from 1 to 25 months and the median was 3.5 months. This duration was significantly longer for cases with infection spread to deeper structures.

We recommend continuing antibiotic therapy, at least until the lesions heal and then for 2 additional months, especially in the cases of deep infection.

Surgery

The place of surgery is controversial. For some authors, surgical debridement along with antimicrobial therapy is usually required for control.[45] For others, surgical debridement should be limited to the cases with criteria known to be associated to a poor prognosis, including steroid injections into the lesion, a persistently draining sinus tract after several months of antimicrobial therapy, and persistent pain.[80] Most of the infections involving deeper structures undergo surgery, which seems reasonable.[81] For the infections limited to skin and soft tissue there is no clear benefit of surgery and surgical side effects are unknown.

Other therapies such as cryotherapy, x-ray therapy, and electrodessication have been reported but have not been evaluated.[46]

EPIDEMIOLOGY AND PREVENTION
Natural Habitats of *M. marinum*

M. marinum has been reported to affect a wide range of freshwater and marine fish species, suggesting an ubiquitous distribution. *M. marinum* is the main mycobacterium isolated from fish, although very little is known about its prevalence and impact on fisheries.[82]

M. marinum is transmitted in fish through the consumption of contaminated feed, cannibalism of infected fish, aquatic detritus, or release of pathogens into the water due to gut or skin lesions or disintegration of infected fish.[38] In this respect, potential sources of infective material are numerous and include the soil and water in which the bacterial cells remain viable for 2 years or more.[38]

M. marinum infection in other aquatic vertebrates may be a source of infection to fish. Frogs, snakes and turtles may become involved in the transmission cycle. Snails are also thought to be a reservoir. Other invertebrate organisms, such as shellfish or water fleas, have been shown to play a role in the transmission of this agent.[38]

A recent study in Italy evaluated the prevalence of nontuberculous mycobacteria in the environment of a swimming pool. Although 88.2% of pool water samples were positive with *M. gordonae*, *M. chelonae* and *M. fortuitum*, *M. marinum* was isolated in only 4.5% of the water samples and pool edges.[83,84]

Epidemiology of M. marinum Infections

Like other NTM infection, *M. marinum* infections are not contagious between humans. Before 1962, most cutaneous *M. marinum* infections reported in the literature involved swimming pool-associated injuries, including 2 large outbreaks involving almost 350 patients.[48,6] A possible explanation of the decline in pool-associated cases is the improvement in swimming pool-water disinfection practices in recent decades. *M. marinum* survives only briefly after exposure to free chlorine concentrations ≥ 0.6 mg/l.

M. marinum skin infection is now often acquired from aquarium maintenance and is called "fish tank granuloma".[85] Since *M. marinum* infection is an important zoonosis, there is a significant risk to all personnel working with fish, aquatic animals or aquaria. *M. marinum* infection may be an occupational hazard for certain professionals (for example for pet shop workers), but many infections occur in people who fancy fish and keep aquariums at home, hence, the name "fish fanciers' finger syndrome".[86] Although infection may be caused by direct injury from the fish fins or bites, most are acquired during the handling of the aquarium such as cleaning or changing the water.[50] Indirect infection has also been described due to a bath that was used to clean out fish tanks.[46,87]

It is expected that the incidence of "fish tank granuloma" will increase[84] due to the increase in fish tank hobbyists and aquarium tourism. For example, in France about 10% of the population has an aquarium at home and business related to fish tank hobbies increased by 3% per year.[44,88]

Frequency of *M. marinum* isolation in laboratories is low and *M. marinum* accounts for less than 1% of the mycobacterial clinical isolates.[89] A recent survey involving 21 laboratories in Spain reported 39 cases from 1991–1998.[90] Less than half of the cases of *M. marinum* infection are bacteriologically confirmed. The incidence of *M. marinum* infection was estimated to be around 0.09 cases per 100,000 inhabitants per year in France[87] and between .05 and .27 per 100,000 in the U.S.A.[90]

Prevention Strategies

For the prevention of swimming pool granuloma, the Centers for Disease Control and Prevention recommend that concentrations of free chlorine in swimming pool water should be kept between 0.4 and 1 mg/l and in spa and hot tub water between 2 and 5 mg/l.[48]

Sanitation, disinfection, and destruction of carrier fish are the primary methods of controlling *M. marinum* infection in fish. This practice is mostly pursued for food fish; however, in expensive fish species, this practice may be difficult to apply. Antimicrobial treatment is not able to eliminate *M. marinum* from affected fish.[91]

Individual prevention is the first line of defense for anyone involved with aquariums, or anyone working or recreating in a marine environment. Preventative strategies should be developed in fish tank related activities as commonsense measures and should include:

1. Wear gloves when cleaning the tank.[51]

2. Bandage or dress any open wound or cut before exposure.

3. Wash hands thoroughly before and after exposure to aquarium water and components. Hydro-alcoholic solutions may be used instead of hand washing.

4. Do not swallow the aquarium water when checking for salinity or siphoning water.

5. Do not overcrowd aquariums since this favors the multiplication of mycobacteria.

6. UV germicide lamps to treat aquarium water are efficient for mycobacteria as long as they are used in clean conditions at the correct flow rate.[92]

7. Do not transfer tank filters or fish in the bath that is used for humans, or carefully clean it with sodium hypochlorite.

8. Exposed populations should be educated to recognize signs of *M. marinum* disease in fish and in humans, so they can inform medical personnel and will expedite the diagnosis.

9. Personnel conducting sale of fish should be educated about the disease and its prevalence. Many tropical fish salesmen ignore "fish tank granuloma." In France, even though 20% of them are at risk of *M. marinum* infection, 95% immerse hands in fish tanks every day without wearing gloves.[93]

Some authors recommend not installing ornamental aquaria in hospital units, particularly in a unit likely to receive immunocompromised patients.

REMAINING PROBLEMS AND CONCLUSION

Treatment evaluation requires large-scale trials probably at an international level. Infection limited to the skin and soft tissue should be distinguished from infections extended to deeper structures. Antibiotics such as tetracyclines, rifampin, and clarithromycin need to be evaluated along with the new fluoroquinolones and linezolid. Surgery needs subsequent evaluation.

Surveillance of *M. marinum* infection, which is expected to increase due to the increase in fish tank hobbyists and aquarium tourism, should be undertaken at least in some highly exposed countries. A simple surveillance could be based on culture-confirmed cases. Bacteriology laboratories, dermatologists, and infectious diseases physicians should play a crucial role for case finding.

Since there is no human-to-human transmission of *M. marinum* infection, the prevention of inoculation from the environment is the main strategy for eradicating the disease. Simple recommendations such as hand protection, hygiene measures, and fish tank and aquaria maintenance need to be widely disseminated and evaluated.

Professionals should also take *M. marinum* risk into account and apply the recommendation for decreasing *M. marinum* infection among farm fish, and among contamination of professionals,handling fish.

Lastly, diagnosis should be expedited:

1. Remember to ask "Do you have a fish tank at home? Who cleans it and how?"

2. Sample the lesion for mycobacteriologic analysis.

3. Inform the laboratory if there is a suspicion of *M. marinum* infection.

4. Incubate at 30°C in addition to 37°C and wait for weeks until smooth photochromogenic colonies appear.

REFERENCES

1. Bataillon E, Moeller A, Terre L. Über die identitat des Bacillus des Karpfens (Bataillon, Dubard et terre) und des bacillus der Blindsschleuche (Moeller). *Zentralblatt für tuberculose*. 1902;3:467–468.

2. Aronson J. Spontaneous tuberculosis in salt-water fish. *J Infect Dis*. 1926;39:315–320.

3. Baker J, Hagan W. Tuberculosis of a Mexican platyfish (*Platypoecilus maculatus*). *J Infect Dis*. 1942;70:248–252.

4. Besse P. Epizootie à bacilles acido-résistants chez des poissons exotiques. *Bulletin de l'académie vétérinaire de France*. 1949;23:151–154.

5. Lacaille F, Blanche S, Bodemer C, et al. Persistent *Mycobacterium marinum* infection in a child with probable visceral involvement. *Ped Infect Dis*. 1990;9:58–60.

6. Linell F, Norden A. *Mycobacterium balnei*. A new acid fast bacillus occuring in swimming pools and capable of producing skin lesions in humans. *Acta Tuberc Scand*. 1954;33:1–54.

7. Ang P, Rattana-Apiromyakij N, Goh CL. Retrospective study of *Mycobacterium marinum* skin infections. *Int J Dermatol*. 2000;39(5):343–347.

8. Ramakrishnan L. *Mycobacterium marinum* infection of the hand. *N Engl J Med*. 1997;28:612.

9. Hale YM, Pfyffer GE, Salfinger M. Laboratory diagnosis of mycobacterial infections: new tools and lessons learned. *Clin Infect Dis*. 2001;33(6):834–846.

10. Helguera-Repetto C, Cox RA, Munoz-Sanchez JL, et al. The pathogen *Mycobacterium marinum*, a faster growing close relative of *Mycobacterium tuberculosis*, has a single rRNA operon per genome. *FEMS Microbiol Lett*. 2004;235(2): 281–288.

11. Stahl D, Urbance J. The division between fast- and slow-growing species corresponds to natural relationships among the mycobacterial. *J Bacteriol*. 1990;172:116–124.

12. Wolinsky E. Mycobacterial diseases other than tuberculosis. *Clin Inf Dis*. 1992;15:1–12.

13. Rogall T, Wolters J, Flohr T, et al. Towards a phylogeny and definition of species at the molecular level within the genus mycobacterium. *J Syst Bac*. 1990;40:323–330.

14. Tonjum T, Welty D, Jantzen E, et al. Differentiation of *Mycobacterium ulcerans, marinum*, and *haemophilum*: mapping of their relationships to *M. tuberculosis* by fatty acid profile analysis, DNA-DNA hybridation, and 16S rRNA gene sequence analysis. *J Clin Microbiol*. 1998;36(4):918–925.

15. Cole ST, Eiglmeier K, Parkhill J, et al. Massive gene decay in the leprosy bacillus. *Nature*. 2001;409(6823):1007–1011.

16. Cole ST, Parkhill J, Garnier T, et al. Deciphering the biology of *Mycobacterium tuberculosis* from the complete genome sequence. *Nature*. 1998;393:537–544.

17. Stinear TP, Jenkin GA, Johnson PD, et al. Comparative genetic analysis of *Mycobacterium ulcerans* and *Mycobacterium marinum* reveals evidence of recent divergence. *J Bacteriol*. 2000;182(22):6322–6330.

18. Chemlal K, Huys G, Fonteyne PA, et al. Evaluation of PCR-restriction profile analysis and IS2404 restriction fragment

length polymorphism and amplified fragment length polymorphism fingerprinting for identification and typing of *Mycobacterium ulcerans* and *M. marinum. J Clin Microbiol.* 2001;39(9):3272–3278.

19. Ucko M, Colorni A, Kvitt H, et al. Strain variation in *Mycobacterium marinum* fish isolates. *Appl Environ Microbiol.* 2002;68(11):5281–5287.

20. Stinear TP, Mve-Obiang A, Small PL, et al. Giant plasmid-encoded polyketide synthases produce the macrolide toxin of *Mycobacterium ulcerans. Proc Natl Acad Sci U S A.* 2004;101(5):1345–1349.

21. Sechi LA, Colorni A, Dupre I, et al. Strain variation in Mediterranean and Red Sea *Mycobacterium marinum* isolates. *New Microbiol.* 2002;25(3):351–356.

22. Ruley KM, Ansede JH, Pritchett CL, et al. Identification of *Mycobacterium marinum* virulence genes using signature-tagged mutagenesis and the goldfish model of mycobacterial pathogenesis. *FEMS Microbiol Lett.* 2004;232(1):75–81.

23. Ramakrishan L, Falkow S. *Mycobacterium marinum* persists in cultured mammalian cells in a temperature-restricted fashion. *Infect Immun.* 1994;62:3222–3229.

24. Talaat AM, Trucksis M. Transformation and transposition of the genome of *Mycobacterium marinum. Am J Vet Res.* 2000;61(2):125–128.

25. Chan K, Knaak T, Satkamp L, et al. Complex pattern of *Mycobacterium marinum* gene expression during long-term granulomatous infection. *Proc Natl Acad Sci U S A.* 2000; 99(6):3920–3925.

26. Ramakrishnan L, Federspiel NA, Falkow S. Granuloma-specific expression of Mycobacterium virulence proteins from the glycine-rich PE-PGRS family [see comments]. *Science.* 2000;288(5470):1436–1439.

27. Prouty MG, Correa NE, Barker LP, et al. Zebrafish-*Mycobacterium marinum* model for mycobacterial pathogenesis. *FEMS Microbiol Lett.* 2003;225(2):177–182.

28. Talaat AM, Reimschuessel R, Wasserman SS, et al. Goldfish, *Carassius auratus,* a novel animal model for the study of *Mycobacterium marinum* pathogenesis. *Infect Immun.* 1998;66(6):2938–2942.

29. Trucksis M. Fishing for mycobacterial virulence genes: a promising animal model. *ASM news.* 2000;66:668–674.

30. Dionne MS, Ghori N, Schneider DS. Drosophila melanogaster is a genetically tractable model host for *Mycobacterium marinum. Infect Immun.* 2003;71(6):3540–3550.

31. Barker L, George K, Falkow S, et al. Differential trafficking of live and dead *Mycobacterium marinum* organisms in macrophages. *Infect Immun.*1997;(1497–1504).

32. El-Etr SH, Yan L, Cirillo JD. Fish monocytes as a model for mycobacterial host-pathogen interactions. *Infect Immun.* 2001;69(12):7310–7317.

33. Gao LY, Groger R, Cox JS, et al. Transposon mutagenesis of *Mycobacterium marinum* identifies a locus linking pigmentation and intracellular survival. *Infect Immun.* 2003;71(2): 922–929.

34. Barker LP, Brooks DM, Small PL. The identification of *Mycobacterium marinum* genes differentially expressed in

macrophage phagosomes using promoter fusions to green fluorescent protein. *Mol Microbiol.* 1998;29(5):1167–1177.

35. Stamm LM, Morisaki JH, Gao LY, et al. *Mycobacterium marinum* escapes from phagosomes and is propelled by actin-based motility. *J Exp Med.* 2003;198(9):1361–1368.

36. Alexander DC, Jones JR, Tan T, et al. PimF, a mannosyl-transferase of mycobacteria, is involved in the biosynthesis of phosphatidylinositol mannosides and lipoarabinomannan. *J Biol Chem.* 2004;279(18):18824–33.

37. Daffe M, Laneelle M, Lacave C. Structure and stereochemistry of mycolic acids of *Mycobacterium marinum* and *Mycobacterium ulcerans. Res Microbiol.* 1991;142:397–403.

38. Decostere A, Hermans K, Haesebrouck F. Piscine mycobacteriosis: a literature review covering the agent and the disease it causes in fish and humans. *Vet Microbiol.* 2004;99(3–4): 159–66.

39. Cernoch P, Enns R, Saubolle M, et al. Laboratory diagnoses of the mycobacterioses. Cumitechs 16A. A. S. Weissfeld, coordinating ed. Washington, D.C: American Society for Microbiology; 1994.

40. Vincent V, Brown-Elliott B, Jost K, et al. *Mycobacterium:* phenotypic and genotypic identification. In: Murray P, ed. Manual of clinical microbiology. 8th ed. Washington, DC: ASM Press, 2003.

41. Alcaide F, Richter I, Bernasconi C, et al. Heterogeneity and clonality among isolates of *Mycobacterium kansasii:* implications for epidemiological and pathogenicity studies. *J Clin Microbiol.* 1997;35(8):1959–1964.

42. Holmes GF, Harrington SM, Romagnoli MJ, et al. Recurrent, disseminated *Mycobacterium marinum* infection caused by the same genotypically defined strain in an immunocompromised patient. *J Clin Microbiol.* 1999;37(9):3059–3061.

43. Tchornobay A, Claudy A, Perot J, et al. Fatal disseminated *Mycobacterium marinum* infection. *Int J Dermatol.* 1992;31: 286–287.

44. Aubry A, Chosidow O, Caumes E, et al. Sixty-three Cases of *Mycobacterium marinum* Infection: Clinical Features, Treatment, and Antibiotic Susceptibility of Causative Isolates. *Arch Intern Med.* 2002;162(15):1746–1752.

45. Gluckman S. *Mycobacterium marinum.* Clinics in dermatology 1995;13:273–276.

46. Edelstein H. *Mycobacterium marinum* skin infections. *Arch Intern Med.* 1994;154:1359–1364.

47. Zenone T, Boibieux A, Tigaud S, et al. Non-tuberculous mycobacterial tenosynovitis: a review. *Scand J Infect Dis.* 1999;31(3):221–228.

48. Philpott JJ, Woodburne A, Philpott O, et al. Swimming pool granuloma : a study of 290 cases. *Arch Dermatol.* 1963;88: 158.

49. Wayne LG, Sramek HA. Agents of newly recognized or infrequently encountered mycobacterial diseases. *Clin Microbiol Rev.* 1992;5(1):1–25.

50. Lewis FM, Marsh BJ, von Reyn CF. Fish tank exposure and cutaneous infections due to *Mycobacterium marinum*: tuberculin skin testing, treatment, and prevention. *Clin Infect Dis.* 2003;37(3):390–7.

51. Jernigan JA, Farr BM. Incubation period and sources of exposure for cutaneous *Mycobacterium marinum* infection: case report and review of the literature. *Clin Infect Dis.* 2000;31(2):439–443.

52. Arend SM, van Meijgaarden KE, de Boer K, et al. Tuberculin skin testing and *in vitro* T cell responses to ESAT-6 and culture filtrate protein 10 after infection with *Mycobacterium marinum* or *M. kansasii. J Infect Dis.* 2002;186(12): 1797–1807.

53. Wallace R, Glassroth J, Griffith D, et al. Diagnostic and treatment of disease caused by nontuberculous mycobacteria. *Am J Respir Crit Care Med.* 1997;156:S1–S25.

54. Pfyffer G, Welscher H, Kissling P. Comparison of the mycobacteria growth indicator tube (MGIT) with radiometric and solid culture for recovery of fast bacilli. *J Clin Microbiol.* 1997;35:364–368.

55. Dauendorffer JN, Guillemin I, Aubry A, et al. Identification of mycobacterial species by PCR sequencing of quinolone resistance-determining regions of DNA gyrase genes. *J Clin Microbiol.* 2003;41(3):1311–1315.

56. Kim BJ, Lee SH, Lyu MA, et al. Identification of mycobacterial species by comparative sequence analysis of the RNA polymerase gene (rpoB). *J Clin Microbiol.* 1999;37(6): 1714–1720.

57. Even-Paz Z, Haas H, Sacks T, et al. *Mycobacterium marinum* skin infection mimicking cutaneous leishmaniasis. *Br J Dermatol.* 1976;94:435–442.

58. Nikaido H. Molecular basis of bacterial outer membrane permeability revisited. *Microbiol Mol Biol Rev.* 2003;67(4): 593–656.

59. Aubry A, Jarlier V, Escolano S, et al. Antibiotic susceptibility pattern of *Mycobacterium marinum. Antimicrob Agents Chemother.* 44(11):3133–3136.

60. Utrup L, Moore T, Actor P, et al. Susceptibilities of nontuberculosis mycobacterial species to amoxicillin-clavulanic acid alone and in combination with antimicrobial agents. *Antimicrob Agents Chemother.* 1995;39(7):1454–1457.

61. Brown-Elliott BA, Crist CJ, Mann LB, et al. *In vitro* activity of linezolid against slowly growing nontuberculous Mycobacteria. *Antimicrob Agents Chemother.* 2003;47(5):1736–1738.

62. Braback M, Riesbeck K, Forsgren A. Susceptibilities of *Mycobacterium marinum* to gatifloxacin, gemifloxacin, levofloxacin, linezolid, moxifloxacin, telithromycin, and quinupristin-dalfopristin (Synercid) compared to its susceptibilities to reference macrolides and quinolones. *Antimicrob Agents Chemother.* 2002;46(4):1114–1116.

63. Rhomberg PR, Jones RN. *In vitro* activity of 11 antimicrobial agents, including gatifloxacin and GAR936, tested against clinical isolates of *Mycobacterium marinum. Diagn Microbiol Infect Dis.* 2002;42(2):145–147.

64. Baker CN, Stocker SA, Culver DH, et al. Comparison of the E Test to agar dilution, broth microdilution, and agar diffusion susceptibility testing techniques by using a special challenge set of bacteria. *J Clin Microbiol.* 1991;29(3):533–538.

65. Biehle J, Cavalieri S, Saubolle M, et al. Evaluation of Etest for susceptibility testing of rapidly growing mycobacteria. *J Clin Microbiol.* 1995;33(7):1760–1764.

66. Flynn C, Kelly C, Barrett M, et al. Application of the Etest to the antimicrobial susceptibility testing of *Mycobacterium marinum* clinical isolates. *J Clin Microbiol.* 1997; 2083–2086.

67. Hoffner S, Klintz L, Olsson-Liljequist B, et al. Evaluation of Etest for susceptibility testing of *Mycobacterium chelonei* and *M. fortuitum. J Clin Microbiol.* 1994;32:1846–1849.

68. Lebrun L, Onody C, Vincent V, et al. Evaluation of the Etest for rapid testing of *Mycobacterium avium* to clarithromycin. *J Clin Microb.* 1996;37:999–1003.

69. Wanger A, Mills K. Testing of *Mycobacterium tuberculosis* susceptibility to ethambutol, isoniazid, rifampicin and streptomycin by using Etest. *J Clin Microbiol.* 1996;34(7): 1672–1676.

70. Werngren J, Olsson-Liljequist B, Gezelius L, et al. Antimicrobial susceptibility of *Mycobacterium marinum* determined by E-test and agar dilution. *Scand J Infect Dis.* 2001;33(8):585–588.

71. Chow S. Correspondence. *The journal of bone and joint surgery.* 1988;70(A n!4):631–632.

72. Forsgren A. Antibiotic susceptibility of *Mycobacterium marinum. Scand J Infect Dis.* 1993;25:779–782.

73. Saito H, Tomioka H, Sato K, et al. *In vitro* and *in vivo* antimycobacterial activities of a new quinolone, DU-6859a. *Antimicrob Agents Chemother.* 1994;38(12):2877–2882.

74. Wallace R, Wiss K. Susceptibility of *Mycobacterium marinum* to tetracyclines and aminoglycosides. *Antimicrob Agents Chemother.* 1981;20(5):610–612.

75. Huminer D, Pitlik S, Block C, et al. Aquarium-borne *Mycobacterium marinum* skin infection. *Arch Dermatol.* 1986;122:698–703.

76. Iijima S, Saito J, Otsuka F. *Mycobacterium marinum* skin infection successfully treated with levofloxacin. *Arch Dermatol.* 1997;133:947–949.

77. Kozin S, Bishop A. Atypical mycobacterium infections of the upper extremity. *J Hand Surger.* 1994;19:480–487.

78. Investigation MRC. Streptomycin treatment of pulmonary tuberculosis. *BMJ.* 1948;2:769.

79. Dautzenberg B, Truffot C, Legris S, et al. Activity of clarithromycin against *Mycobacterium avium* infection in patients with the acquired immune deficiency syndrome. A controlled clinical trial. *Am Rev Respir Dis.* 1991; 144(3 Pt 1):564–569.

80. Chow S, Collins R, Pun W. *Mycobacterium marinum* infection of the hand and wrist. *J Bone Joint Surg.* 1987; 69-A(8):1161–1168.

81. Bhatty MA, Turner DP, Chamberlain ST. *Mycobacterium marinum* hand infection: case reports and review of literature. *Br J Plast Surg.* 2000;53(2):161–165.

82. Heckert RA, Elankumaran S, Milani A, et al. Detection of a new Mycobacterium species in wild striped bass in the Chesapeake Bay. *J Clin Microbiol.* 2001;39(2):710–715.

83. Daffe M, Laneelle MA, Asselineau C, Levy-Frebault V, David H. Taxonomic value of mycobacterial fatty acids: proposal for a method of analysis. *Ann Microbiol (Paris).* 1983 Sep-Oct;134B(2):241–256. French.

84. Leoni E, Legnani P, Mucci MT, et al. Prevalence of mycobacteria in a swimming pool environment. *J Appl Microbiol.* 1999;87(5):683–688.

85. Swift S, Cohen H. Granulomas of the skin due to *Mycobacterium balnei* after abrasions from a fishtank. *N Engl J Med.* 1962;297:1244–1246.

86. Wheeler AP, Graham BS. Atypical mycobacterial infections. *South Med J.* 1989;82(10):1250–1258.

87. Dobos KM, Quinn FD, Ashford DA, et al. Emergence of a unique group of necrotizing mycobacterial diseases. *Emerg Infect Dis.* 1999;5(3):367–378.

88. King AJ, Fairley JA, Rasmussen JE. Disseminated cutaneous *Mycobacterium marinum* infection. *Arch Dermatol.* 1983;119(3):268–270.

89. Good R, Snider D. Isolation of nontuberculosis mycobacteria in the United States. *J Infect Dis.* 1980;146:829–833.

90. Casal M, Casal MM. Multicenter study of incidence of *Mycobacterium marinum* in humans in Spain. *Int J Tuberc Lung Dis.* 2001;5(2):197–199.

91. Astrofsky KM, Schrenzel MD, Bullis RA, et al. Diagnosis and management of atypical *Mycobacterium spp.* infections in established laboratory zebrafish (*Brachydanio rerio*) facilities. *Comp Med.* 2000;50(6):666–672.

92. Dailloux M, Laurain C, Weber M, et al. Water and nontuberculous mycobacteria. *Water Res.* 1999;33(10):2219–2228.

93. Sage R, Derrington A. Opportunisitc cutaneous *Mycobacterium marinum* infection mimicking *Mycobacterium ulcerans* in lymphosarcoma. *Med J Aust.* 1973;2:434–437.

38

Mycobacterium scrofulaceum

Edward A. Horowitz

INTRODUCTION

Mycobacterium scrofulaceum is a member of the Runyon Class II scotochromogenic acid-fast bacilli. It is found widely in nature but is an uncommon human pathogen. It was first described by Prissick and Masson in a preliminary report in 1952[1] and subsequently in more detail.[2,3] It was they who proposed the name, presumably because of its isolation from cervical lymph nodes.

MICROBIOLOGY

M. scrofulaceum is variable in its length on acid-fast stain preparations and may be either longer or shorter than *Mycobacterium tuberculosis*. It is generally thicker and more coarsely beaded than *M. tuberculosis*. It grows slowly on Löwenstein medium. Although occasional strains may develop visible colonies in as little as 10 days, most require 4–6 weeks. Colonies are globular, smooth in consistency, and opaque. Pigmentation is yellow, turning a dark orange with time. Growth is optimal at 37°C, one atmosphere pressure, and under aerobic conditions. Growth is slower at 25° and 35°C. There is no growth at 41°C or higher.

Early work by Wayne and Tsukamura helped to distinguish *M. scrofulaceum* from *Mycobacterium gordonae*.[4–6] The organism is antigenically and biochemically quite similar to *Mycobacterium avium-intracellulare* and for many years was classified with the latter as a complex (MAIS). It usually gives a positive urease reaction that distinguishes it from MAI; however, exceptions can occur,[7] making distinctions difficult. Recent base sequence analysis of the 16S ribosomal RNA confirms that *M. scrofulaceum* is indeed a unique species.[8]

EPIDEMIOLOGY

Sources in Nature

Early reports identified isolates of *M. scrofulaceum* in raw milk, oysters, soil, and water.[9–13] Dunn and Hodgson[14] were able to isolate *M. scrofulaceum*, among other species of nontuberculous mycobacteria (NTM), from raw milk, but not from samples of pasteurized milk. Environmental sources have also been identified in Korea[15] and the water supply system of the Czech Republic.[16]

In the United States, Brooks, et al.[17] isolated *M. scrofulaceum* from the flood plains of 4 eastern rivers. The number of organisms increased with more southerly latitudes. A follow-up study[18] confirmed these findings and showed that environmental factors favoring growth include warm temperature, low oxygen tension, lower pH of soils, and higher water concentrations of zinc, humic acid, and fulvic acid. (The authors did not distinguish between strains of *M. scrofulaceum* and those of the MAI complex). In a study by the same group,[19] analysis of stable DNA plasmids in MAI complex and *M. scrofulaceum* strains showed that isolates from humans and aerosols are more likely to carry plasmids than those strains isolated from soil, dust, sediment, and water. The authors suggest this supports the theory that human disease results from exposure to water aerosols.

Human Isolates

M. scrofulaceum is an uncommon isolate from humans. The first national survey of NTM isolates in the United States was organized by the CDC in 1979.[20] The 763 isolates of *M. scrofulaceum* accounted for approximately 2% of all isolates. There was a predominance of reports from the South Atlantic region, primarily due to 148 isolates from Florida. A follow-up survey in 1980[21] had similar results.

The first survey to collect clinical data was carried out between October, 1981 and September, 1993.[22] *M. scrofulaceum* accounted for 214 (3.9%) of 5469 overall NTM isolates. Forty-seven (22%) of these 214 were considered to represent clinical disease, or 2.2% of all clinically relevant isolates. Twenty-two of the 47 isolates were from sputum samples and one was from lung tissue. Eighteen were from lymph nodes, one was from skin, and 5 were from other tissues or fluids. The mean age of the patients was 38.5 years, the lowest for all of the NTM species reported. Fifteen of the 47 were from patients less than 15 years of age. Patients were predominantly urban. No other geographic data were supplied. Of the NTM isolates from lymph nodes, 81% were MAI complex, 16% were *M. scrofulaceum*, and 3% were *M. kansasii*. This correlates with the change in distribution of isolates from lymph nodes seen by Wolinsky and others (discussed further).

Similar data were reported from South Carolina[23] where 2% of NTM isolates from 210 patients between 1971 and 1980 were *M. scrofulaceum*. Only 4 of 269

NTM isolates at the Cleveland Clinic between 1982 and 1985 were *M. scrofulaceum*.[24]

A number of recent reports have looked at human exposure to *M. scrofulaceum* by analyzing skin test reactions to PPD sensitins derived from that organism. Bruins, et al.[25] found that 7.76% of army recruits in the Netherlands had indurations of 10 mm or greater to *M. scrofulaceum* sensitin. Dascalopoulos, et al.[26] analyzed 8507 Greek armed forces members tested with *M. scrofulaceum* sensitin who lived in or near their birthplaces. Those born in mountainous areas or in seaside areas had positivity rates of 4.1 and 7.1% respectively. Those born on small Aegean islands or on inland plains near large rivers both had rates described as "greater than 8%". The authors concluded these data supported the theory that large bodies of water serve as the principal source of infection. Kwamanga, et al.[27] tested 1015 BCG scar negative children between ages 6 and 13 years in 18 randomly selected areas of Kenya. 22.7% reacted to *M. scrofulaceum* sensitin and 6.1% reacted to PPD-RT. Cross reactivity was 23.8% in children who lived at low altitudes. Similarly, Svandova, et al.[28] found that approximately 15% of 7-year-old children in 2 towns in rural Czechoslovakia were skin test reactors to *M. scrofulaceum* sensitin. The reaction was greater than the simultaneous reaction to PPD-RT in approximately 50%.

These data are all subject to certain limitations. Nevertheless, they are consistent with the theory that *M. scrofulaceum* is widely but unevenly distributed in nature, that humans encounter the organism and develop an immune response in a pattern which reflects this distribution, and that clinical disease is much less common than exposure.

CLINICAL SYNDROMES

Lymphadenitis

As mentioned above, *M. scrofulaceum* was originally isolated from cervical lymph nodes of children and this is the condition most commonly associated with it in the literature.[29–31] Most patients are between 1 and 5 years of age with occasional cases older than 10 years. In cervical lymphadenitis due to all NTM species, girls outnumber boys by 1.3–2.0:1.0. (These data have not been reported specifically for *M. scrofulaceum*). Most cases involve unilateral nodes in the upper cervical chain or just under the mandible. Occasionally, cases of bilateral disease or peripheral node involvement (axillary, inguinal, epitrochlear, mediastinal) have been reported. The children have no systemic signs or symptoms and only occasionally have local symptoms.

The natural history is variable and probably not completely understood. As Wolinsky has noted,[31] we do not know how many cases resolve spontaneously and never come to medical attention. Of the cases seen by physicians, those who are untreated soften, open, and drain, or heal spontaneously with fibrosis or calcification.

The pathophysiology has not been firmly established. The isolation of *M. scrofulaceum* (and also MAI) from tonsils has led to the reasonable speculation that the pharyngeal lymphoid tissue is the portal of entry, with direct drainage into the nodes.[30] In cases of peripheral adenopathy, direct inoculation into the skin by trauma has been documented.[31]

The distribution of mycobacterial species in childhood cervical lymphadenitis has changed over the years. In the preantibiotic era, most cases were due to *M. tuberculosis* or *Mycobacterium bovis*.[32] In the developed countries of the world where tuberculosis (TB) has become a rare disease, the NTM species now predominate.[33] Following the initial reports[1,2] *M. scrofulaceum* was the species most commonly identified. Since 1970, MAI has been more commonly identified than *M. scrofulaceum*.[22,31] Whether this represents a true change, reporting artifact, or more reliable identification by laboratories remains unknown.

Skin testing with mycobacterial antigens is a potentially useful diagnostic strategy. Most children with NTM lymphadenitis have a weak reaction to PPD-S,[31] but react more strongly to antigens derived from NTM strains.[34] The specificity of such comparative testing in this population derives from the relatively small chance that these children have been exposed to *M. tuberculosis*. Unfortunately, these testing agents are not commercially available.

The differential diagnosis includes infection with *M. tuberculosis, M. bovis*, other NTM species, and various viruses (e.g., EBV, CMV, mumps) and deep fungi. Other infections include brucellosis, cat scratch disease, and toxoplasmosis. Noninfectious causes include sarcoidosis, congenital cysts, lymphoma, lipoma, goiter, and drug-induced hyperplasia.

Differentiating NTM lymphadenitis from TB is usually not difficult. Age from 1 to 5 years, unilateral nodes, lack of systemic illness, no history of contact with active TB, normal chest radiograph, no or weak response to 5TU tuberculin skin test, nonreactive tuberculin skin tests in siblings, early suppuration, and no response to antituberculous antibiotics are all points which favor NTM disease. There are no clinical clues, which will distinguish *M. scrofulaceum* from any other NTM species. Ultimately, culture of biopsy or aspirated material is required for definitive diagnosis.

Pulmonary Disease

The vast majority of sputum isolates of *M. scrofulaceum* represent asymptomatic colonization. These are frequently old TB patients being monitored with serial mycobacterial cultures. True invasive disease is seen occasionally, resulting in an indolent, slowly progressive cavitary pneumonitis. All 8 cases reported by Wolinksy[30] had industrial dust or fume exposure, but disease has occurred in the normal host.[35] In this report, Gracey and Byrd described a 48-year-old man with an occasionally productive early morning cough and 25-pound weight loss over 1 year. There was no known TB contact and no industrial exposure. He was afebrile and had posttussive rales over the right lung apex. Chest radiograph had a nodular infiltrate in the right upper lobe with tomography showing a thin-walled cavity. There was an 8 mm indurated reaction to intermediate strength PPD skin testing and a 10 mm reaction to PPD-B. Erythrocyte sedimentation rate and routine laboratory values were normal. Three consecutive sputum samples grew a Group II scotochromogen, further characterized as falling between the *M. scrofulaceum* and *Mycobacterium aquae* subgroups. After 3 months of therapy with isoniazid, para-aminosalicylic acid, streptomycin, cycloserine, and ethionamide, the sputum remained AFB smear positive but culture negative. After 4 months the chest radiograph was unchanged. He did well with surgical resection, although the duration of follow-up was not given. Pathology of the lung tissue showed fibrosis with caseating necrosis. There was no underlying pneumoconiosis. Multiple acid-fast bacilli were seen but mycobacterial and fungal cultures were sterile. This was the only patient of 71 in this series with sputum isolates of Group II scotochromogens thought to have invasive disease due to the organism.

LeMense et al.[36] described 3 pulmonary nodules in a 46-year-old man with a cardiac transplantation for an idiopathic cardiomyopathy. His medications were cyclosporine, azathioprine, trimethoprim-sulfamethoxazole, and acyclovir. He had had episodes of rejection at 7 and 12 months post transplantation. A routine chest radiograph at 15 months showed a left lower lung nodule. He was asymptomatic but remembered a weeklong influenza-like illness one month before. Computed tomography disclosed 3 noncalcified nodules. Wedge biopsy of one of the nodules revealed caseating granulomas and acid-fast bacilli, with *M. scrofulaceum* isolated from culture. The remaining 2 nodules decreased in size during a 6-month course of clarithromycin, ethambutol, and rifampin. Unfortunately, only 3 months of follow-up was reported, during which time the patient remained asymptomatic and the chest radiograph was unchanged.

In a survey of nontuberculous mycobacteria isolated from sputum of HIV-negative South African gold miners in the mid-1990s,[37] 41 of 297 isolates were *M. scrofulaceum*. Thirty-five of these patients had premorbid chest radiographs for comparison, of which 31 (89%) demonstrated new cavitations. The authors calculated the incidence of *M. scrofulaceum* pulmonary disease to be 12 per 100,000 person-years. It therefore appears that pulmonary disease may be more common than previously thought in at least some selected populations.

Extrapulmonary Disease

A small number of extrapulmonary isolates have been reported over the years. Unfortunately, many of the early reports did not speciate the organism beyond the level of scotochromogen.

Bojalil[38] reported an isolate from a spinal cord abscess without clinical details. Yamamoto, et al.[39] reported 6 cases of meningitis due to NTM, 5 of which were due to scotochromogens. There were 4 women and 1 man with an age range of 2–32 years. All were said to have had "clinical manifestations of meningitis". In 2 of the 4 females, disease started after pregnancy. Chest radiographs showed "fibrocaseous lesions with cavity" in 2 patients, miliary lesions in 1, and no findings in 2. The patient with the miliary lesions died. The others were cured with unspecified chemotherapy.

A single case of granulomatous hepatitis has been recognized.[40] This was a 39-year-old man with a 3-year history of mild epigastric pain, diffuse aches, fatigue, and night sweats. An abscess of the left groin had been drained during the first year of illness without culture. His temperature was elevated to 101.5°F, 2–3 times per week. Physical examination showed hepatosplenomegaly. Laboratory showed normal SGOT and bilirubin and an elevated alkaline phosphatase. An intermediate strength PPD was "normal". Chest and spinal radiographs were normal. Liver biopsy demonstrated noncaseating granulomas and culture of the liver tissue grew *M. scrofulaceum*. After 1 year of treatment with isoniazid, rifampin, and cycloserine, the patient was asymptomatic and the alkaline phosphatase had returned to normal. No long-term follow-up was reported.

A recent report[41] describes a case of osteomyelitis/tenosynovitis in the wrist of a 66-year-old diabetic man. He failed to respond to standard antituberculosis therapy. Cultures eventually grew *M. scrofulaceum* and the infection was controlled with the combination of kanamycin, ethambutol, and ethionamide.

A number of reports document multisystem disease with the organism isolated from multiple sites, mimicking miliary TB.[42–54] Some of these patients have had underlying immunodeficiency states, but others have been apparently normal hosts. In retrospect, one wonders about the HIV status of these apparently normal patients reported before the recognition of AIDS. Nonetheless, one recent report[51] documents a patient as being HIV seronegative. That only 11 cases of disseminated disease with *M. scrofulaceum* have been reported in AIDS patients testifies to the low level of the virulence of this organism.

Skin Disease

There are 2 reports of subcutaneous disease.[55,56] The first was a 32-year-old man with corticosteroid dependent systemic lupus erythematosus. Multiple painful subcutaneous abscesses appeared over a 3-week period. He was afebrile and otherwise well. His chest radiograph had calcified granulomata. Skin biopsy demonstrated granulomatous inflammation and acid-fast bacilli. The cultures grew *M. scrofulaceum*. The patient received a 9-month course of isoniazid and rifampin despite *in vitro* resistance to both agents. The lesion healed completely within 5 months and he remained lesion-free for 2 years of follow-up.

Abbott and Smith[57] listed a single renal transplantation patient on prednisone and chlorambucil as having "skin lesions" positive for *M. scrofulaceum* by microscopy and culture. Sowers[58] described a progressive sporotrichoid skin lesion on both hands of a 77-year-old woman whose hands were chronically exposed to aquarium water. The lesion did not respond to a 5-month course of isoniazid, ethambutol, and topical isoniazid 10% cream. Another aquarium water associated case[59] grew both *M. scrofulaceum* and *M. peregrinum*. This patient responded to successive courses of sparfloxacin and minocycline. Finally, a report[60] documents a skin nodule on the index finger of a 59-year-old woman who was seven months postautologous bone marrow transplantation for breast cancer. She had exposure to "thorny roses that had been soaking in slimy water" and had sustained a recent paper cut. Her lesion resolved with a course of azithromycin and rifampin of unspecified duration.

ANTIBIOTIC SENSITIVITY

The sensitivity of *M. scrofulaceum* to antituberculous antibiotics has been reported sporadically. It is one of the most resistant of all NTM species. Unfortunately, few of the reports of clinical isolates describe the methodology used.

The organism is resistant to isoniazid, para-amino-salicylic acid, and kanamycin. Some strains are sensitive to rifampin, rifabutin, ethambutol, streptomycin, cycloserine, amikacin, ethionamide, viomycin, and capreomycin. Using modern broth dilution methods, the minimal inhibitory concentrations of clarithromycin,[61] roxithromycin,[62] and sparfloxacin[63] have recently been shown to be within potentially clinically useful ranges.

TREATMENT

No comparative or controlled treatment trials have ever been reported. A large body of anecdotal evidence suggests that antibiotic therapy has no benefit in lymphadenitis and that node resection usually suffices for complete cure.[29–31] It might be noted that this experience predates the advent of the newer macrolide and fluoroquinolone antibiotics, which possess promising *in vitro* activity.

The experience with systemic disease has simply been too scant and variable to allow any strong recommendations to be made. Certainly a trial of 2 or more agents with demonstrated *in vitro* activity would seem justified in patients with disease, which could not be surgically removed.

REFERENCES

1. Prissick FH, Masson AM. A preliminary report on a study of pigmented mycobacteria [abstract]. *Can J Public Health.* 1952;43:34.
2. Prissick FH, Masson AM. Cervical lymphadenitis in children caused by chromogenic mycobacteria. *Can Med Assoc J.* 1956;75:798–803.
3. Prissick FH, Masson AM. Yellow-pigmented pathogenic mycobacteria from cervical lymphadenitis. *Can J Microbiol.* 1957;3:91–100.
4. Wayne LG, Doubek JR, Diaz GA. Classification and identification of mycobacteria. IV. Some important scotochromogens. *Am Rev Respir Dis.* 1967;96:88–95.
5. Wayne LG. On the identity of *Mycobacterium gordonae* Bojalil and the so-called tap water scotochromogens. *Int J Syst Bacteriol.* 1970;20:149–153.
6. Tsukamura M. Appropriate name for tap water scotochromogens. *Am Rev Respir Dis.* 1970;102:643–644.
7. Good RC. Opportunistic pathogens in the genus *Mycobacterium. Ann Rev Microbiol.* 1985;39:347–369.
8. Rogall T, Wolters T, Flohr T, et al. Towards the phylogeny and definition of species at the molecular level within the genus *Mycobacterium. Int J Syst Bacteriol.* 1990;40:323–330.
9. Chapman JS, Bernard JS, Speight M. Isolation of mycobacteria from raw milk. *Am Rev Resp Dis.* 1965;91:351–355.

10. Hosty TS, McDurmont CI. Isolation of acid-fast organisms from milk and oysters. *Health Lab Sci.* 1975;12:16–19.

11. Wolinsky E, Rynearson TK. Mycobacteria in soil and their relation to disease-associated strains. *Am Rev Respir Dis.* 1968;97:1032–1037.

12. Goslee S, Wolinsky E. Water as a source of potentially pathogenic mycobacteria. *Am Rev Respir Dis.* 1976;113:287–292.

13. Schroder KH, Kazda J, Muller K, et al. Isolation of *Mycobacterium simiae* from the environment. *Int J Med Microbiol Virol Parasitol Infect Dis.* 1992;277:561–564.

14. Dunn BL, Hodgson DJ. "Atypical" mycobacteria in milk. *J Appl Bacteriol.* 1982;52:373–376.

15. Jin BW, Saito H, Yoshii Z. Environmental mycobacteria in Korea. I. Distribution of the organisms. *Microbiol Immunol.* 1984;28:667–677.

16. Kubalek I, Mysak J. The prevalence of environmental mycobacteria in drinking water supply systems in a demarcated region in Czech Republic, in the period 1984–1989. *Eur J Epidemiol.* 1996;12:471–474.

17. Brooks RW, Parker BC, Gruft H, et al. Epidemiology of infection by nontuberculous mycobacteria. V. Numbers in eastern United States soils and correlation with soil characteristics. *Am Rev Respir Dis.* 1984;130:630–633.

18. Kirschner RA Jr, Parker BC, Falkinham JO III. Epidemiology of infection by nontuberculous mycobacteria. *Mycobacterium avium, Mycobacterium intracellulare,* and *Mycobacterium scrofulaceum* in acid, brown-water swamps of the southeastern United States and their association with environmental variables. *Am Rev Respir Dis.* 1992;145:271–275.

19. Meissner PS, Falkinham JO III. Plasmid DNA profiles as epidemiologic markers for clinical and environmental isolates of *Mycobacterium avium, Mycobacterium intracellulare,* and *Mycobacterium scrofulaceum. J Infect Dis.* 1986;153:325–330.

20. Good RC. Isolation of nontuberculous mycobacteria in the United States, 1979. *J Infect Dis.* 1980;142:779–783.

21. Good RC, Snider DE Jr. Isolation of nontuberculous mycobacteria from the United States, 1980. *J Infect Dis.* 1982;146:829–833.

22. O'Brien RJ, Geiter LJ, Snider DE Jr. The epidemiology of nontuberculous mycobacterial diseases in the United States. *Am Rev Respir Dis.* 1987;135:1007–1014.

23. Krajnack MA, Dowda H. Non-tuberculous mycobacteria in South Carolina, 1971–1980. *J S C Med Assoc.* 1981;77:551–555.

24. Woods G, Washington J. Mycobacteria other than *Mycobacterium tuberculosis*: Review of microbiologic and clinical aspects. *Rev Infect Dis.* 1987;9:275–294.

25. Bruins J, Gribnau JH, Bwire R. Investigation into typical and atypical tuberculin sensitivity in the Royal Netherlands Army, resulting in a more rational indication for isoniazid prophylaxis. *Tuber Lung Dis.* 1995;76:540–544.

26. Dascalopoulos GA, Loukas S, Constantopoulos SH. Wide geographic variations of sensitivity of MOTT sensitins in Greece. *Eur Respir J.* 1995;8:715–717.

27. Kwamanga DO, Swai OB, Agwanda R, et al. Effect of nontuberculous mycobacteria infection on tuberculin results among primary school children in Kenya. *East Afr Med J.* 1995;72:222–227.

28. Svandova E, Stastna J, Kubin M. Comparative testing of skin reactions to PPD mycobacterins from *Mycobacterium tuberculosis* and *Mycobacterium scrofulaceum* in school-age children. *J Hyg Epidemiol Microbiol Immunol.* 1984;29:275–281.

29. Lincoln EM, Gilbert LA. Disease in children due to mycobacteria other than *Mycobacterium tuberculosis. Am Rev Respir Dis.* 1972;105:683–714.

30. Wolinsky E. Nontuberculous mycobacteria and associated diseases. *Am Rev Respir Dis.* 1979;119:107–159.

31. Wolinsky E. Mycobacterial lymphadenitis in children: A prospective study of 105 nontuberculous cases with long-term follow-up. *Clin Infect Dis.* 1995;20:954–963.

32. Grzybowski S, Allen EA. History and importance of scrofula. *Lancet.* 1995;346:1472–1474.

33. Allen EA. Tuberculosis and other mycobaterial infections of the lung. In: Thurbeck WM, Chung AM eds. *Pathology of the lung, 2nd ed.* New York, NY: Thieme Medical Publishers; 1995:253–254.

34. Margileth AM. The use of purified protein derivative mycobacterial skin test antigens in children and adolescents: Purified protein derivative skin test results correlated with mycobacterial isolates. *Pediatr Infect Dis.* 1983;2:225–231.

35. Gracey DR, Byrd RB. Scotochromogens and pulmonary disease. Five years' experience at a pulmonary disease center with report of a case. *Am Rev Respir Dis.* 1970;101:959–963.

36. LeMense GP, VanBakel AB, Crumbley AJ III, et al. *Mycobacterium scrofulaceum* infection presenting as lung nodules in a heart transplant recipient. *Chest.* 1994;106:1918–1920.

37. Corbett EL, Hay M, Churchyard GJ, et al. *Mycobacterium kansasii* and *M. scrofulaceum* isolates from HIV-negative South African gold miners: incidence, clinical significance and radiology. *Int J Tuberc Lung Dis.* 1999;3:501–507.

38. Bojalil LF. Frequency and epidemiologic significance of unclassified mycobacteria in Mexico. *Am Rev Respir Dis.* 1961;83:596–599.

39. Yamamoto M, Sudo K, Taga M, et al. A study of diseases caused by atypical mycobacteria in Japan. *Am Rev Respir Dis.* 1967;96:779–787.

40. Patel KM. Granulomatous hepatitis due to *Mycobacterium scrofulaceum*: Report of a case. *Gastroenterology.* 1981;81:156–158.

41. Phoa LL, Khong KS, Thamboo TP, et al. A case of *Mycobacterium scrofulaceum* osteomyelitis of the right wrist. *Ann Acad Med Singapore.* 2000;29:678–681.

42. McCusker JJ, Green RA. Generalized nontuberculous mycobacteriosis: Report of two cases. *Am Rev Respir Dis.* 1962;86:405–414.

43. Joos HA, Hilty LB, Courington D, et al. Fatal disseminated scotochromogenic mycobacteriosis in a child. *Am Rev Respir Dis.* 1967;96:795–801.

44. Zamorano J Jr, Tompsett R. Disseminated atypical mycobacterial infection and pancytopenia. *Arch Intern Med.* 1968;121:424–427.

45. Vinh LT, Duc TV, Nevot P, et al. Infection généralisée mortelle due à une mycobactéria atypique. *Arch Fr Pediatr* 1966;23:1155–1166.

46. McNutt DD, Fudenberg HH. Disseminated scotochromogen infection and unusual myeloproliferative disorder: Report of a case and review of the literature. *Ann Intern Med.* 1971;75:737–744.

47. Dustin P, Demol P, Derks-Jacobovitz D, et al. Generalized fatal chronic infection by *Mycobacterium scrofulaceum* with severe amyloidosis in a child. *Path Res Pract.* 1980;168:237–248.

48. Delabie J, De Wolf-Peeters C, Bobbaers H, et al. Immunophenotypic analysis of histiocytes involved in AIDS-associated *Mycobacterium scrofulaceum* infection: similarities with lepromatous lepra. *Clin Exp Immunol.* 1991;85:214–218.

49. Shafer RW, Sierra MF. *Mycobacterium xenopi, Mycobacterium fortuitum, Mycobacterium kansasii,* and other nontuberculous mycobacteria in an area of endemicity for AIDS. *Clin Infect Dis.* 1992;15:161–162.

50. Sanders JW, Walsh AD, Snider RL, et al. Disseminated *Mycobacterium scrofulaceum* infection: A potentially treatable complication of AIDS. *Clin Infect Dis.* 1995;20:549–556.

51. Hsueh P-R, Hsiue T-R, Jarn J-J, et al. Disseminated infection due to *Mycobacterium scrofulaceum* in an immunocompetent host. *Clin Infect Dis.* 1996;22:156–161.

52. Campos-Herrero MI, Rodriguez H, Lluch J, et al. Infeccion diseminada por *Mycobacterium scrofulaceum*: a proposito de 3 casos. *Enferm Infecc Microbiol Clin.* 1996;14:258–260.

53. Saad MH, Vincent V, Dawson DJ, et al. Analysis of Mycobacterium avium complex serovars isolated from AIDS patients from southeast Brazil. *Mem Inst Oswaldo Cruz.* 1997;92:471–475.

54. Choonhakarn C, Chetchotisakd P, Jirarattanapochai K, et al. Sweet's syndrome associated with non-tuberculous mycobacterial infection: a report of five cases. *Br J Dermatol.* 1998;139:107–110.

55. Murray-Leisure KA, Egan N, Weitekamp MR. Skin lesions caused by *Mycobacterium scrofulaceum. Arch Dermatol.* 1987;123:369–370.

56. Gorse GJ, Fairshter RD, Friedly G, et al. Nontuberculous mycobacterial disease. Experience in a southern California hospital. *Arch Intern Med.* 1983;143:225–228.

57. Abbott MR, Smith DD. Mycobacterial infections in immunosuppressed patients. *Med J Aust.* 1981;1:351–353.

58. Sowers WF. Swimming pool granuloma due to Mycobacterium scrofulaceum. *Arch Dermatol.* 1972;105:760–761.

59. Ishii N, Sugita Y, Sato I, et al. A case of mycobacterial skin disease caused by *Mycobacterium peregrinum* and *Mycobacterium scrofulaceum. Acta Derm Venereol.* 1998;78: 76–77.

60. Kandyil R, Maloney D, Tarrand J, et al. Red nodule on the finger of an immunosuppressed woman. *Arch Dermatol.* 2002;128:689–694.

61. Brown BA, Wallace RJ Jr, Onyi GO. Activities of clarithromycin against eight slowly growing species of nontuberculous mycobacteria, determined by using a broth microdilution MIC system. *Antimicrob Agents Chemother.* 1992;36:1987–1990.

62. Rastogi N, Goh KS, Bryskier A. In vitro activity of roxithromycin against 16 species of atypical mycobacteria and effect of pH on its radiometric MIC. *Antimicrob Agents Chemother.* 1993;37:1560–1562.

63. Yew WW, Piddock LJ, Li MS, et al. In-vitro activity of quinolones and macrolides against mycobacteria. *J Antimicrob Chemother.* 1994;34:343–351.

39

Other Nontuberculous Mycobacteria and Mycobacterium Bovis

Laurel C. Preheim
Marvin J. Bittner

MYCOBACTERIUM BOVIS

Mycobacterium bovis, also known as the bovine tubercle bacillus, belongs to a subset of mycobacteria that includes *M. tuberculosis, M. africanum,* and *M. microti.* A live, attenuated strain of *M. bovis* is used in the Bacille Calmette-Guérin (BCG) vaccine. *M. bovis* was once a major cause of tuberculosis (TB) in the United States and other industrialized nations. The ingestion of raw milk from infected cows was commonly associated with cervical lymphadenitis. Human cases have become rare in this country due to public health legislation mandating tuberculin testing of dairy herds and the routine pasteurization of milk. Reactivation of a primary infection can occur in patients who ingested unpasteurized milk or milk-products in the past.[1–3] Laboratory primates[4] and commercial elk herds[5] can also serve as a reservoir for infection of man. Although human-to-human transmission of disease has become less common, HIV infection and continued immigration from countries with endemic disease, including Mexico, contribute to the persistence of *M. bovis* in the United States.[6] *M. bovis* infections are clinically indistinguishable from those caused by *M. tuberculosis.* Both primary and reactivation infections often involve extrapulmonary sites. Ingested *M. bovis* typically causes cervical adenitis or abdominal TB with peritonitis, mesenteric adenitis, ileocecal involvement, or anorectal disease. The signs and symptoms of abdominal TB can be mistaken for inflammatory bowel disease, appendicitis, or cancer.[7] Children, especially under the age of 2, are at risk for disseminated infections. In this age group miliary disease, including meningitis can develop within 3–9 months of initial infection. In contrast to children, adult extrapulmonary *M. bovis* infections often represent reactivation of disease. The most common sites of involvement have included the GI tract, bones and joints, and central nervous system.[6]

Immunocompromised patients are more susceptible to mycobacterial pathogens, including *M. bovis.* A nosocomial outbreak of multidrug-resistant *M. bovis* was reported among HIV-infected patients in France.[8] Growing numbers of reports have linked *M. bovis* infection to BCG vaccination in patients with AIDS.[9,10] In these patients BCG was isolated from multiple sites, including lymph nodes, abscesses at the vaccination site, blood, urine, sputum, stool, and bone marrow. The time from vaccination to illness has ranged from several days to more than 30 years. The Immunization Practices Advisory Committee of the United States Public Health Service has recommended that, in populations where the risk of TB is low, BCG vaccine be withheld from persons known or suspected to be infected with HIV.[11] Other immunocompromised patients are also at risk of disseminated *M. bovis* infection following BCG vaccination. Meningitis has followed BCG vaccination of children who have leukemia.[12] Intravesicular instillation of BCG, an approved treatment for superficial bladder carcinoma, has been associated with pulmonary *M. bovis* infections in patients with uroepithelial carcinoma who received instillation of BCG into the bladder or renal pelvis.[13] Although *M. bovis* has innate resistance to pyrazinamide, primary resistance to other first-line antituberculous drugs is unusual among strains isolated in the United States.[6] Treatment with 2- or 3-drug combinations of isoniazid, rifampin, ethambutol, and streptomycin has been effective and should continue for a minimum of 9–12 months.

OTHER NONTUBERCULOUS MYCOBACTERIA

Microbiology

The list of clinically important nontuberculous mycobacteria is growing as new species continue to be identified and older ones are found to be pathogenic. More detailed information on these organisms can be found in a number of excellent reviews.[14–19] As a group, these mycobacteria currently cause fewer infections than those species discussed in previous chapters. Some of these organisms are not newly discovered but have heretofore been considered virtually nonpathogenic. Previously many were regarded as contaminants when isolated from clinical specimens. Timpe and Runyon established that these organisms could cause disease in humans and classified them based on pigment production, growth rate, and colonial characteristics. Photochromogens (Group I) grow slowly on culture media (>7 d). Their colonies change from a buff shade to bright yellow or orange after exposure to light. Scotochromogens (Group II) also grow slowly but demonstrate pigmented colonies when incubated in the dark or the light. Group III mycobacteria grow slowly and lack pigment in the dark or light. Rapid growers (Group IV) also lack pigment, but they grow in culture within 3–5 days. Collectively these four groups have been called the "atypical mycobacteria," nontuberculous mycobacteria (NTM), mycobacteria other than tubercle bacilli (MOTT), or "potentially pathogenic environmental mycobacteria"(PPEM).

Epidemiology

Ubiquitous in nature, many NTM have been isolated from ground or tap water, soil, house dust, domestic and wild animals, and birds.[20] Despite their wide distribution, some species are more common in certain geographic locations. Most infections, including those that are hospital-acquired,[21] result from inhalation or direct inoculation from environmental sources. Ingestion may be the source of infection for children with NTM cervical adenopathy and for patients with AIDS whose disseminated infection may begin in the gastrointestinal tract. These infections are not considered contagious since person-to-person transmission is extremely rare.

Pathophysiology

The pathogenic potential for human disease varies among NTM. As a group, these organisms are less virulent for humans than *M. tuberculosis* or *M. bovis* and may colonize body surfaces or secretions without causing disease. Nonetheless, because of reports of invasive disease with such organisms, all mycobacteria should be considered as potentially pathogenic. This is especially true when they are isolated from patients with immunocompromising conditions such as AIDS[22] or cystic fibrosis.[23] In general, disease is slowly progressive, and histopathologic findings resemble those seen in TB.

Diagnosis

The steps taken to diagnose TB generally apply to NTM infections. Standardized, specific skin test antigens for NTM are unavailable. In addition, colonization of asymptomatic individuals and environmental contamination of specimens can yield positive cultures in the absence of clinical infection. NTM disease can be considered present in patients with a cavitary infiltrate on chest radiogram when: (a) two or more sputum (or sputum and a bronchial washing) are smear-positive for acid-fast bacilli and/or

yield moderate to heavy growth on culture; (b) other reasonable causes for the disease process have been excluded, e.g., fungal disease, TB, malignancy, and such like. An additional criterion, (c) failure of the sputum cultures to convert to negative with either bronchial hygiene or 2 weeks of specific mycobacterial drug therapy, is applied in the presence of a noncavitary infiltrate not known to be due to another disease.[24]

The diagnosis is also established if transbronchial, percutaneous, or open lung biopsy tissue reveals mycobacterial histopathologic changes and yields the organism. Extrapulmonary or disseminated disease is confirmed by isolation of the organism from normally sterile body fluids, closed sites, or lesions, and environmental contamination of specimens is excluded. Radiometric culture systems, DNA probes, and polymerase chain reaction assays have increased the speed and accuracy of laboratory diagnosis of pulmonary and extrapulmonary mycobacterial infections; but susceptibility testing is not standardized.[19]

Clinical Disease

NTM cause a broad spectrum of diseases (Table 39-1). It should be noted that therapeutic approaches continue to evolve and therefore remain controversial. Many conventional antituberculous agents have little or no activity against these organisms. Some treatment regimens contain new agents or older antimicrobials newly found to have activity against mycobacteria. Although general guidelines exist for the therapy of infections caused by some of these organisms,[22,24] in most cases the optimal regimen or duration of therapy has not been firmly established. The results of susceptibility testing may be used to select a therapeutic regimen. Immunocompetent patients with clinically significant NTM infections usually should receive 18–24 months of therapy. Infected immunocompromised patients, particularly those with disseminated infection and AIDS, probably should receive therapy as long as their immune systems remain impaired.

Mycobacterium simiae

M. simiae was first isolated from a colony of Macacus rhesus monkeys.[25] A slowly growing photochromogen, its colonies may be only weakly pigmented even after prolonged exposure to light. Unlike other nontuberculous mycobacteria, it produces niacin and thus may be confused with *M. tuberculosis*. Unlike all other known mycobacteria, *M. simiae* contains 16S rRNA sequences that are similar to those found both in slowly growing mycobacteria and in rapidly growing strains. The organism has been isolated from water[26] and human feces.[27]

Table 39-1. Nontuberculous Mycobacterial Infection Sites and Etiologic Species

Site of Infection	Etiologic Species (Runyan Group)*	
	Common	**Less Common**
Lung	*M. avium complex* (III) *M. kansasii* (I) *M. abscessus* (IV) *M. xenopi* (II)	*M. simiae* (I) *M. szulgai* (I/II) *M. malmoense* (III) *M. fortuitum* (IV) *M. chelonae* (IV)
Lymph nodes	*M. avium complex* (III) *M. scrofulaceum* (II)	*M. fortuitum* (IV) *M. chelonae* (IV) *M. abscessus* (IV) *M. kansasii* (I)
Skin or Soft tissue	*M. marinum* (I) *M. fortuitum* (IV) *M. chelonae* (IV) *M. abscessus* (IV) *M. ulcerans* (III)	*M. avium complex* (III) *M. kansasii* (I) *M. terrae* (III) *M. smegmatis* (IV) *M. haemophilum* (III)
Disseminated	*M. avium complex* (III) *M. kansasii* (I) *M. chelonae* (IV) *M. abscessus* (IV) *M. haemophilum* (III)	*M. fortuitum* (IV) *M. xenopi* (II) *M. simiae* (I) *M. gordonae* (II) *M. terrae complex* (III) *M. neoarum* (II) *M. celatum* (III) *M. genavense* (III)

* I = photochromogen; II = scotochromogen; III = nonpigmented; IV = rapid grower

M. simiae can colonize the respiratory tract, and the lung is the most commonly reported site of infection. Most cases of pulmonary disease have been reported from the United States, Thailand, Israel, and Europe.[26,28–30] Findings have included caseating granulomas and chronic progressive pulmonary infiltrates with cavitation. Disseminated disease, osteomyelitis, and renal involvement have been reported.[31] In AIDS patients infections can be localized or disseminated, and blood cultures may be diagnostic.[32] Patients who are clinically infected can be treated initially with a regimen effective for *M. avium-intracellulare* (MAI) pending the results of susceptibility studies.

Mycobacterium genavense

M. genavense is a newly described fastidious pathogen whose identification was based on PCR amplification and sequencing of a 16S rRNA gene fragment.[33,34] The organism does not grow on conventional solid media but can be isolated in liquid (Middlebrook 13 or BACTEC 13A) culture and subcultured to Middlebrook agar supplemented with Mycobactin J[35] or human blood.[36] *M. genavense* appears to have a wide geographic distribution and has been isolated from patients in Europe, the United States, and Australia.[37] It has been recovered from birds, but the source for human infections has not been identified. Originally isolated from HIV-infected patients, *M. genavense* typically causes disseminated disease in those with advanced AIDS.[37–40] Clinically the infection mimics that caused by MAI. Spiking fevers, weight loss, diarrhea, anemia, splenomegaly, and lymphadenopathy are common, whereas pulmonary symptoms are rare. The infection has presented, as a solitary brain abscess in a patient with AIDS.[41] Initial therapy should include clarithromycin combined with two or three other agents effective for MAI infections.

Mycobacterium malmoense

M. malmoense, first described in 1977, is nonchromogenic and slow growing, often requiring at least 6 weeks for primary isolation. It appears to be distributed worldwide and has been isolated from natural waters in Finland and soil in Japan. This organism was initially linked to chronic pulmonary infection in British and northern European adults who had underlying lung disease.[42] Subsequent reports of extrapulmonary disease have described cervical lymphadenopathy, particularly in children, and tenosynovitis.[43,44] Disseminated infection with involvement of the skin, gastrointestinal tract, or lymph nodes has been reported in patients with leukemia or AIDS.[44] Most isolates are susceptible to ethambutol, and many are susceptible to rifampin and streptomycin. A regimen effective against MAI is recommended for initial therapy.[24] A patient with AIDS and disseminated infection was treated successfully with rifabutin, clofazimine, and isoniazid.[44]

Mycobacterium haemophilum

M. haemophilum is nonpigmented, fastidious, slow-growing, and grows optimally at lower temperatures than most mycobacteria. It requires hemin or ferric ammonium citrate for growth. Initially identified as the cause of cutaneous ulcerating lesions in an Israeli woman with Hodgkin's disease,[45] *M. haemophilum* has been isolated from patients in North America, Europe, Africa, and Australia.[46,47] The majority of cases reported to date have involved patients who are immunocompromised by conditions such as organ or bone marrow transplantation, lymphoma, or AIDS.[48] Disease can be focal or widespread. Cutaneous and subcutaneous lesions are most common. They frequently overlie joints and can be nodular, cystic, or papular. Typically they evolve from papules to pustules and can form deep ulcers that may be painful. Other infections have included bacteremia, septic arthritis, osteomyelitis, pneumonitis, sinusitis, and lymphadenitis.[47] Most *M. haemophilum* strains demonstrate *in vitro* susceptibility to p-aminosalicylic acid, amikacin, clofazimine, clarithromycin, fluoroquinolones, and rifamycins. Immuno-compromised adults with multiple cutaneous lesions or osteomyelitis have been successfully treated with regimens that included ciprofloxacin, clarithromycin, and rifampin.[46,49,50] Immunocompetent children with localized lymphadenitis do well with excisional therapy alone.[47]

Mycobacterium xenopi

M. xenopi, first isolated from a toad, is a scotochromogen that grows optimally at 43°C. The organism is able to grow at 45°C and has been recovered from hot-water generators and storage tanks. It is frequently found in both cold and hot water samples from taps and showers. Failure to grow at temperatures below 28°C likely explains its absence in samples from water treatment plants, reservoirs, and distribution systems. A cluster of bronchoscopy-associated *M. xenopi* pseudoinfections was linked to use of tap water for cleaning bronchoscopes.[51] Human exposure to the organism can occur via aerosolization and inhalation or ingestion. *M. xenopi* appears to have a variable geographic distribution. It has been recovered frequently from clinical specimens in Wales, southern England, the northwest coast of Europe, and Toronto, Canada. It was rarely isolated in the United States prior to the AIDS epidemic.[17] Detection of *M. xenopi* in clinical specimens may require prolonged incubation at 37°C or incubation at higher temperatures.

M. xenopi is increasingly recognized as a cause of pulmonary infection. In immunocompetent patients clinical illness typically occurs as an indolent, cavitary lung infection in middle aged men who have underlying chronic pulmonary diseases.[52,53] Less commonly it may infect the spine[54] or joints.[55] *M. xenopi* infections in immunocompromised patients are being reported more frequently. Solid organ transplantation[56,57] and AIDS increase the risk of pulmonary and disseminated disease.[53,58,59] Infections with *M. xenopi* have shown variable responses to drug therapy. Recommendations for initial therapy include isoniazid, rifampin, and ethambutol with or without streptomycin.[24] Isolates may be susceptible to clarithromycin,[55] and pyrazinamide and ciprofloxacin have been included in some successful regimens.[53]

Mycobacterium ulcerans

M. ulcerans is a slowly growing, unpigmented mycobacteria that grows best at 33°C. It produces a heat-stable toxin and is the cause of a chronic necrotizing skin infection (Bairnsdale ulcer or Buruli ulcer). *M. ulcerans* infection was first described in Australia but subsequently has been reported in central and west Africa, Mexico, South America, Southeast Asia, and the central Pacific. Analysis of 16S rRNA sequences of isolates from three continents revealed three subgroups corresponding to the continent of origin.[60] Although unproven, it is a generally accepted assumption that the environment is the source of the organism. The majority of reported infections have occurred in persons living near rivers or stagnant bodies of water. Inoculation appears to occur via trauma to the skin. The trauma may be minor and unrecognized by the patient. Infection has followed snake bite,[61] gun shot wound, or vaccination.[62]

Most lesions occur on the distal parts of a limb and typically begin as a painless papule or subcutaneous swelling. In several weeks the lesion becomes a shallow ulcer with a necrotic base and undermined margins. Prominent involvement of subcutaneous tissue follows, and satellite ulcers and nodules can develop. Ulcers vary in severity and size and may involve joints. Healed lesions leave stellate scars with retraction, and patients with large ulcers may have permanent deformity and disability. Most lesions are widely ulcerated when they are detected and require extensive surgical excision and skin grafting. Early diagnosis and treatment improves outcome. Clumps of acid-fast bacilli are usually visible in material taken from skin lesions, but primary culture of *M. ulcerans* may take several months. The efficacy of antimicrobials has been disappointing, particularly when they are used late in the course of disease. They may be helpful early or when coupled with surgical excision. Regimens have included streptomycin and dapsone with or without ethambutol[14] and various combinations of cotrimoxazole, rifampin, ethambutol, and clarithromycin.[61] Isoniazid, rifampin, and ethambutol for 2 months followed by rifampin and clarithromycin for 5 months was successful therapy in a HIV-infected patient who had a cutaneous ulcer with infection extending to the underlying fascia.[63] Preventive efforts may help reduce the incidence of disease. Wearing long pants appeared to be protective in a case-control study involving Côte D'Ivoire patients who had lower-extremity lesions.[64]

Mycobacterium szulgai

M. szulgai is scotochromogenic at 37°C but photochromogenic at 25°C. The organism has been isolated from patients worldwide, but its presumed environmental source has not been identified.[65] Most reported cases have involved lung disease indistinguishable from that caused by *M. tuberculosis*. Other sites of infection have included the bursa, tendon sheaths, bones, lymph nodes, and skin.[66,67] Therapeutic regimens have included isoniazid, rifampin, ethambutol, and streptomycin.[24,65] A patient with AIDS who had pulmonary infection caused by multidrug-resistant *M. szulgai* responded to therapy with isoniazid, ethambutol, rifampin, and pyrazinamide. The isolate was resistant *in vitro* to isoniazid, kanamycin, capreomycin, and cycloserine but susceptible to ethambutol, rifampin, and ciprofloxacin.[68]

Mycobacterium gordonae

Also known as the "tap water bacillus," the scotochromogen *M. gordonae* (formerly *Mycobacterium aquae*) is ubiquitous in the environment. It is commonly isolated from soil and water sources, including tap water. Its presence in water accounts for its association with numerous nosocomial pseudoinfections and pseudoepidemics.[69–72] *M. gordonae* has long been considered among the least pathogenic mycobacteria, and its presence in clinical cultures is commonly attributed to specimen contamination or even host colonization. In a review of the literature Weinberger et al.[72] concluded that 24 published cases met their criteria for a documented infection caused by *M. gordonae*. These included five cases of disseminated disease with pulmonary and hepatic involvement in four patients, bone marrow involvement in three, and renal and CNS involvement in two each. Four of these five patients had no underlying immunodeficiency, and one had AIDS. Localized sites of infection in the remaining 19 patients included the lung (eight cases), soft-tissue (seven cases), peritoneum (three cases), and cornea (one case).[72] A small but increasing number of reports suggest that *M. gordonae* can not only colonize but also cause disease in patients with AIDS.[73–75] Optimal therapy for a documented *M. gordonae* infection remains undefined. The majority of isolates tested have been resistant *in vitro* to isoniazid and pyrazinamide whereas many are susceptible to ethambutol and rifampin.

Mycobacterium terrae Complex

Members of the *Mycobacterium terrae* Complex include *M. terrae*, *M. nonchromogenicum*, and *M. triviale*. These slow growing, unpigmented mycobacteria rarely cause human infection. Reports have associated them with pulmonary infection.[76–79] They also may cause bone and joint infections, and *M. nonchromogenicum* should be considered in patients who present with tenosynovitis of the hand that is refractory to routine antibiotics and exacerbated by steroid therapy.[80] Although members of the *Mycobacterium terrae* complex are often resistant to many conventional antituberculous agents, susceptibility patterns of isolates vary within and between species. Individual isolates may be susceptible to ethambutol, streptomycin, rifampin, erythromycin, sulfonamides, or fluoroquinolones. Excision with or without antimicrobial therapy may be curative for cutaneous infections due to *M. nonchromogenicum*.

Mycobacterium smegmatis

M. smegmatis is a rapidly growing environmental saprophyte that was initially isolated from syphilitic chancres and smegma in the 1880s. The organism was not recognized as a human pathogen for the next hundred years. Although the first known case of human infection involved the lungs and pleura, the majority of subsequent reports have described chronic cutaneous or soft-tissue infection following injury or surgery.[81,82] *M. smegmatis* has been recovered from soil samples, and a history of a soil-contaminated wound should raise the clinical suspicion of infection with this pathogen. The first reported case of disseminated infection due to *M. smegmatis* involved an 8-year-old girl with inherited interferon-gamma receptor deficiency. Cultures of blood and liver tissue were positive, and the patient died despite antimicrobial therapy.[83] Patients with cutaneous infection usually require extensive surgical debridement followed by skin grafting. Antimicrobial therapy is indicated for severe infections. Isolates are usually resistant to isoniazid and rifampin but may be sensitive to ethambutol, doxycycline, sulfamethoxazole, ciprofloxacin, ofloxacin, streptomycin, amikacin, or imipenem.

Mycobacterium neoarum

M. neoarum is a rapidly growing scotochromogenic mycobacterium found in soil, dust and water. This organism has been isolated from the blood of two immunosuppressed patients, both of whom had indwelling Hickman catheters and clinical signs of infection.[84,85] These isolates frequently show *in vitro* resistance to conventional antituberculous agents. They may be susceptible to a number of antibiotics including amikacin, ticarcillin/clavulanate, tetracycline, cefoxitin, imipenem, ciprofloxacin, erythromycin, clarithromycin, and azithromycin.

Mycobacterium celatum

M. celatum is a slowly growing, nonphotochromogenic species with biochemical and morphologic characteristics resembling those of *M. avium-intracellulare* and *M. xenopi*. It has recently been reported as a cause of pulmonary and disseminated infections in patients with AIDS.[86–88] *M. celatum* isolates have shown variable susceptibility to antimicrobial agents, suggesting that different groups of strains may represent separate clones.[88] Most isolates are resistant to rifampin. Treatment regimens have included various combinations of clarithromycin, ciprofloxacin, pyrazinamide, ethambutol, rifabutin, clofazimine, and amikacin.

Rare NTM Pathogens

A growing number of uncommon NTM are being isolated from clinical specimens. These include *M. shimoidei, M. branderi, M. asiaticum, M. gastri, M. phlei, M. thermoresistibile, M. flavescens, M. intermedium, M. triplex, M. lentiflavum, M. interjectum, M. conspicuum,*

M. heidelbergense, M. heckeshornense, M. bohemicum, and *M. tusciae.* Previously considered nonpathogenic saprophytes or environmental contaminants, many of these strains have been implicated as rare causes of pulmonary, extrapulmonary, or disseminated infections.[14–18,89–91] We can expect to see an increase in the clinical significance of these NTM, particularly in patients who have AIDS or other conditions which diminish host defenses.

REFERENCES

1. Karlson AG, Carr DT. Tuberculosis caused by *Mycobacterium bovis. Ann Intern Med.* 1970;78:979–983.
2. Damsker B, Bottone E, Schneierson S. Human infections with *Mycobacterium bovis. Am Rev Respir Dis.* 1974;110:446–449.
3. O'Donahue WJ, Jr., Sukhdarshan B, Bittner M, et al. Short-course chemotherapy for pulmonary infection due to *Mycobacterium bovis. Arch Intern Med.* 1985;145:703–705.
4. Renner M, Bartholomew WR. Mycobacteriologic data from two outbreaks of bovine tuberculosis in nonhuman primates. *Am Rev Resp Dis.* 1974;109:11–16.
5. Fanning A, Edwards S. *Mycobacterium bovis* infection in human beings in contact with elk (*Cervus elaphus*) in Alberta, Canada. *Lancet.* 1991;338:1253–1255.
6. Dankner WM, Waecker NS, Essey MA, et al. *Mycobacterium bovis* infections in San Diego: A Clinicoepidemiologic study of 73 patients and a historical review of a forgotten pathogen. *Medicine.* 1993;72:11–37.
7. Jakubowski A, Elwood RK, Enarson DA. Clinical features of abdominal tuberculosis. *J Infect Dis.* 1988;158:687–692.
8. Bouvet E, Casalino E, Mendoza-Sassi G, et al. A nosocomial outbreak of multidrug-resistant *Mycobacterium bovis* among HIV-infected patients. A case-control study. *AIDS.* 1993;7:1453–1460.
9. Cornuz J, Fitting JW, Beer V, Chave JP. *Mycobacterium bovis* and AIDS. *AIDS.* 1991;5:1038–1039.
10. Weltman AC, Rose DN. The safety of Bacille Calmette-Guérin vaccination in HIV infection and AIDS. *AIDS.* 1993;7:149–157.
11. Centers for Disease Control. Use of BCG vaccines in the control tuberculosis: a joint statement by the ACIP and the advisory committee for elimination of tuberculosis. *MMWR Morb Mortal Wkly Rep.* 1988;37:663–664 and 37:669–673.
12. Stone MM, Vannier AM, Storch SK, et al. Meningitis due to iatrogenic BCG infection in two immunocompromised children. *N Engl J Med.* 1995;333:561–563.
13. Kristjansson M, Green P, Manning H, et al. Molecular confirmation of Bacillus Calmette-Guérin as the cause of pulmonary infection following urinary tract instillation. *Clin Infect Dis.* 1993;17:228–230.
14. Woods GL, Washington JA, II. Mycobacteria other than *Mycobacterium tuberculosis*: review of microbiologic and clinical aspects. *Rev Infect Dis.* 1987;9:275–294.

15. Wolinsky E. Mycobacterial diseases other than tuberculosis. *Clin Infect Dis.* 1992;15:1–12.
16. Wayne L, Sramek H. Agents of newly recognized or infrequently encountered mycobacterial diseases. *Clin Microbiol Rev.* 1992;5:1–25.
17. Falkinham JO, III. Epidemiology of infection by nontuberculous mycobacteria. *Clin Microbiol Rev.* 1996;9(2):177–215.
18. Brown-Elliott BA, Griffith DE, Wallace Jr RJ. Newly described or emerging human species of nontuberculous mycobacteria. *Infect Dis Clin N Am.* 2002;16:187–220.
19. Hale YM, Pfyffer GE, Salfinger *Mycobacterium*Laboratory diagnosis of mycobacterial infections: New tools and lessons learned. *Clin Infect Dis.* 2001;33:834–846.
20. Primm TP, Lucero CA, Falkinham JO III. Health impacts of environmental mycobacteria. *Clin Microbiol Rev.* 2004;17:98–106.
21. Phillips MS, von Reyn CF. Nosocomial infections due to nontuberculous mycobacteria. *Clin Infect Dis.* 2001;33:1363–1374.
22. Snider D Jr, Hopewell P, Mills J, et al. Mycobacterioses and the acquired immunodeficiency syndrome. *Am Rev Respir Dis.* 1987;136:492–496.
23. Gibson RL, Burns JL, Ramsey BW. Pathophysiology and management of pulmonary infections in cystic fibrosis. *Am J Respir Crit Care Med.* 2003;168:918–951.
24. Wallace RJ Jr, O'Brien R, Glassroth J, et al. Diagnosis and treatment of disease caused by nontuberculous mycobacteria. *Am Rev Respir Dis.* 1990;142:940–953.
25. Weiszfeiler JG, Karasseva V, Karczag E. *Mycobacterium simiae* and related mycobacteria. *Rev Infect Dis.* 1981;3:1040–1045.
26. Lavy A, Yoshpe-Purer Y. Isolation of *Mycobacterium simiae* from clinical specimens in Israel. *Tubercle.* 1982;63:279–285.
27. Portaels F, Larsson L, Smeets P. Isolation of mycobacteria from healthy persons' stools. *Int J Lepr.* 1988;56:468–471.
28. Bell RC, Higuchi JH, Donovan WN, et al. *Mycobacterium simiae* clinical features and follow up of twenty-four patients. *Am Rev Respir Dis.* 1983;127:35–38.
29. Krasnow I, Gross W. *Mycobacterium simiae* infection in the United States. A Case report and discussion of the organism. *Am Rev Respir Dis.* 1985;111:357–360.
30. Sriyabhaya N, Wongwantana S. Pulmonary infection caused by atypical mycobacteria: a report of 24 cases in Thailand. *Rev Infect Dis.* 1981;3:1085–1089.
31. Rose HD, Dorff GI, Lauwasser M, et al. Pulmonary and disseminated *Mycobacterium simiae* infection in humans. *Am Rev Respir Dis.* 1982;126:1110–1113.
32. Huminer D, Dux S, Samra Z, et al. *Mycobacterium simiae* infection in Israeli patients with AIDS. *Clin Infect Dis.* 1993;17:508–509.
33. Hirschel B, Chang HR, Mach N, et al. Fatal Infection with a novel, unidentified mycobacterium in a man with the acquired immunodeficiency syndrome. *N Engl J Med.* 1990;323:109–113.
34. Bottger E, Teske A, Kirschner P, et al. Disseminated "*Mycobacterium genavense*" infection with patients with AIDS. *Lancet.* 1992;340:76–80.
35. Coyle MB, Carlson LDC, Wallis CK, et al. Laboratory aspects of "*Mycobacterium genavense*," a proposed species isolated from AIDS patients. *J Clin Microbiol.* 1992;30:3206–3212.
36. Maier T, Desmond E, McCallum J, et al. Isolation of *Mycobacterium genavense* from AIDS patients and cultivation of the organism of Middlebrook 7H10 agar supplemented with human blood. *Med Microbiol Lett.* 1995;4:173–179.
37. Pechere M, Opravil M, Wald A, et al. Swiss HIV Cohort Study: Clinical and epidemiologic features of infection with *Mycobacterium genavense.* *Arch Intern Med.* 1995;155:400–404.
38. Bessesen MT, Shlay J, Stone-Venohr B, et al. Disseminated *Mycobacterium genavense* infection: clinical and microbiological features and response to therapy. *AIDS.* 1993;7:1357–1361.
39. Maschek H, Georgii A, Schmidt RE, et al. *Mycobacterium genavense* autopsy findings in three patients. *Am J Clin Pathol.* 1994;101:95–99.
40. Gaynor CD, Clark RA, Koontz FP, et al. Disseminated *Mycobacterium genavense* infection in two patients with AIDS. *Clin Infect Dis.* 1994;18:455–457.
41. Berman SM, Kim RC, Haghighat D, et al. *Mycobacterium genavense* infection presenting as a solitary brain mass in a patient with AIDS: case report and review. *Clin Infect Dis.* 1994;19:1152–1154.
42. Banks J, Hunter AM, Campbell IA, et al. Pulmonary infection with *Mycobacterium xenopi*: review of treatment and response. *Thorax.* 1984;39:376–382.
43. Henriques B, Hoffner SE, Petrini B, et al. Infection with *Mycobacterium malmoense* in Sweden: Report of 221 cases. *Clin Infect Dis.* 1994;18:596–600.
44. Zaugg M, Salfinger M, Opravil M, et al. Extrapulmonary and disseminated infections due to *Mycobacterium malmoense*: case report and review. *Clin Infect Dis.* 1993;16:540–549.
45. Sompolinsky D, Lagziel A, Naveh D, et al. *Mycobacterium haemophilum* sp. nov., a new pathogen of humans. *Int J Syst Bacteriol.* 1978;28:67–75.
46. Straus WL, Ostroff SM, Jernigan DB, et al. Clinical and epidemiologic characteristics of *Mycobacterium haemophilum*, an emerging pathogen in immunocompromised patients. *Ann Intern Med.* 1994;120:118–125.
47. Saubolle MA, Kiehn TE, White MH, et al. *Mycobacterium haemophilum*: microbiology and expanding clinical and geographic spectra of disease in humans. *Clin Micro Rev.* 1996;9:435–447.
48. Rogers PL, Wallace RE, Lane HC, et al. Disseminated *Mycobacterium haemophilum* infection in two patients with the acquired immunodeficiency syndrome. *Am J Med.* 1988;84:640–642.
49. White MH, Papadopoulos E, Small TN, et al. *Mycobacterium haemophilum* infections in bone marrow transplant recipients. *Transplantation.* 1995;60:957–960.
50. Plemmons RM, McAllister CK, Garces MC, et al. Osteomyelitis due to *Mycobacterium haemophilum* in a cardiac transplant patient: case report and analysis of

interactions among Clarithromycin, Rifampin, and Cyclosporine. *Clin Infect Dis.* 1997;24:995–997.

51. Bennet SN, Peterson DE, Johnson DR, et al. Bronchoscopy-associated *Mycobacterium xenopi* pseudoinfections. *Am J Respir Crit Care Med.* 1994;150:245–250.

52. Simor AE, Salit IE, Vellend H. The role of *Mycobacterium xenopi* in human disease. *Am Rev Respir Dis.* 1984;129:435–438.

53. Jiva TM, Jacoby HM, Weymouth LA, et al. *Mycobacterium xenopi*: innocent bystander or emerging pathogen? *Clin Infect Dis.* 1997;24:226–232.

54. Miller WC, Perkins MD, Richardson WJ, et al. Pott's disease caused by *Mycobacterium xenopi*: case report and review. *Clin Infect Dis.* 1994;19:1024–1028.

55. Coombes GM, Teh LS, Denton J, et al. *Mycobacterium xenopi*—an unusual presentation as tenosynovitis of the wrist in an immunocompetent patient. *Br J Rheum.* 1996;35:1008–1010.

56. McDiarmid S, Blumberg D, Remotti H, et al. Mycobacterial infections after pediatric liver transplantation: a report of three cases and review of the literature. *J Pediatr Gastroenterol Nutr.* 1995;20:425–431.

57. Weber J, Mettang T, Staerz E, et al. Pulmonary disease due to *Mycobacterium xenopi* in a renal allograft recipient: report of a case and review. *Rev Infect Dis.* 1989;11:961–969.

58. Rigsby MO, Curtis AM. Pulmonary disease from nontuberculous mycobacteria in patients with human immunodeficiency virus. *Chest.* 1994;106:913–919.

59. Jacoby HM, Jiva TM, Kaminski DA, et al. *Mycobacterium xenopi* infection masquerading as pulmonary tuberculosis in two patients infected with the human immunodeficiency virus. *Clin Infect Dis.* 1995;20:1399–1401.

60. Portaels F, Fonteyne PA, DeBeenhouwer HD, et al. Variability in 3′end of 16S rRNA sequence of *Mycobacterium ulcerans* is related to geographic origin of isolates. *J Clin Microbiol.* 1996;34:962–965.

61. Hofer M, Hirschel B, Kirschner P, et al. Disseminated osteomyelitis from *Mycobacterium ulcerans* after a snakebite. *N Engl J Med.* 1993;328:1007–1009.

62. Meyers WM, Tignokpa N, Priuli GB, et al. *Mycobacterium ulcerans* infection (Buruli ulcer): first reported patients in Togo. *Br J Derm.* 1996;134:1116–1121.

63. Delaporte E, Alfandari S, Piette F. *Mycobacterium ulcerans* associated with infection due to the human immunodeficiency virus. *Clin Infect Dis.* 1984;18:839.

64. Marston BJ, Diallo MO, Horsburgh CR Jr, et al. Emergence of Buruli ulcer disease in the Daloa region of Cote D'Ivoire. *Am J Trop Med Hyg.* 1995;52:219–224.

65. Maloney JM, Gregg CR, Stephens DS, et al. Infections caused by *Mycobacterium szulgai* in humans. *Rev Infect Dis.* 1987;9:1120–1126.

66. Stratton CW, Phelps DB, Reller LB. Tuberculoid tenosynovitis and carpal tunnel syndrome caused by *Mycobacterium szulgai*. *Am J Med.* 1978;65:349–351.

67. Gur H, Porat S, Haas H, et al. Disseminated mycobacterial disease caused by *Mycobacterium szulgai*. *Arch Intern Med.* 1984;144:1861–1863.

68. Newshan G, Torres RA. Pulmonary infection due to multidrug resistant *Mycobacterium szulgai* in a patient with AIDS. *Clin Infect Dis.* 1994;18:1022–1023.

69. Steere A, Corrales J, von Graevenitz A. A cluster of *Mycobacterium gordonae* isolates from bronchoscopy specimens. *Am Rev Respir Dis.* 1979;120:214–216.

70. Panwalker AP, Fuhse E. Nosocomial *Mycobacterium gordonae* pseudoinfection from contaminated ice machines. *Infect Control.* 1986;7:67–70.

71. Stine T, Harris A, Rivera L, et al. A pseudoepidemic due to atypical mycobacteria in a hospital water supply. *JAMA.* 1987;258:809–811.

72. Weinberger M, Berg SL, Feuerstein IM, et al. Disseminated infection with *Mycobacterium gordonae*: Report of a case and critical review of the literature. *Clin Infect Dis.* 1992;14:1229–1239.

73. Horsburgh C, Jr, Selik R. The epidemiology of disseminated nontuberculous mycobacterial infection in the acquired immunodeficiency syndrome (AIDS). *Am Rev Respir Dis.* 1989;139:4–7.

74. Barber TW, Craven DE, Farber HW. *Mycobacterium gordonae*: a possible opportunistic respiratory tract pathogen in patients with advanced human immunodeficiency virus, type 1 infection. *Chest.* 1991;100:716–720.

75. Lessnau KD, Milanese S, Talavera W. *Mycobacterium gordonae*: a treatable disease in HIV-positive patients. *Chest.* 1993;104:1779–1785.

76. Tsukamura M, Kita N, Otsuka W, et al. A study of the taxonomy of the *Mycobacterium nonchromogenicum* complex and report of six cases of lung infection due to *Mycobacterium nonchromogenicum*. *Microbiol Immunol.* 1983;27:219–236.

77. Tonner JA, Hammond MD. Pulmonary disease caused by *Mycobacterium terrae* complex. *South Med J.* 1989;82:1279–1282.

78. Peters E, Morice R. Miliary pulmonary infection caused by *Mycobacterium terrae* in an autologous bone marrow transplant patient. *Chest.* 1991;100:1449–1450.

79. Spence TH, Ferris VM. Spontaneous resolution of a lung mass due to infection with *Mycobacterium terrae*. *South Med J.* 1996;89:414–416.

80. Ridderhof JC, Wallace RJ Jr, Kilburn JO, et al. Chronic tenosynovitis of the hand due to *Mycobacterium nonchromogenicum*: use of high-performance liquid chromatography for identification of isolates. *Rev Infect Dis.* 1991;13:857–864.

81. Wallace RJ Jr, Nash DR, Tsukamura M, et al. Human disease due to *Mycobacterium smegmatis*. *J Infect Dis.* 1988;158:52–59.

82. Newton JA, Jr, Weiss PJ, Bowler WA, et al. Soft-tissue infection due to *Mycobacterium smegmatis*: report of two cases. *Clin Infect Dis.* 1993;16:531–533.

83. Pierre-Audigier C, Jouanguy E, Lamhamedi S, et al. Fatal disseminated *Mycobacterium smegmatis* infection in a child with inherited interferon-gamma receptor deficiency. *Clin Infect Dis.* 1997;24:982–984.

84. Davison MB, McCormack JG, Blacklock ZM, et al. Bacteremia caused by *Mycobacterium neoaurum. J Clin Microbiol.* 1988;26:762–764.

85. Holland DJ, Chen SCA, Chew WWK, et al. *Mycobacterium neoaurum* infection of a Hickman catheter in an immunosuppressed patient. *Clin Infect Dis.* 1994;18:1002–1003.

86. Tortoli E, Piersimoni C, Bacosi D, et al. Isolation of the newly described species *Mycobacterium celatum* from AIDS patients. *J Clin Microbiol.* 1995;33:137–140.

87. Zurawski CA, Cage GD, Rimland D, et al. Pneumonia and bactermia due to *Mycobacterium celatum* masquerading as *Mycobacterium xenopi* in patients with AIDS: an under-diagnosed problem? *Clin Infect Dis.* 1997;24:140–143.

88. Piersimoni C, Tortoli E, de Lalla F, et al. Isolation of *Mycobacterium celatum* from patients infected with human immunodeficiency virus. *Clin Infect Dis.* 1997;24:144–147.

89. Tortoli E, Simonetti T. Isolation of *Mycobacterium shimoidei* from a patient with cavitary pulmonary disease. *J Clin Microbiol.* 1991;29:1754–1756.

90. Koukila-Kahkola P, Springer B, Bottger E, et al. *Mycobacterium branderi* sp. nov., a new potential human pathogen. *Int J Syst Bacteriol.* 1995;45:549–553.

91. Fisher PR, Christenson JC, Davis AT, et al. Postoperative *Mycobacterium flavescens* infection in a child. *Infect Dis Clin Practice.* 1997;6:263–265.

INDEX

Page numbers followed by italic *f* or *t* denote figures or tables, respectively.